Palliative Care Nursing

Palliative Care Nursing

Principles and evidence for practice
Third Edition

Edited by Catherine Walshe, Nancy Preston and Bridget Johnston

Open University Press

Open University Press
McGraw-Hill Education
8th Floor, 338 Euston Road
London
England
NW1 3BH

email: enquiries@openup.co.uk
world wide web: www.openup.co.uk

and Two Penn Plaza, New York, NY 10121-2289, USA

First published 2018

A catalogue record of this book is available from the British Library

ISBN-13: 978-0-335-26162-8
ISBN-10: 0-33-526162-0
eISBN: 978-0-335-26163-5

Library of Congress Cataloging-in-Publication Data
CIP data applied for

Typeset by Transforma Pvt. Ltd., Chennai, India

Praise for this book

"I welcome this third edition of Palliative Care Nursing *and congratulations to the new team who have provided us with a dynamic and innovative development of a core text for palliative nursing practice. As the largest workforce in palliative care, and given the changing face of clinical practice for nurses, including increased educational opportunity and expanding roles and responsibilities, this book is timely in its focus on critical issues which frame and scope the reality of palliative care and the nursing contribution to that discipline. The learning exercises, in particular, offer tools for educators and clinicians to reflect on practice and understand new ways of knowing in palliative care. It will be an excellent resource for nursing, both in the UK and Ireland and to the wider international audience, having drawn on the breadth of global nursing expertise to bring this book together.*

Philip Larkin, Professor of Clinical Nursing (Palliative Care), University College Dublin and Our Lady's Hospice and Care Services, Dublin, Ireland; President, European Association for Palliative Care

"This is a book of substance that captures the current status of palliative nursing, including the values and research evidence that underpin it. The changing nature of palliative nursing as an evidence-based specialism is balanced with practical skills and insights from experts, and also considers the needs of those working with, or concerned about, the dying person's well-being.

It covers a range of challenging issues as well as drawing on the wisdom of those who actually undertake this work on a daily basis. I hope that students and practitioners from all disciplines will find this a useful resource to understand the art and craft of good palliative nursing."

Professor Daniel Kelly, Fellow of the Royal College of Nursing and Royal College of Nursing Chair of Nursing Research, Cardiff University, UK

"Palliative Care Nursing: Principles and Evidence for Practice is an important and vital resource for anyone involved in palliative care nursing. This well-written edited volume covers a breadth of important issues for palliative care nursing within a contemporary global context. The division into four key sections is a useful and well-structured approach: starting with a clear focus on the patient and family, examining useful aspects such as patient and family engagement; Part Two focuses on providing palliative nursing care, outlining

the importance of clinical assessment and symptom management; Part Three provides a useful focus on the nurses' role in end of life care and bereavement, concluding with Part Four examining key challenges for contemporary palliative care practice. This is an excellent updated version of this well-known and well-respected textbook for palliative care nursing. All readers will find much to stimulate their thinking, develop their practice and reflect on their overall approach to care."

Professor Sonja McIlfatrick, Professor of Nursing and
Palliative Care, Ulster University, Northern Ireland

"This text is essential reading for nurses and health and social care professionals with an interest in, and commitment to, improving the care of people with life-limiting and life-threatening illness and those at or near the end of life. A contemporary examination of the evidence base for palliative care practice, in an accessible and readable style, this is the first book I reach for when searching for a summary of debates in the field and current thinking on particular topics. In a world now stacked high with open access journal papers this text is an important touchpoint that successfully addresses the meaning and practice of palliative nursing."

Professor Alison Richardson, Professor of Cancer Nursing and
End of Life Care & Director, Southampton Academy of Research,
University of Southampton & University Hospital Southampton
NHS Foundation Trust, UK

"People are living longer, but often with chronic conditions. Palliative care provision is changing in response. This book is for nurses who wish to be aware of current issues in the organisation and delivery of supportive and palliative care. Its comprehensive collection of chapters cover the relevance and delivery of palliative care from diagnosis to end of life.

The book is well-organised, key concepts are defined and important and challenging questions are raised. The guidance provided by authors draws on their own expertise and research evidence. Issues addressed include inequality in access to services, variability in clinical outcomes, support of self-management, coproduction, mental capacity for decision making and the future role of families in care provision. Research, development and innovation are considered in the final chapters and education is identified as a core component of any initiative to improve palliative care worldwide. I found it to be an engaging and thought-provoking read and congratulate the editors in bringing these important contemporary essays together."

Jane B Hopkinson, Professor of Nursing,
Cardiff University, UK

Contents

List of contributors

Samar M. Aoun, Professor of Palliative Care, Palliative Care Unit, School of Psychology and Public Health, La Trobe University, Victoria, Australia.

Mackuline Atieno, Programmes Officer, African Palliative Care Association, Kampala, Uganda.

Lauren Breen, Associate Professor, School of Psychology and Speech Pathology, Curtin University, Perth, Western Australia.

Lynn Calman, Senior Research Fellow in Macmillan Survivorship Research Group (MSRG) in the Faculty of Health Sciences at the University of Southampton, Southampton, UK.

Aileen Collier, Senior Lecturer, Nursing, Faculty of Medical and Health Sciences, University of Auckland, New Zealand.

Michael Connolly, Lecturer, UCD School of Nursing, Midwifery and Health Systems, University College Dublin, Ireland.

Maureen Coombs, Professor – Ahorangi Clinical Nursing (Critical Care), Graduate School of Nursing, Midwifery and Health, Te Kura Tapuhi Hauora Victoria University of Wellington, New Zealand.

John Costello, Associate Professor, University of Manchester, UK, and Nanyang Polytechnic, Singapore.

Josie Dixon, Assistant Professorial Research Fellow, Department of Social Policy, London School of Economics and Political Science, London, UK.

Julia Downing, Chief Executive, International Children's Palliative Care Network, and Professor, Makerere University, Uganda.

Gail Ewing, Senior Research Associate, Centre for Family Research, University of Cambridge, Cambridge, UK.

Morag Farquhar, Senior Lecturer, School of Health Sciences, University of East Anglia, Norwich, UK.

Lise Fillion, Faculté des sciences infirmières, Université Laval, Québec, Canada.

Kate Flemming, Senior Lecturer, Department of Health Sciences, The University of York, York, UK.

Claudia Gamondi, Clinical Director, Palliative and Supportive Clinic, Oncology Institute of Southern Switzerland, Bellinzona, Switzerland.

Sheri Mila Gerson, PhD student, International Observatory on End of Life Care, Lancaster University, Lancaster, UK.

Barbara Gomes, Lecturer and Researcher in Palliative Care, King's College London, London, UK.

Merryn Gott, Professor of Health Sciences, Nursing, Faculty of Medical and Health Sciences. University of Auckland, New Zealand.

Laura Green, Lecturer in Palliative and End-of-Life Care, School of Nursing, Faculty of Health Studies, University of Bradford, Bradford, UK.

Richard Harding, Herbert Dunhill Professor and Director of the Centre for Global Health Palliative Care, Cicely Saunders Institute, Department of Palliative Care, Policy & Rehabilitation, King's College London, London, UK.

Beth Hardy, Lecturer in Nursing, Department of Health Sciences, The University of York, York, UK.

Hamilton Inbadas, Reverend, Research Associate (Wellcome Trust), School of Interdisciplinary Studies, University of Glasgow, Glasgow, UK.

Bridget Johnston, Florence Nightingale Foundation Professor of Clinical Nursing Practice Research, School of Medicine, Dentistry & Nursing, College of Medical, Veterinary & Life Sciences, University of Glasgow, Glasgow, UK.

Catriona Kennedy, QNIS Professor of Community Nursing, School of Nursing and Midwifery, Robert Gordon University, Aberdeen, UK.

Diane Laverty, Nurse Consultant, Palliative Care, St Joseph's Hospice, London, UK.

Deborah Lewis, PhD student, Lancaster University, Lancaster, UK.

Jo Loney, Education Services Manager, Cranford Hospice, Hawke's Bay, New Zealand.

Linda Machin, Honorary Research Fellow, Research Institute for Primary Care and Health Sciences, Keele University, Keele, UK.

Susan McClement, Associate Professor, College of Nursing, University of Manitoba, Winnipeg, Canada.

Dorry McLaughlin, Lecturer in Palliative Care and Chronic Illness, School of Nursing and Midwifery, Queen's University, Belfast, Northern Ireland.

Stuart P. Milligan, Lecturer, School of Health, Nursing and Midwifery, University of West of Scotland, Paisley, UK.

Brian Nyatanga, Senior Lecturer, Academic Lead for Centre for Palliative Care, Institute of Health and Society, Allied Health and Social Sciences & Centre for Palliative Care, University of Worcester, Worcester, UK.

Jane Phillips, Professor of Palliative Nursing, University of Technology, Sydney, Australia.

Nancy Preston, Senior Lecturer and Director of Traditional PhD Programme (C51), International Observatory of End of Life Care, Faculty of Health and Medicine, Furness College, Lancaster University, Lancaster, UK.

Sarah Russell, Head of Research and Clinical Innovation, Hospice UK, London, UK.

Gary Rycroft, Solicitor and Partner, Joseph A. Jones & Co LLP, Lancaster, UK.

Sue Spencer, Practice Development Facilitator, Marie Curie UK, London, UK.

Anna-Marie Stevens, Nurse Consultant, Symptom Control and Palliative Care, Royal Marsden NHS Foundation Trust, London, UK.

Elaine Stevens, Programme Leader and Lecturer in Cancer and Palliative Care, University of the West of Scotland, Glasgow, UK.

Philomena Swarbrick, Specialty Doctor in Palliative Medicine, St John's Hospice, Lancaster, UK.

Vanessa Taylor, Deputy Head of Nursing, Midwifery and Professional Programmes/Chair in Teaching and Learning, Department of Health Sciences, The University of York, York, UK.

Genevieve Thompson, Associate Professor and Research Associate, Manitoba Palliative Care Research Unit, Helen Glass Centre for Nursing, College of Nursing, University of Manitoba, Winnipeg, Canada.

Mary Vachon, Adjunct Professor, Dalla Lana School of Public Health, University of Toronto, Canada.

Catherine Walshe, Professor of Palliative Care, International Observatory on End of Life Care, Lancaster University, Lancaster, UK.

Craig A. White, Divisional Clinical Lead in the Quality and Planning Division of the Healthcare Quality and Strategy Directorate, Scottish Government. Honorary Professor, College of Medical, Veterinary and Life Sciences at the University of Glasgow, Glasgow, UK.

Foreword

Nurses have a vital role in palliative care. In many contexts, they are the main, or even the only, professionals with specialist palliative care expertise. Therefore, it is essential that their knowledge is evidence-based, up-to-date and extensive, combined with professional nursing skills and compassionate attitudes, to deliver care. Honing these three elements of palliative care nursing – knowledge, skills and attitudes – provides the rationale for this book.

Most of us will die in older age with multiple conditions, usually in hospital. Too often dying and the end of life period are enacted in the context of clinical uncertainty with fragmented services and professionals who fail to adequately acknowledge and plan for the possibility of death. This prevents patients and their families having sufficient time to prepare for the end of life, and potentially destroys remaining quality of life, as patients seek increasingly futile, expensive and invasive medical interventions. Thus, with the final period of life comes a frustrating round of impersonal clinic appointments, distressing hospital stays and uncomfortable medical procedures. The imperative to treat often drives patients, families and their physicians to collude in further medical procedures, without due attention to the wider goals and preferences of patients.

Palliative care nursing offers an alternative option, where advanced illness and the end of life period can be supported, dignified and controlled by the preferences and wishes of patients and their families. High quality palliative care can be delivered in any environment; it is not the place but the people delivering care that is pivotal in the experience. While in-patient hospices have pioneered models of excellence in palliative care, some hospitals and nursing homes also provide high quality and sensitive care, in peaceful rooms or wards. Home care is often the preferred option of patients and models of intensive support such as Hospice at Home services demonstrate how this can be delivered in domestic settings. Wherever the patient is, palliative care should be coordinated and integrated with other healthcare and social care services, including volunteer organisations, where these are available.

This book is inspired by a vision to improve palliative care nursing. It is the third edition of a well-known and well-respected textbook, formerly edited by Sheila Payne, Jane Seymour and Christine Ingleton. I am delighted that the new editorial team of Catherine Walshe, Nancy Preston and Bridget Johnston have done an excellent job of revising and completely revamping the book. They have elicited chapters from leading academic and clinical nurses, which challenge taken-for-granted assumptions and introduce contemporary debates and dilemmas. The four-part structure guides the reader to reflect carefully on who can be considered to be a palliative care patient, before presenting key elements of palliative care nursing. The third section highlights the nurse's role around the end of life period, including supporting families in bereavement. Finally, there are a number of fascinating chapters focusing on current topics such as decision-making, assisted dying and change management.

This book offers guidance on how to enable more patients and their families to experience higher quality ends to their lives, as befitting a modern approach to palliative care nursing. I warmly recommend it to you.

Professor Sheila Payne
Emeritus Professor
International Observatory on End of Life Care
Lancaster University
United Kingdom

Part
ONE

WHO IS THE PALLIATIVE CARE PATIENT?

Introduction to Part One

Bridget Johnston

Palliative care as a discipline and concept has grown exponentially in the last few years. *The Global Atlas of Palliative Care* (2014) identifies that palliative care is an essential part of all healthcare systems. Despite this, it is widely acknowledged that there is still inadequate access to hospice and palliative care worldwide. With an ageing population who are going to be living and dying with more complex and often co-morbid conditions, the demand for care is only going to increase in the future. The atlas provides data that each year around 20 million people need end of life palliative care, 6 per cent of whom are children. The estimates are that there are still a large number of people globally with unmet palliative and end of life care needs. More than ever, therefore, there is a need for palliative nursing that is patient-centred and informed by appropriate evidence.

In Chapter 1, Stuart P. Milligan introduces us to the concept of palliative care. He considers the three main criteria by which the palliative patient might be defined (namely, diagnosis, prognosis and level/nature of need). He also explores other important criteria such as suffering and consensus. Stuart also discusses how we identify people with palliative care needs. He explores the issue of whether it is helpful for nurses to use tools to aid prognostication at the end of life as opposed to using clinical judgement alone.

Stuart concludes by posing a challenge, that, due to the rising numbers of people in need of palliative care, solutions could include the extension of the responsibility for the provision of palliative care to a much wider range of professionals, agencies and services than previously. He also considers an increasing emphasis on a public health approach to palliative care that recognises that the latter stages of life are often associated with high symptom burden, challenges to dignity and personhood, and a huge burden of suffering, and suggests that we should develop population-level solutions in response to need.

Chapter 2 by Josie Dixon discusses issues of access and referral to palliative care and, in particular, inequity of access. Inequity issues related to gender, age, ethnicity and geography are explored. She states that not everyone with a palliative care need receives the palliative care they require. She suggests that access is also highly variable across different demographic, social and diagnostic groups. These inequities and gaps in access represent key challenges in the development of palliative care services in future.

Chapter 3 by Barbara Gomes explores where palliative care is provided and how it is changing. She argues that wherever and whenever possible, people suffering from an advanced disease should be cared for and die where they feel it is the right place to be, so that they feel empowered and safe. To help patients achieve their preferences, she proposes that nurses must understand not only how the trends in where we die are evolving but also which factors influence place of death.

Increasingly important in contemporary healthcare is the issue of engaging patients and families in the organisation, care and research of palliative care, and Aileen Collier and Merryn Gott explore these issues in Chapter 4. They explore patient and family engagement and how co-production in healthcare can ultimately improve care.

Patients with life-limiting illness are having to face living with an uncertain prognosis. This issue and how the nurse can support the person with an uncertain prognosis are explored by Lynn Calman in Chapter 5. Lynn also explores the nurse's role in supported self-care, which was an issue postulated by Stuart Milligan in his conclusion in Chapter 1 as an important future role of the nurse.

The final chapter in Part One explores the nurse's role in clinical assessment and outcome measurement. Kate Flemming, Beth Hardy and Vanessa Taylor argue that clinical assessment is the cornerstone of individualised patient care. They suggest that nurses should adopt a comprehensive assessment process that requires making accurate observations, gathering data about physical, psychological, spiritual, social and cultural aspects and making judgements to determine the care and treatment needs of the patient, and state this can enhance communication between patients, families and professionals, and also between members of the multi-professional team. Clinical assessment, incorporating the use of patient reported outcome measures, is being advocated in palliative care clinical practice as an approach that enables the patient's perspective to inform clinical decision-making at both an individual and population level.

Who is the palliative care patient?

Stuart P. Milligan

Introduction

The history of palliative care and the development of the role of nurses within the discipline make for fascinating and inspiring reading. From modest beginnings, palliative care has grown into a truly world-wide movement. Nurses today find themselves engaged in many, increasingly sophisticated, facets of palliative care practice, including symptom management, psychosocial interventions, enhanced communication and existential support. However, at the heart of all of this activity stands the patient, and this chapter sets out to discover what palliative care is by understanding more about who it is for.

When searching for a definition of the palliative care patient, a useful starting place would appear to be the definition of palliative care itself. According to the World Health Organization (WHO 2016):

> Palliative care is an approach that improves the quality of life of patients and their families facing the problems associated with life-threatening illness, through the prevention and relief of suffering by means of early identification and impeccable assessment and treatment of pain and other problems, physical, psychosocial and spiritual.

However, a cursory review of this and other definitions will reveal a lack of consensus about exactly who the palliative care patient is. According to which definition is used, he or she could be someone who has a 'life-threatening illness', a 'serious life-limiting illness' or a disease which is 'not responsive to curative treatment'.

Patients, and the public generally, also struggle to understand who palliative care is for. Three-quarters of people who responded to a recent survey admitted that they had little or no knowledge of the meaning of the term 'palliative care' and a similar picture is evident across a range of developed and developing countries (McIlfatrick et al. 2013).

Similar levels of uncertainty appear to exist in patient populations, including those likely to require palliative care in the near future (Zimmermann et al. 2016). Interestingly, however, when people with advanced, life-limiting illnesses are better informed of the role that palliative care can play, at least some regard themselves as suitable candidates for that option (Fortnum, Grennan and Smolonogov 2015).

A lack of consensus over who the palliative care patient is, is also apparent in palliative care research (Van Mechelen et al. 2013). The problem is particularly apparent in (but by no means confined to) studies involving patients with non-malignant diseases. This disagreement results in a lack of comparability between studies and a reduction in the likelihood that the results they produce will be translated into clinical practice.

Learning exercise 1.1

- Consider the potential benefits of a greater consensus around who the palliative care patient is.
- Can you think of benefits for patients, the public generally, nurses and other professionals?
- Make a list, then compare it with what follows.

It should be apparent that uncertainty over who the palliative care patient is can lead to undesirable consequences, such as limited patient choice and delay in accessing appropriate care. Some of the benefits of better defining the palliative care patient might be:

- ensuring that palliative care can be provided to all those patients for whom it would be appropriate;
- enabling palliative care nurses and other practitioners to develop their practice to better reach those who need them most;
- supporting ethical decision-making over the withholding or withdrawal of inappropriate interventions;
- helping agree ceilings of care and promoting realistic medicine;
- creating intelligent local, national and international policy to address the needs of those who fall under the title of 'the palliative patient';
- effectively communicating with and educating the public about what palliative care is and who should be accessing it;
- enabling patients to make informed decisions about their future care;
- better defining study populations, enabling consistent research which produces transferable findings.

The task is daunting, but this chapter will consider the three main criteria by which the palliative patient might be defined (namely, diagnosis, prognosis and level/nature of need). It will also explore other potential criteria such as suffering and consensus.

Diagnosis

It has already been stated that the palliative care patient is likely to have a 'life-threatening illness', a 'serious life-limiting illness' or a disease which is 'not responsive to curative treatment'. However, patients with certain diseases (principally non-cancer) can be difficult to sort into these categories and can consequently find their access to palliative care restricted or delayed (Zheng et al. 2013; Rosenwax et al. 2016).

Precisely which disease the palliative patient was suffering from seemed to matter little to the early pioneers of the care of people with life-limiting or life-threatening diseases. For instance, Francis Bacon's call (published in the 1770s) for doctors to 'mitigate the pains and torments of disease [. . . even . . .] when all hope of recovery [. . . is . . .] gone' was not limited to any particular diagnostic group (Vanderpool 2015). Similarly, John Gregory's statement from the same period that 'It is as much the business of a physician to alleviate pain, and to smooth the avenues of death, when [. . . death is . . .] unavoidable, as [. . . it . . .] is to cure diseases' was presumably intended to refer to all dying people (Vanderpool 2015). As those early shoots of palliative care began to lengthen in the eighteenth and nineteenth centuries, with the establishment of various homes and other institutions dedicated to the care of the dying, there was little evidence of discrimination on the basis of disease (Lewis 2006). Nevertheless, as these institutions gave way to the modern hospices of the 1960s and thereafter, particular emphasis began to be placed on the care of people with advanced, incurable cancer. The reasons for this development are complex and have been rehearsed elsewhere (Clark et al. 2005). However, the result was that in the 1960s, the 1970s and beyond, palliative care in the minds of both professionals and the public, at least in the UK, became inextricably linked with cancer (Clark 2007; Overy and Tansey 2012).

Concerted national and international efforts have been made to challenge this belief and argue that palliative care should be available to patients on the basis of need, not diagnosis. For instance, when defining palliative care nursing, Johnston et al. (2014) stated:

> All life-threatening illnesses – be they cancer, neuro-logical, cardiac or respiratory disease – have implications for physical, social, psychological and spiritual health, for both the individual and their family. The role of palliative nursing is therefore to assess needs in each of these areas and to plan, implement and evaluate appropriate interventions. It aims to improve the quality of life and to enable a dignified death.

However, concerns continue to be expressed that people with non-malignant conditions are missing out on palliative care because they have the 'wrong' diagnosis (Calanzani, Higginson and Gomes 2013; Marie Curie 2015a).

A definition of palliative care simply based on pathologies which have no curative treatment options would clearly be too wide as it would encompass conditions where palliative care has little relevance, such as endometriosis, osteoarthritis and low back pain (Van Mechelen et al. 2013). Instead, a consensus group represented by Weissman and Meier (2011) has produced the following, useful definition of what a 'potentially life-limiting or life-threatening condition' might refer to:

> Any disease/disorder/condition that is known to be life-limiting (e.g., dementia, COPD, chronic renal failure, metastatic cancer, cirrhosis, muscular dystrophy, cystic fibrosis) or that has a high chance of leading to death (e.g., sepsis, multi-organ failure, major trauma, complex congenital heart disease). Medical conditions that are serious, but for which recovery to baseline function is routine (e.g., community-acquired pneumonia in an otherwise healthy patient) are not included in this definition.

Such moves towards a definition of palliative care based firmly on a broad range of diagnoses rather than cancer alone are very much to be welcomed. And, in practice, tremendous strides have been made in growing the evidence base for palliative care in some important non-malignant conditions such as advanced kidney disease, chronic obstructive pulmonary disease, advanced heart failure and HIV/AIDS (Douglas et al. 2009; Boland et al. 2013; Merlin et al. 2013; NHS Improving Quality 2014).

Dementia is an interesting case in point, with consistent calls for the principles of palliative care to be applied wholesale to this debilitating, progressive disease (Sampson 2010; European Association for Palliative Care 2013). The need still exists for empirical evidence to support the use of palliative care in this patient group and to define exactly what best practice is (Sampson et al. 2005; Candy et al. 2015). Long-term developments could include dementia-specific palliative care strategies and better integration of palliative care and dementia care (Mehta et al. 2012).

Another interesting example is general frailty, which is increasingly being discussed in terms of the role that palliative care might play in its management. It is suggested that older people who have no specific diagnosis may still benefit from good symptom management, psychosocial support, enhanced communication and other elements of palliative care as they progress towards death (De Lepelaire et al. 2009; Gardiner et al. 2013).

One of the challenges of attempting to define the palliative patient on the basis of his or her underlying diagnosis is the variability in the trajectories that different terminal diseases follow. Palliative care has mainly developed to address the familiar cancer trajectory which is characterised by relatively predictable phases and usually a very obvious terminal decline (Mitchell et al. 2015). People dying with organ failure or with a dementia or general frailty can be more difficult to identify, and their trajectories more difficult to predict (Murray et al. 2005). It can therefore be extremely difficult to classify such people into either 'palliative' or 'active treatment' categories (Figure 1.1). You will note that other chapters such as Chapter 4 and Chapter 5 also refer to these trajectories. Consider how relevant they are to your nursing practice.

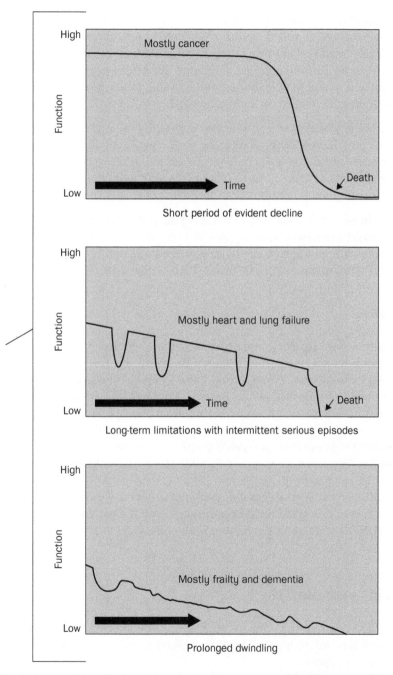

Figure 1.1 Typical trajectories displayed by people dying from or with different conditions
Source: Lynn and Adamson (2003).

The use of palliative care lists (such as the cancer/palliative care registers advocated by the Gold Standards Framework) can be of some help. Indeed, Dale et al. (2009), while acknowledging the lack of evidence on their efficacy at improving patient outcomes, nevertheless identified significant benefits of maintaining a list of palliative care patients. These included better quality of palliative care, better communication within the primary care team and reduced likelihood that patients would be 'missed' (although people with non-malignant conditions were notably much more likely to be omitted than people with cancer) (Courtney and Callow 2014).

There is evidence, however, that the imperative to extend the definition of palliative care to populations other than those with cancer is gaining ground. For instance, a recent review of randomised controlled trials in palliative care found that 34 per cent of the populations studied (where a diagnosis was mentioned) were characterised by having non-malignant conditions (Van Mechelen et al. 2013).

As has been shown, one way of defining the palliative care patient is by specifying that they must have a particular diagnosis. In practice, this is not always possible. Also, many people with an appropriate diagnosis may still not be suitable because of some other factor coming into play. One of these, to be discussed next, is prognosis.

Prognosis

If the palliative care patient cannot be defined on the basis of his or her diagnosis, perhaps prognosis would be a better indicator. Traditionally, palliative care was often introduced when 'nothing more could be done' and when death was expected to follow within a defined period of time (Meier and Brawley 2011). Setting an arbitrary life expectancy limit of, say, 6 months or one year is therefore one approach that has been tried, to attempt to identify who might be most appropriate for palliative care. For instance, in the United States, someone can receive hospice care through the Medicare scheme if two doctors agree that they have less than 6 months to live (should the disease follow its usual course) (US Department of Health and Human Services 2016). However, entitlement to general palliative care services is not restricted in such a way and can be claimed by any patient for whom it is considered appropriate, even if they are expected to make a full recovery (US Department of Health and Human Services 2015).

Learning exercise 1.2

- Think about the concept of waiting until someone has an agreed period of time left to live before introducing palliative care. How feasible is such an approach?
- How reasonable do you think it is to withhold palliative care until that point?
- How else might we decide when someone is 'ready' for palliative care?

Being at the point where no further curative treatment is indicated would, on first consideration, appear to be a convenient way to define the palliative care patient. However, this approach has been found wanting, primarily because it is so difficult to reach agreement on what the ceiling of treatment for a particular individual should be and whether it has been reached (Starkweather 2016). Another drawback of withholding palliative care until an arbitrary period of life is left is that patients can potentially miss out on palliative care that they would have benefited from while 'waiting to be ill enough' (Filbet 2008).

The current version of the World Health Organization's definition of palliative care includes the caveat 'is applicable early in the course of illness, in conjunction with other therapies that are intended to prolong life' (WHO 2016). Furthermore, recent research has suggested that timely referral to palliative care can deliver considerable benefits in terms of improved quality of life, less consumption of resources, greater likelihood of dying at home and even a longer prognosis (Temel et al. 2010; Hui et al. 2014; Humphreys and Harma 2014).

Increasingly, palliative care is being seen as having a role to play earlier in the disease process than was previously believed. It is also becoming widely accepted that the 'trajectory model' (where palliative care is introduced progressively as curative care is withdrawn) is much preferable to the traditional 'transition model' (where palliative care begins once curative efforts have ceased) (Lynn and Adamson 2003; Van Mechelen et al. 2013) (Figure 1.2). Nevertheless, some clinicians still struggle with this concept, and are consequently slow to refer to appropriate services (Akashi, Yano and Aruga 2012; Zheng et al. 2013; Gomes 2015).

The reasons why some people are not considered 'palliative care patients' even when their condition would benefit from the addition of palliative care are often quite legitimate. Disease trajectories may be difficult to predict or prognostic data may be inconclusive (Gomes 2015). There may be concerns about how the patient may react to a change in management or genuine uncertainty about the role that palliative care can play (Meier and Brawley 2011). Patients and families may need time to adjust to a change from predominantly active to predominantly palliative care (Waldrop, Meeker and Kutner 2015). The term 'palliative care' itself may be a barrier. For instance, a survey carried out by Fadul et al. (2009) demonstrated that referring clinicians preferred the term 'supportive care' when offering people with progressive cancer the addition of care intended to preserve quality of life.

There clearly remains a need for earlier identification of who needs palliative care (who the 'palliative care patient is') in order to match services to the most appropriate individuals at the most appropriate time points (Zheng et al. 2013). The use of dying trajectories to envisage how people with different diagnoses might die has helped this process (Penrod et al. 2011; Gardiner et al. 2015). So too has the identification of 'phases of illness' where desired outcomes are revised (and the most appropriate interventions implemented) according to which phase of his or her deterioration a particular person has reached (Witt et al. 2014).

Prognostic indicators have received a lot of attention in the literature and in government policy documents of late (Maltoni et al. 2012; Brown et al. 2013; The Scottish

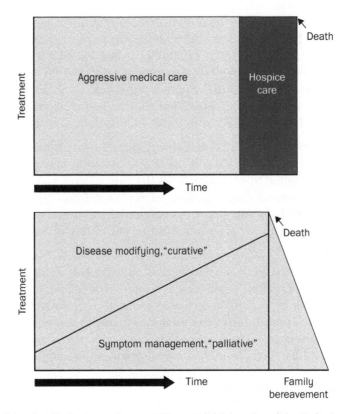

Figure 1.2 Models of palliative care: the transition model (above) and the trajectory model (below)
Source: Lynn and Adamson (2003).

Government 2015; NHS England 2016). Those with the greatest utility, such as the Palliative Prognostic Index and the Palliative Performance Scale, do not rely solely on physiological markers to estimate prognosis but look at function, deterioration and progression as helpful indicators (Glare et al. 2015). As a convenient and accessible tool, the GSF Prognostic Indicator Guidance has usefully brought together much of what is recognised as good practice in prognostication (National Gold Standards Framework Centre England 2008).

The Supportive and Palliative Indicators Tool (SPICT) is an internationally accepted, convenient and validated tool for identifying people at risk of deteriorating and dying in all care settings (Highet et al. 2013). It places particular emphasis not just on detecting the patient's deteriorating condition but also on the identification of his or her supportive and palliative care needs (Dunphy et al. 2016). It also takes special cognisance of the different indicators for the different life-limiting diseases, thus addressing the very real inequity which continues to result in the palliative care needs of people with non-malignant diseases being less likely to be recognised or recognised later than those of people with cancer (Zheng et al. 2013).

Evidence is accumulating to suggest that prognostic tools are more effective at predicting who might be dying (and therefore might potentially be requiring of palliative care) than intuition and clinical judgement alone (Mitchell et al. 2016). However, one of the most popular and widely used prognostic tools continues to be the surprise question: 'Would I be surprised if this person was to die within the next 6/12 months?' (Lynn 2005). It has been shown to be effective in the early identification of people dying of cancer (Moroni et al. 2014). It also has some value in the identification of people with COPD and heart failure nearing the end of life, although its use in isolation is not advised (Murray and Boyd 2011).

The surprise question, while having its limitations, has the advantage of being a simple and easily applied tool for triggering the commencement of palliative care. Other specific triggers have been proposed and include:

- complex or persistent symptoms such as pain or breathlessness;
- high levels of unplanned hospital use;
- multiple co-morbidities;
- anorexia, malnourishment and weight loss;
- need for supplementary feeding or ventilatory support;
- diagnosis of a new, life-limiting condition;
- high levels of palliative care needs as indicated by an appropriate screening tool.

(Marie Curie 2015b)

What should be becoming clear is that there is no easy way to identify or define the palliative care patient simply on the basis of prognosis (Mitchell et al. 2013). Indeed, Mitchell et al. (2016) have suggested that an over-emphasis on accurate death prediction may not be serving potential beneficiaries of palliative care well. A more appropriate approach might be to use evidence of increasing disease burden to trigger holistic needs assessment, proactive consultations with patients and their families and anticipatory care planning (Rocker, Downar and Morrison 2016). The remainder of this chapter will examine these issues.

Need

If the palliative care patient cannot be adequately defined in terms of diagnosis or prognosis, a third option is to identify him or her in terms of his or her need for palliative care. At this point it is necessary, briefly, to consider levels of palliative care. A patient may 'need' palliative care, but can find that all of his or her needs can be met by those already involved in his or her care. Another patient may have needs which require the additional input of specialists in palliative care. In Europe, three levels of provision are recognised (Gamondi, Larkin and Payne 2013, p. 87):

1   *Palliative care approach*: A way to integrate palliative care methods and procedures in settings not specialised in palliative care. This is practised by general practitioners and staff in general hospitals, as well as nursing services and nursing home staff.

2   *General palliative care*: Provided by primary care professionals and specialists treating patients with life-threatening diseases who have good basic palliative care skills and knowledge. This is also practised by professionals who are involved more frequently in palliative care, such as oncologists or geriatric specialists, but who do not provide palliative care as the main focus of their work.

3   *Specialist palliative care*: Provided in services whose main activity is the provision of palliative care. These services generally care for patients with complex and difficult needs but whose needs are not adequately covered by other treatment options.

These distinctions are important in the present context because they highlight the fact that the level of palliative care needs that an individual has can determine whether they are regarded as an appropriate patient to be referred to a particular service. For instance, the Association for Palliative Medicine of Great Britain and Ireland (APM) has recommended that referral to specialist palliative care should be based on the following criteria:

1   The patient has active, progressive advanced disease, a limited prognosis, and the focus of care is on quality of life.
2   The patient has unresolved complex needs that cannot be met by the caring team. These needs may be physical, psychological, social and/or spiritual.
3   The patient consents to referral (where the patient has capacity for this consent).
(APM 2012, pp. 13–14)

Certainly it is a positive step that such criteria recognise the importance not just of assigning a diagnostic label, but also of recognising the severity, complexity, burden and impact of the symptoms experienced by that individual (Skilbeck and Payne 2005). Indeed, it is crucial that any needs assessment recognises that the palliative care patient is not just a collection of symptoms (albeit potentially highly complex and burdensome) but an individual (often existing in the context of a wider 'family') with uniquely complex and dynamic needs (Ryan et al. 2013). This is amply illustrated by Weissman and Meier (2011), who listed triggers for palliative care assessment which may be recognised in hospital-based patients. These include factors related to their previous care setting (such as limited social support or the absence of advance care planning), circumstances around the actual admission (such as whether it was precipitated by a worsening symptom or a recurring cause) and factors which can crop up unexpectedly on any particular day (such as difficult-to-control physical or psychological symptoms or family distress).

What might be referred to as person-centred needs can sometimes be overlooked in the presence of complex physical symptom burdens. This might particularly be the case in people with non-malignant diseases such as dementia where social and psychological burden can be particularly extreme (Ryan et al. 2013). It can also be the case in certain settings such as intensive care where the predominant focus is on supporting vital functions (Holms, Milligan and Kydd 2014; Davies and Vora 2016). Pringle, Johnston and

Buchanan (2015) and others have drawn attention to the need for dignity-conserving and person-centred care, particularly in hospitalised patients (Milligan 2012). They highlight the fact that people with palliative care needs are particularly at risk of having their dignity compromised. Therefore, in addressing the question 'Who is the palliative care patient?', part of the answer may be 'someone who has particularly acute needs for dignity enhancing and preserving care'.

Care must also be taken not to overlook the needs of the family. The palliative care patient will often be surrounded by a network of individuals, each suffering in his or her own way. Each may also be struggling with the developmental transition, from 'living with' a life-limiting disease to 'dying from' it, that accepting palliative care may signal (Waldrop, Meeker and Kutner 2015). Carers' needs can be subtle and include the need for restorative care and for recognition of the emotional labour associated with the carer's role (Sampson et al. 2014). They may also need knowledge and skills to enable them to play a role which is often unexpected and unprepared for (Connolly and Milligan 2014). Early evidence suggests that implementation of a comprehensive assessment of carer needs can deliver significant benefits such as lower levels of early grief and better psychological and physical health (Grande et al. 2014).

Defining the palliative care patient according to need is fraught with difficulties. Needs are often complex, and always unique to the individual concerned. Whereas the reason for assessing need is sometimes the requirement to determine suitability for referral to specialist services, nevertheless where needs assessment is applied early, perhaps linked to prognostic estimation, there is the potential to identify the need for and facilitate vitally important palliative interventions. These may include the commencement of strong opioids, referral for specialist palliative care input and fast-tracking for financial allowances (Farquhar et al. 2002). They may also include exploration of care goals, anticipatory care planning and support for carers (Highet et al. 2013).

Dialogue and consensus

In practice, the point at which an individual becomes suitable for palliative care (i.e. becomes a 'palliative care patient') is to a certain extent influenced by the person themselves, their family and their care team. Patients and families may resist being given a palliative diagnosis because of concerns that it will signal loss of hope, acceptance of defeat and withdrawal of other care options (Weissman and Meier 2011). Professionals may delay arriving at that diagnosis out of sensitivity to these feelings, out of unwillingness to forgo active treatment or out of misconceptions about the role that palliative care could play (Cheang et al. 2015). And yet reaching a consensus is crucial if the benefits of palliative care are to be experienced by more patients and at an earlier stage. Perhaps it is time to place less emphasis on an arbitrary prognostic threshold for the commencement of palliative care and more on an individualised one which triggers when patient, family and professionals reach a fully informed consensus (Van Mechelen et al. 2012).

Conversations about choosing palliative care are often extremely challenging, and professionals are sometimes reluctant to take part in them (Sleeman 2013). However, there is evidence that patients and families want to have these conversations (although they may wish to negotiate how much is discussed and when), especially if they are facilitated by a familiar and trusted health professional (Parker et al. 2007). Further-more there is evidence that shared decision-making is possible and, if adequate informa-tion and preparation are provided, patients can play a full part in deciding the course of their future care (Fortnum, Grennan and Smolonogov 2015).

Conclusion

It seems inevitable that as the scope of palliative care broadens, as prognostic tools improve, as the ability to define and meet palliative care needs increases and as commu-nication between professionals and patients becomes more sophisticated, the number of people classified as 'palliative care patients' will increase. Not only will the overall number increase, but due to the trend towards earlier identification, the lengths of time individuals find themselves in receipt of palliative care will also rise. This scenario has profound implications in terms of the demand likely to be placed on existing resources. Some of the solutions that will no doubt have to be explored will include the extension of the responsibility for the provision of palliative care to a much wider range of profes-sionals, agencies and services than ever before, and the increasing facilitation of patient and family self-care. Another potential solution may be to move the focus of palliative and end of life care away from diagnostic labels for individuals and towards greater emphasis on a public health approach (Skilbeck and Payne 2005). This would recognise that the latter stages of life are often associated with high symptom burden, challenges to dignity and personhood, and a huge burden of suffering, and then population-level solutions should be developed in response.

References

Akashi, M., Yano, E. and Aruga, E. (2012) Under-diagnosis of pain by primary physi-cians and late referral to a palliative care team. *BMC Palliative Care*, 11(7). doi: 10.1186/1472-684X-11-7.

APM (Association for Palliative Medicine of Great Britain and Ireland) (2012) *Commis-sioning Guidance for Specialist Palliative Care: Helping to Deliver Commissioning Objectives*. Guidance document published collaboratively with the Association for Palliative Medicine of Great Britain and Ireland, Consultant Nurse in Palliative Care Reference Group, Marie Curie Cancer Care, National Council for Palliative Care, and Palliative Care Section of the Royal Society of Medicine, London, UK. Southampton: APM. Available at: http://www.ncpc.org.uk/sites/default/files/Commissioning GuidanceforSpecialistPalliativeCare.pdf

Boland, J., Martin, J., Wells, A.U. and Ross, J.R. (2013) Palliative care for people with non-malignant lung disease: summary of current evidence and future direction. *Palliative Medicine*, 27(9): 811–16.

Brown, M.A., Sampson, E.L., Jones, L. and Barron, A.M. (2013) Prognostic indicators of 6-month mortality in elderly people with advanced dementia: a systematic review. *Palliative Medicine*, 27(5): 389–400.

Calanzani, N., Higginson, I.J. and Gomes B. (2013) *Current and Future Needs for Hospice Care: An Evidence-Based Report*. London. Help the Hospices Ltd.

Candy, B., Elliott, M., Moore, K. et al. (2015) UK quality statements on end of life care in dementia: a systematic review of research evidence. *BMC Palliative Care*, 14(51). doi: 10.1186/s12904-015-0047-6.

Cheang, M.H., Rose, G., Cheung, C-C. and Thomas, M. (2015) Current challenges in palliative care provision for heart failure in the UK: a survey on the perspectives of palliative care professionals. *Open Heart*, 2(1). doi: 10.1136/openhrt-2014-000188.

Clark, D. (2007) From margins to centre: a review of the history of palliative care in cancer. *Lancet Oncology*, 8: 430–8.

Clark, D., Small, N., Wright, M. et al. (2005) *A Little Bit of Heaven for the Few? An Oral History of the Modern Hospice Movement in the United Kingdom*. Lancaster: Observatory Publications.

Connolly, J. and Milligan, S. (2014) Knowledge and skills needed by informal carers to look after terminally ill patients at home. *End of Life Journal*, 4(2): 1–14.

Courtney, R. and Callow, A. (2014) Audit of palliative care patient identification in general practice (poster). *BMJ Supportive and Palliative Care*, 4(1): A98.

Dale, J., Petrova, M., Munday, D. and Thomas, K. (2009) A national facilitation project to improve primary palliative care: impact of the Gold Standards Framework on process and self-ratings of quality. *Quality and Safety in Health Care*, 18(3). doi: 10.1136/qshc.2007.024836.

Davies, J. and Vora, V. (2016) Experience of providing palliative care in critical care settings. *BMJ Supportive and Palliative Care*. Published Online First 12 January 2016. doi: 10.1136/bmjspcare-2015-000900.

De Lepelaire, J., Iliffe, S., Mann, E. and Degryse, J.M. (2009) Frailty: an emerging concept for general practice. *British Journal of General Practice*, 59(562): e177–e182. doi: 10.3399/bjgp09X420653.

Douglas, C., Murtagh, F.E., Chambers, E.J. et al. (2009) Symptom management for the adult patient dying with advanced chronic kidney disease: a review of the literature and development of evidence-based guidelines by a United Kingdom Expert Consensus Group. *Palliative Medicine*, 23(2): 103–10.

Dunphy, E.J., Conlon, S.C., O'Brien, S.A. et al. (2016) End-of-life planning with frail patients attending general practice: an exploratory prospective cross-sectional study. *British Journal of General Practice*. Online First 15 July 2016. doi: 10.3399/bjgp16X686557.

European Association for Palliative Care (2013) Recommendations on palliative care and treatment of older people with Alzheimer's disease and other progressive dementias. Available at: http://www.eapcnet.eu/LinkClick.aspx?fileticket=SouPo-_uNLw%3D

Fadul, N., Elsayem, A., Palmer, J.L. et al. (2009) Supportive versus palliative care: what's in a name? A survey of medical oncologists and midlevel providers at a comprehensive cancer center. *Cancer*, 115(9): 2013–21.

Farquhar, M., Grande, G., Todd, C. and Barclay, S. (2002) Defining patients as palliative: hospital doctors' versus general practitioners' perceptions. *Palliative Medicine*, 16: 247–50.

Filbet, M. (2008) Who's afraid of palliative care? (Editorial). *European Journal of Palliative Care*, 15(3): 109.

Fortnum, D., Grennan, K. and Smolonogov, T. (2015) End-stage kidney disease patient evaluation of the Australian 'My Kidneys, My Choice' decision aid. *Clinical Kidney Journal*, 8(4): 469–75.

Gamondi, C., Larkin, P. and Payne, S. (2013) Core competencies in palliative care: an EAPC White Paper on palliative care education – Part 1. *European Journal of Palliative Care*, 20(2): 86–91.

Gardiner, C., Gott, M., Ingleton, C. and Richards, N. (2013) Palliative care in frail older people: a cross-sectional survey of patients at two hospitals in England. *Progress in Palliative Care*, 21(5): 272–7.

Gardiner, C., Ingleton, C., Gott, M. and Ryan, T. (2015) Exploring the transition from curative care to palliative care: a systematic review of the literature. *BMJ Supportive and Palliative Care*, 5: 335–42. doi: 10.1136/bmjspcare-2010-000001rep.

Glare, P., Sinclair, C.T., Stone, P. and Clayton, J.M. (2015) Predicting survival in patients with advanced disease. In Cherney, N., Fallon, M., Kaasa, S. et al. (eds) *Oxford Textbook of Palliative Medicine* (5th edn). Oxford: Oxford University Press.

Gomes, B. (2015) Palliative care: if it makes a difference, why wait? (Editorial). *Journal of Clinical Oncology*, 60: 5386.

Grande, G.E., Austin, L., Ewing, G. et al. (2014) Assessing the impact of a Carer Support Needs Assessment Tool (CSNAT) intervention in palliative home care: a stepped wedge cluster trial. *BMJ Supportive and Palliative Care*. Published Online First. doi: 10.1136/bmjspcare-2014-000829.

Highet, G., Crawford, D., Murray, S.A. and Boyd, K. (2013) Development and evaluation of the Supportive and Palliative Care Indicators Tool (SPICT): a mixed-methods study. *BMJ Supportive and Palliative Care*, 4(3). doi: 10.1136/bmjspcare-2013-000488.

Holms, N., Milligan, S. and Kydd, A. (2014) A study of the lived experiences of registered nurses who have provided end-of-life care within an intensive care unit. *International Journal of Palliative Nursing*, 20(11): 549–56.

Hui, D., Kim, S.Y., Roquemore, J. et al. (2014) Impact of timing and setting of palliative care referral on quality of end-of-life care in cancer patients. *Cancer*, 20(11): 1743–9.

Humphreys, J. and Harma, S. (2014) Late referral to palliative care consultation service: length of stay and in-hospital mortality outcomes. *Journal of Community and Supportive Oncology*, 12(4): 129–36.

Johnston, B., Rogerson, L., Macijauskiene, J. et al. (2014) An exploration of self-management support in the context of palliative nursing: a modified concept analysis. *BMC Nursing*, 13(21). Available at: http://www.biomedcentral.com/1472-6955/13/21

Lewis, M.J. (2006) *Medicine and care of the dying: A modern history*; Oxford University Press, Oxford.

Lynn, J. (2005) Living long in fragile health: the new demographics shape end of life care. *Hastings Center Report. Special Report*, 35(6): S14–S18.

Lynn, J. and Adamson, D.M. (2003) Living well at the end of life: adapting health care to serious chronic illness in old age. Rand White Paper. Santa Monica, CA: Rand Corporation. Available at: https://www.rand.org/content/dam/rand/pubs/white_papers/2005/WP137.pdf

Maltoni, M., Scarpi, E., Pittureri, C. et al. (2012) Prospective comparison of prognostic scores in palliative care cancer populations. *Oncologist*, 17(3): 446–54.

Marie Curie (2015a) *Equity in the Provision of Palliative and End of Life Care in the UK*. London: Marie Curie UK.

Marie Curie (2015b) *Triggers for Palliative Care*. London. Marie Curie UK. Available at: https://www.mariecurie.org.uk/globalassets/media/documents/policy/policy-publications/june-2015/triggers-for-palliative-care-executive-summary.pdf

McIlfatrick, S., Hasson, F., McLaughlin, D. et al. (2013) Public awareness and attitudes toward palliative care in Northern Ireland. *BMC Palliative Care*, 12(34). doi: 10.1186/1472-684X-12-34. Available at: http://bmcpalliatcare.biomedcentral.com/articles/10.1186/1472-684X-12-34

Mehta, Z., Giorgini, K., Ellison, N. and Roth, M.E. (2012) Integrating palliative medicine with dementia care. *Aging Well*, 5(2): 18.

Meier, D.E. and Brawley, O.W. (2011) Palliative care and the quality of life. *Journal of Clinical Oncology*, 29(20): 2750–2.

Merlin, J.S., Tucker, R.O., Saag, M.S. and Selwyn, P.A. (2013) The role of palliative care in the current HIV treatment era in developed countries. *Topics in Antiviral Medicine*, 21(1): 20–6.

Milligan, S. (2012) Optimising palliative and end of life care in hospital. *Nursing Standard*, 26(41): 48–56.

Mitchell, G., Senior, H., Rhee, J. et al. (2016) Using intuition or a formal palliative care needs assessment screening pathway in general practice to predict death within twelve months: a randomized controlled trial (Oral Presentation abstract). Presented at conference: The evolving role of primary care in cancer, 4 March 2016. Western Centre for Health Research and Education, Sunshine Hospital, Melbourne. Available at: https://s3-ap-southeast-2.amazonaws.com/ap-southeast-2.accounts.ivvy.com/account8357/events/83457/files/56d3e5dacbe01.pdf

Mitchell, H., Noble, S., Finlay, I. and Nelson, A. (2015) Defining the palliative care patient: its challenges and implications for service delivery. *BMJ Supportive and Palliative Care*, 5: 46–52.

Moroni, M., Zocchi, D., Bolognesi, D. et al. on behalf of the SUQ-P Group (2014) The 'surprise' question in advanced cancer patients: a prospective study among general practitioners. *Palliative Medicine*, 28(7): 959–64.

Murray, S.A. and Boyd, K. (2011) Using the 'surprise question' can identify people with advanced heart failure and COPD who would benefit from a palliative care approach. *Palliative Medicine*, 25(4): 382.

Murray, S.A., Kendall, M., Boyd, K. and Sheikh, A. (2005) Illness trajectories and palliative care. *British Medical Journal*, 33: 1007–11.

National Council for Palliative Care (2015) Palliative care explained. Available at: http://www.ncpc.org.uk/palliative-care-explained

National Gold Standards Framework Centre England (2008) National Gold Standards Framework Prognostic Indicator Guidance, Revised Vs 5. September 2008. National

Gold Standards Framework Centre England. Available at: http://www.gov.scot/resource/doc/924/0092227.pdf

NHS England (2016) Commissioning person-centred end of life care: a toolkit for health and social care. Updated April 2016. London. NHS England. Available at: https://www.england.nhs.uk/wp-content/uploads/2016/04/nhsiq-comms-eolc-tlkit-.pdf

NHS Improving Quality (2014) End of life care in heart failure: a framework for implementation. NHS Improving Quality. Available at: http://www.nhsiq.nhs.uk/media/2574509/end-of-life-care-in-heart-failure-framework-for-implementation.pdf

Overy, C. and Tansey, E.M. (2012) *Palliative Medicine in the UK, c.1970–2010*. London: University of London Queen Mary College.

Parker, S.M., Clayton, J.M., Hancock, K. et al. (2007) A systematic review of prognostic/end-of-life communication with adults in the advanced stages of a life-limiting illness: patient/caregiver preferences for the content, style, and timing of information. *Journal of Pain and Symptom Management*, 34(1): 81–93.

Penrod, J., Hupcey, J.E., Baney, B.L. and Loeb, S.J. (2011) End-of-life caregiving trajectories. *Clinical Nursing Research*, 20(1): 7–24.

Pringle, J., Johnston, B. and Buchanan, D. (2015) Dignity and patient-centred care for people with palliative care needs in the acute hospital setting: a systematic review. *Palliative Medicine*, 29(8): 675–94.

Rocker, G., Downar, J. and Morrison, R.S. (2016) Palliative care for chronic illness: driving change. *Canadian Medical Association Journal*. First published 22 August 2016. doi: 10.1503/cmaj.151454.

Rosenwax, L., Spilsbury, K., McNamara, B.A. and Semmens, J.B. (2016) A retrospective population-based cohort study of access to specialist palliative care in the last year of life: who is still missing out a decade on? *BMC Palliative Care*, 15(46). doi: 10.1186/s12904-016-0119-246.

Ryan, T., Ingleton, C., Gardiner, C. et al. (2013) Symptom burden, palliative care need and predictors of physical and psychological discomfort in two UK hospitals. *BMC Palliative Care*, 12(11). doi: 10.1186/1472-684X-12-11.

Sampson, E.L. (2010) Palliative care for people with dementia. *British Medical Bulletin*, 96(1): 159–74.

Sampson, E.L., Finlay, I., Byrne, A. et al. (2014) The practice of palliative care from the perspective of patients and carers. *BMJ Supportive and Palliative Care*, 4(1): 291–8.

Sampson, E.L., Ritchie, C.W., Raven, P.W. and Blanchard, B.R. (2005) A systematic review of the scientific evidence for the efficacy of a palliative care approach in advanced dementia. *International Psychogeriatrics*, 17(1): 31–40.

Skilbeck, J.K. and Payne, S.A. (2005) End of life care: a discursive analysis of end of life care nursing. *Journal of Advanced Nursing*, 51(4): 325–34.

Sleeman, K.E. (2013) End-of-life communication: let's talk about death (Editorial). *Journal of the Royal College of Physicians of Edinburgh*, 43: 107–9.

Starkweather, A. (2016) Palliative care in the emergency department. In Dahlin, C., Coyne, P.J. and Ferrell, B.R. (eds) *Advanced Practice Palliative Nursing*. Oxford: Oxford University Press.

Temel, J.S., Greer, J.A., Muzikansky, A. et al. (2010) Early palliative care for patients with metastatic non-small-cell lung cancer. *New England Journal of Medicine*, 363(8): 733–42.

The Scottish Government (2015) *Strategic Framework for Action on Palliative and End of Life Care 2016–2021*. Edinburgh: The Scottish Government Available at: http://www.gov.scot/Resource/0049/00491388.pdf

US Department of Health and Human Services (2015) CMS announces Medicare Care Choices Model awards (Press release). Available at: http://www.hhs.gov/about/news/2015/07/20/cms-announces-medicare-care-choices-model-awards.html

US Department of Health and Human Services (2016) *Medicare Hospice Benefits*. Baltimore, MD: Centers for Medicare & Medicaid Services. Available at: https://www.medicare.gov/Pubs/pdf/02154.pdf

Vanderpool, H.Y. (2015) *Palliative Care: The 400 Year Quest for a Good Death*. Jefferson, NC: McFarland and Company.

Van Mechelen, W., Aertgeerts, B., De Ceulaer, K. et al. (2013) Defining the palliative care patient: a systematic review. *Palliative Medicine*, 27(3): 197–208.

Waldrop, D., Meeker, M.A. and Kutner, J.S. (2015) The developmental transition from living with to dying from cancer: hospice decision-making. *Journal of Psychosocial Oncology*, 33(5): 576–98.

Weissman, D.E. and Meier, D.E. (2011) Identifying patients in need of a palliative care assessment in the hospital setting: a consensus report from the Center to Advance Palliative Care. *Journal of Palliative Medicine*, 14: 17–23.

Witt, J., Murtagh, F.E.M., de Wolf-Linder, S. et al. (2014) *Introducing the Outcome Assessment and Complexity Collaborative (OACC) Suite of Measures: A Brief Introduction*. London: King's College, London. Available at: https://www.kcl.ac.uk/lsm/research/divisions/cicelysaunders/attachments/Studies-OACC-Brief-Introduction-Booklet.pdf

WHO (World Health Organization) (2016) Definition of palliative care. Available at: http://www.who.int/cancer/palliative/definition/en/

Zheng, L., Finucane, A.M., Oxenham, D. et al. (2013) How good is primary care at identifying patients who need palliative care? A mixed methods study. *European Journal of Palliative Care*, 20(50): 216–22.

Zimmermann, C., Swami, N., Krzyzanowska, M. et al. (2016) Perceptions of palliative care among patients with advanced cancer and their caregivers. *Canadian Medical Association Journal*. Early release, published at www.cmaj.ca on 18 April 2016. doi: 10.1503/cmaj.151171.

Issues of referral to and accessing palliative care

Josie Dixon

Palliative care is not provided by a single service or type of provider. Rather, it is provided by many different care providers, delivering different types of care at different points in time and within different care settings. It is provided both by generalist palliative care providers, such as general practitioners or care home staff, as well as by palliative care specialists, often working together in multi-disciplinary teams. Providing palliative care is complex, dynamic, time-critical and relies on highly effective coordination, between providers and across settings.

This chapter focuses on access to palliative care services. See Chapter 1 in this volume for an explanation of the three levels of palliative care provision. In this chapter we consider the role of generalist and specialist providers, how they work together and how people access these services. In particular, we will consider the role of generalists as providers of palliative care, the support that is provided to them for this role and the evidence concerning access to generalist palliative care. We will go on to look at specialist palliative care and evidence on access to these services. And we will consider how all of this provision is coordinated and the potential of poor coordination to lead to gaps in provision. Finally, we will explore the evidence concerning equitable access to palliative care services.

Generalist palliative care services

The role of generalists in palliative care provision

Generalist providers of palliative care are those who provide day-to-day care to chronically and seriously ill people. These cover a wide range of different professionals, including general practitioners and district and general nurses (see Box 2.1). These providers are not specialists in palliative care, although they may have specialist skills in their own fields. Some will have more substantial roles in providing palliative care than others but, together, these professionals provide the majority of palliative care that is delivered to patients and their families.

Box 2.1   Generalist (non-specialist) providers of palliative care

- General practitioners
- District or community nurses
- Hospital consultants
- Care home staff
- Care assistants
- Health assistants
- Social workers
- Social care staff
- Domiciliary care workers
- Occupational therapists
- Counsellors
- Hospital chaplains, spiritual and religious support
- Volunteers

Among these different professionals, general practitioners are key. They have a central role in identifying patients who may benefit from palliative care and, working alongside other generalists, such as district nurses and social workers, they deliver palliative care directly to patients in the community. They also play a key role in referring people to specialist palliative care services where palliative care needs are complex and cannot readily be managed solely by the usual healthcare team. Non-palliative hospital consultants, also generalist providers of palliative care, may also refer patients to specialist palliative care teams, working either in the hospital or in the community. This is likely to occur in situations where the focus of care changes from curative to palliative and the prognosis is limited, or where there are complex specialist palliative care needs and the aim is stabilisation and subsequent discharge. Generalist providers may also call on specialist palliative care teams for advice, support and, in some cases, training.

Support for generalists providing palliative care

While generalist providers of palliative care are not specialists in palliative care, they should have competencies, of a type and level appropriate to their role, to support them in working with people with serious illness or at the end of life (see Box 2.2).

***

Box 2.2   Palliative care competencies for generalist providers

The National Council of Palliative Care states that generalist providers of palliative care, in all settings, should be able to do the following:

- assess the care needs of each patient and their family across the domains of physical, psychological, social, spiritual and information needs;
- meet those needs within the limits of their knowledge, skills, competence in palliative care;
- know when to seek advice from or refer to specialist palliative care service.

Source: National Council for Palliative Care website:
http://www.ncpc.org.uk/palliative-care-explained

***

To support the development and maintenance of these competencies among generalists, the NHS National End of Life Care Programme (NHS NEOLCP), which was established to help implement the National End of Life Care Strategy in England (Department of Health 2008), produced a range of support and guidance. This included the *Routes to Success in End of Life Care* series of publications, which provided practical guidance to generalist staff providing care to people at the end of life in acute hospitals (NHS NEOLCP 2010; NHS England 2015), for care homes (NHS IQ 2010a), for ambulance services (NHS NEOLCP 2012), for domiciliary care (NHS NEOLCP 2011a), for social work (NHS IQ/CSW 2012), for occupational therapy (NHS NEOLCP/COT 2011), for prisons (NHS IQ 2011a) and for general nursing (NHS NEOLCP/RCN 2011), as well as for particular groups of people, including lesbian, gay, bi-sexual and transgender (LGBT) people (NHS IQ 2012), people with learning disabilities (NHS IQ 2011b) and people who are homeless (NHS IQ 2010b). The NHS NEOLCP also published guidance on advance care planning, a process of discussing and recording preferences for future care, for generalist healthcare and social care staff (NHS NEOLCP 2011b).

Support for generalist providers of palliative care has focused primarily on professionals working in the community, with a particular focus on general practitioners and district nurses. This reflects the fact that, over the last decade or so, healthcare policy has supported a shifting of care from acute hospitals to the community, with the aims of delivering care closer to home, reducing avoidable hospital admissions and readmissions, reducing the average length of hospital stay, increasing patient choice and making better use of healthcare resources (NHS 2014). There has consequently been considerable policy support for general practitioners taking a clear lead in identifying and meeting the palliative care needs of their patients in the community. A key initiative here was introducing, as of 2006, palliative care registers, and an associated 3-monthly multidisciplinary meeting about people on the register, as a quality and outcome framework (QOF) measure (QOF is a system for the performance management and payment of general practitioners in the National Health Service) (NHS England 2016). It is intended that the register includes all patients, both with cancer and non-cancer conditions, who are thought to be in their last year of life and who are therefore likely to have palliative care needs. In order to identify the patients who should be on the register, general practitioners are encouraged to ask themselves 'the surprise question': 'Would you be surprised if this patient died in the next 6–12 months?', although there are also a range of prognostic indicator and risk stratification tools available (Walsh et al. 2015).[1] It is recommended that the palliative care register and multi-disciplinary meetings are implemented within the context of the Gold Standards Framework, a coordinated programme of care for those in the last 12 months of life (NHS England 2016). The QOF measure is complemented by the *Find Your 1%* campaign. This is hosted by the Dying Matters Coalition, working with Macmillan Cancer Support, the Royal College of General Practitioners (RCGP) and others. It provides general practitioners with a range of information and resources to help them identify the, on average, 1 per cent of their patients who are likely to die within the next 12 months and to support them to help their patients achieve a good death. The competencies of general practitioners and others in palliative and end of life care are also supported by professional and clinical training, guidance and tools developed by, for example, the Royal College of Nursing (RCN),[2] the Royal College of General Practitioners (RCGP),[3] and the General Medical Council (GMC).[4]

Access to generalist palliative care

Despite the fact that generalists are important providers of palliative care, there is currently limited information available about access to generalist palliative care services. The *Independent Palliative Care Funding Review* (Hughes-Hallet et al. 2011) estimated that around 355,000 people annually in England would benefit from palliative care at the end of their life, with around 171,000 known to be receiving care from palliative care specialists. Of the remainder, the review estimated that maybe 92,000 people receive palliative care solely from generalist providers and 92,000 receive no palliative care at all, although these estimates of generalist-only and no care are necessarily based on very limited evidence (Hughes-Hallet et al. 2011). Similarly, while we know that 97.6 per cent of general practices met the QOF palliative care measures in 2014/2015 (HSCIC 2015), we do not know how actively these practices used their palliative care registers to improve access to palliative care, with studies showing that, commonly, only around a third of deceased patients are on the palliative care register, with many of these entered in the last weeks and days of life (Harrison et al. 2012; Gadoud et al. 2014).

While undoubtedly there is much excellent palliative care provided by general practitioners and other generalists, available evidence suggests that there remain gaps in provision and concerns about the quality of care provided. Results from the most recent National Survey of Bereaved People, for example, based on a sample of almost 50,000 bereaved people, reports that 30 per cent of respondents thought care provided by general practitioners in the last 3 months of their friend's or relative's life was only fair (17.5 per cent) or poor (12.5 per cent), rather than good (35.7 per cent) or excellent (34.2 per cent) (ONS 2016a). This was almost the poorest rating given to different types of service provider, poorer than that for hospital doctors and nurses, for example, and only better than the rating for urgent care services. In this case, 37.5 per cent of respondents rated urgent care services received by their friend or relative in the last 3 months of their life as poor (16.4 per cent) or fair (23.1 per cent), rather than good (37 per cent) or excellent (25.5 per cent). Care from district and community nurses, however, was rated more highly, with less than 20 per cent of respondents thinking that the care received by their friend or relative was only poor (6.6 per cent) or fair (12.6 per cent).

Research studies also suggest that there are difficulties and challenges in the provision of generalist palliative care services, which effectively limit access. In a systematic review of research exploring the views of patients, carers and primary care staff concerning the provision of palliative care for non-cancer patients in the community, Oishi and Murtagh (2014) found that, although general practitioners were generally acknowledged to have the lead role in providing end of life and palliative care for people in the community, in practice they often struggled to allocate sufficient time to this role and commonly expected nurses and others to take a greater lead. Lack of resources and lack of palliative care expertise were also identified as barriers. In another study involving nearly 60 generalist healthcare staff in England, Gott et al. (2012) found that many respondents struggled to define palliative care, did not recognise themselves as palliative care providers and were unfamiliar with the term 'generalist palliative care'. And, as in the Oishi and Murtagh study, many generalist providers reported difficulty in integrating palliative care responsibilities into their workload. This picture is also reflected in findings from a 2008 consultation study conducted with 210 invited participants, including generalist healthcare and social care staff, specialist palliative care providers, commissioners, policy-makers, academics and representatives from user and voluntary groups (Shipman et al. 2008). The report from the study noted that generalists usually cared for relatively few people nearing the end of life and did so in the context of many competing responsibilities. Many general practitioners were also thought to be 'disengaged', while condition-specific expertise among general practitioners and nurses was often thought to be limited, particularly in non-cancer conditions. The problems of incorporating palliative care responsibilities into a generalist workload were also highlighted.

Learning exercise 2.1

Reflect on your practice.

- Do you see difficulties in accessing palliative care services?
- Are there groups that have inequity of access? (See, for instance, Chapter 13 in this volume.)
- Is there anything you do in your area to increase referrals and ensure more equity of access?

Specialist palliative care services

The role of specialist palliative care services

Current policy and practice in NHS England is that local clinical commissioning groups (CCGs) commission a range of specialist palliative care services, across settings and for patients at different stages in their illness (see Box 2.3). These services are provided by specialist palliative care professionals who have undergone extensive specialist training. They usually work as part of multi-disciplinary teams consisting of palliative consultants and palliative care nurse specialists working alongside allied professionals such as physiotherapists, occupational therapists, dieticians, pharmacists, social workers and those able to give spiritual and psychological support.

Box 2.3   Specialist palliative care services

- Specialist in-patient facilities within hospices or hospitals.
- The provision of specialist advice, working alongside generalist providers to support someone in hospital or at home.
- Coordinated home support for patients with complex needs and more extensive 'hospice at home' services, involving palliative medical, nursing, social and emotional support.
- Specialist palliative out-patient services, working alongside the primary care team.
- Specialist day care facilities, providing assessment services, a range of physical, social and psychological therapies, complementary therapies and social and creative activities.
- Bereavement support services.
- Education, training and continuing professional development in palliative care.

Adapted from National Council of Palliative Care
website which is now part of Hospice UK.

Not everyone with a palliative care need will require specialist palliative care services. Specialist palliative care services are intended for people with complex needs, primarily relating to symptom management, that cannot be met by the existing healthcare and social care team. National standards set by the National Institute for Health and Care Excellence (NICE) state that specialist palliative care services should be available to people approaching the end of life who may require it, 'in a timely way, appropriate to their needs and preferences, at any time of day or night' (NICE 2011, updated 2016).

Access to specialist palliative care services

The Minimum Data Set (MDS) for Specialist Palliative Care Services is the main source of information about access to specialist palliative care.[5] It was first developed in 1995 to provide quality, comprehensive annual statistics and data on palliative care services in the UK. The National Council for Palliative Care collects data annually.

In 2012/13 there were, in total, around 451 organisations providing specialist palliative care in around 1,500 services across a range of different settings in England, Wales and Northern Ireland (NCPC/PHE 2014). In standardised analyses, there has been an increase in the number of patients seen across all settings: 29.7 per cent in hospital support from 2008/09 to 2013/14, 29.3 per cent in day care and 8.9 per cent for in-patient settings (NCPC/PHE/Hospice UK 2015). There remain, however, inequities in who accesses these different services, which are discussed in later sections of this chapter.

Coordination and integration of provision

Integrated and coordinated care is vital in order to provide effective palliative care to patients across different providers and as they move between care settings. Coordination of care was a key focus for the National End of Life Care Strategy (Department of Health 2008). This sought to bring about, 'a step change in access to high quality care for all people approaching the end of life' by promoting a 'whole systems and care pathway approach' for commissioning and providing integrated services and improving coordination (Shipman et al. 2008). This is formalised in national standards for end of life care for adults set by the National Institute for Health and Care Excellence (NICE 2011, updated 2016), which require that

> people approaching the end of life receive consistent care that is coordinated effectively across all relevant settings and services at any time of day or night, and delivered by practitioners who are aware of the person's current medical condition, care plan and preferences.

NICE quality standards are for use by the NHS in England and do not have formal status in the social care sector. However, social care commissioners and providers are encouraged and supported to take account of them in order to promote effective joint working. Coordination is also one of the six ambitions in *Ambitions for Palliative and End of Life Care: A National Framework for Local Action 2015–20* (National Palliative and End of Life Care Partnership 2015). Internationally, the World Health Assembly (World Health Organization 2014) also states that palliative care needs to be fully integrated into mainstream health and social care.

What is meant by integration, however, is not entirely clear in policy or practice. Murray identifies several different understandings of the concept (Murray 2016). These include integration, and coordination, across different providers, across different care settings and, holistically, across different palliative care needs. It may also refer to the integration of palliative care into the early stages of serious illness, delivered alongside active treatments. Integration and coordination are particularly important to ensure consistent and seamless care between hospitals and community settings, between healthcare and social care services and between generalist and specialist providers. However, in guidance to commissioners, NHS England (2016) identify a very wide range of services that need to coordinate their provision to ensure the effective delivery of palliative and end of life care (Box 2.4).

Box 2.4 Services that need to be coordinated to provide effective end of life care

- Specialist palliative care providers
- Primary and community providers – general practitioners, district nurses, and out-of-hours services
- The cross-service and sector-integrated multi-disciplinary team
- The rapid response team
- Adult social care services – both in and out of hours
- Other providers of palliative and end of life care services: statutory and voluntary
- Providers of acute care
- Urgent and emergency care services, including 111 and ambulance services
- Providers of paediatric palliative care
- Public health
- Providers of services for individuals with long-term conditions.

Source: NHS England (2016b).

Data-sharing is a key aspect in effective coordination of palliative care services. Palliative care services have to deal with a number of complex issues regarding the use and sharing of patient information, including issues of capacity (under the Mental Capacity Act 2005) and issues of sharing information with carers and family members. Locality-wide registers were introduced in the National End of Life Care Strategy (Department of Health 2008) as a way of achieving greater coordination. These registers were renamed EPaCCS (Electronic Palliative Care Coordination Systems) and, in March 2012, an information standard for new EPaCCS (SCCI 1580) was established. In 2013, 64 CCGs had operational systems. Further development of EPaCCS faces a range of challenges, including changes in the commissioning landscape for end of life care services and the realisation that EPaCCS need to be adapted to wider coordination needs such as managing the care of people with long-term chronic health conditions (WSP 2016). Consequently, they are still very much in development in most areas of England (WSP 2016).

Research studies suggest that coordination can frequently be poor. For example, in their systematic review, Oishi and Murtagh found evidence of a lack of clarity about roles and poor communication and collaboration between different professionals, concluding that, 'on the whole, inter-professional work in primary palliative care settings is relatively ineffective despite the importance of collaboration having been repeatedly emphasised' (2014, p. 1094). Shipman et al. (2008), in their consultation study, similarly found that poor integration between health and social care was considered a key factor limiting continuity and completeness of care. Gott et al. (2012) argue that while the balance between generalist care and specialist care, with its focus on complex cases and providing support to generalist providers, may be understood in policy, this has not always been translated effectively into practice on the ground.

There is also evidence of poor collaboration between hospital consultants and palliative care teams, with generalist clinicians sometimes seeing specialist palliative care as only for patients for whom active treatment is no longer an option (Gott et al. 2012). The Amber Care model is a promising approach to ensure that those with uncertain illness trajectories yet being actively treated have the same access to specialist palliative care services, where needed, as those who are no longer being actively treated (Box 2.5).

Box 2.5   Amber Care Bundle

One model that has so far had good results is the Amber Care Bundle (AMBER – **A**ssessment **M**anagement **B**est practice **E**ngagement of patients and carers for patients whose **R**ecovery is uncertain). The Amber Care Bundle is used in hospitals and ensures that people being actively treated but where recovery is uncertain gain timely access to appropriate palliative care. It provides a framework for non-palliative consultants and the palliative care team to share responsibility for a patient, pursuing curative treatments while, at the same time, putting in place palliative care support and preparing for possible deterioration and, potentially, end of life. The approach was developed at the Guy's and St Thomas' NHS Foundation Trust, London, and is now being implemented more widely, nationally and internationally. It is also a key plank of the Transform Programme, which encourages hospital trusts to develop a strategic approach to improve the quality of end of life care.

See the Transform Programme, available at: http://www.nhsiq.nhs.uk/improvement-programmes/long-term-conditions-and-integrated-care/end-of-life-care/acute-hospital-care/more-about-the-transform-programme.aspx

---

Poor coordination and integration between different providers translate into poor and fragmented access, as well as poor continuity of care, for patients and their families. The National Survey of Bereaved People 2015 release (ONS 2016a) reports that respondents thought hospital services 'worked well together' with general practitioners and other services outside the hospital in only 30.5 per cent of cases. Respondents thought these services worked well together 'to some extent' in a further 36.1 per cent of cases and poorly in 33.4 per cent of cases. When patients were being cared for at home, services were experienced as working better together, with 40 per cent of respondents saying services worked well together, with only 16.4 per cent of respondents saying that coordination was poor. Poor coordination is widely identified as a key reason for failures and omissions in palliative and end of life care, including, for example, by the Parliamentary and Health Service Ombudsman, the independent organisation responsible for investigating complaints about the NHS (PHSO 2015).

Evidence of inequity in access to palliative care

There is evidence that suggests that there is differential access to palliative care services, both generalist and specialist, for different groups of patients. A key area of inequity of access is that of diagnosis, with people with non-cancer diagnoses experiencing less access overall and less access to specialist and other high-quality palliative care when compared to people with cancer. Addressing this inequity has been an important focus for recent end of life care policy. Older people, including the 'oldest old' (people over 85), also receive proportionately less access to palliative care than people in younger age groups, although, as with diagnosis, the gap has slightly narrowed in recent years. People from black Asian and minority ethnic (BAME) groups are commonly thought to have less access to palliative care, although the evidence is more mixed than is generally thought. There is also evidence that access to timely and good quality palliative care is less for people who live in the most deprived areas, for care home residents, for people who are cared for and/or die in hospital and for people without partners or spouses. Relevant indicators of access include receipt of services, but also outcomes measures that suggest sufficiency of palliative and end of life care, such as effective pain control or death in usual place of residence. These issues are discussed in further detail below.

People with non-cancer diagnoses

A wide range of research studies have shown that people with non-cancer conditions are likely to have similarly distressing symptoms and as much need for palliative care as those with cancer (Dixon et al. 2015). Even though cancer accounts for just 29 per cent of all deaths, Murtagh et al. (2013) estimate that as many as 82 per cent of deaths in high-income countries are likely to have preceding palliative care needs. This, however, is not currently reflected in either palliative care registers or referrals to specialist palliative care services. Harrison et al. (2012), for example, found that 68 per cent of people entered on the palliative care registers of six general practices had a cancer diagnosis. In another study, only 7 per cent of decedents with heart failure were found to be on the palliative care register compared to 48 per cent of decedents with cancer (Gadoud et al. 2014). The patients with heart failure were also placed on the register much later, often days or a few weeks before death (Gadoud et al. 2014).

Currently only around 20 per cent of referrals to specialist palliative care are for people with conditions other than cancer (NCPC/PHE 2014; NCPC/PHE/Hospice UK 2015). This is up from 5 per cent in 2000 and 12 per cent in 2008. People undergoing active cancer treatment and with haematological cancer are also less likely to get a specialist referral. Furthermore, studies have found that people with conditions other than cancer in their last months of life also have considerably less contact time with generalists, including their general practitioner and district nurses, than people with cancer (Burt et al. 2010; Georghiou and Bardsley 2014). Secondary analyses of data from the National Survey of Bereaved People (using multivariate regression models to control for age, sex, deprivation, ethnicity, whether person has a spouse) also found that people with non-cancer conditions had less access to a range of community- and home-based support, including Marie Curie Nurses, other community-based nurses, spiritual and emotional care, hospice at home, rapid response services and home help/meals on wheels and, more generally, sufficient help and support from health-care and social services to be cared for at home (Dixon et al. 2015). This study also found that people with cancer were more likely to die in their usual place of residence, to have pain relieved 'completely, all the time' when being cared for at home and to experience care that their relatives considered to be 'excellent' or 'outstanding' (Dixon et al. 2015).

There is likely to be a range of reasons for this disparity. These include that non-cancer conditions tend to have far less predictable disease trajectories, making it harder to make a prognosis or identify a terminal stage (Dixon et al. 2015). Additionally, non-cancer conditions may present unique challenges. For example, in dementia, identification of palliative care need is complicated by communication difficulties and concerns about ethical, regulatory and legal issues. See Chapter 7 in this volume for more information on this (Birch and Draper 2008; Davies et al. 2014). However, it also reflects the fact that there is commonly a lack of condition-specific expertise and information among palliative care providers and a lack of appropriate models of care for people with non-cancer conditions (Shipman et al. 2008; Gott et al. 2012; Murtagh et al. 2014; Dixon et al. 2015).

Age

People aged 85 or over account for 39 per cent of deaths but just 16 per cent of referrals to specialist palliative care services, although this figure is up from 11 per cent in 2012 (NCPC/PHE 2014). In the most recent report, it is found that younger people (aged 64 and under) account for 13.5 per cent of deaths but, looking at each different setting separately, always are at least 23.8 per cent of people accessing any specialist palliative care (NCPC/PHE/Hospice UK 2015). There is considerable evidence that there is no difference in clinical need that would explain such a disparity (Walshe et al. 2009), although one study involving a multivariate analysis of data from a survey of 252 people with lung cancer found that age was not associated with access to specialist palliative care services, although measures of clinical need and where treatment was provided were (Burt et al. 2010). There is some evidence that the palliative care needs of people in this age group may be systematically under-identified by healthcare professionals. For example, in a study of 514 older hospital patients, 36 per cent were found to meet the criteria for palliative care need according to the

Gold Standards Framework (GSF) prognostic indicator, while medical staff estimated that only 15.5 per cent had palliative care needs and nursing staff estimated that only 17.4 per cent had palliative care needs (Gardiner et al. 2013; Gott et al. 2013). It was suggested that this may be because illness and death are more expected in old age and that, potentially, older people may also tend to under-report their symptoms.

The evidence on pain control for older patients is equivocal. Secondary analyses of data from the National Survey of Bereaved People – involving multivariate regression analysis that controlled for factors such as diagnosis and area deprivation – showed that respondents believed pain to be well controlled in this age group (Dixon et al. 2015). However, studies involving more objective measures have suggested this may not be the case. For example, in a study involving data from 29,825 patients, Higginson and Gao (2012) found that people over 60, when compared to those under 50, had measurably less access to opoids.

Ethnicity

Around 7 per cent of new people accessing palliative care are from black, Asian and minority ethnic (BAME) groups (NCPC/PHE 2014). This appears lower than might be expected given that 14 per cent of the population in England is from a BAME group. This has led to a view that BAME groups are under-represented among specialist palliative care referrals. However, the age profile of the BAME population is significantly younger – just 4.8 per cent of over 65-year-olds in England are from BAME groups (Dixon et al. 2015). As BAME populations age, we would expect the proportion of BAME people referred to specialist palliative care to increase proportionately (Calanzani et al. 2013b). There is some limited evidence that some BAME groups may have different disease profiles, although this difference is likely to be small and also reducing over time (Calanzani et al. 2013b).

In secondary analyses of data from the National Survey of Bereaved People (using multivariate regression models to control for age, sex, deprivation, ethnicity, whether person has a spouse), Dixon et al. (2015) found that BAME groups had access to similar types of community-based service (such as Marie Curie nurses or hospice at home services) as people of white ethnicity, although it is unknown whether they received the same level of service or whether the care provided was of the same quality. People from BAME groups were also found to be as likely as people of white ethnicity to die at home (Dixon et al. 2015). However, notably, relatives of decedents from BAME backgrounds reported poorer quality of care, especially in care homes, than relatives of people of white ethnicity (Dixon et al. 2015). They were also more likely to die in hospital than a care home, when compared to people of white ethnicity (Dixon et al. 2015). However, other research has found a very small but statistically significant effect of being from a BAME group on the likelihood of dying in hospital, as well as more hospital admissions and longer hospital stays (Bardsley et al. 2016), and that first-generation BAME groups, if not people from BAME backgrounds in general, are more likely to die in hospital than at home (Koffman et al. 2014).

Learning exercise 2.2

In your experience as a nurse, have you found it harder for certain groups to access palliative care services? In terms of geography, what areas tend to have more or less services?

Geography and area deprivation

In recent analyses of data from the Minimum Data Set (MDS) for Specialist Palliative Care Services, it is reported that 'variation in the number of services per 1,000 deaths in each region suggest differing patterns of service provision across the country', varying between 4.05 services for every 1,000 deaths in East of England to 1.83 services per 1000 deaths in London (NCPC/PHE 2014, p. 21). There are also differences by area deprivation (as measured by Index of Multiple Deprivation, IMD, quintiles). Secondary analyses of data from the National Survey of Bereaved People find that people from more deprived areas have similar access to a range of community-based palliative and end of life services (Marie Curie nurses, other community-based nurses, home help or meals on wheels, hospice at home or rapid response services), although the level and quality of the services received are unknown (Dixon et al. 2015). However, these secondary analyses did show that people from more deprived areas were less likely to think that help and support from healthcare and social services to care for the decedent at home was sufficient (Dixon et al. 2015). Findings from the National Survey of Bereaved People also show that people from more deprived areas are less satisfied with the care they receive, especially from general practitioners, and are less likely to feel treated with dignity by all of the professionals involved in their care (ONS 2013). They also more frequently die in hospital than at home or in their care home (ONS 2013). Finally, we also know that hospices, whose provision is consistently considered to be of a very high quality, tend to be concentrated in less deprived areas (Gatrell and Wood 2012). We also know that, in the least deprived quintile, 7 per cent of people die in a hospice compared to just 5 per cent in the most deprived quintile (ONS 2013).

Care homes

Care homes have become increasingly important providers of end of life care. Currently, around 22 per cent of all deaths occur in care homes (ONS 2016b), although this figure varies between care homes (NAO 2007). In the last decade or two, care home residents have become increasingly frail (British Geriatrics Society 2010). They also increasingly have dementia, with around 55 per cent of people with dementia now likely to die in a care home (Sleeman et al. 2014). We know too that the proportion of people who die within a year of moving to a care home has increased, from around 28 per cent in 1997 (Sidell et al. 1997) to 47 per cent in 2006 (Froggatt and Payne 2006) and to 56 per cent in 2014 (Kinley et al. 2014). All of this suggests the need for increased palliative care expertise within, and available to, care homes.

However, evidence suggests that many care homes may not be finding it easy to respond to this increasing need. Research studies show that the level of external health-care support to care homes, both generalist and specialist, is highly variable, with confusion about the respective roles and responsibilities of care home staff and external healthcare providers and particular difficulties of coordination where residents' prognosis is uncertain (Seymour et al. 2011; Handley et al. 2014; Kinley et al. 2014). In one study covering 38 homes implementing the Gold Standards Framework for Care Homes (GSFCH) and 2,444 residents, the vast majority of residents were found to have been seen by a general practitioner in their last months of life. However, far fewer were attended by specialist palliative care nurses and there were fewer visits from clinical nurse specialists or the mental health team than might be reasonably expected, given the diagnostic profile of residents (Kinley et al. 2014). In a survey of over 180 care homes, Seymour et al. (2011) found that the reluctance of general practitioners to prescribe appropriate medication, lack of out of hours support, difficulties in obtaining syringe drivers and a lack of training were identified as the key barriers to providing effective palliative care to residents. Kinley et al. (2014, p. 378) have argued that 'care homes acting as isolated providers of care is not an option if residents' health and social care needs are to be met'.

Hospitals

In some parts of the world there is limited access to face-to-face specialist palliative care for hospital in-patients. A national audit in the UK conducted by the Royal College of Physicians (2014) found that only 21 per cent of hospitals provide access 7 days a week despite national recommendations that they do so, with only 2 per cent providing round-the-clock access. There is also, perhaps surprisingly, often limited training in end of life care for staff and evidence of poor communication with patients about their care, as well as a failure to address the needs of carers (Royal College of Physicians 2014). Hospital end of life care is also consistently judged to be of poorer quality than that in other settings, with only 33.4 per cent of bereaved relatives rating care in hospitals as 'outstanding' or 'excellent', compared to 49.2 per cent of respondents whose relative died at home, 50 per cent whose relative died in a care home and 52.2 per cent whose relative died in a hospice (ONS 2016a). This, however, shows some improvement on figures from earlier years. For example, in 2013, only 32.7 per cent rated care in hospitals as 'outstanding' or 'excellent', compared to 53.2 per at home, 50.8 per cent in a care home and 59 per cent in a hospice (ONS 2014).

Having a spouse or partner

In adjusted secondary analyses of data from the National Survey of Bereaved People, those without a spouse or partner were found to be less likely to receive home-based services, to die at home, have their pain well-controlled or receive care that their families considered to be high quality (Dixon et al. 2015). These results may reflect the fact that people with spouses or partners are those most able to be cared for and die at home (Murtagh et al. 2012). Spouses or partners can also help to ensure high quality care by informally coordinating the care of different professionals, by acting as advocates and by providing care directly, such as administering medicines (Dixon et al. 2015).

Conclusion

As we have seen, notwithstanding the fact that we know there to be much excellent palliative care provided in a coordinated and timely way to many people with serious illness and their families, the evidence also suggests that access to high quality palliative and end of life care is far from comprehensive or equitable. Not everyone with a palliative care need receives the palliative care they require, whether this is from generalist or specialist providers, with access being dependent upon timely, pro-active and effective identification; the quality and availability of skilled and engaged generalists; effective coordination and integration across providers and care settings; the criteria and processes for specialist referrals and on the availability of appropriate specialist services. Access is also highly variable across different demographic, social and diagnostic groups. These inequities and gaps in access represent key challenges in the development of palliative care services in future.

Notes

1 Royal College of General Practitioners (RCGP), palliative care toolkit, available at: http://www.rcgp.org.uk/clinical-and-research/toolkits/palliative-and-end-of-life-care-toolkit.aspx
2 Royal College of Nursing, *Getting It Right Every Time: Fundamentals of Nursing Care at End of Life*, available at: http://rcnendoflife.org.uk/
3 Royal College of General Practitioners (RCGP), palliative care toolkit, available at: http://www.rcgp.org.uk/clinical-and-research/toolkits/palliative-and-end-of-life-care-toolkit.aspx
4 General Medical Council (GMC), *End of Life Care Guidance*, available at: http://www.gmc-uk.org/guidance/ethical_guidance/end_of_life_guidance.asp
5 Minimum Dataset for Specialist Palliative Care Services, available at: http://www.ncpc.org.uk/minimum-data-set

References

Bardsley, M., Georghiou, T., Spence, R. and Billings, J. (2016) Factors associated with variation in hospital use at the end of life in England. *BMJ Support Palliative Care*. Available at: www.bmjspcare-2015-000936.

Birch, D. and Draper, J. (2008) A critical literature review exploring the challenges of delivering effective palliative care to older people with dementia. *Journal of Clinical Nursing*, 17(9): 1144–63.

British Geriatrics Society (2010) Palliative and End of Life Care for Older People. Available at http://www.bgs.org.uk/good-practice-guides/resources/goodpractice/palliativecare

Burt, J., Plant, H., Omar, R. and Raine, R. (2010) Equity of use of specialist palliative care by age: cross-sectional study of lung cancer patients. *Palliative Medicine*, 24(6): 641–50.

Calanzani, N., Higginson, I.J. and Gomes, B. (2013a) *Current and Future Needs for Hospice Care: An Evidence-Based Report*. London: Help the Hospices Commission. Available at: www.helpthehospices.org.uk/commission

Calanzani, N., Koffman, J. and Higginson, I. (2013b) *Palliative and End of Life Care for Black, Asian and Minority Ethnic (BAME) Groups in the UK: Demographic Profile and the Current State of Palliative and End of Life Care*. London: Marie Curie Cancer Care. Available at: https://www.mariecurie.org.uk/.../palliative-care-bame_full-report.pdf

Davies, N., Maio, L., Vedavanam, K. et al. for the IMPACT research team (2014) Barriers to the provision of high-quality palliative care for people with dementia in England: a qualitative study of professionals' experiences. *Health and Social Care in the Community*, 22(4): 386–94.

Department of Health (2008) *The End of Life Care Strategy for England: Promoting High Quality Care for All Adults at the End of Life*. London: Department of Health.

Dixon, J., King, D., Matosevic, T. et al. (2015) *Equity in Palliative Care in the UK*. London: PSSRU, London School of Economics/Marie Curie.

Froggatt, K. and Payne, S. (2006) A survey of end-of-life care in care homes: issues of definition and practice. *Health & Social Care in the Community*, 14(4): 341–8.

Gadoud, A., Kane, E., MacLeod, U. and Johnson, M. (2014) Palliative care among heart failure patients in primary care: a comparison to cancer patients using English family practice data. *PLoS ONE*, 9(11): e113188.

Gardiner, C., Gott, M., Ingleton, C. et al. (2013) Extent of palliative care need in the acute hospital setting: a survey of two acute hospitals in the UK. *Palliative Medicine*, 27(1): 76–83.

Gatrell, A.C. and Wood, D.J. (2012) Variation in geographic access to specialist inpatient hospices in England and Wales. *Health & Place*, 18(4): 832–40.

Georghiou, T. and Bardsley, M. (2014) *Exploring the Cost of Care at the End of Life*. London: The Nuffield Trust.

Gott, M., Ingleton, C., Gardiner, C. et al. (2013) Transitions to palliative care for older people in acute hospitals: a mixed-methods study. *Health Services Delivery Research*, 1(11).

Gott, M., Seymour, J., Ingleton, C. et al. (2012) 'That's part of everybody's job': the perspectives of health care staff in England and New Zealand on the meaning and remit of palliative care. *Palliative Medicine*, 26(3): 232–41.

Handley, M., Goodman, C., Froggatt, K. et al. (2014) Living and dying: responsibility for end-of-life care in care homes without on-site nursing provision – a prospective study. *Health Soc Care Community*, 22: 22–29. doi:10.1111/hsc.12055.

Harrison, N., Cavers, D., Campbell, C. and Murray, S.A. (2012) Are UK primary care teams formally identifying patients for palliative care before they die?, *British Journal of General Practice*, 62(598): e344–52.

Higginson, I.J. and Gao, W. (2012) Opioid prescribing for cancer pain during the last 3 months of life: associated factors and 9-year trends in a nationwide United Kingdom cohort study. *Journal of Clinical Oncology*, 30(35): 4373–9.

HSCIC (Health and Social Care Information Centre) (2015) Quality and Outcomes Framework (QOF), 2014–15. Available at: http://digital.nhs.uk/catalogue/PUB18887

Hughes-Hallet, T., Craft, A. and Davies, C. (2011) *Palliative Care Funding Review: Funding the Right Care and Support for Everyone.* London: Department of Health.

Kinley, J., Hockley, J., Stone, L. et al. (2014) The provision of care for residents dying in U.K. nursing care homes. *Age and Ageing*, 43(3): 375–9.

Koffman, J., Ho, Y.K., Davies, J. et al. (2014) Does ethnicity affect where people with cancer die? A population-based 10 year study. *PloS One*, 9(4): e95052.

Murray, S. (2016) Session Abstract: Integrated palliative care: an international perspective. Can palliative care now go viral? 11th Palliative Care Congress.

Murtagh, F.E., Bausewein, C., Petkova, H. et al. (2012) *Understanding Place of Death for Patients with Non-Malignant Conditions: A Systematic Literature Review.* Service Delivery and Organisation Programme, National Institute for Health Research. Available at: https://www.nihr.ac.uk

Murtagh, F.E., Bausewein, C., Verne, J. et al. (2014) How many people need palliative care? A study developing and comparing methods for population-based estimates. *Palliative Medicine*, 28(1): 49–58.

NAO (National Audit Office) (2007) *End of Life Care: Report by the Comptroller and Auditor General*, HC 1043, session 2007–2008. London: NAO.

National Palliative and End of Life Care Partnership (2015) *Ambitions for Palliative and End of Life Care: A National Framework for Local Action 2015–20.* Available at: www.ncpc.org.uk

NCPC/PHE (National Council of Palliative Care/Public Health England) (2014) *The National Survey of Patient Activity Data for Specialist Palliative Care Services: MDS Full Report for the Year 2012–13 (Covering England, Wales and Northern Ireland).* Available at: www.ncpc.org.uk

NCPC/PHE (National Council of Palliative Care/Public Health England/Hospice UK) (2015) *National Survey of Patient Activity Data for Specialist Palliative Care Services: MDS Full Report for the Year 2013–2014 (Covering England, Wales and Northern Ireland).* Available at: www.ncpc.org.uk

NHS (2014) *Five Year Forward View.* Available at: https://www.england.nhs.uk/wp-content/uploads/2014/10/5yfv-web.pdf

NHS England (2015) *Transforming End of Life Care in Acute Hospitals: The Route to Success 'How To' Guide.* Available at: https://www.england.nhs.uk/wp-content/uploads/2016/01/transforming.

NHS England (2016a) General Medical Services (GMS) Contract Quality and Outcomes Framework (QOF): Guidance for GMS Contract 2016/17. Available at: https://www.england.nhs.uk/gp/gpfv/investment/gp-contract/2016-2017

NHS England (2016b) *Specialist Level Palliative Care: Information for Commissioners.* Available at: www.londoncanceralliance.nhs.uk/.../rm-partners-palliative-care

NHS IQ (NHS Improving Quality) (2010a) *The Route to Success in End of Life Care: Achieving Quality in Care Homes.* Available at: https://www.slideshare.net/NHSIQlegacy/the-route-to-success-in-end

NHS IQ (NHS Improving Quality) (2010b) *The Route to Success in End of Life Care: Achieving Quality in Hostels and for Homeless People.* Available at: https://www. slideshare.net/NHSIQlegacy/the-route-to-success-in-end

NHS IQ (NHS Improving Quality) (2011a) *The Route to Success in End of Life Care: Achieving Quality in Prisons and for Prisoners.* Available at: https://www.slideshare. net/NHSIQlegacy/the-route-to-success-in-end

NHS IQ (NHS Improving Quality) (2011b) *The Route to Success in End of Life Care: Achieving Quality for People with Learning Disabilities.* Available at: https://www. slideshare.net/NHSIQlegacy/the-route-to-success-in-end

NHS IQ (NHS Improving Quality) (2012) *The Route to Success in End of Life Care: Achieving Quality for Lesbian, Gay, Bisexual and Transgender People.* Available at: https://www.slideshare.net/NHSIQlegacy/the-route-to-success-in-end

NHS IQ/CSW (NHS Improving Quality/College of Social Work) (2012) *The Route to Success in End of Life Care: Achieving Quality for Social Work.* Available at: https:// www.slideshare.net/NHSIQlegacy/the-route-to-success-in-end

NHS NEOLCP (NHS National End of Life Care Programme) (2010) *The Route to Success in End of Life Care: Achieving Quality in Acute Hospitals.* Available at: https:// www.slideshare.net/NHSIQlegacy/the-route-to-success-in-end

NHS NEOLCP (NHS National End of Life Care Programme) (2011a) *The Route to Success in End of Life Care: Achieving Quality in Domiciliary Care.* Available at: https:// www.slideshare.net/NHSIQlegacy/the-route-to-success-in-end

NHS NEOCLP (NHS National End of Life Care Programme) (2011b) *Capacity, Care Planning and Advance Care Planning in Life Limiting Illness: A Guide for Health and Social Care Staff.* Available at: https://www.slideshare.net/NHSIQlegacy/ the-route-to-success-in-end

NHS NEOLCP (NHS National End of Life Care Programme) (2012) *The Route to Success in End of Life Care: Achieving Quality in Ambulance Services.* Available at: https:// www.slideshare.net/NHSIQlegacy/the-route-to-success-in-end

NHS NEOLCP COT (NHS National End of Life Care Programme College of Occupational Therapists) (2011) *The Route to Success in End of Life Care: Achieving Quality for Occupational Therapy.* Available at: https://www.slideshare.net/NHSIQlegacy/ the-route-to-success-in-end

NHS NEOLCP RCN (NHS National End of Life Care Programme Royal College of Nursing) (2011) *The Route to Success: The Key Contribution of Nursing to End of Life Care.* Available at: https://www.slideshare.net/NHSIQlegacy/the-route-to-success-in-end

NICE (National Institute for Health and Care Excellence) (2011, updated 2016) *Quality Standard QS13: End of Life Care for Adults.* Available at: https://www.nice.org.uk/ guidance/QS13

Oishi, A. and Murtagh, F. (2014) The challenges of uncertainty and interprofessional collaboration in palliative care for non-cancer patients in the community: a systematic review of views from patients, carers and health-care professionals. *Palliative Medicine,* 28(9): 1081–98.

ONS (Office for National Statistics) (2013) *Statistical Bulletin: National Bereavement Survey (VOICES) by Area Deprivation, 2011*. Newport: ONS.

ONS (Office for National Statistics) (2014) *National Survey of Bereaved People (VOICES): 2013*. Newport: ONS.

ONS (Office for National Statistics) (2016a) *National Survey of Bereaved People (VOICES): England, 2015: Quality of Care Delivered in the Last 3 Months of Life for Adults who Died in England*. Newport: ONS.

ONS (Office for National Statistics) (2016b) *All Deaths and Deaths Occurring at Usual Residence (Numbers of Deaths and Indicator), England: Deaths Registered between Q4 2010/11 and Q3 2015/16*. Newport: ONS.

PHSO (Parliamentary and Health Service Ombudsman) (2015) *Dying Without Dignity. Investigations by the Parliamentary and Health Service Ombudsman into Complaints about End of Life Care*. London: PHSO.

RGP (Royal College of Physicians) (2014) *National Care of the Dying Audit for Hospitals, England*. London: RGP.

Seymour, J.E., Kumar, A. and Froggatt, K. (2011) Do nursing homes for older people have the support they need to provide end-of-life care? A mixed methods enquiry in England. *Palliative Medicine*, 25(2): 125–38.

Shipman, C., Gysels, M., White, P. et al.. (2008) Improving generalist end of life care: national consultation with practitioners, commissioners, academics, and service user groups. *British Medical Journal*, 337: 848–51.

Sidell, M., Katz, J. and Komaromy, C. (1997) *Death and Dying in Residential and Nursing Homes for Older People: Examining the Case for Palliative Care*. Milton Keynes: School of Health and Social Welfare, Open University.

Sleeman, K., Ho, Y.K., Verne, J. and Higginson, I.J. (2014) Reversal of English trend towards hospital death in dementia: a population-based study of place of death and associated individual and regional factors, 2001–2010. *BMC Neurology*, 14: 59.

Walsh, R.I., Mitchell, G., Francis, L. and van Driel, M.L. (2015) What diagnostic tools exist for the early identification of palliative care patients in general practice? A systematic review. *Journal of Palliative Care*, 31(2): 118–23.

Walshe, C., Todd, C., Caress, A. and Chew-Graham, C. (2009) Patterns of access to community palliative care services: a literature review. *Journal of Pain and Symptom Management*, 37(5): 884–912.

WHO (World Health Organization) (2014) *World Health Assembly, 134th Session. EB134.R7, Agenda Item 9.4. Strengthening of Palliative Care as a Component of Integrated Treatment Within the Continuum of Care*. 23 January 2014. Available at: http://apps.who.int/gb/ebwha/pdf_files/EB134/B134_R7-en.pdf

WSP (Whole Systems Partnership) (2016) *Independent Evaluation of Palliative Care Coordination Systems (EPaCCS) in England: Final Report*. Available at: www.endoflifecare-intelligence.org.uk/.../epaccs_in_england

Where is palliative care provided and how is it changing?

Barbara Gomes

Palliative care should be provided to all in need irrespective of place. Wherever and whenever possible, people suffering from an advanced disease should be cared for and die where they feel it is the right place to be, so they feel empowered and safe. To help patients achieve their preferences, nurses must understand how the trends in where we die are evolving and what factors influence the place of death. This is what this chapter intends to discuss.

Emerging transition pattern in places of death

For most of history, the majority of people died at home surrounded by their family, often from infectious diseases and with minimal medical input once the disease was in its last stages, with the exceptions of accidents and wars (Rothman 2014). This norm began to change in the mid-twentieth century. Hospitals became the locus of healthcare and providers of cures from previously serious diseases such as syphilis. They became modern places for dying when curative efforts failed, instead of shelters for the poor and pilgrims as before. This change was not immediate; the shift from dying at home with family to dying in hospital alone is what Ariès (1974) called the 'displacement of site of death'. This occurred slowly but steadily over decades, amplified by urbanisation and immigration. By the late 1970s and 1980s, in several nations, more than half of all deaths occurred in hospitals (Broad 2013).

In the last three decades, however, the global scenario has changed. The nearly universal hospitalisation trend has been replaced by multiple realities, with several countries shifting towards dying in the community. Some began to see a drop in hospital deaths and a rise in home deaths – the US in the 1980s (Flory et al. 2004), Canada in the 1990s

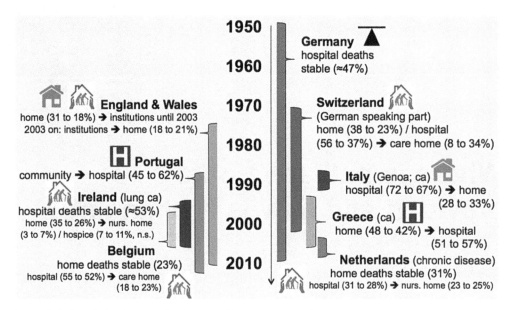

Figure 3.1 Trends in place of death in ten European countries
Sources: England and Wales (Gomes and Higginson 2008; Gomes et al. 2012a), Portugal (Sarmento et al. 2016), Ireland (Sharp et al. 2010), Belgium (Houttekier et al. 2011), Germany (Simon et al. 2012), Switzerland (Fischer et al. 2004), Italy (Costantini et al. 1993), Greece (Mystakidou et al. 2009), the Netherlands (van der Velden et al. 2009).

(Wilson 2009), and the UK in the 2000s (Gomes. Calanzani and Higginson 2012). Others are seeing a shift away from hospitals into care homes, e.g. Switzerland (Fischer et al. 2004), Germany (Dasch, Blum and Bausewein 2015), the Netherlands (van der Velden et al. 2009), and Belgium (Houttekier et al. 2011) (Figure 3.1). In some countries. the hospitalisation trend persists, e.g. Greece (Mystakidou et al. 2009), Portugal (Sarmento et al. 2016), Japan (Yang, Sakamoto and Marui 2006), and Korea (Yun et al. 2006).

In-patient hospices have a relatively small weight as places of death, even in countries where they have mostly developed, for instance, around 6 per cent of all deaths in England occur in free-standing hospices (Sleeman et al. 2016).

Due to ageing and increased mortality from chronic diseases, the need for palliative care is now greater than ever before. Estimates of the proportion of people who die from diseases who would benefit from palliative care currently range from 38 per cent to 84 per cent (Murtagh et al. 2014; Morin et al. 2016). Home and care homes have been shown to be the two places of death with the highest prevalence of palliative care need (Morin et al. 2016).

Preferences

The emerging transition pattern towards a 'dehospitalisation of death' seems to align with people's preferences. Survey findings of the population about their preferences

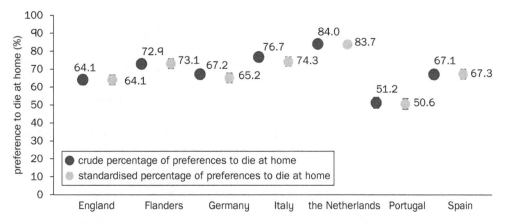

Figure 3.2 Preferences for place of death in seven European countries

for place of death in seven European countries (Figure 3.2) (Gomes, Higginson and Calanzani 2012), similar surveys in African countries (Downing et al. 2014; Powell et al. 2014) and a systematic review of preferences for dying at home (Gomes et al. 2014) show that, despite some heterogeneity, most adults would prefer dying at home in a scenario of advanced illness. Qualitative studies revealed that being at home makes patients feel empowered and safe (Collier, Phillips and Iedema 2015). Home is closely related to feelings of safety, privacy, sense of identity and social connection, in particular with family life (Gomes et al. 2014; Collier, Phillips and Iedema 2015). Overall, hospitals are the least preferred places, followed by care homes (Calanzani, Moens and Cohen 2014).

However, there have been concerns that when faced with the reality of illness progression towards death and complications, preferences may change, leading many to go into hospital. This is far from being a resolved issue in science. There is very little evidence on how people's preferences evolve over time in relation to their experiences of places and this is a critical gap. Out of 1,395 participants across 10 studies that examined individual changes (identified through systematic reviewing) (Gomes et al. 2013b), 20 per cent switched preferences, but this ranged from 2 per cent to 80 per cent and the direction varied – most commonly from hospital to home, home to hospice or home to hospital. One study found that preferences for both the place of care (asked a mean of >6 times) and place of death (asked a mean of >4 times) changed for patients (28 per cent and 30 per cent respectively) and carers (31 per cent and 30 per cent, respectively) (Agar et al. 2008). However, this study was conducted with 71 dyads of patients and family caregivers in a randomised controlled trial of an outreach visiting and case conferencing in palliative care. The preferences of other groups might change further, depending on their experiences of care in different places.

Furthermore, there is a substantial minority for whom home is not first choice; usually, hospices and palliative care units are the second most preferred places. This warns of diversity in views.

Learning exercise 3.1

- In your experience, do these reviews and trials relate to what you see in your everyday practice?
- If people's preferred place of care is home, can we match this with appropriate care?
- What are the implications for receiving care at home for both nursing care and families?

Children and adolescents

Much less is known about the preferences of children and adolescents and their parents, partially because of the challenges of conducting research on this topic with this population. A recent systematic review found nine studies in which the majority of parents reported a preference for death at home (Bluebond-Langner et al. 2013). Only one study examined changes over time. Among 164 families (cancer patients aged 4 months to 19 years), the family preference for home death increased from 68 per cent at enrolment to 80 per cent by the last month of life (Vickers et al. 2007). However, this was also a study conducted in the context of outreach palliative care provision (in the UK). One study examined the preferences of adolescent patients (with HIV/AIDS; age: 14–21 years); 90 per cent thought it was very or somewhat important to stay home (Lyon et al. 2010). No study has yet assessed the preferences of children, although it is ethically appropriate to ask a child with a complex chronic condition from the age of 6 (school entry) onwards where she/he prefers to be cared for (but not about place of death). In the USA, trends of place of death for children and adolescents with complex chronic conditions have shifted towards death at home, similarly to adults (Feudtner et al. 2007). In England, for example, home deaths have remained stable, at 40 per cent for those dying from cancer (Gao et al. 2016).

The family perspective

It is important that the nurse knows the family perspective about where care is provided because the patient and the family function as a unit of care, and palliative care aims to help with decisions that will be best for the whole unit. Indeed, it is very difficult for a patient to die at home if the family disagrees (Grande and Ewing 2008; Gomes et al. 2013a). Because family preferences are important to patients, they may consider the views of relatives when making choices. Families have therefore a crucial role in decision-making processes regarding place of care and place of death, not just because of their involvement in caregiving but also because the decision may have consequences for them, for example, in terms of how they cope with their bereavement.

Some studies suggest that family caregivers prefer the patient to die at home less often than patients, although the evidence was not found to be conclusive in a systematic review (Gomes et al. 2013b). More recently, a mortality follow-up survey of bereaved relatives due to cancer showed a lower home preference from relatives compared to patients (Gomes et al. 2015). Most relatives said that their own preferences were stable in the last 3 months before the patient died, with less than a fifth changing their mind during this period. Early conversations about preferences involving patients and families seem, therefore, appropriate, provided they are well conducted and preferences are monitored over time.

Learning exercise 3.2

- Look at Chapters 15 and 16 in this volume. Consider using advanced care plans to record both patient and family wishes.
- How else can nurses record or assess family wishes? Look at Chapter 12 for other ways to do this.

Is dying at home better than dying in hospital?

In order to meet patient preference at no expense of the best possible outcomes, it is crucial for nurses to find out whether death at home is better for patients and families. There is some evidence showing better results on psychological, social, and holistic measures of well-being in the last weeks or days of life for patients dying at home compared to hospital (Higginson et al. 2014). However, findings on symptoms and family outcomes are inconsistent, particularly for two widely researched outcomes: pain and grief. In 2015, a new study filled in this critical gap by providing novel knowledge suggesting that dying at home is better than hospital for peace and grief, with no difference in the levels of pain experienced in the last week of life. This study by QUALY-CARE was a comprehensive population-based study of factors and outcomes associated with dying at home compared to hospital, and included over 350 people who had died from cancer and their relatives in the largest metropolitan area in the UK (Gomes et al. 2015). In addition, in 2016, a multicentre study from Japan showed that cancer patients who died at home lived some more days than those who died in hospitals (both groups receiving specialist palliative care), even after adjusting for patients' demographic and clinical characteristics (Hamano et al. 2016).

Such an encouraging reality reflects multiple factors, which include the work of nurses on the ground, particularly of those working in the community, to ensure that patients and families are adequately supported at home. Yet, the research findings highlight the need to do more. There are some people for whom death at home is not peaceful and pain-free, and there are relatives who are left in a state of intense grieving. Input from a comprehensive range of community healthcare and social care services is essential to guarantee a patient with an advanced disease who wants to die at home that they will achieve their wish with quality care.

How can nurses help a patient die comfortably at home?

Nurses play a central role in ensuring each of their individual patients spends their last days where they wish. They are often the key professional point of contact whom patients and families rely on to get things done throughout their illness experience (Gomes et al. 2015). Having this key contact point is a protective factor against transition to hospital (Gomes et al. 2015; Bone et al. 2016). Therefore, nurses are indispensable partners in the wider societal vision of meeting preferences regarding where to die for more than just a few in the future. It is important they know the risks and what can help.

The network of factors that increase people's chances of dying at home is complex and multifaceted but there is an evidence-based conceptual model that can help improve nursing practice (Figure 3.3) (Gomes and Higginson 2006). The model shows that place of death results from interactions between three main groups of factors: those related to the illness, the individual, and the environment, the latter found to be the most important. There is good evidence for the effect of 17 factors, of which six are strongly associated with home death: patients' low functional status (adjusted odds ratios (AORs) range from 2.29 to 1.11), their preferences (2.19 to 5.47), home care (1.37 to 5.1) and its intensity (1.06 to 8.65), living with relatives (1.78 to 7.85), and extended family support (2.28 to 5.47).

More recently, the QUALYCARE study found that receiving a comprehensive home care package makes a big difference for patients who want to die at home (Gomes et al. 2015). Specialist palliative care services and community/district nurses are essential to help achieve death at home. General practitioners (GPs) and Marie Curie nurses are also important (Marie Curie nurses care for people at home in the last few months or weeks of their lives, with the core service being one-to-one overnight nursing). Clinical practice should therefore focus on ways of empowering families, as well as intensifying home care and risk assessment.

Most of these factors have been shown to have strong and significant associations with death at home internationally (Gomes and Higginson 2006). Aspects of the model are further supported by experimental research such as the effect of home palliative care services (Gomes et al. 2013b). However, most of the model is based on retrospective or cross-sectional data and associations; these may or may not be causal relationships. Moreover, it is difficult to identify some of the factors prospectively. Finally, it is important to note that the model was developed for cancer. A systematic review of factors in non-malignant conditions flags additional factors (Murtagh et al. 2012). For example, having a diagnosis of heart disease, chronic obstructive pulmonary disease or dementia increases the odds of home death. The existence of comorbidities decreases the odds of dying at home.

The algorithm in Figure 3.4 might help nurses to approach discussions about place of care and place of death with patients and their relatives. Responding to the diversity of disease stages and settings in which clinical encounters take place, the algorithm is based on QUALYCARE findings (Gomes et al. 2015). It is intended to be a flexible prompt responding to concerns from clinicians working in primary and palliative care with the

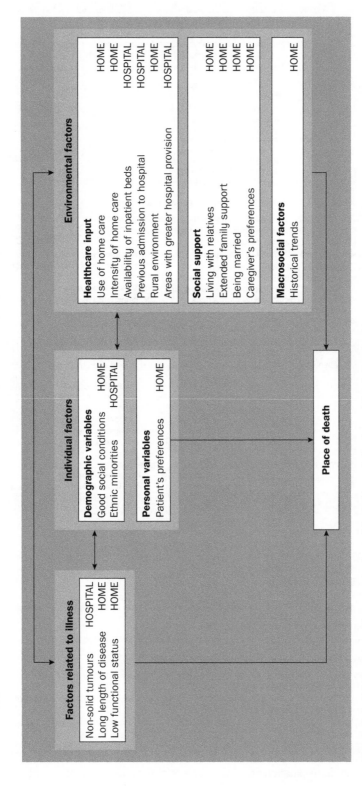

Figure 3.3 Evidence-based conceptual model of place of death and its determinants

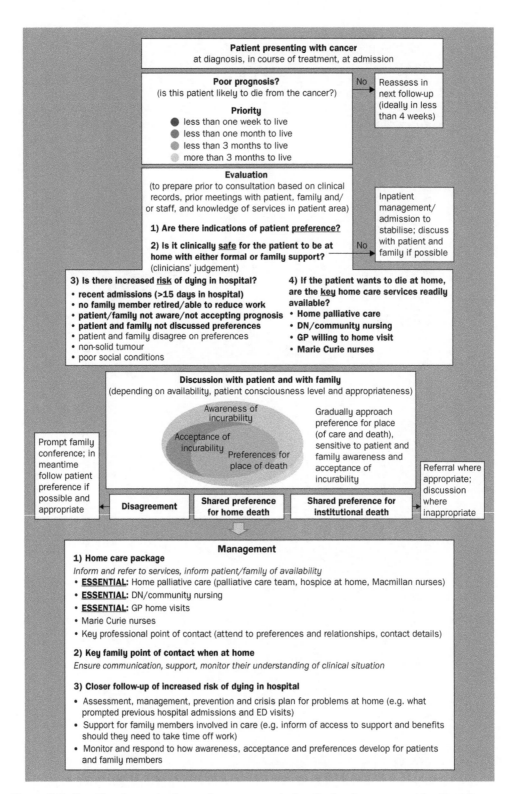

Figure 3.4 Algorithm for evaluation and management of patients who may want to die at home

increased pressure to record and audit preferences for place of death for all patients, regardless of whether it is appropriate or feasible (Munday, Petrova and Dale 2009). It may also be used in multi-disciplinary team meetings and by palliative care specialists when training others.

When exploring patients' and families' preferences for place of care and place of death, it is important to find out what are the intentions behind those preferences. Often choices for place of care and place of death are considered by patients and families as enablers of fulfilling other life goals. For example, preferring to die at home has been associated with wanting to involve family in decisions and prioritising keeping a positive attitude above other things, including symptom control (Higginson et al. 2014). Hence, looking at the priorities and goals behind these preferences is crucial in order to meet wishes because there may be several ways of meeting those priorities and goals even if dying in the preferred place is not possible.

Nurses should keep in mind that none of the risks and opportunities for meeting preferences for place of care and place of death are to be regarded in isolation. It is rare for someone to present only with risks and no opportunities for dying at home. It is more frequent but also rare for someone to present with only opportunities and no risks. Having spent the last 2 weeks in hospital does not necessarily mean that Mr Brown will die in hospital. The fact that Mrs Smith's GP visits her at home once a week does not guarantee she will die at home. Therefore, the role of nurses working with other health-care and social care professionals in minimising risks and maximising opportunities is of utmost importance.

What we know less about

There are important gaps in the knowledge about the places where palliative care is provided and the circumstances of dying for certain groups of patients. Less is known about people suffering from non-malignant conditions, children and adolescents. Most of the existing evidence is from high-income countries. We know very little about specific places where palliative care service penetration is very thin, although innovative care models are developing in prisons, shelters for the homeless and psychiatric hospitals for the people with psychiatric disorders including dementia, for example (see Chapter 13 in this volume).

Although we still know little about the economics associated with different places of care and death, there is increasing evidence that care at home shifts costs from healthcare services to the family (Yu, Guerriere and Coyte 2015). Added financial burden may impact on employment and extend beyond bereavement. Nurses should, therefore, bear any potential costs in mind, particularly for patients and families with poorer social conditions who are known to have less chance of experiencing death at home. There is a key role for nurses here in terms of assessing the costs of care financially as well as emotionally for families.

Also, there is an important distinction between place of care and place of death. Although the former determines the latter, patients often move between care settings, particularly within the last few months of life. Little is still known about the individual pathways and last transitions leading someone to die in a specific place, though interest has risen following research from the USA with a random sample of 848,303 Medicare beneficiaries aged 66 years and over, showing that while deaths in acute care hospitals increased, intensive care unit use and transitions between places in the last 90 days of life increased between 2000 and 2009 (Teno, Gozalo and Bynum 2013). This study warns of finer differences in care patterns that we are unable to discern if we only examine place of death. However, an important research question remains unanswered: are these transitions aligned with the preferences of patients and their family members? Even if it is impossible or not appropriate to avoid a terminal admission into hospital, there is much to be done to help maximise the time patients spend at home in their last months of life (Groff, Colla and Lee 2016).

The future

It is hard to predict what might happen in the future in terms of where palliative care is provided. There are now more places to consider beyond the classic dichotomy of home/hospital; care homes, in-patient hospices and palliative care units are increasingly important providers of care towards the end of life and places where people die. The global pattern that seems to be emerging towards death in the community must be put in the context of a fast-growing need of a changed social world with limited care resources. Worldwide, deaths are set to rise from 57 million in 2015 to 70 million in 2030 (World Health Organization 2016). There is a combination of societal and health-care forces that may hinder the sustainability of the emerging transition pattern into the twenty-first century. These include ageing (affecting both patients and caregivers), changes in family structure and location (towards smaller and more dispersed families, and with increased migration there may be more requests to return to die in homeland country, for example), and treatment advances (particularly in heart diseases and cancers, which are leading causes of death worldwide).

Conclusion

Where people die is a complex phenomenon that can only be understood by bringing together the best available evidence (quantitative and qualitative) and the best possible clinical care for each individual patient. Nurses are best placed to talk to patients and their families about place of care and place of death, assess barriers and facilitators and help organise care at the right place for them. But there are tough challenges ahead related to where people die that nurses must prepare for in order to continue providing the best care for patients and families in the future.

Acknowledgements

I am grateful to the Calouste Gulbenkian Foundation for funding, and to Despina Anagnostou and Emma Murphy for comments on an earlier draft.

References

Agar, M., Currow, D.C., Shelby-James, T.M. et al. (2008) Preference for place of care and place of death in palliative care: are these different questions? *Palliative Medicine*, 22(7): 787–95.

Ariès, P. (1974) *Western Attitudes Toward Death From the Middle Ages to the Present*. Baltimore, MD: Johns Hopkins University Press.

Bluebond-Langner, M., Beecham, E., Candy, B. et al. (2013) Preferred place of death for children and young people with life-limiting and life-threatening conditions: a systematic review of the literature and recommendations for future inquiry and policy. *Palliative Medicine*, 27(8): 705–13.

Bone, A., Gao, W., Gomes, B. et al. (2016) Factors associated with transition from community settings to hospital as place of death for adults aged 75 and older: a population-based mortality follow-back survey. *Journal of the American Geriatrics Society*, 9 September. doi: 10.1111/jgs.14442. [Epub ahead of print].

Broad, J.B., Gott, M., Kim, H., et al. (2013) Where do people die? An international comparison of the percentage of deaths occurring in hospital and residential aged care settings in 45 populations, using published and available statistics. *International Journal of Public Health*, 58(2): 257–67.

Calanzani, N., Moens, K., Cohen, J. et al. on behalf of PRISMA (2014) Choosing care homes as the least preferred place to die: a cross-national survey of public preferences in seven European countries. *BMC Palliative Care*, 13: 48.

Collier, A., Phillips, J.L. and Iedema, R. (2015) The meaning of home at the end of life: a video-reflexive ethnography study. *Palliative Medicine*, 29(8): 695–702.

Costantini, M., Camoirano, E., Madeddu, L. et al. (1993) Palliative home care and place of death among cancer patients: a population-based study. *Palliative Medicine*, 7(4): 323–31.

Dasch, B., Blum, K. and Bausewein, C. (2015) Place of death: trends over the course of a decade: a population-based study of death certificates from the years 2001 and 2011. *Deutsches Ärzteblatt International*, 112(29–30): 496–504.

Downing, J., Gomes, B., Gikaara, N. et al. (2014) Public preferences and priorities for end-of-life care in Kenya: a population-based street survey. *BMC Palliative Care*, 14(13): 4.

Feudtner, C., Feinstein, J.A., Satchell, M. et al. (2007) Shifting place of death among children with complex chronic conditions in the United States, 1989–2003. *JAMA*, 297(24): 2725–32.

Fischer, S., Bosshard, G., Zellweger, U. and Faisst, K. (2004) Place of death: 'Where do people die in Switzerland nowadays?' *Zeitschrift für Gerontologie und Geriatrie*, 37(6): 467–74.

Flory, J., Yinong, Y.X., Gurol, I. et al. (2004) Place of death: US trends since 1980. *Health Affairs*, 23(3): 194–200.

Gao, W., Verne, J., Peacock, J. et al. (2016) Place of death in children and young people with cancer and implications for end of life care: a population-based study in England, 1993–2014. *BMC Cancer*, 16: 727.

Gomes, B., Calanzani, N., Curiale, V. et al. (2013a) Effectiveness and cost-effectiveness of home palliative care services for adults with advanced illness and their caregivers. *Cochrane Database of Systematic Reviews*, Issue 6, Art. No.: CD007760. doi: 10.1002/14651858.CD007760.pub2.

Gomes, B., Calanzani, N., Gysels, M, et al. (2013b) Heterogeneity and changes in preferences for dying at home: a systematic review. *BMC Palliative Care*, 12(1): 7.

Gomes, B., Calanzani, N. and Higginson, I.J. (2012a) Reversal of the British trends in place of death: time series analysis 2004–2010. *Palliative Medicine*, 26(2): 102–7.

Gomes, B., Calanzani, N., Koffman, J. and Higginson, I.J. (2015) Is dying in hospital better than home in incurable cancer and what factors influence this? A population-based study. *BMC Medicine*, 13: 235.

Gomes, B. and Higginson, I.J. (2006) Factors influencing death at home in terminally ill patients with cancer: systematic review. *BMJ*, 332(7540): 515–21.

Gomes, B. and Higginson, I.J. (2008) Where people die (1974–2030): past trends, future projections and implications for care. *Palliative Medicine*, 22(1): 33–41.

Gomes, B., Higginson, I.J., Calanzani, N. et al. on behalf of PRISMA (2012b) Preferences for place of death if faced with advanced cancer: a population survey in England, Flanders, Italy, Germany, the Netherlands, Portugal and Spain. *Annals of Oncology*, 23(8): 2006–15.

Gomes, B., Calanzani N., Higginson, I.J. et al. (2014) Benefits and costs of home palliative care compared with usual care for patients with advanced illness and their family Caregivers. *JAMA*, 311(10): 1060–1061. doi:10.1001/jama.2014.553.

Grande, G. and Ewing, G. (2008) Death at home unlikely if informal carers prefer otherwise: implications for policy. *Palliative Medicine*, 22(8): 971–2.

Groff, A.C., Colla, C.H. and Lee, T.H. (2016) Days spent at home: a patient-centered goal and outcome. *New England Journal of Medicine*, 375: 1610–12.

Hamano, J., Yamaguchi, T., Maeda, I. et al. (2016) Multicenter cohort study on the survival time of cancer patients dying at home or in a hospital: does place matter? *Cancer*, 122(9): 1453–60.

Higginson, I.J., Gomes, B., Calanzani, N. et al. on behalf of Project PRISMA (2014) Priorities for treatment, care and information if faced with serious illness: a comparative population-based survey in seven European countries. *Palliative Medicine*, 28(2): 101–10.

Higginson, I.J., Sarmento, V.P., Calanzani, N. et al. (2014) Dying at home – is it better? A narrative appraisal of the state of the science. *Palliative Medicine*, 27(10): 918–24.

Houttekier, D., Cohen, J., Surkyn, J. and Deliens, L. (2011) Study of recent and future trends in place of death in Belgium using death certificate data: a shift from hospitals to care homes. *BMC Public Health*, 11: 228.

Lyon, M., Garvie, P., Briggs, L. et al. (2010) Do families know what adolescents want? An end-of-life (EOL) survey of adolescents with HIV/AIDS and their families. *Journal of Adolescent Health*, 1: S4–S5.

Morin, L., Aubry, R., Frova, L. et al. (2016) Estimating the need for palliative care at the population level: a cross-national study in 12 countries. *Palliative Medicine*, 28 September. doi: 10.1177/0269216316671280 [Epub ahead of print].

Munday, D., Petrova, M. and Dale, J. (2009) Exploring preferences for place of death with terminally ill patients: qualitative study of experiences of general practitioners and community nurses in England. *BMJ*, 338: b2391.

Murtagh, F.E.M., Bausewein, C., Petkova, H. et al. (2012) Understanding place of death for patients with non-malignant conditions: a systematic literature review. Final report. NIHR Service Delivery and Organisation programme. Available at: www.netscc.ac.uk/hsdr/files/adhoc/annual-review-2010.pdf

Murtagh, F., Bausewein, C., Verne, J. et al. (2014) How many people need palliative care? A study developing and comparing methods for population-based estimates. *Palliative Medicine*, 28(1): 49–58.

Mystakidou, K., Parpa, E., Tsilika, E. et al. (2009) Where do cancer patients die in Greece? A population-based study on the place of death in 1993 and 2003. *Journal of Pain Symptom Management*, 38(2): 309–14.

Powell, R.A., Namisango, E., Gikaara, N. et al. (2014) Public priorities and preferences for end-of-life care in Namibia. *Journal of Pain and Symptom Management*, 47(3): 620–30.

Rothman, D.J. (2014) Where we die. *New England Journal of Medicine*, 370(26): 2457–60.

Sarmento, V.P., Higginson, I.J., Ferreira, P.L. and Gomes, B. (2016) Past trends and projections of hospital deaths to inform the integration of palliative care in one of the most ageing countries in the world. *Palliative Medicine*, 30(4): 363–73.

Sharp. L., Foll, P., Deady, S. et al. (2010) Where do people with lung cancer die and how is this changing? *Irish Medical Journal*, 103(9): 262–5.

Sleeman, K., Davies, J.M., Verne, J. et al. (2016) The changing demographics of inpatient hospice death: population-based cross-sectional study in England, 1993–2012. *Palliative Medicine*, 30(1): 45–53.

Teno, J., Gozalo, P.L., Bynum, J.P.W. et al. (2013) Change in end-of-life care for Medicare beneficiaries. *JAMA*, 309(5): 470–7.

van der Velden, L.F., Francke, A.L., Hingstman, L. et al. (2009) Dying from cancer or other chronic diseases in the Netherlands: ten-year trends derived from death certificate data. *BMC Palliative Care*, 8: 4.

Vickers, J., Thompson, A., Collins, G.S. et al. (2007) Place and provision of palliative care for children with progressive cancer: a study by the Paediatric Oncology Nurses' Forum/United Kingdom Children's Cancer Study Palliative Care Working Group. *Journal of Clinical Oncology*, 25(8): 4472–6.

Wilson, D., Truman, C.D., Thomas, R. et al. (2009) The rapidly changing location of death in Canada, 1994–2004. *Social Science & Medicine*, 68(10): 1752–8.

World Health Organization (2015) World Health Organization Fact Sheet: Projections of mortality and causes of death, 2015 and 2030. Available at: http://www.who.int/healthinfo/global_burden_disease/projections/en/ (accessed 15 November 2016).

Yang, L., Sakamoto, N. and Marui, E. (2006) A study of home deaths in Japan from 1951 to 2002. *BMC Palliative Care*, 5: 2.

Yu, M., Guerriere, D.N. and Coyte, P.C. (2015) Societal costs of home and hospital end-of-life care for palliative care patients in Ontario. *Health and Social Care in the Community*, 23(6): 605–18.

Yun, Y.H., Lim, M.K., Choi, K.S. and Rhee, Y.S. (2006) Predictors associated with the place of death in a country with increasing hospital deaths. *Palliative Medicine*, 20(4): 455–61.

Engaging patients and families in the organisation, care and research of palliative care

Aileen Collier and Merryn Gott

Introduction

Recently we have seen a significant shift in healthcare practice, policy and research away from viewing the patient role as passive to acknowledging that it should be more active. Progress towards patient engagement is highlighted as a priority area in international policy with expectations that they should be: proactive in the self-care management of their chronic illness, responsible for their role in 'shared decision-making', 'empowered' by managing their own symptoms, able to record preferences for their end of life care, and involved in co-designing both healthcare services and research. So, what does this mean for patients and families, nurses and other clinicians and organisations? What does it mean for the research we carry out, participate in, or seek to apply in practice?

From these questions, more emerge: Who do we seek to engage? Do they want to engage, and how? What if patients and families want to engage (or not) in a way that conflicts with us as nurses or researchers? How will we know if we are engaging effectively?

We seek in this chapter to try to address these questions by critically examining the complexities of 'engagement' in a palliative care context. We identify key concepts related to patient engagement and critically appraise these concepts as they relate to palliative care. We consider engagement at both a micro-level of patient care and the macro-levels of health service development and research, including understanding, promoting and providing palliative care. Ultimately, we argue that the engagement agenda for palliative care needs to be conceived from the perspectives of patients, families, and citizens themselves, as well as nurses and other professionals.

Learning outcomes

This chapter will enable you to do the following:

- Define and describe key concepts related to patient and family engagement in contemporary healthcare.
- Consider and critique these concepts as they relate to the context of palliative care.
- Reflect on patient and family engagement in your own work context.
- Critique the role of patients and families in palliative care research.

Patient and family engagement: key concepts

Contemporary policy and healthcare documents, along with academic literature, are replete with terms and concepts to describe the increasing focus on people's interactions with health care. At its simplest perhaps is the Center for Advancing Health (2010, p. 2) definition, which states that patient engagement is the 'actions individuals must take to obtain the greatest benefit from the health care services available to them'. However, other related concepts also abound, for example, patient participation; patient experience; patient-centred care; patient involvement; patient empowerment; patient activation; shared decision-making; self-care; self-management; co-production; co-design; and public and patient involvement (PPI) (Fumagalli et al. 2015). Many of these terms have multiple meanings, are used interchangeably and, sometimes, are misunderstood. Although it is not within the scope of this chapter to present an extensive concept map, we provide an overview of definitions in Table 4.1 as a frame of reference and to foreshadow our discussion of patient engagement that follows. Notwithstanding the array of terms used, they all assume a need for informed patients and families who actively participate in their own care.

Since the 1990s, a number of factors have driven this shift. As the population ages and health technologies continue to expand, there is a continuing and increasing demand on our healthcare systems, together with a push for efficiency in the context of limited resources. Engaging patients and families more actively at all levels of healthcare is, to a large extent, seen as a way of making contemporary health systems more sustainable. At the same time, people are living for longer periods with cancer and other chronic illnesses, hospital stays have become shorter, and care in outpatient settings has become increasingly complex (Jenerette and Mayer 2016). As a result, patients and their families are required to take on a significant role in aspects of care previously held within the domain of nurses. In addition, there has been a move away from a paternalistic approach to healthcare towards one that at least, rhetorically, increases patient autonomy and power, by emphasising people's capacities and abilities

Table 4.1 Concepts and definitions

Concept	Definition
Engagement	Patients, families, their representatives, and health professionals working in active partnership at various levels across the healthcare system – direct care, organizational design and governance, and policymaking – to improve health and healthcare. (Carman and Workman 2016, p. 25)
Patient-centred care	Care that is respectful of and responsive to individual patient preferences, needs, and values and ensuring that patient values guide all clinical decisions. (Institute of Medicine 2001)
Empowerment	The ability of people to gain understanding and control over personal, social, economic and political forces in order to take action to improve their life situations. (Israel et al. 1994, p. 152)
Patient participation	Used interchangeably with patient involvement, user participation and user involvement and at micro and macro levels. (Castro et al. 2016)
Patient activation	Refers to the extent of the individual's understanding of the need to play an active role in managing their own health, and the scope of their capacity to be able to fulfill that role including their knowledge, skill, and confidence for doing so. (Hibbard and Mahoney 2010)
Shared decision-making	A process in which clinicians and patients work together to select tests, treatments, management or support packages, based on clinical evidence and the patient's informed preferences. It involves the provision of evidence-based information about options, outcomes and uncertainties, together with decision support counselling and a system for recording and implementing patients' informed preferences. (Coulter and Collins 2011, p. vii)
Self-management	The successful outcome of the person and all appropriate individuals and services working together to support him or her to deal with the very real implications of living the rest of their life with one or more long-term conditions. (The Long-Term Conditions Alliance Scotland: People Not Patients, 2008, p. 5)
Co-production	Co-production means delivering public services in an equal and reciprocal relationship between professionals, people using services, their families and their neighbours. Where activities are co-produced in this way, both services and neighbourhoods become far more effective agents of change. (Boyle and Harris 2009, p. 11)
Experience-based co-design	A user-focused design process that is focused on user experiences to design services that are experiences rather than designing services without considering the patient experience. (Bate and Robert 2007)

rather than their needs and deficits (Castro et al. 2016) . However, despite this growing movement promoting patient involvement, research on the topic remains limited (Snyder and Engstrom 2015).

Reality or rhetoric: patient and family engagement in palliative care

Engagement: the heart of palliative care

On the face of it, engaging patients and families in palliative care appears to sit at the heart of its philosophy. Historically the modern hospice movement was born out of what Cicely Saunders regarded as the marginalisation of patients with life-limiting illness and their resultant suffering and she prioritised 'the freedom of each individual to make his or her own journey towards their ultimate goals' (Saunders 1996, p. 319). Thus, any efforts towards engaging patients and families in palliative care would, at the outset, seem both laudable and consistent with palliative care philosophy. When we begin to dig deeper, however, the engagement of patients and families starts to become more complex. We turn now to explore some of these complexities.

Do patients and families want to engage?

The shift from the role of 'patient' to active healthcare consumer requires 'open awareness' of one's dying and is predicated on coming to terms with illness, putting one's affairs in order, acknowledging impending dying and death, including making decisions about end of life care and preferred place of death (Pastrana et al. 2008). However, not everyone, especially older patients, necessarily wants or seeks full disclosure (Gott et al. 2008; Richards et al. 2013) or to take on the role of 'engaged expert' (Fox et al. 2005), particularly when their expertise is not acknowledged by healthcare workers, who to a large extent seek to hold on to power (Henwood et al. 2003; Fox et al. 2005). We reflect further on the ways in which palliative care nurses enact power in relationships with patients, families and other clinicians as we now consider shared decision-making.

Shared decision-making in palliative care

A shared decision-making (SDM) approach requires both healthcare professionals and patients to share their knowledge, preferences and values about healthcare choices and to work towards beneficial outcomes (Marjolein et al. 2016). SDM is currently largely based on models, such as that outlined by Elwyn et al. (2012) of: introducing choice (choice talk); discussing various treatment options, including benefits and harms (option talk), and 'reaching a decision together, by helping patients explore preferences'. Despite potential positive outcomes, SDM remains an aspiration rather than everyday practice (Couet et al. 2013) and patient health outcomes of SDM in palliative care remain uncertain (Belanger et al. 2010) and potentially contingent upon age, gender and socio-economic status (Legare et al. 2014). Some kind of intervention appears helpful, however, and those targeting both patients and healthcare professionals seem to show more potential than those focused on one or the other (Legare et al. 2014). This raises the important question of whether nurses are appropriately equipped to engage in SDM and whether organisations and services are able to promote environments conducive to SDM (Snyder and Engstrom 2015).

Self-management and palliative care

Applying a palliative nursing framework, self-management in palliative care is defined as 'assessing, planning, and implementing appropriate care to enable the patient to live until they die and supporting the patient to be given the means to master or deal with their illness or the effects of their illness themselves' (Johnston et al. 2014, p. 1). For people requiring palliative care, however, the expectations of self-management in the context of multiple co-morbidities, increasing technology and complexities of treatment may be problematic. For example, Benner et al. (2003, p. 558) argue that the very process of dying itself may limit people's capacity to engage, particularly where cognitive impairment is present. Furthermore, nurses need to consider cultural differences as well as styles of decision-making where a person's preference, for example, might be to engage through a family member (Hsiung et al. 2007).

Gulbrandsen et al. (2016) have argued that greater attention to the emotional and relational dimensions of engagement in SDM are needed, given the inherent uncertainty, vulnerability, and lack of power of people who are seriously unwell. In addition, patients and families are not always happy with the decision-making roles that clinicians attribute to them (Steinhauser et al. 2000; van der Eerden 2016). Moreover, as Kaufman (2005, p. 74) puts it: 'Patients and families are not unencumbered actors making treatment choices in social isolation or in isolation to webs of power.' Thus, we argue for a reframing of care – one that recognises people are interconnected with each other and act in creative and productive ways in response to one another. In essence, therefore, 'There is no intrinsically "superior" or "preferred" form of engagement as this necessarily depends on what a specific patient desires in a specific situation' (Fumagalli et al. 2015). Engagement also depends on the capacity, desire or need of people (patients, families, nurses, researchers and service providers) to engage at any particular time and in any particular place or setting. Crucially, recognising the role of the clinician in this way is important to move beyond a focus on what clinicians want patients, families and communities to do. Tang and Smith (2016) propose the following questions to support this shift:

- How do we build a health system in which people want to engage?
- How do we build a system that defines value through the lens of the people it serves – a system that helps people define the health goals they want to achieve and then provides the data, knowledge, and tools to support them in the process of achieving those goals?
- How do we engage the communities in which people live to promote an environment of healthy living?

Learning exercise 4.1

You may find it helpful to read Chapter 7 along with this chapter. Reflect on your own engagement with patients and families as we embark on the first practice example.

Practice example 1: Shared decision-making in palliative care

George Paladoplis is a 79-year-old Greek gentleman with extensive head and neck cancer currently living at home with his wife who has mild dementia. He has three adult sons. George has an extensive foul-smelling fungating wound eroding his face. The district nurse attends to the wound daily but George is a very private man and finds it difficult to accept that he needs nursing visits and is also reluctant to accept help from his sons. Senior palliative care nurse Angela, along with the palliative care registrar, have visited George at home to introduce the service. George is polite but firmly states that he doesn't want visits from the palliative care team. Angela closes the case file according to the policy of the area health service. She feels a little uneasy about this, knowing the extent of George's issues so she calls back the following week. Again George states 'no thank you' to having specialist palliative care visits at home. A week later Angela is on a day off and one of George's sons Nigel calls the service in distress. This time the call is picked up by Pauline (another of the senior nurses). Nigel is anxious about his father, saying that he appears to want to die at home but he is in severe pain and seems a little 'mixed up'. He explains that the GP has told them just to call an ambulance if George becomes unwell but George is adamant that he does not wish to return to hospital. Nigel explains that he also had a bad experience in hospital when a doctor entered the room and demanded of his brothers: 'Why have you let your father languish in this state?' Pauline feels that she should support Nigel as best she can and talks through his concerns on the phone.

1   What would you take into consideration if you were Pauline in this situation? How would you approach decision-making? Should anyone else be involved?
2   Select a model of shared decision-making and critique the applicability of the model in relation to the care of George, his family and Pauline. How helpful was it? What were the limitations?

Engaging patients and families in the organisation of palliative care

Co-production and palliative care

The critical idea underpinning co-production is that people who use services are hidden resources and untapped assets rather than a burden to healthcare systems (Boyle

Table 4.2 Types of co-production

Project and purpose	Who was involved and the outcome
A co-produced strategy to improve the care and experience of children with a life-limiting illness in Cornwall (Parent Carer Council Cornwall 2012)	Three parent carers with personal experience were recruited via social media and employed to work on the strategy together with the Parent Carer Council for Cornwall.
	Together they initiated a workshop to include all stakeholders followed by a survey to establish strategic priorities.
St Margaret's Hospice, Somerset, UK, is leading the 'Fit for Future' review	A wide range of representative voices from the community, including patients, doctors, health managers, and the Church.
	Complete redesign of hospice services at St Margaret's in Somerset, based on patient consultation.
To design, develop and deliver an improvement programme for specialist dementia units across Scotland.	Led by the Focus on Dementia team in Healthcare Improvement Scotland, applying experience-based co-design – involves specialist dementia unit staff as well as people with dementia and their families and carers to work as equal partners to agree what is important to them, design solutions and make improvements. http://blogs.iriss.org.uk/ebcd/dementia/
Public and patient involvement (PPI)	Doing research with or by the public rather than to, about or for the public (Hanley et al. 2004).

and Harris 2009). This is arguably creating 'the most important revolution in public services since the Beveridge report' (Boyle and Harris 2009, p. 3) and is an approach now enshrined in policy in many countries, including England and Australia (Australian Commission for Safety and Quality in Healthcare 2011).

Most of us would find it difficult to dispute the need for recipients of palliative care to informed service provision and policy. Indeed, it could be argued that the hospice movement has, by default, developed out of co-production, with many services evolving from community-driven advocacy groups and funded from the charitable sector. Co-production, as a concept, has also found its way into palliative and end of life care policy documents. For example, the National Council for Palliative Care has guidelines on 'Involving patients, carers and the public in palliative care and end of life care services' (The National Council for Palliative Care 2009). Table 4.2 provides some examples of co-production in a palliative care context.

A public health approach and health-promoting palliative care

At a macro level, the drive towards 'open awareness' now extends beyond those living with serious illness to all of society's citizens more generally. We are encouraged to have discussions about death, dying and bereavement whoever we are and whatever our circumstances. Indeed, the 'public health approach to palliative care' (PHAPC), of which such thinking is a key component, is becoming embedded in policy internationally. Palliative Care Australia (2005, p. 24), for example, proposes: 'Community and public health initiatives in palliative care [as] joint programs developed by palliative care services in partnership with their local communities to reduce these possible harms' (associated with death and dying). Similarly a more recent strategic policy document in Scotland: 'support[s] greater public and personal discussion of bereavement, death, dying and care at the end life, partly through commissioning work to facilitate this' (Scottish Government 2015, p. 4). Intuitively this approach would seem to support a power shift in favour of patients and families as it positions those living with the experience of life-limiting illness, rather than health professionals, as the 'experts' in their care and support-related needs. However, arguably, more critical thinking is required in order for the full benefits of the model to be realised, particularly for the marginalised groups we highlighted previously. In particular, there is a lack of clarity regarding both by what is meant by PHAPC, with three different interpretations currently evident within the palliative care literature (Dempers and Gott 2016) and lack of definitional clarity of key concepts underpinning the model, including 'community', 'empowerment' and 'social capital'.

This lack of conceptual clarity evidently has very practical implications for how engagement is understood within a PHAPC context. Perhaps of most interest to explore in this regard is the question of engagement with whom and by whom? Writing within PHAPC is clear that the focus of any intervention informed by this approach has to be wider than 'the patient' or 'carer'. Rather, we are urged to look to the wider community as a focus of 'capacity-building' activities. However, to do this, do we not need to be clear about what we mean by community? While we agree with Horsfall et al. (2011) that an individual community should be defined from the perspective of the person with a life-limiting illness and their significant others, this may be less helpful at a policy and planning level. Indeed, literature from other disciplines reminds us that communities can be of place, or interest, or of identity (James et al. 2015). Within a PHAPC context, which of these is being invoked is rarely made clear. However, each would require a different method of engagement. Similarly, we would argue the need to critically consider which individuals typically comprise the active community members required to be 'partners in care'.

Similarly, the concept of empowerment, while highly appealing, can again be argued to be under-theorised within a PHAPC context. For example, Paul and Sallnow (2013, p.196) argue that this approach should 'focus on empowering people, families and communities [to] allow them to draw on their own resources and community supports to adapt and cope'. However, it is unclear how we should understand 'empowerment' within this context and, moreover, is there not a risk that those with access to limited resources and community supports are further disadvantaged and marginalised by this approach? It would be fruitful for future research and commentary to draw on previous work critiquing the concept of empowerment from feminist and wider health promotion perspectives, for example, Gore (2003) or Rissel (1994).

Engaging patients and families in the research of palliative care

By now you will not be surprised to learn that there are a number of terms referring to patient, family and public involvement in research and how they are defined. For example, Oliver et al. (2015) use the term 'involvement' to describe 'people's participation in a shared research task' and 'engagement' to describe their intellectual focus on research or researchers. How people are involved in research is often described in terms of a continuum from no involvement or tokenistic involvement to service users leading and making decisions (Oliver et al. 2015). For example, if researchers believe or take the view that lay partners are unable to understand or are uninterested in their research, they are less likely to draw on and engage with them as partners (Supple et al. 2015). Further, the role and positioning of patients in research encompass everything from 'data' to patient as researcher and co-investigator whereby patients are trained in established research methods, for example, interviewing other research participants (Vrijhoe 2015).

There are moral, ethical, political and practical imperatives for engaging all stakeholders, including patients and families in healthcare research. Publicly funded research should be transparent and be accountable to the public (Thompson et al. 2014; Oliver et al. 2015). Involving people with experience of health issues and of services is considered likely to lead to research questions that are relevant and applicable and to improve recruitment and accurate data and findings of influence. Of key significance is that having service users drive the research agenda is an important predictor of whether or not findings are applied (Lomas 2000). Involving patients in the design of information for clinical trials, for example, results in information that is more readable, relevant and better understood. These imperatives are recognised by advisory bodies in most western countries, including INVOLVE (the National Institute for Health Research) in the UK (NHS: National Institute for Health Research 1996), the US Patient-Centered Outcomes Research Institute (PCORI) (Patient-Centered Outcomes Research Institute 2011), and the World Health Organization's Patients for Patient Safety programme (World Health Organization 2017).

User involvement is now a condition of funding bodies in a number of jurisdictions and academic researchers are judged on their capacity to include this. In the UK, for example, involving patients and families in research is a requirement as part of the Research Excellence Framework. Most critically perhaps is that user involvement is purported to lead to research that is ethically sound (Staley and Minogue 2006). Some bioethicists take this even further, arguing that patients as well as all other stakeholders have an ethical obligation to contribute to healthcare research and learning (Faden et al. 2013).

The NIHR identifies five key stages of research where service users could potentially contribute to studies: (1) development of the grant application; (2) design and management of the research; (3) the undertaking of the research; (4) the analysis of research data; and (5) the dissemination of findings. Exactly how patients should be engaged in research continues to be debated, however, including the acceptability and feasibility of engaging them and the effectiveness of doing so (Shipee et al. 2013; Domecq et al. 2014; Oliver et al. 2015). So what are the implications of these imperatives for both patients and families requiring palliative care as well as for nurse researchers of palliative care?

The potential benefits of patient and public involvement (PPI) in palliative care research may have far-reaching benefits. For example, PPI can provide an important life purpose and a means of re-creating aspects of identity and self for people with chronic illness (Thompson et al. 2014). PPI provides an opportunity to demystify and raise awareness of palliative care and its role in healthcare with the public (Daveson et al. 2015). Also, crucially, PPI can support the conduct of research which is potentially more responsive to the views and preferences of service users themselves. However, many questions about what current practice is, and ought to be, remain. Most fundamentally, what do we know about how palliative care researchers engage patients and families in all stages of research? More philosophically, how should patients and public be engaged in palliative care research? How might palliative care researchers engage patients, families and the public without becoming tokenistic? And how will researchers know if they are successfully engaging patients and public in research? These questions raise important opportunities as well as issues for researchers.

However, an evolving evidence base for patient and public participation in healthcare research and more specifically palliative care research does now exist to guide us. What is increasingly clear is that the success of PPI is much less about linear numerical and predetermined individual outcome measures and more about relationships. For example, an ethnographic case study of a study funded by CLAHRC (Collaborations for Leadership in Applied Health Research and Care for Northwest London) demonstrated that collaborative relationships between diverse stakeholders resulting in what were often unanticipated positive effects were what determined success of PPI (Marston and Renedo 2013). It is also increasingly apparent that, in attempts to measure and justify PPI, there is a danger of omitting the voices and experiences of those patients and public involved.

Palliative care research, of course, brings its own challenges as people deteriorate and may die before the completion of a project. There is also the potential for PPI to have negative consequences, such as adding to the emotional burden for patients and families as well as those involved becoming disillusioned with the process and outcomes of the research project (Staley 2009). Despite these challenges, however, exemplars from previous studies are available for us to build on. For instance, INVOLVE describes how a PPI advisory group worked with the research team throughout the course of the Transitions to Palliative Care for Older People in Acute Hospitals study, including the dissemination phase (Gott et al. 2013).

Overall, there is a need for us as researchers to be flexible and creative in how, where and when we engage people. For example, Daveson et al. (2015) suggest engaging different users at different stages of a research project if necessary and applying different methods for different purposes, for example, facilitating a focus group may be useful to generate research ideas whereas email may be more appropriate for refining a grant application. Daveson et al. (2015) provide a helpful summary of essential elements for an optimal model of PPI:

- Promote and emphasise the contribution of patients and public and the difference they make; part of achieving this is articulating clearly what is meant by palliative care; patients and public should be encouraged to add value to the research.
- Involve people as early as possible in the project and preferably at the inception of any project. This is necessary to improving the relevance and quality of the research as well as its productivity.
- Accommodate a high degree of flexibility and diversity of methods, given the fluctuation of the disease process and deterioration along with caregiver priorities.

In terms of creativity and flexibility, we argue that as palliative care researchers we need to develop and advance complementary research methodologies and knowledge paradigms alongside more traditional ones requiring participants to fit into strictly defined research methods. Our own experience of qualitative and participatory methods is that by positioning participants centrally as experts in our respective studies and seeking to engage with people on their terms, we are able to discover new knowledge together (Collier and Wyer 2015; Williams et al. 2017).

In this respect, we argue that as palliative care researchers we might need to think even more creatively about how to involve and engage patients, families and the public more fully in the research process. For example, there is now a movement to include patients in health conferences. Yet patients, family and public keynote speakers, abstract presenters and workshop leaders are notably absent from palliative care conferences. Should we be asking, for example, how many palliative care specific journals are patients and families able to access free of charge and/or have patient and family representatives sit on their editorial boards or act as peer reviewers?

Learning exercise 4.2

Practice example 2

Alice Thompson is the nursing director of Sunnyside, one of a dozen aged care facilities owned and run by a not-for-profit company. The executive group is committed to improving palliative care across the organisation. They want to initiate some changes to the environment and the model of care delivery across the organisation. They know Alice is reaching the end of her Master's studies in palliative care and want to commence these changes at Sunnyside. Alice is committed to delivering good care and wants to involve the residents but is not quite sure where to begin. She also believes that any changes need to be properly evaluated.

1   Alice approaches you for advice about how to involve residents and their families in the proposed changes at Sunnyside. What advice would you give her about 'where to begin'? What resources might you direct her to?

2   Alice asks you whom she might approach to help her evaluate the proposed changes and what you think is important in helping her to decide who to involve. What would you suggest?

3   Alice is excited that several residents and family members have expressed an interest in contributing to the planning group but the executive of the organisation just wants to press ahead with plans. She has asked for your help in presenting them with evidence and justification for taking a co-design approach. How will you help her?

Conclusion

In this chapter, we have explored the potential for patient, family and public engagement in palliative care at both micro and macro levels, including direct patient care, healthcare organisation and development and research. At face value, patient and family engagement appears consistent with the philosophy and principles of palliative care and an inherent good. We hope to have shown, however, that engagement is not without significant challenges, both philosophical and practical, and the research evidence related to outcomes for patients, families and the public is scarce. We have posited that if nurses, health and social professionals as well as policy-makers and researchers continue down the path of engagement, then we should be aware of the potential for unintended consequences, including the further marginalisation of those groups requiring palliative care but who do not receive it. Thus, we argue that those whom we engage, whether patients, families and/or the public, should themselves have opportunities to voice or indeed to 'not voice' how engagement in the context of palliative care might proceed. The challenge is how as practitioners, researchers, health service managers and policy-makers, we move beyond the rhetoric to reality of engagement.

Web resources

http://www.ahrq.gov/professionals/education/curriculumtools/shareddecision-
making/tools/tool-2/index.html

https://www.caresearch.com.au/caresearch/tabid/3866/Default.aspx

http://www.coproductionscotland.org.uk/
http://www.dyingtoknowday.org/
http://www.fit4future.org.uk/
http://www.healthcodesign.org.nz/
http://healthtalk.org/peoples-experiences/improving-health-care/patient-and-
    public-involvement-research/what-patient-and-public-involvement-and-why-
    it-important?utm_content=bufferfe6bbandutm_medium=socialandutm_
    source=twitter.comandutm_campaign=buffer
http://www.nationalvoices.org.uk/our-work/five-year-forward-view/new-model-
    partnership-people-and-communities?platform=hootsuite Six principles for
    engaging people and communities
http://patientfamilyengagement.org
https://patientsincluded.org/http://personcentredcare.health.org.uk/http://www.
    scie.org.uk/publications/guides/guide51/what-is-coproduction/

References

Australian Commission for Safety and Quality in Healthcare (ACSQHC) (2011) *National Safety and Quality Health Service Standards.* Sydney: ACSQHC.

Bate, P. and Robert, G. (2007) *Bringing User Experience to Healthcare Improvement: The Concepts, Methods and Practices of Experienced-Based Design.* Oxford: Radcliffe Publishing.

Belanger, E., Rodriguez, C. and Groleau, D. (2010) Shared decision-making in palliative care: a systematic mixed studies review using narrative synthesis. *Palliative Medicine,* 25(3): 242–61.

Benner, P., Kerchner, S., Corless, I. and Davies, B. (2003) Attending death as a human passage: core nursing principles for end of life care. *American Journal of Critical Care,* 12: 558–61.

Boyle, D. and Harris, M. (2009) The challenge of co-production: how equal partnerships between professionals and the public are crucial to improving health services. Available at: http://www.scdc.org.uk/media/resources/documents/The_Challenge_of_Co-production.pdf

Carman, K.L. and Workman, T.A. (2016) Engaging patients and consumers in research evidence: applying the conceptual model of patient and family engagement. *Patient Education and Counselling,* 100(1): 25–9.

Castro, E.M., Regenmortel, T.V., Vanhaecht, K. et al. (2016) Patient empowerment, patient participation and patient centredness in hospital care: a concept analysis based on a literature review. *Patient Education and Counselling,* 99(12): 1923–39.

Center for Advancing Health (2010) *A New Definition of Patient Engagement: What is Engagement and Why is It Important?* Washington, DC: Center for Advancing Health.

Collier, A. and Wyer, M. (2015) Researching reflexively with patients and families: two studies using video-reflexive ethnography to collaborate with patients and families in patient safety research. *Qualitative Health Research*, 26(7): 979–93.

Couet, N., Desroches, S., Robitalille, H. et al. (2013) Assessments of the extent to which health-care providers involve patients in decision making: a systematic review of studies using the OPTION instrument. *Health Expectations*, 18: 542–61.

Coulter, A. and Collins, A. (2011) *Making Shared Decision-Making a Reality: No Decision About Me Without Me*. London: King's Fund.

Daveson, B.A., De Wolf-Linder, S., Witt, J. et al. (2015) Results of transparent expert consultation on patient and public involvement in palliative care research. *Palliative Medicine*, 29: 939–49.

Dempers, C. and Gott, M. (2016) Which public health approach to palliative care? An integrative literature review. *Progress in Palliative Care*, 25(1): 1–10.

Domecq, J.P., Prutsky, G., Elraiyah, T. et al. (2014) Patient engagement in research: a systematic review. *BMC Health Services Research*, 14: 89.

Elwyn, G., Frosch, D., Thomson, R. et al. (2012) Shared decision making: a model for clinical practice. *Journal of General Internal Medicine*, 27: 1361–7.

Faden, R., Kass, N.E., Goodman, S.N. et al. (2013) An ethics framework for a learning health care system: a departure from traditional research ethics. *The Hastings Center Report*, 43: S16–S27.

Fox, N.J., Ward, K.J. and O'Rourke, A.J. (2005) The 'expert patient': empowerment or medical dominance? The case of weight loss, pharmaceutical drugs and the internet. *Social Science and Medicine*, 60: 1299–309.

Fumagalli, L.P., Radaelli, G., Lettieri, E. et al. (2015) Patient empowerment and its neighbours: clarifying the boundaries and their mutual relationship. *Health Policy*, 119: 384–94.

Gore, J. (2003) What we can do for you! What can 'we' do for 'you'?: Struggling over empowerment in critical and feminist pedagogy. In Darder, A., Baltodano, M. and Torres, R.D. (eds) *The Critical Pedagogy Reader*. London: RoutledgeFalmer.

Gott, M., Ingleton, C., Gardiner, C. et al. (2013) Transitions to palliative care for older people in acute hospitals: a mixed methods study. *Health Services and Delivery Research*, 1(11).

Gott, M., Small, N., Barnes, S. et al. (2008) Older people's views of a good death in heart failure: implications for palliative care provision. *Social Science and Medicine*, 67: 1113–21.

Gulbrandsen, P., Clayman, M.L., Beach, M.C. et al. (2016) Shared decision-making as an existential journey; aiming for restored autonomous capacity. *Patient Education and Counselling*, 99(9): 1505–10.

Hanley, B., Bradburn, J., Barnes, M. et al. (2004) Involving the public in NHS, Public Health and Social Care Research: Briefing notes for researchers. (second edition). Eastleigh: INVOLVE Support Unit.

Henwood, F., Wyatts, S., Hart, A. and Smith, J. (2003) 'Ignorance is bliss sometimes': constraints on the emergence of the 'informed patient' in the changing landscapes of health information. *Sociology of Health and Illness*, 25: 589–607.

Hibbard, J.H. and Mahoney, E. (2010) Toward a theory of patient and consumer activation. *Patient Education and Counselling*, 78: 377–81.

Horsfall, D., Noonan, K. and Leonard, R. (2011) *Bringing our Dying Home: Creating Community at End of Life.* Sydney: University of Western Sydney.

Hsiung, Y., Ferrans, Y. and Estwing, C. (2007) Recognising Chinese Americans' cultural needs in making end-of-life treatment decisions. *Journal of Hospice and Palliative Nursing,* 9: 132–40.

Institute of Medicine (2001) *Crossing the Quality Chasm: A New Health System for the 21st Century.* Washington, DC: Institute of Medicine.

Israel, B., Checkoway, B., Schulz, A. et al. (1994) Health education and community empowerment: conceptualising and measuring perceptions of individual, organisational, and community control. *Health Education Quarterly,* 21: 149–70.

James, P., with Magee, L., Scerri, A. and Steger, M. (2015) *Urban Sustainability in Theory and Practice: Circles of Sustainability.* New York, Routledge.

Jenerette, C.M. and Mayer, D.K. (2016) Patient-provider communication: the rise of patient engagement. *Seminars in Oncology Nursing,* 32: 134–43.

Johnston, B., Rogerson, L., Macijauskiene, J. et al. (2014) An exploration of self–management support in the context of palliative nursing: a modified concept analysis. *BMC Nursing,* 13.

Kaufman, S.R. (2005) *. . . and a Time to Die: How American Hospitals Shape the End of Life.* Chicago: University of Chicago Press.

Legare, F., Stacey, D., Turcotte, S. et al. (2014) Interventions for improving the adoption of shared decision making by health professionals. *Cochrane Database of Systematic Reviews.* No. 9, CD006732.

Lomas, J. (2000) Using 'linkage and exchange' to move research into policy at a Canadian foundation. *Health Affairs,* 19: 236–40.

Marjolein, H.J., Pol, V.D., Fluit, C.R.M.G. et al. (2016) Expert and patient consensus on a dynamic model for shared decision-making in frail older patients. *Patient Education and Counselling,* 99: 1069–77.

Marston, C. and Renedo, A. (2013) Understanding and measuring the effects of patient and public involvement: an ethnographic study. London School of Hygiene and Tropical Medicine research.

NHS (National Institute for Health Research) (1996) *INVOLVE.* Available: http://www.invo.org.uk/ (accessed 3 March 2017).

Oliver, S., Liabo, K., Stewart, R. and Rees, R. (2015) Public involvement in research: making sense of the diversity. *Journal of Health Services Research and Policy,* 20: 45–51.

Palliative care Australia (2005) *A Guide to Palliative Care Service Development: A Population-based Approach.* Deakin West, ACT: Palliative Care Australia. Available at: http://palliativecare.org.au/wp-content/uploads/2015/05/A-guide-to-palliative-care-service-development-a-population-based-approach.pdf.

Parent Carer Council Cornwall (2012) Parent Carer Council Cornwall: co-production in developing a palliative care strategy. *NHS Parent Carer Participation Case Study.* Cornwall.

Pastrana, T., Junger, S., Ostgathe, C. et al. (2008) A matter of definition: key elements identified in a discourse analysis of definitions of palliative care. *Palliative Medicine,* 22: 222–32.

Patient-Centered Outcomes Research Institute (2011) Available at: http://www.pcori.org/ (accessed 3 March 2017).

Paul, S. and Sallnow, L. (2013) Public health approaches to end-of-life care in the UK: an online survey of palliative care services. *BMJ Supportive and Palliative Care,* 3: 196–9.

Richards, N., Ingleton, C., Gardiner, C. and Gott, M. (2013) Awareness contexts revisited: indeterminacy in initiating discussions at the end-of-life. *Journal of Advanced Nursing*, 69: 2654–64.

Rissel, C. (1994) Empowerment: the holy grail of health promotion. *Health Promotion International*, 9: 39–48.

Saunders, C. (1996) Guest contribution: hospice. *Mortality*, 1: 317–22.

Scottish Government (2015) *Strategic Framework for Action on Palliative and End of Life Care, 2016–2021*. Edinburgh: The Scottish Government.

Shipee, N.D., Garces, J.P.D., Prutsky Lopez, G.J. et al. (2013) Patient and service user engagement in research: a systematic review and synthesised framework. *Health Expectations*, 18(5): 1151–66.

Snyder, H. and Engstrom, J. (2015) The antecedents, forms and consequences of patient involvement: a narrative review of the literature. *International Journal of Nursing Studies*, 53: 351–78.

Staley, K. (2009) *What Impact Does Patient and Public Involvement Have on Health and Social Care Research? A Literature Review*. Eastleigh: INVOLVE.

Staley, K. and Minogue, V. (2006) User involvement leads to more ethically sound research. *Clinical Ethics*, 1(2): 95–100.

Steinhauser, K.E., Clipp, E.C., Mcneilly, M. et al. (2000) In search of a good death: observations of patients, families and providers. *Annals of Internal Medicine*, 132: 825–32.

Supple, D., Roberts, A., Hudson, V. et al. (2015) From tokenism to meaningful engagement: best practices in patient involvement in an EU project. *Research Involvement and Engagement*, 1: 5.

Tang, P.C. and Smith, M. (2016) Democratization of health care. *JAMA*, 316(16): 1663–4.

The Long-Term Conditions Alliance Scotland: People Not Patients (2008) *'Gaun yersel!' The Self-Management Strategy for Long Term Conditions in Scotlan*d. Edinburgh: The Scottish Government.

The National Council for Palliative Care (2009) *A Guide to Involving Patients, Carers and the Public in Palliative and End of Life Care Service*s. London: The National Centre for Involvement, NHS.

Thompson, J., Bissell, P., Cooper, C.L. et al. (2014) Exploring the impact of patient and public involvement in a cancer research setting. *Qualitative Health Research*, 24: 46–54.

van Der Eerden, M. (2016) Patient-centred care: how far should patients be 'active collaboration' partners? EAPC blog. Available at: https://eapcnet.wordpress.com/2016/08/22/patient-centred-care-how-far-should-patients-be-active-collaboration-partners/ (accessed 16 December 2016).

Vrijhoe, H.J. (2015) Patient engagement is the new hard currency in health care. *International Journal of Care Co-ordination*, 18: 3–4.

Williams, L., Gott, M., Moeke-Maxwell, T. et al. (2017) Death, dying and digital stories. In Beresford, P. and Carr, S. (eds) *Social Policy First Hand*. Bristol: Policy Press.

World Health Organization (2017) *Patients for Patient Safety*. Available at: http://www.who.int/patientsafety/patients_for_patient/en/ (accessed 3 March 2017).

Living with an uncertain prognosis

Lynn Calman

Introduction

Living with disease is an area of palliative care which is changing across a number of conditions. The survival rates of people living with diseases have been improving over the past few decades. Considering specifically cancer first of all, now more than 50 per cent of all cancer patients in the UK are surviving for more than 10 years, and this rate has doubled since the 1970s when it was 24 per cent (CRUK 2016). These improvements have been due to screening, earlier diagnosis and improvement in and access to treatment. However, cancer is still the leading cause of preventable deaths in England and in Wales. In England, 40 per cent of all preventable deaths are caused by cancer (ONS 2016). While incidence and mortality rates for most cancers are decreasing in western countries, they are increasing in less developed and economically transitioning countries. Cancers, such as lung cancer, are increasing as populations engage in less healthy behaviour and lifestyles associated with economically developed countries (Jemal et al. 2010; Hashim et al. 2016).

The number of people dying from coronary heart disease (CHD) has more than halved from 166,000 in 1961 to about 80,000 in 2009 (Scarborough et al. 2011) and in Europe there has been a downward trend in death for chronic obstructive pulmonary disease (COPD) (López-Campo et al. 2013). However, a different picture is emerging for dementia/Alzheimer's disease, potentially due to improved awareness, early recognition of symptoms and diagnosis, with increasing prevalence and mortality reported.

The overall improvement in mortality has led to a number of implications for both patients and health services. A growing number of people are experiencing long-term conditions, for example cancer, not as life-limiting 'incurable' diseases, but as life-changing and long-term conditions with a number of phases. Patients are living for longer with the consequences of their disease and its treatment, and this has an impact on health and well-being in the short, medium and long terms. The time for patient referral to palliative care may be longer as people experience prolonged periods of living with advanced disease. Specialist palliative care services increasingly have to work alongside other services delivering active treatment and surveillance for disease.

Another significant change in the experience of patients receiving palliative care is that many people are living with one or more co-morbidities. The number of people with co-morbidities is set to increase in England from 1.9 million in 2008 to 2.9 million by 2018 (Department of Health 2014). This is one of the most significant issues currently facing health systems in the developed world. Patients living with multiple long-term conditions is becoming the norm in ageing populations and an approach to disease management that focuses on single diseases cannot adequately address the issues (Department of Health 2014).

Uncertainty is a multidimensional concept that has been described in the healthcare literature for around 30 years (Mishel 1981). Uncertainty arises from the interaction between a number of different factors. The characteristics of uncertain experiences have been described as complexity, unpredictability, ambiguity, lack of information, unfamiliarity, vagueness (lack of details) and inconsistency (Etkind and Koffman 2016). In a concept analysis of uncertainty in illness, McCormick (2002) describes three attributes of uncertainty itself: (1) probability (the likelihood that something might happen); (2) temporality (what does the future hold? This includes duration, pace and frequency); and (3) perception (understanding based on previous experience). The interrelatedness of uncertainty to other concepts makes it complex to understand and research. For example, although loss of control is related to uncertainty (McCormick 2002), it is not considered the same thing; perceived control is a personality factor; and how 'in control' people feel can influence uncertainty. Feeling loss of control can also lead to the same outcomes as uncertainty.

The negative outcomes of uncertainty in illness have been well documented and include emotional distress, anxiety and depression (McCormick 2002). Positive outcomes and responses to living with uncertainty in life-limiting conditions, such as resilience (Molina et al. 2014), have been of more recent interest to researchers and clinicians and offer an interesting reconceptualisation of the experience of life-limiting diseases.

Etkind and Koffman (2016) highlight that there are additional aspects of uncertainty of life-limiting conditions, in particular, the uncertainty around prognosis, which will be discussed later in this chapter. Strategies to help manage uncertainty include:

- the development of complex care packages;
- education interventions for both patients and healthcare professionals to enhance communication;

- introducing psychological approaches to patients such as cognitive behavioural therapy;
- mindfulness or patient activation models to support patients in engaging in care (Etkind and Koffman 2016).

Living with complexity and uncertainty is a key feature of living with a life-limiting condition and this chapter aims to introduce the patient experience of living with uncertainty, prognostication, changing disease trajectories and the increasing importance of self-management support.

Changing trajectories

Improvements in mortality and treatment options have resulted in the emergence of new patient populations (Lobb et al. 2013), such as cancer patients living for extended periods with advanced disease. Living with uncertainty with cancer over a long period poses a unique challenge to patients and their families and is experienced often with contradictory responses; avoiding thinking about the illness, while trying to minimise the impact of the disease, maintaining normality and focusing on the positive but placing an importance on the outcome of palliative treatments and surveillance regimes (Lobb et al. 2013). This tension between maintaining normality and the involvement of healthcare is complex. Clinic appointments and clinicians 'keeping an eye on them' are highly valued by patients, but patients do not necessarily see themselves as passive but are highly skilled at managing everyday changes to their life to maintain normality and live well.

There has been a significant change in the way people experience illness. Improvements in early diagnosis, treatment and monitoring have changed trajectories of those living with life-limiting conditions. A particularly stark example of this is HIV/AIDS. In the late 1990s, delaying the onset of AIDS was the clinical goal and life expectancy was around 12 years from infection. Developments in antiretroviral treatments have turned HIV into a chronic condition with patients potentially living long and fulfilled lives and a near normal lifespan, if diagnosed early after infection (Yin et al. 2014).

Survival improvements in cancer have also been marked over the past 40 years. The UK 10-year survival rate for breast cancer is now nearly 80 per cent for breast cancer and 84 per cent for prostate cancer (CRUK 2016). Increases in life expectancy are to be celebrated but there is a more complex picture behind these survival data. There is still poor prognosis in some cancer groups which have changed little since the 1970s, for example, lung cancer survival remains very poor (5 per cent survival at 10 years and 10 per cent survival at 5 years (CRUK 2016)). More than a quarter of all people with a cancer diagnosis die within a year of diagnosis (Maddams et al. 2011).

Living longer does not always mean living well. Data has emerged in the last five years that builds a more complex picture of living with and beyond cancer. The burden of co-morbidities and the consequences of cancer and its treatment are now being understood. A large retrospective study of cancer patients, including nearly 140,000 patients in the UK highlights that one in five women with breast cancer and one in four men with prostate cancer will survive for 7 years and in good health but the majority will be living with one or more co-morbidities, such as heart, liver or kidney disease, or have a cancer recurrence or spread (Macmillan Cancer Support 2014a). Aaronson et al. (2014) provide an overview of physical and psychological impacts of living with cancer; they include pain and pain management, cancer-related fatigue, psychosocial and psychological distress. Macmillan Cancer Support (2013b) have estimated that of the 2 million people living with and beyond cancer in the UK, there are at least 500,000 people living with one or more physical or psychosocial consequences of their cancer or its treatment that affects their lives on a long-term basis. These consequences have an impact on the way people live their lives.

One way to understand the complexity of living with a life-limiting disease is to try to describe the typical trajectories people face living with life-limiting conditions. Trajectories of dying have long been recognised in the literature (Glaser and Strauss 1968) and four trajectories of dying are identified in Figure 5.1 (Lunney et al. 2003; Murray et al. 2005; Murtagh et al. 2008).

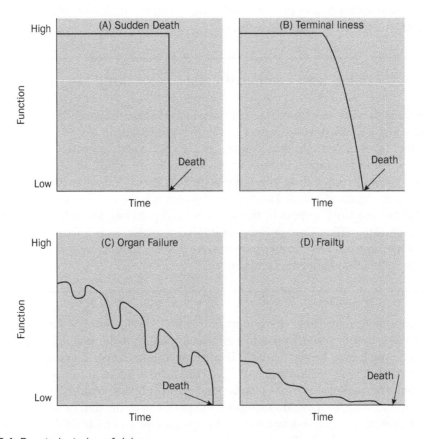

Figure 5.1 Four trajectories of dying

The first of the trajectories is sudden death which can occur without a prior diagnosis or symptoms (Figure 5.1A). In the second, we see a period of relative good function followed by a rapid decline in the advanced stages (Figure 5.1B), this trajectory is considered typical of a patient diagnosed with cancer. The third trajectory is one of acute episodes, which may require hospital admission, with recovery but function may not be to the level previously experienced (Figure 5.1C). The patient is eventually likely to die during one of these episodes. This pattern is typical of patients with organ failure, such as end-stage cardiac or respiratory disease. The final trajectory (Figure 5.1D) is one of gradual decline typically seen in the very elderly and those patients with diseases such as dementia.

There are some limitations to this model of understanding phases of illness. These trajectories have not been supported by research evidence in all conditions and are largely theoretical in some areas of practice, such as kidney failure (Murtagh et al. 2008). New evidence, for example, suggests that the trajectories associated with cancer are not quite as straightforward, as many people are living with the consequences of disease and treatment. Patients may move between these trajectories depending on treatment options (stopping or starting treatment). The impact of co-morbidities is not incorporated into this model but may play a significant part in decline – for instance, it may not be a person's cancer that drives the trajectory but their dementia – so seeing the whole picture of a person's health is vital.

Box 5.1   Living with complexity and uncertainty: lung cancer

Most patients with lung cancer (69 per cent) in the UK are diagnosed with advanced disease (CRUK 2016). Lung cancer patients have higher levels of symptom burden than other cancer patients (Vainio et al. 1996), which are often uncontrolled, and frequently symptoms present as clusters (Cooley 2008). Patients are, in the main, elderly, living with co-morbidities and incidence is higher for those living in the most deprived areas. Two-thirds of patients have cancer complications or morbidities requiring in-patient treatment and 55 per cent die within 6 months of diagnosis (Macmillan Cancer Support 2014b). Despite high levels of symptoms and active disease, lung cancer patients can live for months or sometimes years, usually on continuous systemic therapy.

Despite limitations, there are important clinical implications of these trajectories. They can help with forward planning and understanding the inevitability of decline and death, which may be particularly important in non-cancer conditions where it is known that predicting decline and palliative care need is difficult (Shipman et al. 2008). Acknowledging patients are on a dying trajectory allows healthcare professionals, patients and families to honestly recognise the pathway of the patient and resulting priorities of care which may be empowering for the patient and their family (Murray et al. 2005; Murtagh et al. 2008). These trajectories are useful for understanding patterns of decline but are a generalisation and an individual's disease trajectory may be uncertain. People diagnosed with life-limiting conditions increasingly experience personal journeys, relationships and clinical pathways characterised by complexity.

A longitudinal qualitative exploration (Murray et al. 2005) comparing the experiences of dying of lung cancer and heart failure highlights in more detail the lived experiences of different dying trajectories and the impact these have on the individual, including understanding of the disease trajectory, support for family, psychological well-being and access to healthcare services.

Learning exercise 5.1

There have been many accounts of the experiences of how patients live with cancer and life-limiting chronic disease in the literature.

- Conduct a literature search to identify published research which explores the experience of people living with a type of chronic or life-limiting illness.
- Does reading about the experience of care, the challenges and/or rewards experienced, from the patient's perspective, make you think differently about nursing a patient with this condition?

Some things to think about:

- How did you go about searching for the type of research, what key words did you use?
- What type of research methodology did the researcher use?
- What questions did they ask and was the research guided by a theoretical perspective?
- How might you critique the quality of the research?
- If you can identify more than one paper exploring the experience of the illness, do the findings differ? If so, how might you explain this?
- Could you compare living with the condition you have chosen to the experience of another chronic or life-limiting condition – how do they differ?

People will be living with the consequences of their disease and its treatment through the disease trajectory with many patients living with advanced disease or consequences for prolonged periods. It has been argued that managing the time for transition to supportive and palliative care is arguably more of a challenge than identifying people who are in the last days of life (Boyd and Murray 2010). It is generally agreed that early palliative care interventions are supportive to the patients and caregivers and lead to better outcomes, such as choice of place of death (Ravi et al. 2013; Ali et al. 2015; Dionne-Odom et al. 2015). Some emerging evidence in the USA has also highlighted a potential survival benefit for patients accessing early palliative care for lung cancer, although this has yet to be replicated in other healthcare systems (Temel et al. 2010).

Uncertainty presents major challenges for people living with advanced illnesses and for the professionals caring for them (Kimbell et al. 2016). Living with uncertainty and the unpredictability of a disease course is challenging and complex and requires psychological adjustment (this is the focus of Chapter 9 in this volume). But uncertainty has also been seen as an opportunity. Acknowledging uncertainty can be the basis of communication and shared decision-making as a person's health declines (Kimbell et al. 2016). Research on resilience and positive psychological consequences is a growing area and offers an opportunity to understand why some patients cope well in the face of deteriorating health and death (Molina et al. 2014).

Prognostication

Understanding the potential trajectory of disease can be helpful in determining prognosis. Although most healthcare teams in the western world would now disclose a diagnosis of cancer, issues of prognosis may be less commonly discussed (Butow et al. 2002). Many of the factors identified as important to patients at the end of life focus on planning ahead and preparation for the end of life (Steinhauser et al. 2000). Accurate prognostication has been identified as a central aspect of oncology and palliative care practice (Maltoni et al. 2005; Mendis et al. 2015).

As described above, uncertainty is a major cause of emotional distress for patients, while talking about diagnosis and prognosis can be therapeutic and give relief from uncertainty (Girgis and Sanson-Fisher 1998). A qualitative study (Butow et al. 2002) has explored what cancer patients with metastatic disease want to know about prognosis. Seven themes were identified including: (1) communication within a caring, trusting, long-term relationship; (2) open and repeated negotiations for patient preferences for information; (3) clear, straightforward presentation of prognosis where desired; (4) strategies to ensure patient understanding; (5) encouragement of hope and a sense of control; (6) consistency of communication within the multi-disciplinary team; and (7) communication with other members of the family.

It may be important for patients and families to have information about their prognosis to allow them to put affairs in order and make the most of the life they have left. People nearing the end of life often wish to know how long they have got left to live, although not all want this to be communicated as a number of weeks or months to live (Finlay and Casarett 2009). Many patients do not have a good understanding of their disease or prognosis and can have difficulty remembering information they have been given (Lobb et al. 1999).

Despite differences in trajectories in early disease, cancer patients often have a more predictable pattern of decline in the advanced phase (Finlay and Casarett 2009). Despite this, clinicians often have difficulty in predicting survival. There is a robust body of evidence that suggests physicians are inaccurate in their estimations of survival in cancer patients and in the main estimates tend to be overly optimistic, although accuracy improves the closer the patient is to death (Mendis et al. 2015). This is particularly problematic when discussion of prognostication comes about in the context of making treatment decisions when prognosis can be an important factor in weighing up quality and quantity of life in the face of toxic and lengthy treatments, and it has been mooted that oncologists' bias for giving anti-cancer treatments can result in more optimistic prognosis. A study by Weeks et al. (1998) found that patients made different treatment choices based on their perceived prognosis of 6 months or more. Those who believed they had at least a 10 per cent chance of dying within 6 months were less likely to choose life-extending therapies that those who expected to be alive in 6 months.

Inaccurate prognostication can also have implications for appropriate use of resources and referral to palliative care at an early point in the pathway. Prognostication may be particularly important in insurance-based health systems when it may trigger transition between care settings (Finlay and Casarett 2009). In some insurance systems in the USA, for example, it is a requirement that patients give up access to anti-cancer treatments to enrol in hospice care, although there is no such restriction on hospital-based palliative care. Enrolment in hospice care in insurance-based health systems may require the patient to meet specific criteria, including a prognosis of less than 6 months. In some state-funded health and welfare systems (with increasingly limited budgets and increasing demands), prognosis can be an eligibility criterion for some welfare benefits.

Attempts to increase the accuracy of prognostication have led to the development of a number of tools and frameworks to aid prognosis in advanced cancer (Finlay and Casarett 2009). These are multi-faceted and do not rely solely on clinical predictions of survival that have proved to be inaccurate.

Gwilliam et al. (2011) identified a range of variables that can help in prediction of prognosis in advanced cancer and these are summarised in Box 5.2.

Box 5.2 Factors that have prognosis utility

- Observed presence of symptoms (including pain, breathlessness and loss of appetite)
- Performance status
- Global health status
- Clinical observations – weight and height
- Cognitive status (to identify confusion)
- Clinician prediction (from multiple sources) of survival (in days, weeks, months or years)
- Demographic, disease and treatment-rated variables
- Co-morbidity
- Laboratory variables (to analyse haematological and biochemical factors).

Adapted from Gwilliam et al. (2011).

Examples of prognostic tools include the palliative prognostic score (Pirovano et al. 1999), which uses a number of variables, clinical assessment, performance status, symptoms and blood results to predict prognosis – the result is three levels of prediction: >70 per cent chance, 30–70 per cent chance or a <30 per cent chance of surviving for at least one month. The Palliative Prognosis Index (Morita et al. 1999) uses palliative and performance status and symptoms to predict survival of <3 weeks, <6 weeks or >6 weeks. Tools have been tested through research and resulted in more accurate prognosis but they are still not a perfect predictor of survival.

The three prognostic tools above are complex and are generally embedded in specialist cancer services. Judging prognosis is particularly difficult for non-cancer patients due to the paucity and limitations of prognostic indicators to inform decision-making (Shipman et al. 2008; Boyd and Murray 2010).

For life-limiting conditions other than cancer, as we have seen above, trajectories are often less predictable and are managed not in specialist services but in primary care. In the UK context., there have been moves to improve palliative care by generalist primary care staff and the Gold Standards Framework (GSF), a service improvement tool (GSF 2016), which was developed over a decade ago to enable primary care staff to proactively manage palliative care in the community. Snapshot audit data (RCGP and RCN 2012) has suggested that only a minority of patients on a GP's register who died were included on the GP's register of palliative care, and the register was heavily weighted to cancer patients. One aspect of the GSF has been to support early identification of patients with palliative care needs and this includes determining prognosis with the aim of placing patients on a supportive care pathway and determining preferences (advanced care planning) at early identification of increasing needs rather than giving patients accurate timescales.

The GSF prognostic indicator guidance was published in 2011 (Thomas 2011) to try to support the 1 per cent of a GP's population who will die each year. The guidance suggests three triggers that could indicate that a patient is nearing the end of life (last 12 months):

- the surprise question: 'Would you be surprised if this patient were to die in the next few months, weeks, days?';
- general indicators of decline, including: decreasing activity, functional performance score decreasing, limited self-care, in bed or chair 50 per cent of day, decreasing response to treatments, choice to have no further active treatment, weight loss, repeated unplanned/crisis admissions;
- specific clinical indicators of decline related to certain conditions (cancer, organ failure, renal disease, general and specific neurological disease and frailty/dementia).

The GSF framework also recommends needs-based coding to prioritise need to give the right care at the right time in the right place. The key to successful identification of patients who may require palliative care is regular assessment and planning care in collaboration with patients and their families. For further discussion on prognostic tools see Chapter 6.

Communicating prognosis

It is acknowledged that there are two parts to communicating prognostication: foreseeing and foretelling (Krawczyk and Gallagher 2016). Foreseeing is the skill to estimate the course of the illness and foretelling the communication of the prognosis to the patient. Both are skills that come with experience and knowledge. The experiences of family members reflecting on how uncertainty about the end of life was communicated in the hospital setting is revealing about foretelling (Krawczyk and Gallagher 2016). In this research, conducted in Canada, family members reported that they lacked the understanding that death was the possible outcome and felt there was lack of communication about prognosis. There was confusion in the paradox of acute care treatments being given up to the point of death, the inappropriate use of euphemisms, such as 'not doing too well', and the provision of false hope.

Despite many patients and families wanting information on prognosis, and improvements in accuracy of prognosis through the development of tools, conveying this information is challenging. Patients want accurate information delivered honestly and sensitively by people they trust and ideally have a relationship with (Finlay and Casarett 2009; Gwilliam et al. 2011). The need for honest disclosure may be balanced by the patient's need for hope, therefore, understanding the type and level of information people want is complex, and this is likely to change over time (Finlay and Casarett 2009). Kutner et al. (1999) identified that patients were often in conflict between wanting to know what is going on and fearing bad news. A number of studies have looked at characteristics that may predict preferences for disclosure of prognosis but there is no clear agreement in these studies, although age and cultural beliefs may have an impact on preferences. Therefore, clinicians must have a flexible, individualised approach to talking about prognosis, that is directed by the patient and family. Research has demonstrated that clinical staff may be reluctant to discuss prognosis. Barriers to discussion include:

- concerns that a doctor's prognosis may be wrong and that patients will lose faith in them;
- the difficulty of the balance between being honest and hopeful;
- lack of skills in managing personal emotional reaction as well as that of the patient and family;
- lack of communication skills training;
- limited time to spend with patients in clinics.

These barriers, in the main, can be overcome with training and support to develop an individual approach to giving a prognosis. Communication with patients and families is the subject of Chapter 7 in this volume and will be discussed further there, but is it important to acknowledge the contextual issues such as time and resources required to support staff, patients and families after disclosing prognosis.

Survivorship: living with and beyond cancer

In response to the increasing number of people living with the impact of cancer and its treatment, there has been a focus over the last few decades on cancer survivorship or living with and beyond cancer. The number of people living with and beyond cancer in the UK is set to double, to an estimated four million, by 2030 (Maddams et al. 2012). However, as we have seen above, cancer and its treatment can have a considerable and long-term impact on everyday life (Hewitt et al. 2003; Corner et al. 2007; Foster et al. 2009). Cancer survivors may face a range of challenges that can have a significant impact on all aspects of daily life and may last over the life course (Foster et al. 2009).

Although cancer treatments have improved, have become more targeted and have resulted in significant improvement in survival for some types of cancer, the effects of radiotherapy, chemotherapy and surgery do have an impact on well-being over the long term. Of the two million people living with and beyond cancer in the UK, it has been estimated that a quarter are facing poor health or disability (Macmillan Cancer Support 2013a). At least 200,000 are living with moderate to severe pain after curative treatment, 150,000 are affected by urinary problems such as incontinence, and 90,000 are experiencing gastrointestinal problems, including faecal incontinence, diarrhoea and bleeding (Macmillan Cancer Support 2013a). Some consequences may not become apparent until five or ten years after treatment but can have a significant impact, for example, some chemotherapy can increase the risk of heart disease and long-term hormone therapy is related to osteoporosis (Macmillan Cancer Support 2013a).

Patients have highlighted the need for support to manage the impact of cancer on everyday life (Corner et al. 2007). People can be unprepared for the impact that cancer and its treatment can have on their lives, may feel vulnerable and experience loss of confidence, and may struggle to access care and support (Hewitt et al. 2005; Jefford et al. 2008; Foster et al., 2009; Foster and Fenlon 2011). There is a growing recognition that healthcare services need to adapt to the rapidly growing number of people living with and beyond cancer. There has been a significant focus on aftercare of patients, with, for example, risk stratification models developed (Foster 2015), and this will have an impact on how care is managed at different parts of the disease trajectory.

Learning exercise 5.2

- What do you understand by the term 'survivorship'?
- What is the nurse's role in survivorship?
- Are there aspects of supportive and palliative care that apply to survivorship and aftercare?

The term survivorship is a contested concept, an identity not endorsed by all patients (Khan et al. 2012). It developed from cancer activism in the mid-1980s in the USA (Bell and Ristovski-Slijepcevic 2013) and the concept has gained legitimacy through inclusion in health policy, service developments and research. Survivorship not only encompasses those living disease-free but all stages of illness from diagnosis to end of life care. In the UK, the National Cancer Survivorship Initiative (NCSI) workstream on active and advanced disease focuses on keeping well, accessing support services, re-entering the healthcare system, i.e. for cancer recurrence or further treatment, and the progression of illness to end of life.

Living with and beyond cancer (cancer survivorship) encompasses both physical and psychological impacts of cancer and has its roots in a number of theoretical positions, including biological sciences, psychological theories of coping and self-efficacy (Lent 2007) and social role and identity, such as disrupted and new identities (Bury 1982). Foster and Fenlon's (2011) conceptual model of recovery of health and well-being following cancer treatment attempts to draw these factors together with their own research findings, focusing on the views and priorities of patients. They hypothesise that health and well-being of those living with and beyond cancer are positively associated with presence of support for the individual and the patient's confidence (self-efficacy) to manage problems faced as a consequence of their cancer and its treatment (Foster and Fenlon 2011).

Since 2014, the initiative has become the Living With and Beyond Cancer (LWBC) programme (www.ncsi.org.uk), focusing on putting the recommendations and priorities identified by the NCSI into service development and provisions. The LWBC programme is focusing on:

- ensuring all cancer patients have access to holistic needs assessment, treatment summary, cancer care review and a patient education and support event – the 'Recovery Package';
- developing and commissioning risk-stratified pathways of post-treatment management;
- promoting health and well-being, including physical activity;
- understanding and commissioning for improved management of the consequences of treatment.

Survivorship initiatives, such as the NCSI, have been the driver for systems change in service delivery and significant changes in recognising needs and supporting patients and their families living with and beyond cancer. Much of the evidence that has been used to develop services (such as self-management support) has been based on long-term conditions and translated to the oncology setting. As we have seen above, there is a significant imperative in integrating cancer services with long-term conditions, although evidence for managing the care of patients with multi-morbidity is limited (Smith et al. 2012). A future challenge is to integrate survivorship initiatives into the management in multi-morbidity, particularly at the end of life.

Self-management support

Most of the time, people living with life-limiting disease, in collaboration with those close to them, such as family and friends, manage their own health and well-being at home without the input of health professionals. There is a growing view that cancer can be managed as a chronic illness (McCorkle et al. 2011). Self-management support is embedded in UK health policy and there is increasing evidence that supporting people to manage their own health has positive outcomes, including improved quality of life and reduced use of health services (Health Foundation 2015).

Self-management support is multi-faceted and there is some ambiguity in its definition (Johnston et al. 2014). It requires knowledge, skills and confidence to develop and maintain control of care. For people with long-term conditions, it can be defined as (Health Foundation 2015, p. 5):

- being active partners in determining outcomes that are important to them and how to achieve them, working in collaboration with healthcare professionals;
- being supported to build knowledge, skills, confidence and resilience to manage the impact of their symptoms and limitations so they can live a full and meaningful life;
- being enabled to access the support they need within and beyond health services to better manage their own health and well-being on an ongoing basis.

Self-management support, as seen above, has more recently become an important component of cancer care. There has been a growing recognition that cancer survivors have to manage the impact of cancer and its treatment but that current methods of aftercare do not meet their needs (Armes et al. 2009). Cancer patients have highlighted the need for support in managing the impact of cancer on everyday life (Corner et al. 2007). The UK National Cancer Survivorship Initiative was established to investigate new models of aftercare (Department of Health, Macmillan Cancer Support and NHS Improvement 2010), with an increasing focus on self-management support as a key element of aftercare for cancer patients. For cancer survivors, self-management support includes managing consequences of cancer and its treatment, such as symptoms, seeking support when appropriate, recognising and reporting signs and symptoms of possible disease progression, and making lifestyle changes to promote health, well-being and survival (Foster 2015).

The evidence base to inform self-management support in people living with advanced disease and palliative care is limited. Much of the evidence for supported self-management in cancer care relates to patients during active treatment that is potentially curative (Fenlon and Foster 2009). There has been a very limited amount of research that explores the role of self-management support in advanced cancer (Johnston et al. 2009). Johnston et al. (2014) conducted a concept analysis of self-management support in palliative nursing to develop a clear conceptual understanding of the topic. Their proposed definition was based on current published literature, most of which was based on chronic disease management:

> Supportive self-management in palliative nursing is: assessing, planning, and implementing appropriate care to enable the patient to live until they die and supporting the patient to be given the means to master or deal with their illness or their effects of their illness themselves.
>
> (Johnston et al. 2014, p. 8)

We need further evidence to understand the contribution self-management support makes (and could potentially make) to the health and well-being of people living with life-limiting conditions, acknowledging that not all patients will want to or be able to engage in self-management activities. We need to identify the challenges people face in doing this, the factors that enable and inhibit engagement in self-management, as well as the implications for those closest to them and the HCPs involved. We need to prepare and support patients to self-manage, to more effectively use their own strategies or be supported to develop new strategies. A significant source of support for many comes from personal social networks (such as partners, family and friends) and these are recognised as having an important role in self-management (Vassilev et al. 2014). Other sources of support, e.g. community groups, also have involvement in support but are not always acknowleged in the healthcare setting. It is important to consider the impact of consequences of cancer and its treatment beyond the patients and on those who support the patient following treatment.

The Health Foundation guide to self-managed support suggests that elements of a model of self-managed care include:

- embedding self-management support in commissioning and planning so this is complementary to medical care;
- supporting patient, families and networks to develop skills, knowledge and confidence to manage health;
- supporting health professionals to have the skills, both communication and clinical, to be collaborative in their approach;
- having the organisation processes to support patients and professionals in self-management;
- developing peer and community support to bring people together with similar experiences.

There is evidence that patients with advanced cancer wish to maintain independence and normality and maintain control over their lives (Hopkinson et al. 2006; McCorkle et al. 2011; Johnston et al. 2012). Although the evidence on how self-managed support is operationalised in palliative care is an emerging area, it is important for professionals working in the area to understand that many patients, particularly those with chronic diseases, will be moving through the trajectory of their illness by self-managing their condition. In cancer care, for example, risk stratification of aftercare is becoming commonplace. It is expected that a proportion of the growing population of survivors in the UK will be self-managing their condition with support. New models of aftercare, such as patient-triggered follow-up are being developed and tested. Palliative care professionals need to develop skills to support patients to self-manage, to make often small adaptations to their lives to maintain their quality of life. Understanding patient priorities becomes crucial and may require a different type of consultation which can be challenging for the healthcare system.

> ### Learning exercise 5.3
>
> *Reflection*
>
> - What kinds of everyday activities might patients seek support with?
> - What communication skills are required by nurses to support self-management?
> - What resources might you need to support patients?

The changing relationships between healthcare and those experiencing ill health

We have seen that the exponential rise in people living with chronic and life-limiting conditions and with co-existing co-morbidity has placed a significant burden on patients and on healthcare. Management of chronic and life-limiting illness involves work, not to cure, but to identify and prevent recurrence, changing lifestyle, manage exacerbations, complexity and uncertainty. Increasingly patients are held accountable for this work (May et al. 2014). The change in the experience of the patients due to the extension of life, but living with morbidity from diseases and treatment and often multiple co-morbidity, has led to a re-evaluation of what it is to be a patient in contemporary healthcare.

Being a patient involves 'managed engagement with multiple healthcare practices' due to the increased number of people living with chronic and life-limiting conditions and developments in medicines and technological and life sciences innovations and the shift of care from the hospital to the community (May et al. 2014). This is set within the context of debates about who is responsible for health, the individual or the state (or the healthcare provider in insurance-based healthcare systems). As described above, self-care, management and monitoring are the central tenets of current healthcare practices.

May et al. (2014) propose a new model 'the burden of treatment theory', a contemporary understanding of the relationship between sick people, social networks and healthcare. They argue that it is not just the patient but the wider social network that has to be engaged with healthcare providers and responsible for managing health. The burden of treatment theory aims to understand how people's *capacity* (their ability to engage with healthcare, access to social network support, the constraints of the health systems and access to healthcare) interacts with *patient work* (sense-making, engaging others – professionals and social networks – mobilising collective action and reflexive monitoring). This is a highly complex process and can be used to understand variations in healthcare use and adherence across different services and health contexts (May et al. 2014).

This results in significant challenges to healthcare, and in how the interactions between services and contexts in the hospital and community are managed. There has been a call to redesign healthcare using the principle of what has been described as minimally disruptive medicine (May et al. 2009). This whole systems change, as the authors acknowledge, is very complex (May et al. 2014). Minimally disruptive medicine aims for whole systems change that puts the patient at the centre of healthcare and acknowledges the patient (and social network) perspective and work that contributes to managing the illness.

Conclusion

Patients face a number of challenges as they transition through phases of an illness trajectory towards death. Much of that journey is uncertain and it takes considerable effort on the part of the patients and their social network to manage different healthcare settings and the burden of their treatment or care. Patients may be active in the management of disease, treatment and its consequences and need to be supported to have the confidence and skills to do so. Patients may wish clear information about their prognosis to be delivered in an individualised way with sensitivity, in a manner that maintains hope and with a focus on well-being. Healthcare professionals also face challenges in working with patients living in uncertainty; it is emotionally challenging and requires skill and commitment. This chapter signposts professionals towards resources to support their practice.

References

Aaronson, N., Mattioli, V., Minton, O. et al. (2014) Beyond treatment: psychosocial and behavioural issues in cancer survivorship research and practice. *European Journal of Cancer Supplements*, 12(1): 54–64. http://dx.doi.org/10.1016/j.ejcsup.2014.03.005.

Ali, M., Capel, M., Jones, P. and Gazt, T. (2015) The importance of identifying preferred place of death. *BMJ Supportive and Palliative Care*. doi: 10.1136/bmjspcare-2015-000878.

Armes, J., Crowe, M., Colbourne, L. et al. (2009) Patients' supportive care needs beyond the end of cancer treatment: a prospective, longitudinal survey. *Journal of Clinical Oncology*, 27(36): 6172–9.

Bell, K. and Ristovski-Slijepcevic, S. (2013) Cancer survivorship: why labels matter. *Journal of Clinical Oncology*, 21(4): 409–11.

Boyd, K. and Murray, S. (2010) Recognising and managing key transitions in end of life care. *BMJ*, 341: c4863.

Bury, M. (1982) Chronic illness as biographical disruption. *Sociology of Health and Illness*, 4(2): 167–82.

Butow, P., Dowsett, S., Hagert, R. et al. (2002) Communicating prognosis to patients with metastatic disease: what do they really want to know? *Supportive Care in Cancer*, 10: 161–8. doi: 10.1007/s005200100290.

Cooley, M.E. (2008) Symptoms in adults with lung cancer: a systematic research review. *Journal of Pain Symptom Management*, 19: 137–53.

Corner, J., Wright, D., Hopkinson, J. et al. (2007) The research priorities of patients attending UK cancer treatment centres: findings from a modified nominal group study. *British Journal of Cancer*, 96: 875–81.

CRUK (2016) Cancer statistics. Available at: http://www.cancerresearchuk.org/health-professional/cancer-statistics (accessed August 2016).

Department of Health (2014) *Comorbidities: A Framework of Principles for System-Wide Action*. Available at: https://www.gov.uk/government/publications/better-care-for-people-with-2-or-more-long-term-conditions (accessed August 2016).

Department of Health, Macmillan Cancer Support and NHS Improvement (2010) *The National Cancer Survivorship Initiative Vision*. Available at: http://www.dh.gov.uk/en/Publicationsandstatistics/Publications/PublicationsPolicyAndGuidance/DH_111230

Department of Health, Macmillan Cancer Support and NHS Improvement (2013) *Living with and Beyond Cancer: Taking Action to Improve Outcomes*. London: DoH. Available at: http://www.ncsi.org.uk/wp-content/uploads/Living-with-and-beyond-2013.pdf

Dionne-Odom, J.N., Azuero, A., Lyons, K.D. et al. (2015) Benefits of early versus delayed palliative care to informal family caregivers of patients with advanced cancer: outcomes from the ENABLE III randomized controlled trial. *Journal of Clinical Oncology*, 33: 1446–52.

Etkind, S.N. and Koffman, J. (2016) Approaches to managing uncertainty in people with life-limiting conditions: role of communication and palliative care. *Postgraduate Medical Journal*, 92: 412–17. doi: 10.1136/postgradmedj-2015-133371.

Fenlon, D. and Foster, C. (2009) Self-management support: a review of the evidence. Working document to support the National Cancer Survivorship Self-management workstream. Macmillan Research Unit, University of Southampton.

Finlay, E. and Casarett, D. (2009) Making difficult discussions easier: using prognosis to facilitate transitions to hospice. *CA: A Cancer Journal for Clinicians*, 59(4): 250–63. doi: 10.3322/caac.20022. Epub 17 June 2009.

Foster, C. (2015) Survivorship and self-management in cancer care. In Wyatt, D. and Hubert-Williams, N. (eds) *Cancer and Cancer Care*. London: Sage.

Foster, C., Wright, D., Hill, H. (2009) Psychosocial implications of living 5 years or more following a cancer diagnosis: a systematic review of the research evidence. *European Journal of Cancer Care*, 18(3): 223–47.

Foster, C. and Fenlon, D. (2011) Recovery and self-management support following primary cancer treatment. *British Journal of Cancer*, 105(Suppl. 1): S21–S28.

Girgis, A. and Sanson-Fisher, R.W. (1998) Breaking bad news. 1: Current best advice for clinicians. *Behavioral Medicine*, 24(2): 53–9.

Glaser, B. and Strauss, A. (1968) *A Time for Dying*. Chicago: Aldine Publishing Co.

GSF (2016) Gold Standards Framework. Available at: http://www.goldstandardsframework.org.uk/ (accessed August 2016).

Gwilliam, B., Keeley, V., Todd, C. et al. (2011) Development of Prognosis in Palliative care Study (PiPS) predictor models to improve prognostication in advanced cancer: prospective cohort study. *BMJ*, 343: d4920.

Hashim, D., Boffetta, P., La Vecchia, C. et al. (2016) The global decrease in cancer mortality: trends and disparities. *Annals of Oncology*, 27(5): 926–33. doi: 10.1093/annonc/mdw027.

Health Foundation (2015) *A Practical Guide to Self-Management Support: Key Components for Successful Implementation*. London: Health Foundation.

Hewitt, M., Greenfield, S. and Stovall, E. (2005) *From Cancer Patient to Cancer Survivor: Lost in Transition*. Washington, DC: National Academies Press.

Hewitt, M., Rowland, J.H. and Yancik, R. (2003) Cancer survivors in the United States: age, health, and disability. *Journals of Gerontology A: Biological Sciences and Medical Sciences*, 58(1): 82–91.

Hopkinson, J., Wright, D. and Corner, J. (2006) Exploring the experience of weight loss in people with advanced cancer. *Journal of Advanced Nursing*, 54(3): 304–12.

Jefford, M., Karahalios, E., Pollard, A. et al. (2008) Survivorship issues following treatment completion: results from focus groups with Australian cancer survivors and health professionals. *Journal of Cancer Survivorship*, 2(1): 20–32.

Jemal, A., Center, M., DeSantis, C. and Ward, E. (2010) Global patterns of cancer incidence and mortality rates and trends. *Cancer Epidemiology, Biomarkers and Prevention*, August 2010, 19: 1893–907.

Johnston, B., McGill, M., Milligan, S. et al. (2009) Self care and end of life care in advanced cancer: literature review. *European Journal of Oncology Nursing*, 3(5): 386–98.

Johnston, B., Rogerson, L., Macijauskiene, J. and Blaževi Cholewka, P. (2014) An exploration of self-management support in the context of palliative nursing: a modified concept analysis: *BMC Nursing*, 13: 21. doi: 10.1186/1472-6955-13-21.

Johnston, B.M., Milligan, S., Foster, C. and Kearney, N. (2012) Self-care and end of life care: patients' and carers' experience a qualitative study utilising serial triangulated interviews. *Supportive Care in Cancer*, 20: 1619–25.

Khan, N.F., Harrison, S., Rose, P.W. et al. (2012) Interpretation and acceptance of the term 'cancer survivor': a United Kingdom-based qualitative study. *European Journal of Cancer Care*, 21(2): 177–86. doi: 10.1111/j.1365-2354.2011.01277.x.

Kimbell, B., Murray, S., Macpherson, S. and Boyd, K. (2016) Embracing inherent uncertainty in advanced illness. *BMJ*, 354: i3802. doi: http://dx.doi.org/10.1136/bmj.i380.

Krawczyk, M. and Gallagher, R. (2016) Communicating prognostic uncertainty in potential end-of-life contexts: experiences of family members. *BMC Palliative Care*, 15: 59. doi: 10.1186/s12904-016-0133-4.

Kutner, J.S., Steiner, J.F., Corbett, K.K. et al. (1999) Information needs in terminal illness. *Social Science and Medicine*, 48: 1341–52.

Lent, R.W. (2007) Restoring emotional well-being: a theoretical model. In Feuerstein, M. (ed.) *Handbook of Cancer Survivorship*. New York: Springer, pp. 231–48.

Lobb, E., Butow, P.N., Kenny, D.T. and Tattersall, M.H. (1999) Communicating prognosis in early breast cancer: do women understand the language used? *Medical Journal of Australia*, 171(6): 290–4.

Lobb, E., Lacey, J., Kearsley, J. et al. (2013) Living with advanced cancer and an uncertain disease trajectory: an emerging patient population in palliative care? *BMJ Supportive and Palliative Care*. Available at: bmjspcare-2012-000381.

López-Campo, J., Ruiz-Ramos, M. and Soriano, J. (2013) Mortality trends in chronic obstructive pulmonary disease in Europe, 1994–2010: a joinpoint regression analysis. *The Lancet Respiratory Medicine*, 2(1): 54–62.

Lunney, J.R., Lynn, J., Foley, D.J. et al. (2003) Patterns of functional decline at the end of life. *JAMA*, 289: 2387–92.

Macmillan Cancer Support (2013a) *Cured But at What Cost?* London: Macmillan Cancer Support. Available at: http://www.macmillan.org.uk/documents/aboutus/newsroom/consequences_of_treatment_june2013.pdf (accessed August 2016).

Macmillan Cancer Support (2013b) *Throwing Light on the Consequences of Cancer and Its Treatment*. London: Macmillan Cancer Support. Available at: http://www.ncsi.org.uk/wp-content/uploads/MAC14312_CoT_Throwing-light_report_FINAL.pdf (accessed August 2016).

Macmillan Cancer Support (2014a) *Cancer's Unequal Burden*. London: Macmillan Cancer Support. Available at: http://www.macmillan.org.uk/documents/cancersunequalburden_2014.pdf (accessed August 2016).

Macmillan Cancer Support (2014b) *Routes from Diagnosis*. London: Macmillan Cancer Support. Available at: http://www.macmillan.org.uk/_images/routesfromdiagnosisreport_tcm9-265651.pdf (accessed August 2016).

Maddams, J., Utley, M. and Möller, H. (2011) A person-time analysis of hospital activity among cancer survivors in England. *British Journal of Cancer*, 105: S38–S45. doi: 10.1038/bjc.2011.421.

Maddams, J., Utley, M. and Möller, H (2012) Projections of cancer prevalence in the United Kingdom, 2010–2040. *British Journal of Cancer*, 107(7): 1195–202.

Maltoni, M., Caraceni, A., Brunelli, C. et al. and the Steering Committee of the European Association for Palliative Care (2005) Prognostic factors in advanced cancer patients: evidence-based clinical recommendations: a study by the Steering Committee of the European Association for Palliative Care. *Journal of Clinical Oncology*, 23(25): 6240–8.

May, C., Eton, D., Boehmer, K. et al. (2014) Rethinking the patient: using Burden of Treatment Theory to understand the changing dynamics of illness. *BMC Health Services Research*, 14: 281. doi: 10.1186/1472-6963-14-281.

May, C., Montori, V.M. and Mair, F.S. (2009) We need minimally disruptive medicine. *British Medical Journal*, 339: b2803.

McCorkle, R., Ercolano, E., Lazenby, M. et al. (2011) Self-management: enabling and empowering patients living with cancer as a chronic illness. *CA: A Cancer Journal for Clinicians*, 61(1): 50–62. doi: 10.3322/caac.20093.

McCormick, K.M. (2002) A concept analysis of uncertainty in illness. *Journal of Nursing Scholarship*, 34: 127–31. doi: 10.1111/j.1547-5069.2002.00127.x.

Mendis, R., Soo, W.K., Zannino, D. et al. (2015) Multidisciplinary prognostication using the palliative prognostic score in an Australian cancer center. *Palliative Care*, 9: 7–14. doi: 10.4137/PCRT.S24411. eCollection 2015.

Mishel, M.H. (1981) The measurement of uncertainty in illness. *Nursing Research*, 30: 258–63. doi: 10.1097/00006199-198109000-00002.

Molina, Y., Yi, J., Martinez-Gutierrez, J. et al. (2014) Resilience among patients across the cancer continuum: diverse perspectives. *Clinical Journal of Oncology Nursing*, 18(1): 93–101. doi: 10.1188/14.CJON.93-101.

Morita, T., Tsunoda, J., Inoue, S. and Chihara, S. (1999) The Palliative Prognostic Index: a scoring system for survival prediction of terminally ill cancer patients. *Supportive Care in Cancer*, 7: 128–33.

Murray, S., Kendall, M., Boyd, K. and Sheikh, A. (2005) Illness trajectories and palliative care. *BMJ*, 330: 1007.

Murtagh, F., Murphy, E. and Sheerin, N. (2008) Illness trajectories: an important concept in the management of kidney failure. *Nephrology Dialysis Transplantation*, 23(12): 3746–8. doi: 10.1093/ndt/gfn532.

ONS (Office of National Statistics) (2016) *Avoidable Mortality in England and Wales: 2014.* Available at: https://www.ons.gov.uk/peoplepopulationandcommunity/healthandsocialcare/causesofdeath/bulletins/avoidablemortalityinenglandandwales/2014#main-points (accessed August 2016).

Pirovano, M., Maltoni, M., Nanni, O. et al. (1999) A new palliative prognostic score: a first step for the staging of terminally ill cancer patients. Italian Multicenter and Study Group on Palliative Care. *Journal of Pain Symptom Management*, 17: 231–9.

Ravi, B., Parikh, A.B., Kirch, R.A. et al. (2013) Early specialty palliative care: translating data in oncology into practice. *New England Journal of Medicine*, 369: 2347–51.

RCGP and RCN (2012) *Matters of Life and Death.* Available at: http://www.rcgp.org.uk/~/media/Files/CIRC/Matters per cent20of per cent20Life per cent20and per cent20 Death per cent20FINAL.ashx

Scarborough, P., Wickramasinghe, K., Bhatnagar, P. and Rayner, M. (2011) *Trends in Coronary Heart Disease 1961–2011.* London: British Heart Foundation.

Shipman, C., Gysels White, P., Worth, A. et al. (2008) Improving generalist end of life care: national consultation with practitioners, commissioners, academics, and service user groups. *BMJ*, 337: a1720.

Smith, S.M., Soubhi, H., Fortin, M. et al. (2012) Managing patients with multimorbidity: systematic review of interventions in primary care and community settings. *BMJ*, 345: e5205.

Steinhauser, K.E., Christakis, N.A., Clipp, E.C. et al. (2000) Factors considered important at the end of life by patients, family, physicians, and other care providers. *JAMA*, 284(19): 2476–82. doi: 10.1001/jama.284.19.2476.

Temel, J.S., Greer, J.A., Muzikansky, A. et al (2010) Early palliative care for patients with metastatic non-small-cell lung cancer. *New England Journal of Medicine*, 363(8): 733–42. doi: 10.1056/NEJMoa1000678.

Thomas, K. (2011) *Prognostic Indicator Guidance (PIG)* (4th edn). Shrewsbury: The National Gold Standards Framework Centre in End of Life Care CIC.

Vainio, A. and Auvinen, A. (1996) Prevalence of symptoms among patients with advanced cancer: an international collaborative study. *Journal of Pain Symptom Management*, 12: 3–10.

Vassilev, I., Rogers, A., Kennedy, A. and Koetsenruijter, J. (2014) The influence of social networks on self-management support: a metasynthesis. *BMC Public Health*, 14: 719.

Weeks, J.C., Cook, E.F., O'Day, S.J. et al. (1998) Relationship between cancer patients' predictions of prognosis and their treatment preferences. *JAMA*, 279(21): 1709–14.

Yin, Z., Brown, A.E., Hughes, G. et al. (2014) *HIV in the United Kingdom 2014 Report: Data to End 2013*. London: Public Health England.

Clinical assessment and outcome measurement

Kate Flemming, Beth Hardy and Vanessa Taylor

Clinical assessment is the cornerstone of individualised patient care. Adopting a systematic, continuous and interactive process between the patient and the nurse enables the individual patient's needs and concerns to be identified. For the professional, a comprehensive assessment process requires making accurate observations, gathering data about physical, psychological, spiritual, social and cultural aspects and making judgements to determine the care and treatment needs of the patient. Using a structured approach to undertake mini, comprehensive, focused or on-going clinical assessments can enhance communication between patients, families and professionals, and also between members of the multi-professional teams and services involved in the delivery of integrated palliative care services to enable continuity and monitoring of the effectiveness and quality of care.

More recently, as part of the assessment and monitoring process, the use of patient reported outcome measures (PROMs) has become increasingly widespread in healthcare with interest growing in the use of PROMs to inform individual patient care and manage the performance of healthcare providers. In the UK National Health Service, for example, the routine collection of PROMs was introduced in 2009 to measure and improve clinical quality for specific areas of practice. While clinical assessment is a continuous process, PROMs assess the quality of care delivered from the patient's perspective by measuring a patient's health status or health-related quality of life at a single point in time (NHS Digital n.d.). A review of 27 papers, drawing on international evidence, suggested that the systematic use of information from PROMs can lead to better communication and decision-making between doctors and patients, and improve patient satisfaction with their care (Chen et al. 2013). In palliative care, PROMs are also being seen as increasingly significant when incorporated into routine clinical practice with evidence of improved patient outcomes at an individual patient and systems level (Antunes et al. 2014; Currow et al. 2015).

This chapter aims to examine clinical assessment and PROMs in palliative care, exploring what these mean in palliative care clinical practice for practitioners. The benefits of clinical assessment and outcome measurement are explored. Potential facilitators and barriers to clinical assessment and the implementation of PROMs are discussed. A series of activities are included, focused on enabling practitioners to consider the benefits and challenges for clinical assessment and PROMs within their own practice.

Why assess and measure?

> *We have to prove the quality of the care that we deliver, account for the resources that are allocated and verify that patients are receiving the best possible care in relation to these resources.*
>
> (Radbruch 2011, p. iii)

Measurement is fundamental to the role of palliative care, the goal of which is:

> [to] improve quality of life for patients and their families facing the problems associated with life-threatening illness, through the prevention and relief of suffering by means of *early identification and impeccable assessment* and treatment of pain and other problems, physical, psychosocial and spiritual.
>
> (WHO 2015)

Measurement and clinical assessment are applicable throughout the trajectory of a life-limiting disease, in conjunction with other therapies that are intended to prolong or improve quality of life, such as chemotherapy or radiation therapy. Measurement includes those investigations which are needed to better understand the nature and cause of and to manage distressing clinical complications.

What do we mean by clinical assessment and outcome measurement in the context of palliative care?

Clinical assessment in palliative care is broad and involves establishing the needs of a patient and their family in relation to physical, psychological, social, cultural and spiritual aspects of care. It includes the assessment of care needs as well as the adequacy of available resources (Cherney 2015).

Outcome measurement, by contrast, captures 'change in health status' as a consequence of healthcare or interventions (Donabedian 1980). In palliative care, the use of outcome measures is central to improving the quality, efficiency and availability of palliative care. Using outcome measures to establish how a patient's health has changed over time, and alongside this determining the reasons for those changes, can help inform the quality of services (Bausewein 2011). As policies such as the End of Life Care Strategy in England and Wales have matured, and as international work in the field has developed, so has understanding of how best to measure good outcomes in end of life care (Department of Health 2008; Bausewein et al. 2011). Death in the Usual Place of Residence (DIUPR) has been used as a useful proxy measure, but is limited in that it does not give insight into the quality and experience of care. DIUPR has also been useful as a driver of change and service redesign. There is, however, increasing dissatisfaction with it as a proxy measure for quality as it fails to give insight into the deceased person's quality and experience of care (National Palliative and End of Life Care Partnership 2015; Pollock 2015).

There is, however, no consensus regarding the way in which outcomes can be measured in palliative care, resulting in a lack of widely accepted standards and a large number of scales and measurement tools available (Radbruch 2011), many of which are locally developed for the purpose (Dy et al. 2015). Alongside this variation in approach is a seam of debate as to whether measuring outcomes is appropriate within the patient-centred ethos of palliative care, resulting in a restriction of creativity of clinical practice and detracting from the benefits patients receive from particular interventions (Bausewein et al. 2011). It is, however, the perceived advantages of the employment of outcome measures in clinical palliative care that this chapter will focus on, namely, that the use of outcome measures does the following:

- helps to assess symptoms of significance to an individual;
- provides an evidence-based support to the resources required for patient-centred, high quality and accountable care;
- enables the identification of effective clinical interventions for individual patients.

(Bausewein et al. 2011)

Who benefits from clinical assessment and outcome measurement?

The patient

Done well, a thorough and well-thought-out clinical assessment should help identify current issues that are a source of concern or distress to the patient and will enable a focus on the current and future goals of care.

Issues that may be of concern to a patient include their current disease status, disease progression and prognosis, symptoms, level of function, ability to manage essential activities of daily living, spiritual, cultural or existential matters. Assessing these concerns with validated pain and symptom assessment tools provides a baseline from which communication around future plans with health professionals can be based, the effectiveness (or not) of which can assessed using an appropriate outcome measure (Mularski et al. 2007; Cherney 2015). The way assessment is undertaken is of relevance to outcomes also. An empathetic and caring approach to assessment paves the way for the development of positive and trusting relationships between practitioner and patient, the existence of which is known to contribute to more accurate reporting of symptoms by patients (Flemming et al. 2012).

The patient's family/carer

It is essential to involve a patient's family not only in the assessment process of the patient themselves, but separately, to ensure that the needs of family members, who commonly have a significant caring role, are identified. It is important to establish factors which not only directly affect the carer themselves but that subsequently may indirectly affect their ability to continue to provide care (Table 6.1). Assessment of carer well-being and their caring burden is essential in the maintenance of positive and sustainable caring roles, which subsequently may affect the ability of a patient to remain in their preferred place of care. Specific tools have been developed to identify the support that carers need to help facilitate their role when providing palliative home care (for example, the Carer Support Needs Assessment Tools, Ewing et al. 2013; Ewing et al. 2016).

Family and caregivers of people with advanced illness may additionally experience anticipatory grief or low levels of preparedness for the impending death of the patient. It is an additional 'symptom' that is worthy of assessment as it is common that symptoms of anticipatory grief may manifest themselves as depression, anxiety or pain (Shore et al. 2016) and go unsupported. A number of assessment scales exist and include questions on practical tasks, thoughts, and feelings of the impending death and plans for the future as well. As with the assessment of other symptoms, there is lack of congruity between scales; a review of assessment tools found substantial variation between them, although all scales contained a core focus on the caregiver's emotional status (Nielsen et al. 2016). It is recommended that to provide the support that key family members or caregivers require, health professionals should systematically and repeatedly assess caregivers' grief and preparedness (Nielsen et al. 2016).

Organisations and teams

In order to improve care, it is important to have a detailed understanding of the current level of the quality of care using valid and reliable instruments to record this; triangulating these data with patient and carer experience; and undertaking, where relevant and present, comparisons with local and national benchmarks.

Table 6.1 Some essential elements to consider in family assessment

Family understanding of nature and extent of the patient's illness
How family understanding matches patient's understanding
Expectations arising from any treatment or interventions
Psychological concerns
Any medical problems related to the individual
Willingness to take on a caring role
Expectations of themselves in a caring role

Developed from Cherney et al. (2015).

Palliative care organisations and teams have not routinely collected quality improvement data, or where they have, have used locally developed and non-validated instruments (Dy et al. 2015). Increasingly service providers are required to be accountable to their users and to those who fund them and need to demonstrate that services are both efficient and of high quality (Bausewein et al. 2011). Palliative care services are no exception to this and need to engage in the use of outcome measures in order to enhance quality assurance, maintain on-going quality improvement and strengthen the learning capacity of the organisation. Recent work has, however, looked to develop specific outcome measures and quality indicators for palliative care from both a European (Bausewein et al. 2011) and a US perspective (Dy et al. 2015).

What to assess and measure

Assessment is required to discover what care a person needs. The core principles of assessment in palliative care are no different to assessment in other disciplines of nursing. The nursing process (Assess, Plan, Implement and Evaluate), a fundamental aspect of nursing practice since its introduction in the UK and Europe in the 1970s (Castledine 2011), highlights the essential nature of assessment as part of nursing care. Without appropriate assessment, patient needs remain unidentified and therefore unaddressed: person-centred care is compromised with the potential to cause distress and suffering for patients and families (Maher and Hemming 2005; NHS 2010).

Assessment may take a variety of forms and will gather, and make sense of, information from a range of sources, depending on the purpose and context. Objective and subjective information is collected using observation, physical assessment, conversation, questioning, and use of clinical assessment tools and PROMs. There are four types of assessment (Dougherty, Lister and West-Oram 2015): (1) mini; (2) comprehensive; (3) focused; and (4) on-going. Mini assessments provide a snapshot overview, and are based on visual and physical assessment – they aim to establish level of consciousness, vital signs and mental status prior to assessment of the major presenting problems. Comprehensive (often referred to as 'holistic') assessment aims to gather information from patients and their significant others to develop an understanding about an individual's overall health and well-being support needs. This assessment focuses on the whole person, taking a bio-psychosocial perspective, thus considering physical, emotional, spiritual, social and environmental factors (NCSI 2013). Effective comprehensive assessment will enable the nurse to discover what is important to the individual and to identify and explore their goals for care so that care planning and delivery are aligned with the individual's own values and aspirations. Comprehensive assessment in palliative care is an opportunity to ascertain the individual's own understanding of their illness and personal situation. This understanding will directly inform how the nurse works with, and responds to, that individual. Focused, specific symptom or situation-orientated assessments will build on the core assessment once issues have been identified as significant to the individual concerned. On-going assessment occurs as part of monitoring the effectiveness of interventions, and identifies changes in the patient or carer situation requiring new assessment.

Table 6.2 Possible patient issues requiring assessment in palliative care

Quality of life	Nausea and vomiting
Fatigue	Skin integrity
Pain	Mobility
Functional status	Dyspnoea
Elimination	Home assessment
Nutrition and hydration	Medication
Carer support needs	Wishes and preferences for future care (advance/future care planning)
Self-care support needs	Psychological well-being
Depression	Social support needs
Distress	Spiritual well-being
Occupational issues	Disability
Sleep	Lymphoedema

The range of possible issues that a patient may be experiencing that can be assessed by nurses are identified in Table 6.2.

Assessment tools and PROMs

Numerous tools exist to support assessment and measurement. A systematic literature review undertaken by Hudson et al. (2016) identified 90 clinical assessment tools that they appraised for their applicability in an Australian specialist palliative care setting, and many more exist that could be used in the generalist environment. The range of tools reflects not only the complexity of palliative care and care needs themselves, but also the variety of care contexts in which care for people requiring a palliative approach occurs.

Assessment tools can be valuable resources when used correctly. There are a significant number of considerations when choosing whether or not to use an assessment tool, and then which tool, or set of tools, to use. Doctors and nurses delivering palliative care across Europe and Africa, for example, report access to freely available, validated and translated tools that allow for a coordinated and cohesive approach to practice, as well as cross-national research, as being important considerations. They prioritise multi-dimensional and brief patient outcome measures and PROMs, and are influenced by the availability of outcome measurement training, information and guidance (Daveson et al. 2012). Nurses may also vary in their abilities to elicit information from patients, as patients do in their abilities to voice their concerns (Richardson et al. 2007). Tools can support the information exchange between nurse and patient, but should not be seen as a substitute for other forms of nursing assessment and communication. Assessment tools and PROMs should, therefore, have an evidence base for their effectiveness; they should be valid (they assess/measure what they purport to assess/measure) and reliable (they achieve similar results when administered in similar conditions). They also need to be feasible, for example, can they be completed in the time available? Are they acceptable, for example, is the recipient happy to use the tool? Does the nurse have time to use the tool as intended? These are questions nurses and doctors should consider when choosing tools for use in their clinical setting or service.

Using assessment tools and PROMs can also support information exchange within and across organisations, particularly if information is available digitally and accessible where and when clinically required. Information recorded within a tool should be easy to extract and this availability can reduce unnecessary multiple assessments, improve continuity and timeliness of care as well as generally improving the flow of information. Information from objective quantitative measures may also be used for audit and research purposes. The MORECare project (Higginson et al. 2013), which aimed to improve research quality in palliative and end of life care, highlighted the importance of outcome measures for research and clinical practice:

> To enable the wide application and interpretation of outcome measures in palliative and EOL care, the measurement properties need to be validated for this population, capture multidimensional components, and be broadly applicable across health systems, popular science, disease trajectories (including post-death for bereaved carers), languages, and cultures. The best measures have essential properties of simplicity of use and good interpretability, the ability to measure clinical change.
>
> (Evans et al. 2013, p. 935)

Thus, important considerations for the selection of a tool are whether the organisation supports the use of specific tools, which tools neighbouring organisations use, what training and support are available to ensure correct use of the tool, and whether the information collected is intended to be used as an outcome measure for research purposes in addition to clinical practice . Examples of some commonly reported assessment tools and PROMs used in palliative care are outlined in Table 6.3.

Prognostic indicators

> *Early identification of people nearing the end of life leads to better planning and better care.*
>
> (GSF 2011)

Assessment of prognosis will occur at various stages of a person's experience of living with advanced disease. These stages include transition to a palliative approach to care, as they enter the last year of life, and as they approach the last days of life. In line with person-centred approaches to care, individuals may choose whether or not they wish to have this information, and nurses, along with the wider

Table 6.3 Examples of assessment tools and PROMs used in palliative care

Focus of tool	Tool name	Description
Holistic assessment	Holistic common assessment of supportive and palliative care needs for adults requiring end of life care (NHS 2010)	This guidance contains five broad domains: background information and assessment preferences; physical needs; social and occupational needs; psychological well-being; spiritual well-being and life goals. Additional sub-domains contribute to exploring the complexity of living with palliative and supportive care-related needs
Holistic assessment	PEPSI COLA aide-mémoire	Aide-mémoire covering Physical, Emotional, Personal, Social Support, Information and Communication, Control and Autonomy, Out of Hours, Living with Illness and After Care support needs. Tool includes prompt questions and suggested resources (GSF 2011)
Palliative care support needs	Palliative care Outcome Scale (POS)	A suite of tools to measure physical symptoms, emotional, psychological, spiritual, informational support needs (Cicely Saunders Institute 2012)
Pain assessment	Visual Analogue Scale (VAS)	A line, usually 10 cms long and labelled with the extremes of pain, with 0 being no pain and 10 being the worst possible pain. The patient marks on the line where their pain is
Pain assessment	Numerical Rating Scale (NRS)	The patient is asked to verbally rate their pain from 0–10, or 100, with 0 being no pain and 10 or 100 being the worst possible pain
Symptom assessment	Edmonton System Assessment System Revised (ESAS-r)	A self-report numerical tool of symptom intensity based on nine common symptoms with one patient-specific option (Watanabe et al. 2011)
Functional impairment assessment	Karnofsky Performance Scale (KPS)	Ten-point index that enables classification of patients' functional impairment
Carer support	Carer Support Needs Assessment Tool (CSNAT)	A brief 14-domain self-completed tool, with additional 'anything else' option. Explores support needed to help the carer in their caring role, and support needed for carers themselves (Ewing et al. 2013; Ewing et al. 2016)
Prognostic indicator	The GSF Prognostic Indicator Guidance	Guidance which includes three triggers that suggest a patient might be nearing the end of life: (1) 'the surprise question'; (2) general indicators of decline; (3) specific clinical indicators for certain conditions (GSF 2011)
Prognostic indicator	Supportive and Palliative Care Indicators Tool (SPICT™)	A guide to identifying people at risk of deterioration and dying who need further assessment of holistic care needs (Highet et al. 2014)

multi-disciplinary team (MDT), need to be skilled in assessing the person's current level of understanding and managing the sensitive nature of conversations about prognosis (NICE 2015).

There are numerous benefits to formal identification of prognosis. Patients and their significant others have time to deal with the news in keeping with their own views and preferences and have a chance to plan for the future; patients are less likely to receive invasive treatments of limited clinical value; care can be planned to ensure that it is consistent with patients' values rather than reactive in response to crisis; well-planned care can reduce hospital admission and increase the likelihood of death at home in line with patient choice, also leading to reduced care costs (Sleeman 2013; Walczak et al. 2014; Dying Matters Coalition 2016).

Nurses should be aware of disease-specific prognostic signs and clinical tools for assessing prognosis in their particular clinical area. Some prognosis decisions will be made as part of the MDT, such as transition to a palliative approach to care, and diagnosing dying. Others, such as a family asking whether a patient is near death, may be made by a nurse observing physical changes in a person's breathing or other symptoms. Examples of tools to support prognosis decisions are shown in Table 6.3.

Assessment within person-centred and relationship-centred care

Person-centred and family-centred care are seen as a fundamental principle of palliative care. In person-centred care, the 'patient' is respected as an individual who is more than a collection of symptoms or behaviours. They are a person with unique abilities, attributes and preferences and seen as a partner in care (including the assessment). As previously mentioned, the family (however that is defined to the individuals themselves) are recognised as also being affected by illness, and have an important role in the health and well-being of the patient, and where appropriate should be involved with patient assessment.

Assessment tools and PROMs are not a panacea for quality assessment. The nursing assessment occurs within a particular paradigm, a specific core set of beliefs and values, which guide the actions and decisions that are made. Good quality assessment relies partly on the information obtained through conversation and is largely dependent on the skills of the nurse to establish and maintain a therapeutic relationship with the patient and family (Maher and Hemming 2005); nurses need to consider how best to develop such relationships and engage with individuals as partners in care. Relationship-centred care, or relational practice, takes the principles of person-centred care one step further. Championed as an approach for gerontological nursing (Nolan et al. 2004), the principles are also particularly relevant within palliative care. This approach recognises the impact of the relationship between the nurse (and other healthcare staff) and the individuals with whom they work, and highlights the importance of a supportive, well-resourced care environment to enable 'appreciative caring conversations' to take place (Dewar and Nolan 2013).

Who contributes to the assessment and implementation of PROMs?

In order to meet their needs, the delivery of palliative care may be the responsibility of practitioners from diverse disciplines who all play fundamental roles contributing to the complex assessment and delivery of care, ultimately influencing patient and family outcomes across teams, services and organisations.

The delivery of palliative care is described as occurring at three levels (for more information, see Chapter 1 in this volume):

1   *Palliative care approach*: this is intended as a way to integrate palliative care methods and procedures in general settings of care.
2   *General palliative care*: intended for professionals frequently involved with palliative care patients or acting as a resource person for palliative care in their setting of care, but for whom palliative care is not the main focus of their clinical practice.
3   *Specialist palliative care*: intended for professionals working solely in the field of palliative care and whose main activity is devoted to dealing with complex problems requiring specialised skills and competencies.

(Gamondi et al. 2013a, 2013b)

The individual patient's healthcare and social care team is responsible for ensuring that clinical assessment takes place. For continuity, however, it has been recommended that, where multiple team members or teams are involved, one team member is identified as responsible for comprehensive assessment of the patient's needs or for ensuring that an assessment is carried out (NHS Improving Quality 2010; Travers and Taylor 2016). In selecting an appropriate assessor, the principles for teams to consider include a professional who:

- has an appropriate level of knowledge of the patient's condition, treatment and likely prognoses;
- has achieved an agreed level of competence in the assessment process;
- is in accordance with the preferences a patient has expressed for communicating with professionals;
- has access to up-to-date information about local healthcare and social care providers, referral criteria and support services;
- has an understanding of advance care planning.

This approach acknowledges the skills and expertise of individual members of the multi-professional team. The assessment process should include a review of previous assessments, including those from other healthcare and social care settings, and take account of the needs identified in them. Through the assessment process, patients and their families/carers may have identified a range of holistic needs, including the need to discuss end of life care decisions and develop advance care plans. Although doctors are traditionally regarded as the lead for directing end of life discussions, this role and responsibility can be led by nurses (Department of Health 2008). Indeed, nurse participants, in a study by Garner et al. (2013), reported that lack of empowerment of nursing staff led to delayed discussions or deferral to other healthcare providers, resulting in an abrupt or conflict-laden transition to end of life care. Ensuring people receive the care they need, therefore, requires palliative and end of life care to be considered the business of all paid carers and clinicians at every level of palliative care. Furthermore, among an ageing population of patients with increasing multiple co-morbidities (World Health Assembly 2014), ensuring appropriate team-working and a successful multi-professional approach through joined-up working, shared goals and clear documentation is paramount (National Voices 2015).

Working in teams and across services has been an integral part of the philosophy of palliative and end of life care, enshrined in its philosophy and embedded in its practice (WHO 2016). In contemporary practice, delivering quality integrated palliative care services requires those providing palliative care to have an expectation of, and a process for, collaboration. This involves having an understanding of how each discipline, team, service and organisation might approach the care to avoid conflicting advice, timelines and goals, and collaborating for the benefit of patients and their families.

A review of 31 papers exploring the facilitators and barriers to the implementation of PROMs determined that implementation needs to be tailored according to the clinical setting and team where the PROMs are to be used. Key to successful use of PROMs is developing an understanding of the interpersonal relationships that occur between team members. Also established was that clinical decision-making is enhanced by timely feedback on outcomes that are relevant to the patient, and that communication not only between patient and clinician but also within the multi-disciplinary team is enhanced (Antunes et al. 2014).

Furthermore, groups such as the National Palliative and End of Life Care Partnership (2015) have reinforced the need for organisations to learn to work collaboratively and differently, and to demonstrate the improvements in end of life care outcomes, including people's experiences and quality of care, whatever the setting. Education, training, organisational and professional support with local leadership and accountability are all advocated to achieve the following outcomes:

- shared understanding and purposes for end of life care;
- inequity and variations in practice are addressed;
- integrated systems are developed that support efficient and effective palliative and end of life care (National Palliative and End of Life Care Partnership 2015).

Learning exercise 6.1

Consider the following questions:

- What level of palliative care do you and your team/service deliver?
- Who do you, your team and service collaborate with in the delivery of an integrated palliative care service?

- How do you and your team identify who will lead assessment or coordinate the clinical assessment of your patients' palliative care needs?
- What education and training needs do you, your team and service have to enhance the clinical assessment of patients' palliative care needs?

As discussed earlier in this chapter, the use and systematic collection of PROMs, using validated questionnaires, is considered beneficial in palliative care settings to focus on the priorities of individual patients and families, as well as capturing their effectiveness for meeting population needs. To recap, the use of patient reported outcomes measures:

1 facilitates identification and screening of physical, psychological, spiritual and social unmet needs;
2 provides information on disease progression and the impact of prescribed treatment;
3 facilitates patient/family/carer–clinician communication promoting a model of patient-centred care by shared decision-making and advance care planning;
4 enables monitoring of outcomes as a strategy for improvement of the quality of care provided and its costs;
5 provides data demonstrating service performance and outcomes for commissioners/funding agencies.

(Antunes et al. 2014)

The use of outcome measures can inform and illustrate how to meet the contractual requirements for funding, organisational quality assurance standards and issues for service improvement and future service directions. In addition, the European Association for Palliative Care (EAPC) Task Force on Outcome Measurement suggests that introducing outcome measurement into practice will enable national and international comparisons and is key to understanding different models of care (Bausewein et al. 2016). The EAPC has developed recommendations for implementing outcome measurement in palliative care for teams, services and organisations (Table 6.4).

Delivering an integrated palliative care service is complex, involving organisations representing healthcare and social care, statutory and voluntary bodies, and people with personal and professional experience working collaboratively at different levels of palliative care aiming to ensure effective patient and family access to a cohesive palliative care service system (National Palliative and End of Life Care Partnership 2015). Collaboration is acknowledged as challenging, while the benefits for the team and patient care, and the opportunities for evaluating and developing care models have also been recognised. A review of evidence relating to views on the provision of palliative care for non-cancer patients by primary care providers, for example, found that patients expect community-based doctors to provide compassionate care, have appropriate knowledge and play a central role in coordinated care (Oishi and Murtagh 2014). However, uncertainty regarding the illness trajectory, unclear definition of the role of

Table 6.4 EAPC Task Force on Outcome Measurement (Bausewein et al. 2016)

1	Use PROMs that have been validated with relevant populations requiring palliative care ensuring these are sufficiently brief and straightforward and that they allow for proxy reports when the patient is unable to self-report
2	Use multidimensional measures that capture the holistic nature of palliative care
3	Use outcome measures to assess the needs of unpaid caregivers alongside the needs of patients
4	Use measures that have sound psychometric properties
5	Use measures that are suited to the clinical task being delivered and also suited to the aims of your clinical work and the population you work with
6	Use valid and reliable measures in research that are relevant to the research question and consider patient burden when using measures
7	Use change management principles, facilitation and communication to embed outcomes measurement into routine clinical practice and evaluate the implementation process to ensure sustained use that penetrates practice within the organisation
8	Relate outcome measurement to quality indicators
9	Establish and use quality improvement systems to sustain routine practice of outcome measurement and institute electronic systems to ensure integration of measures and across settings
10	Use measures that allow for comparisons across care settings and throughout Europe
11	Advance the field of palliative and end of life care through establishing national and international outcome collaborations that work towards benchmarking to establish and improve care standards
12	To improve and monitor palliative care practice, policy-makers should recommend routine collection of outcome data

professionals and lack of collaboration between professionals were recognised as barriers to effective primary palliative care. Managing these challenges required the clear role definitions of each professional and effective interprofessional collaboration alongside more in-depth evaluation of existing care models in order to demonstrate how they work and what impact they have on multi-disciplinary teams to inform future policymaking (Oishi and Murtagh 2014). Similarly, Albers et al. (2016) identified that limited knowledge and understanding of what other disciplines offer, a lack of common practice and a lack of communication between disciplines and settings were considered barriers to collaboration between palliative care and geriatric medicine. Multi-disciplinary team working, integration, strong leadership and recognition of both disciplines were considered facilitators of collaborative working, with strategic collaboration in education and policy needed.

The implementation of PROMs in different palliative care settings for routine practice is similarly acknowledged as an on-going, iterative and continuous process. Services need to identify and address potential barriers to a successful implementation, using appropriate facilitators, tailored to the characteristics of each setting

(Antunes et al. 2014). For example, there is a need to acknowledge interpersonal relationships between members of the clinical team and the emotional and cognitive processes that arise for each individual. Fear of change, feelings of being assessed and that own work is open to criticism due to the results of PROMs, as well as concerns about additional workload are some of the issues that lead to behaviour which opposes change. Building on the findings from a systematic review and narrative analysis exploring the facilitators and barriers to implementing PROMs, Antunes et al. (2014) developed a three-phase guidance model for implementing PROMs in palliative care clinical practice, aimed at improving practice and the quality of care provided by assisting clinical decision-making at management, healthcare practitioner and patient levels (Table 6.5).

Table 6.5 Recommendations for implementation of PROMs in clinical practice

Phase of implementation	Level of implementation
1 Preparation	**Management level includes:** Exploring feasibility of implementation of a measure; appraising resources; developing data collection methods, analysis and presentation of results; training of clinical staff; establishing a programme evaluation system and implementation plan; investing in computerised systems and organisational support; identifying a coordinator and cascade system
	Healthcare practitioner level includes: Education programme delivered promoting understanding why measure is needed and will benefit practice, understanding measures to be implemented, role play to explain their use to patients, exploring interpretation of results at patient and population levels, storage and management of data, understanding evaluation, mechanisms for sharing information across services and caregivers
2 Implementation	**Management level** – maintaining strategy of reminders to incorporate use of PROMs in practice, encouragement to ensure implementation is successful, creating space/time to discuss implementation process/issues
	Healthcare professional level – every team member who should be using outcome measure does so and contributes to discussing process of implementation, feedback on monitoring patient's progress and disease management at agreed assessment points (daily, weekly, at each appointment), interpretation of results used in practice
	Patient level – education and motivation of patients could improve compliance
3 Assessment and improvement	**Management level** – collected items reviewed as being clinically relevant and not burdensome to collect
	Healthcare professional level – collected items reviewed as being clinically relevant and not burdensome to collect, assessing and improving documentation to highlight needs
	Patient level – assess if patient benefits in achieving better outcomes

Adapted from Antunes et al. (2014).

Learning exercise 6.2

Consider the implementation of PROMs in the delivery of palliative care in your clinical practice. Using the three-phase approach recommended by Antunes et al. (2014), reflect on, develop or evaluate your implementation plan (Table 6.6).

Table 6.6 Implementation of PROMs in the delivery of palliative care

Phase of implementation	Level of implementation	What you will do
Preparation	Management level Healthcare professional level Patient level	
Implementation	Management level Healthcare professional level Patient level	
Assessment and improvement	Management level Healthcare professional level Patient level	

Based on Antunes et al. (2014).

Conclusion

Clinical assessment, incorporating the use of PROMs, is being advocated in palliative care clinical practice as an approach that enables the patient's perspective to inform clinical decision-making at both an individual and a population level. In this chapter, we have examined how, at an individual level, clinical assessment and PROMs can be used to improve communication between patients, families and practitioners, promote patient-centred care and shared decision-making. Additionally, in the delivery of integrated palliative care services, PROMs can enhance communication between teams, services and organisations and enable auditing of patient and service outcomes to improve the quality of care. A structured approach to clinical assessment and PROMs in palliative care requires local leadership and commitment from every organisation, service, team and professionals involved in palliative care delivery to overcome any individual barriers, address inequity and variation in palliative and end of life care, and develop systems for effective service delivery.

References

Albers, G., Froggatt, K., Van den Block, G. et al. (2016) A qualitative exploration of the collaborative working between palliative care and geriatric medicine: barriers and facilitators from a European perspective. *BMC Palliative Care*, 15: 47.

Antunes, B., Harding, R. and Higginson, I. (2014) Implementing patient-reported outcomes measures in palliative care clinical practice: a systematic review of facilitators and barriers. *Palliative Medicine*, 28(2): 158–75.

Bausewein, C., Daveson, B., Benalia, H. et al. (2011) *Outcome Measurement in Palliative Care: The Essentials.* London: PRISMA.

Bausewein, C., Daveson, B.A., Currow, D.C. et al. (2016) EAPC White Paper on outcome measurement in palliative care: improving practice, attaining outcomes and delivering quality services. Recommendations from the European Association for Palliative Care (EAPC) Task Force on Outcome Measurement. *Palliative Medicine*, 30(1): 6–22.

Castledine, G. (2011) Updating the nursing process. *British Journal of Nursing*, 20(2): 131.

Chen, J., Ou, L. and Hollis, S.J. (2013) A systematic review of the impact of routine collection of patient reported outcome measures on patients, providers and health organisations in an oncologic setting. *BMC Health Services Research*, 13: 211.

Cherney, N.I. (2015) The problem of suffering and the principles of assessment in palliative medicine. In Cherney, N.I., Fallon, M.T., Kaasa, S. et al. (eds) *The Oxford Textbook of Palliative Medicine.* Oxford: Oxford University Press.

Cicely Saunders Institute (2012) Palliative Care Outcome Scale website. Available at: http://pos-pal.org/ (accessed 12 October 2016).

Currow, D.C., Allingham, S., Yates, P. et al. (2015) Improving national hospice/palliative care service symptom outcomes systematically through point of care data collection, structured feedback and benchmarking. *Supportive Care in Cancer*, 23(2): 307–15.

Daveson, B.A., Simon, S.T., Benalia, H. et al. (2012) Are we heading in the same direction? European and African doctors' and nurses' views and experiences regarding outcome measurement in palliative care. *Palliative Medicine*, 26(3): 242–9.

Department of Health (2008) *End of Life Care Strategy: Promoting High Quality Care for Adults at the End of Their Life.* London: Department of Health.

Dewar, B. and Nolan, M. (2013) Caring about caring: developing a model to implement compassionate relationship-centred care in an older people care setting. *International Journal of Nursing Studies*, 50(9): 1247–58.

Donabedian, A. (1980) *Explorations in Quality Assessment and Monitoring: The Definition of Quality and Approaches to Its Assessment*, vol. I. Ann Arbor, MI: Health Administration Press.

Dougherty, L., Lister, L. and West-Oram, A. (2015) *The Royal Marsden Manual of Clinical Nursing Procedures* (9th edn). Chichester: John Wiley & Sons Ltd.

Dy, S., Kiley, K., Ast, K. et al. (2015) Measuring what matters: top ranked quality indicators for hospice and palliative care from the American Academy of Hospice and Palliative Medicine and Hospice and Palliative Nurses Association. *Journal of Pain and Symptom Management*, 49(4): 773–81.

Dying Matters Coalition (2016) Identifying end of life patients. Available at: www.dyingmatters.org (accessed 20 August 2016).

Evans, C., Benalia, H., Preston, N. et al. (2013) The selection and use of outcome measures in palliative and end of life care research: the MORECare international consensus workshop. *Journal of Pain and Symptom Management*, 46(6): 925–37.

Ewing, G., Austin, L. and Grande, G. (2016) The role of the Carer Support Needs Assessment Tool in palliative home care: a qualitative study of practitioners' perspectives of its impact and mechanisms of action. *Palliative Medicine*, 30(4): 392–400.

Ewing, G., Brundle, C. and Payne, S. (2013) The Carer Support Needs Assessment Tool (CSNAT) for use in palliative and end-of-life care at home: a validation study. *Journal of Pain and Symptom Management*, 46(3): 395–405.

Flemming, K., Closs, S.J., Bennett, M.I. and Foy, R. (2012) Educational interventions for symptom management in advanced disease: synthesis of qualitative research examining health care professionals' perceived knowledge, attitudes and ability. *Journal of Pain and Symptom Management*, 43(5): 885–901.

Gamondi, C., Larkin, P. and Payne, S. (2013a) Core competencies in palliative care: an EAPC White Paper on palliative care education – part 1. *European Journal of Palliative Care*, 20(2): 86–91.

Gamondi, C., Larkin, P. and Payne, S. (2013b) Core competencies in palliative care: an EAPC White Paper on palliative care education – part 2. *European Journal of Palliative Care*, 20(3): 140–5.

Garner, K.K., Goodwin, J.A., McSweeney, J.C. et al. (2013) Nurse executives' perceptions of end-of-life care provided in hospitals. *Journal of Pain and Symptom Management*, 45(2): 235–43.

Gold Standards Framework (2011) The GSF Prognostic Indicator Guidance. Available at: http://www.goldstandardsframework.org.uk/cd-content/uploads/files/General% 20Files/Prognostic%20Indicator%20Guidance%20October%202011.pdf (accessed 3 September 2016).

Higginson, I., Evans, C., Grande, G. et al. (2013) Evaluating complex interventions in end of life care: the MORECare statement on good practice generated by a synthesis of transparent expert consultations and systematic reviews. *BMC Medicine*. Available at: www.biomedcentral.com/1741-7015/11/111 (accessed 31 March 2017).

Highet, G., Crawford, D., Murray, S. and Boyd, K. (2014) Development and evaluation for the Supportive and Palliative Care Indicators Tool (SPICT): a mixed-methods study. *BMJ Supportive and Palliative Care*, 4(3): 285–90.

Hudson, P., Collins, A., Bostanci, A. et al. (2016) Towards a systematic approach to assessment and care planning in palliative care: a practice review of clinical tools. *Palliative and Supportive Care*, 14: 161–73.

Maher, D. and Hemming, L. (2005) Understanding patient and family holistic assessment in palliative care. *British Journal of Community Nursing*, 10(7): 318–22.

Mularski, R.A., Dy, S.M., Shugarman, L.R. et al. (2007) A systematic review of measures of end of life care and its outcomes. *Health Services Research*, 42(5): 1848–70.

National Palliative and End of Life Care Partnership (2015) *Ambitions for Palliative and End of Life Care: A National Framework for Local Action 2015–2020*. Available at: http://endoflifecareambitions.org.uk/wp-content/uploads/2015/09/Ambitions-for-Palliative-and-End-of-Life-Care.pdf (accessed 12 October 2016).

National Voices (2015) *Every Moment Counts: A Narrative for Person Centred Coordinated Care for People Near the End of Life*. London: National Voices and the National Council for Palliative Care, in partnership with NHS England.

NCSI (2013) Assessment and care planning definitions. Available at: http://www.ncsi. org.uk/what-we-are-doing/assessment-care-planning/assessment-care-planning-definitions/ (accessed 4 August 2016).

NHS (2010) Holistic common assessment of supportive and palliative care needs for adults requiring end of life care. Available at: http://www.nhsiq.nhs.uk/media/2566496/holistic_common_assessment.pdf (accessed 12 October 2016).

NHS Digital (n.d.) Patient Reported Outcome Measures (PROMs). Available at: http://content.digital.nhs.uk/proms (accessed 12 October 2016).

NHS Improving Quality (2010) Holistic common assessment of supportive and palliative care needs for adults requiring end of life care. Available at: http://www.nhsiq.nhs. uk/media/2566496/holistic_common_assessment.pdf (accessed 12 October 2016).

NICE (National Institute for Health and Care Excellence) (2015) *Care of Dying Adults in the Last Days of Life*. NICE Guideline, 31. Available at: https://www. nice.org.uk/guidance/ng31/resources/care-of-dying-adults-in-the-last-days-of-life-1837387324357 (accessed 5 September 2016).

Nielsen, M.K., Neergaard, M.A., Jensen, A.B. et al. (2016) Do we need to change our understanding of anticipatory grief in caregivers? A systematic review of caregiver studies during end-of-life caregiving and bereavement. *Clinical Psychology Review*, 44: 75–93.

Nolan, M., Davies, S., Brown, J. et al. (2004) Beyond person centred care: a new vision for gerontological nursing. *International Journal of Older People Nursing*, 13(3a): 45–53.

Oishi, A. and Murtagh, F.E.M. (2014) The challenges of uncertainty and interprofessional collaboration in palliative care for non-cancer patients in the community: a systematic review of views from patients, carers and health-care professionals. *Palliative Medicine*, 28(9): 1081–98.

Pollock, K. (2015) Is home always the best and preferred place of death? *BMJ*, 351: h4855.

Radbruch, L. (2011) Foreword. In Bausewein, C., Daveson, B., Benalia, H. et al. (eds) *Outcome Measurement in Palliative Care: The Essentials*. London: PRISMA.

Richardson, A., Medina, J., Brown, V. and Sitzia, J. (2007) Patients needs assessment in cancer care: review of assessment tools. *Supportive Care in Cancer*, 15(10): 1125–44.

Shore, J.C., Gelber, M.W., Koch, L.M. and Sower, E. (2016) Anticipatory grief: an evidence-based approach. *Journal of Hospice and Palliative Nursing*, 18(1): 15–19.

Sleeman, K. (2013) Caring for a dying patient in hospital. *BMJ*, 346: f2174.

Travers, A. and Taylor, V. (2016) What are the barriers to initiating end-of-life conversations with patients in the last year of life? *International Journal of Palliative Nursing*, 22(9): 454–62.

Walczak, A., Butow, P., Clayton, J. et al. (2014) Discussing prognosis and end-of-life care in the final year of life: a randomised controlled trial of a nurse-led communication support programme for patients and caregivers. *BMJ Open*, 4(6): e005745.

Watanabe, S., Nekolaichuk, C., Beaumont, C. et al. (2011) A multi-centre comparison of two numerical versions of the Edmonton Symptom Assessment System in palliative care patients. *Journal of Pain and Symptom Management*, 41: 456–68.

World Health Assembly (2014) *Strengthening of Palliative Care as a Component of Integrated Treatment within the Continuum of Care.* Available at: http://tinyurl.com/l29n975

WHO (World Health Organization) (2015) Palliative Care Fact Sheet 402. Available at: http://www.who.int/mediacentre/factsheets/fs402/en/ (accessed 31 August 2016).

WHO (World Health Organization) (2016) *Definition of Palliative Care.* Available at: http://www.who.int/cancer/palliative/definition/en/ (accessed 12 October 2016).

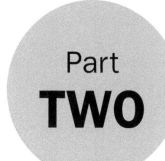

Part
TWO

PROVIDING PALLIATIVE NURSING CARE

Introduction to Part Two

Bridget Johnston, Nancy Preston and
Catherine Walshe

Nurses are frequently core members of teams providing palliative care, both where this is a central element of the post and where caring for those at the end of their lives is a part of the role. Fundamental to the way that nurses enact that role are elements of valuing the care given and the people for whom care is given, connecting with and empowering people, doing for others, and enabling people to find meaning in these challenging situations, often through the vehicle of developing relationships (Davies and Oberle 1990; Mok and Chiu 2004). Nursing care is also frequently offered to family caregivers, as part of a person-centred approach to care (Mead and Bower 2000; Candy et al. 2011; Chi and Demiris 2014). In Part Two, we explore different aspects of the nursing role in palliative and end of life care, exploring how nurses can contribute to symptom management, the importance of communication and person-centred care, how to reach out to those who find palliative care hard to access, and debating nursing roles.

Integral to good nursing care is how we communicate with our patients (Wittenberg-Lyles et al. 2011). In Chapter 7, Elaine Stevens explores this in palliative care where she recognises that communication at the end of life is particularly difficult. She covers the key areas of communication but also gives recommendations and ideas for practice. Using useful reflections, she presents areas nurses can reflect upon to look at their own practice and think about how this might be modified based upon recommendations in the chapter. In Chapter 8, Diane Laverty and Anna-Marie Stevens give a comprehensive overview of the key symptoms patients face at the end of life, namely, pain, breathlessness, constipation and fatigue. They present the key role of nurses in supporting patients with these symptoms which links to assessment in Chapter 6. These pharmacological and physical support systems build upon the central role of communication discussed in Chapter 7.

Palliative nursing is widely recognised as attending not only to the physical needs of patients but also to their psychological and spiritual needs (Johnston 2006). In Chapter 9,

Craig White explores the nurse's role in psychological assessment and care management. In addition, in a thoughtful chapter (Chapter 10), Hamilton Inbadas explores the importance of spiritual issues in end of life care and how nurses can help and support patients. He reminds us that Cicely Saunders, the founder of the modern hospice movement, recognised that spiritual pain is a significant part of patients' experience at the end of life. She coined the term 'total pain' acknowledging the physical, psychological, social and spiritual aspects of suffering. Hamilton also suggests that as nurses we also consider our own self and spiritual caring. In Chapter 11, Susan McClement and Genevieve Thompson, Canadian nurse academics, explore important issues of identity, person-centred care and dignity, issues we know are central to effective palliative nursing (McCormack and McCance 2016). They explore the idea that to alleviate suffering in patients receiving palliative care, nurses need to consider how identity and sense of self are supported. They suggest part of our nursing role is to ensure that individuals feel whole and that their dignity is bolstered or remains intact as they near the end of life.

Palliative care is not simply provided to those who are at the end of their lives, but also focuses on friends and family, the so-called 'informal caregivers' who can frequently be central to care provision (Hudson and Payne 2011). We know that their needs are important, and not always met well (Bee et al. 2008; Docherty et al. 2008). In Chapter 12, Samar Aoun and Gail Ewing explore the key role of carers, assessing care needs, and supportive interventions for carers in palliative care. They suggest that evidence-based, holistic assessment processes are essential, but that there is little evidence on the effectiveness of many interventions developed for carers.

Equity in access to palliative care services is intuitively appropriate. There is clear evidence that access appears to be influenced by issues such as age, gender and diagnosis (Burt and Raine 2006; Walshe et al. 2009; Dixon et al. 2015), but Chapter 13 by Dorry McLaughlin and Brian Nyatanga specifically explores the issues of palliative care nursing provision for two groups in society known to struggle to access healthcare – those with intellectual disabilities and the homeless. They recommend that a focus on integrating palliative care with other care provision may be a way forward to address some of the issues these groups face.

There is an increasing demand for palliative and supportive care to meet the needs of populations who are ageing, with multi-morbidity, and receiving increasingly complex and sophisticated healthcare interventions (Gomez-Batiste et al. 2014; Murtagh et al. 2014). In Chapter 14,Catriona Kennedy and Michael Connolly explore how the development of advanced and extended nursing roles can be facilitated to enable nursing to be best placed to meet these changing needs. They argue that these roles need definition, development and personal and organisational preparation if they are to be optimally effective.

References

Bee, P., Barnes, P. and Luker, K.A. (2008) A systematic review of informal caregivers' needs in providing home-based end-of-life care to people with cancer. *Journal of Clinical Nursing*, doi: 10.1111/j.1365-2702.2008.02405.x.

Burt, J. and Raine, R. (2006) The effect of age on referral to and use of specialist palliative care services in adult cancer patients: a systematic review. *Age and Ageing*, 35(5): 469–76.

Candy, B., Jones, L., Drake, R. et al. (2011) Interventions for supporting informal caregivers of patients in the terminal phase of a disease. *Cochrane Database of Systematic Reviews*, 6: CD007617.

Chi, N.-C. and Demiris, G. (2014) A systematic review of telehealth tools and interventions to support family caregivers. *Journal of Telemedicine and Telecare*, doi:10:1177/1357633X14562734.

Davies, B. and Oberle, K. (1990) Dimensions of the supportive role of the nurse in palliative care. *Oncology Nursing Forum*, 17(1): 87–94.

Dixon, J.K., Matosevic, D., Clark, T. and Knapp, M (2015) *Equity in the Provision of Palliative Care in the UK: Review of Evidence*. London: London School of Economics.

Docherty, A., Owens, A., Sadi-Lari, M. et al. (2008) Knowledge and information needs of informal caregivers in palliative care: a qualitative systematic review. *Palliative Medicine*, 22(2): 153–71.

Gomez-Batiste, X., Martinez-Munoz, M., Blay, C. et al. (2014) Prevalence and characteristics of patients with advanced chronic conditions in need of palliative care in the general population: a cross-sectional study. *Palliative Medicine*, 28(4): 302–11.

Hudson, P. and Payne, S. (2011) Family caregivers and palliative care: current status and agenda for the future. *Journal of Palliative Medicine*, 14(7): 864–9.

Johnston, B. (2006) Overview of nursing developments. In Lugton, J. and McIntyre, R. (eds) *Palliative Care: The Nursing Role*. Edinburgh: Elsevier.

McCormack, B. and McCance, T. (eds) (2016) *Person-Centred Practice in Nursing and Health Care: Theory and Practice*. Chichester: John Wiley and Sons.

Mead, N. and Bower, P. (2000) Patient-centredness: a conceptual framework and review of the empirical literature. *Social Science and Medicine*, 51(7): 1087–110.

Mok, E. and Chiu, P.C. (2004) Nurse–patient relationships in palliative care. *Journal of Advanced Nursing*, 48(5): 475–83.

Murtagh, F.E., Bausewein, C., Verne, J. et al. (2014) How many people need palliative care? A study developing and comparing methods for population-based estimates. *Palliative Medicine*, 28(1): 49–58.

Walshe, C., Todd, C., Caress, A. and Chew-Graham, C. (2009) Patterns of access to community palliative care services: a literature review. *Journal of Pain and Symptom Management*, 37(5): 884–912.

Wittenberg-Lyles, E., Goldsmith, J. and Ragan, S. (2011) The shift to early palliative care: a typology of illness journeys and the role of nursing. *Clinical Journal of Oncology Nursing*, 15(3): 304–10.

Communication and palliative care nursing

Elaine Stevens

Introduction

This chapter introduces the reader to the role communication plays in high quality palliative care before outlining challenges that prevent nurses meeting the information needs of people in their care. Communication skills competences will be summarised before therapeutic relationships are discussed. Finally, practical guidance on communication challenges that test palliative care nurses will be provided. These are: conducting an interview, breaking bad news and collusion.

The World Health Organization (WHO) (2016) recognises palliative care as an endeavour where people are united within a healing journey (Hutchison et al. 2011). This partnership should not divide people into body, mind and spirit for the purpose of care provision but must engage with them as an integrated whole. This whole-person approach is a crucial element of quality healthcare (Morgan and Yoder 2012) and a central tenet of palliative care. However, individuals are not islands and are situated within their cultural worldview, family system, personal identity, value systems and vision for the future (Witt Sherman and Free 2015). Thus, working in a person-centred partnership means nurses need both the knowledge and skills to communicate with people effectively.

The role of communication

Person-centred palliative care engages with the person and their family to create and maintain therapeutic relationships grounded in mutuality, openness and honesty (Norton et al. 2013). Within such relationships members of the multi-professional team work in partnership with the individual and their family to explore their issues. For example, ill people and their families have a range of questions related to care provision and what to expect from services. McEwan and Harris (2010) suggest people have a range of information needs, from requiring simple information about their illness through to the exploration of complex issues of advanced disease and end of life care. The Department of Health (DoH) (2004) National Health Service (NHS) Knowledge and Skills Framework recommends communication skills development is shaped by specific professional roles and provides guidance on the core communication skills that professionals working in the NHS should possess. Notwithstanding the fact that a considerable amount of palliative care is provided outside of the NHS, this guidance provides a benchmark for communication skills in healthcare.

Challenges to effective communication

In contrast to the ideal outlined above, not all professionals have the knowledge, skills and attributes to communicate with ill people and their families in an effective way (Chan et al. 2016). Inadequate communication skills may result in distancing, which prevents the development of therapeutic relationships and leads to feelings of isolation, especially in people coming to the end of life (Kellehear 2014). Furthermore substandard communication skills may lead to missed opportunities to engage in advance care planning and may prohibit both people nearing the end of life and their families from making sound future decisions (Ahluwalia et al. 2015). Jenkins and Fallowfield (2016) propose poor information-giving leaves people with a flawed understanding about their illness, which leads them to seek information from less reliable sources such as the internet. Lack of confidence in communicating potentially distressing news stems from the idea that this is not a task undertaken regularly enough to build such confidence. Also less experienced professionals are less confident in communicating (Moir et al. 2015), which reinforces the belief that palliative care should be delivered by a team that is comprised of experienced and novice practitioners with complementary skills.

Communication skills training

Palliative care professionals should attend communication skills training regularly. This ought to include explorations of culturally sensitive communication skills, tailored to individual learners' needs (Goldsmith et al. 2012). Furthermore, teaching should focus on attitudes and behaviours in order for professionals to develop therapeutic relationships with ill people and their families and to enhance cooperation between professionals and others providing care and support to the person (Verschuur et al. 2014).

Communication courses should be delivered over an extended period of time to enable sustained changes in communication skills practices to emerge. This is reinforced by a systematic review by Barth and Lannen (2011), although they also note that shorter courses enable small positive changes in communication skills. Indeed, the post-evaluation of a focused 3-hour training course discovered skills and confidence had increased, although further long-term evaluation is required (Connolly et al. 2014).

The majority of training takes place in the classroom, using a combination of didactic approaches and learner-centred activities (Yoo and Park 2015). This use of case-based reflection, role play and simulation away from practice seems to enhance communication behaviours and skills (Hendricks-Ferguson et al. 2015). However, a challenge remains in that even though professionals display required behaviours and skills in the classroom, these are not always translated into practice due to organisational culture and time constraints (Brown 2010). Shadowing and role-modelling in practice allow dovetailing of theories with real-life situations to increase confidence when communicating in complex situations (Brown 2010). Indeed, a sizeable evidence base indicates that communication skills training, which integrates communication theories and experiential techniques, empowers professionals and enables them to conquer their reservations about communicating with people with advanced illness and their families (Barth and Lannen 2011).

Communication competences

Recognising effective communication as crucial to optimal palliative care has guided the development of numerous communication frameworks and competencies, and, although developed to guide best practice, such documents are often discipline-specific or are created for single health systems and consequently may not meet the requirements of a range of palliative care providers and individual professionals. Thus, in 2010, the European Association for Palliative Care developed a competency framework that could be used to benchmark best practice in palliative care globally (Gamondi et al. 2013a). Within their framework, Gamondi et al. (2013b, p. 142) suggest professionals require a range of communication skills to enable them to do the following:

- Demonstrate ways of building a therapeutic relationship with patients and family carers.
- Foster greater communication within the team and with other professional colleagues.
- Choose appropriate methods of relating and interacting according to age, wishes and intellectual abilities, verifying the understanding of decisions taken.
- Interpret the different types of communication (for example, verbal, non-verbal, formal and informal) of patients and family carers appropriately.
- Use guidelines for breaking bad news, where available.
- Adapt language to the different phases of the illness, be sensitive to cultural issues and avoid the use of medical jargon.
- Support people's informed decisions regarding the level of information they wish to receive and share with their family.
- Pace the provision of information according to the preferences and cognitive abilities of patients and family carers.

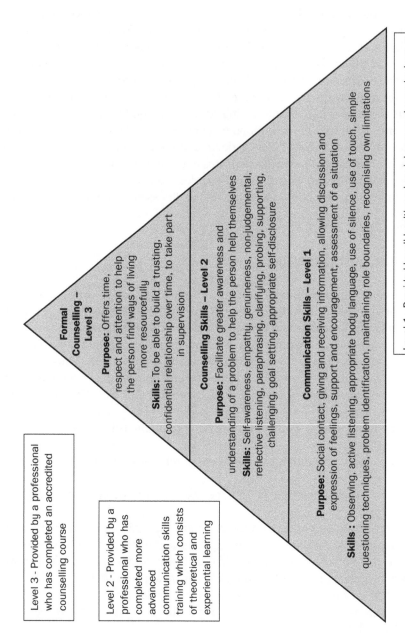

Level 3 - Provided by a professional who has completed an accredited counselling course

Level 2 - Provided by a professional who has completed more advanced communication skills training which consists of theoretical and experiential learning

Formal Counselling – Level 3

Purpose: Offers time, respect and attention to help the person find ways of living more resourcefully

Skills: To be able to build a trusting, confidential relationship over time, to take part in supervision

Counselling Skills – Level 2

Purpose: Facilitate greater awareness and understanding of a problem to help the person help themselves

Skills: Self-awareness, empathy, genuineness, non-judgemental, reflective listening, paraphrasing, clarifying, probing, supporting, challenging, goal setting, appropriate self-disclosure

Communication Skills – Level 1

Purpose: Social contact, giving and receiving information, allowing discussion and expression of feelings, support and encouragement, assessment of a situation

Skills : Observing, active listening, appropriate body language, use of silence, use of touch, simple questioning techniques, problem identification, maintaining role boundaries, recognising own limitations

Level 1 - Provided by all health and social care workers who have a role in caring for people requiring palliative care. Requires the completion of a course on the fundamental communication skills outlined in the model.

Figure 7.1 Range of communication skills required to care for patients with palliative care needs

While these competencies provide general guidance, it is recognised the information needs of patients and their families range widely, and consequently it may be useful for these to be used in conjunction with other frameworks, such as the one developed to depict the range of communication skills required by those working in palliative care (Figure 7.1).

Level 1 outlines a range of communication skills that all those in contact with ill people and their families in a work role should possess to show compassion and understanding. Such skills may be taught as part of an induction programme, as part of ongoing professional development or as part of an undergraduate training course. All workers should revisit their knowledge and skills regularly to enable them to perform effectively (Gamondi et al. 2013a).

Level 2 communication skills can only be acquired once the first level ones have been developed. Such skills would be more likely to be required by professional carers as they include skills of counselling, although not used within a formal counselling framework (Amis 2011). Indeed, the majority of complex communication with patients and their families is provided by proficient clinicians who have gained higher levels of communication skills (Department of Health 2004). Second level communication and simple counselling skills may be taught in short training sessions, focusing on one specific issue, such as breaking bad news (Brown and Bylund 2008). However, more advanced counselling skills are learned by taking part in training which includes a range of theories and experiential activities and takes place over a period of time. This should be delivered by teachers who have completed a trainer's course, to enable the learner to apply theories to practice (Wilkinson et al. 2008).

Level 3 of the framework represents the role of the counsellor, i.e. a person who holds a recognised counselling qualification and who works within a formal framework (Amis 2011). Such counsellors may be required to meet the needs of some people and their families who have complex needs (National Institute of Clinical Excellence 2004). Consequently, the professional team should be aware of when their skills have been exhausted and when to refer the person with complex needs on to a more expert practitioner. Indeed, over-confidence in one's abilities may lead to errors in information giving and damage the therapeutic relationship.

Learning exercise 7.1

Reflect on your communication skills, abilities and behaviours in relation to your role. Make some notes about how well you currently communicate and how much more you know about the theories of communication. Revisit the communication skills outlined in Figure 7.1 and explore the communication competencies developed by the EAPC (Gamondi et al. 2013a) and the NHS Knowledge and Skills Framework (Department of Health 2004). Tie all of these reflections together and develop a personal learning plan of how you can close the gap between what the guidance suggests and your current abilities.

Feedback

Your knowledge and skills of communication will vary depending on your role in palliative care. However, this activity should give you a clearer idea of what you need to do to enhance these. It is hoped that the remainder of this chapter will provide some of the theory required to understand the importance of communication to the nurse in palliative care. It will also provide some practical information on more complicated communication issues that apply specifically to palliative care nursing. In addition, explore communication skills training sessions that are available in your local area. This will enable you to dovetail theoretical and practical advice to the communication skills taught within experiential learning environments.

The palliative care nurse and the therapeutic relationship

The essence of palliative care nursing is to provide compassionate and comforting care in which patients and their families are able to discuss their deepest worries (Dobrina et al. 2014). Thus, the aim is to develop a non-judgemental, mutually respectful relationship with patients and families, which takes into account their values and family history, and concentrates on developing an understanding of how illness is experienced by them all (Reed 2010). This therapeutic relationship improves patient outcomes through the process of mutual goal-setting, the promotion of patient autonomy and the improvement of the symptoms associated with advanced illness (Canning et al. 2007). However, it may be challenging to develop relationships with patients and families when time is short; so making the most of each interaction is essential. Indeed, relationships may become strained if the patient and family have different views on the future and treatments to be offered (Roe and Leslie 2010), and consequently using techniques such as active listening are imperative in the development of such relationships (Stickley and Freshwater 2006). To build a trusting relationship with patients and families, nurses must first of all know themselves and how their perceptions and prejudices affect the situations they encounter in practice. Thus, it is the combination of effective communication skills, such as those outlined in Figure 7.1, and the effective use of the self that enables the nurse to build a secure therapeutic relationship with patients and their families.

Self-awareness and emotional intelligence

Self-awareness and emotional intelligence are two intertwined concepts that determine how well individuals know themselves and how competent they are in dealing with the emotional aspects of relationships. Only humans have a conscious awareness of the 'self' that allows them to appraise themselves in relation to the world around them (Leary 2004). Indeed, Rungapadiachy (2008) suggests all humans have an unconscious store of self-knowledge based on life experiences, although they are often unaware of the impact such knowledge has on behavioural responses. Thus, self-awareness is the ability to bring this unconscious self-knowledge into the conscious and to have a dialogue with one's self on how thoughts, feelings and behaviours impact on relationships individuals have with others. Leary (2004) suggests such self-discovery allows people to determine the type of person they are, make decisions about how to control their behaviour, evaluate and make changes to themselves, decode the meaning of the world around them and understand how other people may be feeling in particular situations. This self-awareness enables nurses to reflect on the biases they bring to their role and allows them to become more empathetic. It is only once personal beliefs and values are examined and understood by nurses that therapeutic relationships can be developed.

Sharma et al. (2016, p. 203) define emotional intelligence (EI) as 'a cluster of traits or abilities relating to the emotional side of life'. It is worth noting that although individuals have a core identity, they may also have other personal and professional characteristics that come to the fore when they are in different circumstances. For example, a nurse may display more nursing characteristics when at work but when at home the characteristics of a parent come to the fore. However, they are still the same core person and as such need to be emotionally intelligent in order to display appropriate emotional characteristics in specific situations (Kozub et al. 2016). Thus, being emotionally intelligent is being competent to evaluate one's own and other people's emotions by recognising the emotions being displayed, understanding their impact and by managing these positively so that the aims of the interaction are realised (Schutte et al. 2013). Therefore, emotional intelligence is an attribute that enables nurses to provide compassionate care within recognised nursing values (Snowden et al. 2015).

To work on this aspect of communication, the nurse must first assess their own level of EI. This may be achieved by completing a checklist such as the one developed by Schutte et al. (1998) as described in Learning exercise 7.2.

Learning exercise 7.2

Measuring your emotional intelligence

Conduct an internet search for Schutte et al. (1998). In this article you will find the Schutte Self-Report Emotional Intelligence Scale (SSEIT). Answer all 33 questions honestly using the following rating scale:

Rating scale: 1 = Strongly Disagree–5 = Strongly Agree

Score your own emotional intelligence using the guidance below:

- In most questions 1 = 1; 2 = 2; 3 = 3; 4 = 4; 5 = 5.
- However, in questions 5, 28 and 33, which are in reverse order, 1 = 5; 2 = 4; 3 = 3; 4 = 2; 5 = 1.

- Add all 33 scores together and you will have a score between 33 and 165.
- The lower the score, the lower your EI.

(Schutte et al. 2009)

Schutte et al. (2013) suggest that EI can be enhanced by attending EI training which can lead to feelings of increased life and job satisfaction, improvements in overall health and in personal relationships. Such training is often mapped against Goleman's (1998) five components of EI:

1   Self-awareness
2   Self-regulation
3   Internal motivation
4   Empathy
5   Social skills.

Thus, it may include: how to recognise emotions, how these impact on the dimensions of a person's life and how emotions can be accepted and managed (Sabzevar et al. 2016). In addition, sessions on self and social awareness as well as how relationships can be managed may be part of emotional intelligence training (Sharma et al. 2016).

Conducting an interview

Nurses interact with patients and their families for many reasons, ranging from informal social discourse through to in-depth explorations of specific problems. Within this, the interview may be defined as an optimal way of gaining a complete set of information about a person which can be used to develop a person-centred package of care based on their needs (Srivastava 2014). However, even those people with finely tuned communication skills find some interviews difficult, especially when the topics may be emotionally sensitive. Indeed, De Graaf et al. (2012) propose that clinicians, including nurses, are not good at identifying the needs of diverse groups of people with end of life needs.

Before embarking on the interview, the nurse should ensure they have all the required information (Chovan et al. 2014), so they can focus on the right issues with the right people, at the right time and in the right place. To guide development of an optimal interviewing technique, it may be fruitful to use an interview framework. The best known of these is the Calgary Cambridge Guide (Silverman et al. 2013) and although nurses have different relationships with patients from doctors, this tool can guide the nurse in the development of interviewing skills. The Calgary Cambridge Guide is divided into six discrete sections:

- Initiating the session.
- Gathering information.

- Providing structure.
- Building relationship.
- Explanation and planning.
- Closing the session.

In each of these stages the nurse should take the lead and attend to the timing and structure of the interview (McEwan and Harris 2010). By gathering information first, the nurse can build the relationship with the interviewee by individually tailoring information to their needs. Such a skill will ensure that the needs of dying patients and their families are identified in a timely manner and that an individualised plan of care is developed in keeping with their wants and wishes. When explaining and planning care, time should be taken to allow information to sink in and jargon should be avoided to aid understanding (Chovan et al. 2014). An interview should always close following a summary of the main points and the plan for the future, if one has been mutually agreed.

Breaking bad news

Palliative care nursing necessitates caring for people at a time when their health status is declining and death may be approaching. Such change results in uncertainties for the patient, their family and the professional team, which provides ideal territory for anxiety and fear in patients and families and stress in professionals (Rosenfield et al. 2014). The antidote to this is the provision of individually tailored information which is delivered with honesty. One element of information giving is disclosing bad news, although sometimes nurses erroneously believe they do not break bad news but that this is left to their medical colleagues. Bad news, however, is not only information about major life-changing events but also includes any information that has a detrimental effect on the future well-being of the person receiving the news (Pereira et al. 2013).

Thus, the nurse must first and foremost reflect on how such news may affect the recipient's future and be prepared to deliver information in a way that acknowledges that it may be perceived as 'bad'. The use of a standardised approach to breaking bad news, such as the Spikes Protocol presented in Box 7.1 (Baile et al. 2000), allows professionals to remember a best practice format even when they are working in stressful circumstances.

Box 7.1   The Spikes Protocol for breaking bad news

- **S**etting up – getting the environment right and all the information you might need.
- **P**erception – finding out what the patient and family already know.
- **I**nvitation – let patients and family members choose how much they wish to hear and how much information they require.

- **K**nowledge – give the information in a simple clear way. No jargon!
- **E**motions – bad news causes emotions which need to be expressed. Stay close if needed. If not, leave the family to one other – once emotions have subsided, carry on with the discussion.
- **S**trategy and summary – work out a future plan with the patient and family. If the situation is too emotional, you may need to come back later. Always finish with information about availability of staff should any questions arise.

Adapted from Baile et al. (2000)

Preparation required for the bad news interview mirrors that for all interviews, however, Caillier (2010) adds that here the nurse must also rehearse how the news will be given and prepare for the different reactions to the news. For this reason, Pereira et al. (2013) suggest the nurse considers who should attend the interview to support the interviewees, thus, more than one professional may be required to attend. While some interviews may take place with one interviewee, it is recommended that the recipient of bad news has the opportunity to be accompanied by someone who can support them (Caillier 2010).

The nurse should be guided by interviewees in determining their current understanding of the situation and in gauging how much information should be disclosed. This is important as people wish to have a gradual disclosure of bad news and although they value honesty, few want the 'whole' truth, especially about impending death (Deschepper et al. 2008).

Baile et al. (2000) suggest the news should be given in simple language to aid understanding. This may be preceded by what is termed a warning shot that allows the interviewee(s) to be aware something unpleasant may be coming (Morar 2005). An example of a warning shot may be, 'We have the results of your tests and they are more complicated than we thought' or 'I am sorry but what I have to speak to you about today is very serious.'

Once news has been disclosed, emotional upset should be acknowledged and the interview paused (Caillier 2010). Baile et al. (2000) suggest remaining close by and maintaining an empathetic manner. However, some people will wish to be alone and, if this is the case, the nurse should make it known they will return so interviewees do not feel abandoned. Only once emotions have subsided, can the final stage of the interview take place. It is important for the nurse to ensure interviewees are ready for the next stage of the interview so they can take full part in the final part of the interview (Baile et al. 2000).

To close the interview, the nurse should always provide interviewees with information on next steps and develop a mutual plan. Kurer and Zekri (2008) suggest written material may help decision-making processes, while contact details of support groups may also be useful. It may also be supportive for the nurse to offer to speak to others who did not attend the interview as this may be too difficult for the interviewees to do. Finally, the nurse should ensure that interviewees know who is best placed to answer any further questions in the short term (Caillier 2010). This is especially important if the nurse is going off shift and/or is not due on duty again for a few days.

Truth-telling and collusion

Fallowfield et al. (2002) observe that there are differences in what patients and families want to know and what professionals think they want to know, and some professionals believe patients and families do not want to hear upsetting information. However, for most people, open and sensitive disclosure, set within the context of an equal relationship with professionals, is their preferred method of receiving information. Chatuverdi et al. (2009) suggest, although truthful news may be upsetting, it is more beneficial for the patient and family to hear this than for it to be withheld. Indeed, open and honest communication is the preferred option for most patients and families, and thus professionals should assess everyone in their care on an on-going basis to enable an individually tailored disclosure to take place (Parker et al. 2007).

The counter term to truth-telling is collusion. This is when the truth is fully or partially withheld from one or more people for a deceitful purpose (Chatuverdi, Loiselle and Chandra 2009); although, in palliative care, the primary reason for collusion is to protect others from distressing information (De Caesteker 2012). Collusion usually results from a failure to disclose information to the patient about some or all of the facts of their illness, resulting in a collusive partnership between the professionals and the family. However, collusion also occurs in a partnership between the professionals and the patient, when the patient does not wish the family to know that they are going to die (Chatuverdi, Loiselle and Chandra 2009). However, collusion does not exist when a person has made an informed decision not to be given information and a third person is identified as the receiver of this. This highlights the need for accurate documentation of people's needs so the whole professional team understands the care strategy and who knows what (Jellis 2010).

Partnership between professionals and the family

Baile and Parker (2010) acknowledge that historically it was acceptable to allow families to decide whether patients should be given information, and indeed this remains the custom in some cultures. However, Al-Amri (2013) insists that culture itself should not be a barrier to honest communication with patients and that information should be given in keeping with best practice guidance, such as legislation, ethical and professional standards. Nevertheless, there are still situations when family members are given information first and wish to withhold it from the patient. For example, if the patient is thought to be near death but then recovers sufficiently to take part in such discussions. Another example of professional/family collusion may arise when communication practices, in which relatives are traditionally given information first, remain part of the professional practice or organisational culture. Indeed, Kurer and Zekri (2008) note that doctors from cultures where it is customary for the family to take control of information may be more willing to develop a collusive relationship with the family, even though the family may have never lied to their loved one before. However, despite the reasons for this type of collusion, it leads to false hope in patients and prevents them from making decisions about their future care and to say goodbye to their loved ones (Parker et al. 2007).

Partnership between professionals and the patient

Professionals cannot legally disclose a competent patient's information without their consent (Al-Amri 2013). Thus, a patient may wish to protect the family from the distress of knowing they are going to die and while the professionals may discuss the decision, ultimately it is the patient's own choice. However, McEwan and Harris (2010) suggest that non-verbal communication often gives the game away and as such families may recognise that something is not right. Such a breakdown in communication leads to strained relationships, anxiety and fear as the information needs of families exceed those of patients as the end of life approaches, and this may lead to poor end of life care planning and may have an impact on the family in their bereavement (Worden 2009).

Managing collusion

The key to preventing collusive relationships being established is through communication skills training which covers the impact of collusion and provides experiential activities to enhance the knowledge and skills of professionals. In addition, Graham et al. (2005) suggest clinical supervision, structured team reflection and debriefing sessions can help prevent collusive events. However, managing established collusive relationships is complex and apart from general guidance on how to remain open and honest with patients and their families, there has been no formal guidance on the management of established collusion since that of Faulkner (1998). This suggests that established collusion may be ended by openly discussing the issues with all those involved. The strategy involves a three-interview process:

- *Interview 1 – with the colluder(s).* The aim is for the nurse to sensitively determine the reasons for collusion and to negotiate access to the person who is having the truth withheld from them. The nurse should promise not to tell this person the truth, however, there is a caveat to this statement which the nurse should explain clearly. The caveat is: if person being kept in the dark shows they know the truth, then this will be confirmed. The nurse should make it clear that they will not lie to the person.
- *Interview 2 – with the person from whom information is being withheld.* This can only take place if the nurse has successfully negotiated access to this person. This may take more than one attempt with the colluders to achieve this, as they need to understand the benefits of an open and honest relationship.

The aim of this interview is to find out what facts the person knows about the current situation.

- *Interview 3 – with all parties.* This can be difficult for the nurse to facilitate as strong feelings and emotions may emerge when the deceit is revealed. Although this may be short-lived when the person realises collusion has occurred out of feelings of love and protection, it may also be difficult for all parties to discuss the issues that have been hidden. At this stage the nurse may have to do little, but support people as they talk about the issues that have been avoided. This shows empathy, compassion and respect for each of them as individuals.

Finally, Faulkner (1998) notes collusion cannot always be broken because of the wishes and beliefs of those involved. Furthermore, if the situation has been in place for a long time, or if the person who has not received information is close to death, it may not be wise to break collusion since there may not be time to deal with all the resulting issues. In this situation, clinical supervision and reflection may help the nurse to reflect on the issues and to develop a practice plan for the future.

Conclusion

In conclusion, it is nurses who spend most time with patients and their families and, as such, have varied and valued roles within palliative care. It is, therefore, of the utmost importance that individual nurses have the required communication skills and knowledge to provide high quality palliative care in an effective manner. However, while many nurses believe they communicate effectively, evidence would suggest this is not always the case. It has been shown that effective communication can be learned through training that combines theory, experiential learning and the opportunity to practise this in the clinical setting. The use of such communication skills allows the nurse to build and maintain therapeutic relationships and it is recognised these are based on openness, honesty and trust. However, it is the nurse's responsibility to ensure such relationships are based on the information needs of individuals and not those of the nurse or the professional team. Palliative care nurses experience complex communication issues, however, using best practice guidance and enhanced communication skills should enable the nurse to succeed in dealing with such situations with confidence.

References

Ahluwalia, S.C., Bekelman, D.B., Alexis. K. et al. (2015) Barriers and strategies to an iterative model of advance care planning communication. *American Journal of Hospice & Palliative Medicine*, 32(8): 817–23.

Al-Amri, A.M. (2013) Ethical issues in disclosing bad news to cancer patients: reflections of an oncologist in Saudi Arabia. In Surbone, A., Zwitter, M., Rajer, R. and Stiefel, R. (eds) *New Challenges in Communication with Cancer Patients*. New York: Springer.

Amis, K. (2011) *Becoming a Counsellor: A Student Companion*. London: Sage.

Baile, W.F., Buckman, R., Lenzi, R. et al. (2000) SPIKES: a six-step protocol for delivering bad news: application to the patient with cancer. *The Oncologist*, 5: 302–11.

Baile, W.F. and Parker, P.A. (2010) Breaking bad news. In Kissane, D., Bultz, B., Butow, P. and Finlay, I. (eds) *Handbook of Communication in Oncology and Palliative Care*. Oxford: Oxford University Press.

Barth, J. and Lannen, P. (2011) Efficacy of communication skills training courses in oncology: a systematic review and meta-analysis. *Annals of Oncology*, 22: 1030–40.

Brown, J. (2010) Transferring clinical communication skills from the classroom to the clinical environment: perceptions of a group of medical students in the United Kingdom. *Academic Medicine*, 85(6): 1052–9.

Brown, R.F. and Bylund, C.L. (2008) Communication skills training: describing a new conceptual model. *Academic Medicine*, 83(1): 37–44.

Caillier, R. (2010) Breaking bad news to patients: this valuable communication skill will reward you in the end. *Podiatry Management*, January: 123–4.

Canning, D., Rosenberg, J.P. and Yates, P. (2007) Therapeutic relationships in specialist palliative care nursing practice. *International Journal of Palliative Nursing*, 13(5): 222–9.

Chan, R.J., Webster, J. and Bowers, A. (2016) End of life pathways for improving outcomes in care of the dying. *Cochrane Database of Systematic Reviews* 11. Available at: http://doi.wiley.com/10.1002/14651858.CD008006.pub4 (accessed 22 August 2016).

Chatuverdi, S.K., Loiselle, C.G. and Chandra, P.S. (2009) Communication with relatives and collusion in palliative care: a cross-cultural perspective. *Indian Journal of Palliative Care*, 15(1): 1–8.

Chovan, J.D., Cluxton, D. and Rancour, P. (2014) Principles of patient and family assessment. In Ferrell, B.R., Coyle, N. and Paice, J.A. (eds) *The Oxford Textbook of Palliative Nursing* (4th edn). Oxford: Oxford University Press.

Connolly, M., Thomas, J.M., Orford, J.A. et al. (2014) The impact of the SAGE & THYME Foundation Level Workshop on factors influencing communication skills in health care professionals. *Journal of Continuing Education in the Health Professions*, 34(1): 37–46.

De Caesteker, S. (2012) Communication skills. In Faull, C., De Caesteker, S., Nicholson, A. and Black, F. (eds) *Handbook of Palliative Care*. Chichester: Wiley-Blackwell.

de Graaf, F.M., Franckec, A.L., van den Muijsenberghe, M.E.T.C. and van der Geesta, S. (2012) Understanding and improving communication and decision-making in palliative care for Turkish and Moroccan immigrants: a multi-perspective study. *Ethnicity and Health*, 17(4): 363–84.

Department of Health (2004) *NHS Knowledge and Skills Framework (NHSKSF) and the Development Review Process*. London: Department of Health.

Deschepper, R., Bernheim, J.L., Vander Stichele, R. et al. (2008) Truth-telling at the end of life: a pilot study on the perspective of patients and professional caregivers. *Patient Education and Counselling*, 71: 52–6.

Dobrina, R., Tenze, M. and Palese, A. (2014) An overview of hospice and palliative care nursing models and theories. *International Journal of Palliative Nursing*, 20(22): 75–81.

Fallowfield, L.J., Jenkins, V.A. and Beveridge, H.A. (2002) The truth hurts but deceit hurts more: communication in palliative care. *Palliative Medicine*, 16: 297–303.

Faulkner, A. (1998) *Effective Interaction with Patients* (2nd edn). Edinburgh: Churchill Livingstone.

Gamondi, C., Larkin, P. and Payne, S. (2013a) Core competencies in palliative care: an EAPC White Paper on palliative care education – Part 1. *European Journal of Palliative Care*, 20(2): 86–91.

Gamondi, C., Larkin, P. and Payne, S. (2013b) Core competencies in palliative care: an EAPC White Paper on palliative care education – Part 2. *European Journal of Palliative Care*, 20(3): 140–5.

Goldsmith, J., Ferrell, B., Wittenberg-Lyles, E. and Ragan, S.L. (2012) Palliative care communication in oncology nursing. *Clinical Journal of Oncology Nursing*, 17(2): 163–7.

Goleman, D. (1998) *Working with Emotional Intelligence*. London: Bloomsbury.

Graham, C., Robson, C. and Whitford, S. (2005) Collusion in palliative care: a reflective account. *Journal of Community Nursing*, 19(6): 4–8.

Hendricks-Ferguson, V.L., Sawin, K.J., Montgomery, K. et al. (2015) Novice nurses' experiences with palliative and end-of-life communication. *Journal of Pediatric Oncology Nursing*, 32(4): 240–52.

Hutchison, T.A., Mount, B.M. and Kearney, M. (2011). The healing journey. In Hutchison, T.A. (ed.) *Whole Person Care: A New Paradigm for the 21st Century*. New York: Springer.

Jellis, V. (2010) Effective communication in teams. In Kraszewski, S. and McEwan, A. (eds) *Communication Skills for Adult Nurses*. Maidenhead: McGraw-Hill/Open University Press.

Jenkins, V.A. and Fallowfield, L.J. (2016) No man's land: information needs of men with metastatic castrate resistant prostate cancer. *Supportive Care in Cancer*. Available at: http://dx.doi.org/10.1007/s00520-016-3358-0 (accessed 22 August 2016).

Kellehear, A. (2014) *The Inner Life of the Dying Person*. New York: Columbia University Press.

Kozub, E., Brown, A. and Ecoff, L. (2016) Strategies for success: cultivating emotional competence in the clinical nurse specialist role. *AACN Advanced Critical Care*, 27(2): 145–51.

Kurer, M.A. and Zekri, J.M. (2008) Breaking bad news: can we get it right? *The Libyan Journal of Medicine*, 3: 200–3.

Leary, M. (2004) *The Curse of the Self: Self-awareness, Egotism and the Quality of Human Life*. Oxford: Oxford University Press.

McEwan, A. and Harris, G. (2010) Communication: fundamental skills. In Kraszewski, S. and McEwan, A. (eds) *Communication Skills for Adult Nurses*. Maidenhead: McGraw-Hill/Open University Press.

Moir, C., Roberts, R., Martz, K. et al. (2015) Communicating with patients and their families about palliative and end-of-life care: comfort and educational needs of nurses. *International Journal of Palliative Nursing*, 21(3): 109–12.

Morar, P. (2005) Breaking bad news. *British Medical Journal*, 330: 1131.

Morgan, S. and Yoder, L.H. (2012) A concept analysis in person-centred care. *Journal of Holistic Nursing*, 30(1): 6–15.

NICE (National Institute for Clinical Excellence) (2004) *Supportive and Palliative Care for Adults with Cancer*. London: NICE.

Norton, S.A., Metzger, M., De Luca, J. et al. (2013) Palliative care communication: linking patients' prognoses, values and goals of care. *Research in Nursing & Health*, 36: 582–90.

Parker, S.M., Clayton, J.M., Hancock, K. et al. (2007) A systematic review of prognostic/ end of-life communication with adults in the advanced stages of a life-limiting illness: patient/caregiver preferences for the content, style, and timing of information. *Journal of Pain and Symptom Management*, 34(1): 81–93.

Pereira, A.T.G., Fortes, I.F.L. and Mendes, J.M.G. (2013) Communication of bad news: systematic literature review. *Journal of Nursing UFPE Online*. doi: 10.5205/ reuol.3049-24704-1-LE.0701201331 (accessed 9 August 2016).

Reed, S.M. (2010) A unitary-caring conceptual model for advanced practice nursing in palliative care. *Holistic Nursing Practice*, 24(1): 23–34.

Roe, J.W.G. and Leslie, P. (2010) Beginning of the end? Ending the therapeutic relationship in palliative care. *International Journal of Speech-Language Pathology*, 12(4): 304–8.

Rosenfield, D., Ridge, D. and Von Lob, G. (2014) Vital scientific puzzle or lived uncertainty? Professional and lived approaches to the uncertainties of ageing with HIV. *Health Sociology Review*, 23(1), 20–32.

Rungapadiachy, D.M. (2008) *Self-Awareness in Health Care: Engaging in Helping Relationships*. Basingstoke: Palgrave.

Sabzevar, A.V., Sarpoosh, H.R., Esmaeili, F. and Khojeh, A. (2016) The effect of emotional intelligence training on employed nurses. *Journal of Nursing and Midwifery Sciences*, 3(3): 46–53.

Schutte, N.S., Malouff, J.M. and Bhullar, N. (2009) The assessing emotions scale. In Stough, C., Saklofske, D. and Parker, J. (eds) *The Assessment of Emotional Intelligence*. New York: Springer.

Schutte, N.S., Malouff, J.M. and Thornsteinsson, E.B. (2013) Increasing emotional intelligence through training: current status and future directions. *International Journal of Emotional Education*, 5(1): 56–72.

Schutte, N.S., Malouff, J.M., Hall, L.E. et al. (1998) Development and validation of a measure of emotional intelligence. *Personality and Individual Differences*, 25: 167–77.

Sharma, V.S., Das, K., Malhi, P. and Ghai, S. (2016) A pre experimental study to assess the effect of emotional intelligence skill training on emotional intelligence of undergraduate nursing students. *International Journal of Nursing Education*, 8(2): 203–8.

Silverman, J.D., Kurtz, S.M. and Draper, J. (2013) *Skills for Communicating with Patients* (3rd edn). Oxford: Radcliffe Medical Press.

Snowden, A., Stenhouse, R., Young, J. et al. (2015) The relationship between emotional intelligence, previous caring experience and mindfulness in student nurses and midwives: a cross-sectional analysis. *Nurse Education Today*, 35: 152–8.

Srivastava, S.B. (2014) The patient interview. In Lauster, C.D. and Srivastava, S.B. (eds) *Fundamental Skills for Patient Care in Pharmacy Practice*. Burlington, VT: Jones and Bartlett.

Stickley, T. and Freshwater, D. (2006) The art of listening in the therapeutic relationship. *Mental Health Practice*, 9(5): 12–18.

Verschuur, E.M.L., Groot, M.M. and van der Sande, R. (2014) Nurses' perceptions of pro-active palliative care: a Dutch focus group study. *International Journal of Palliative Nursing*, 20(5): 241–5.

Wilkinson, S., Perry, R., Blanchard, K. and Linsell, L. (2008) Effectiveness of a three-day communication skills course in changing nurses' communication skills with cancer/palliative care patients: a randomised controlled trial. *Palliative Medicine*, 22: 365–75.

Witt Sherman, D. and Free, D. (2015) Cultural and spirituality as domains of quality palliative care. In Matzo, M. and Witt Sherman, D. (eds) *Palliative Care Nursing: Quality Care to the End of Life* (4th edn). New York: Springer, pp. 170–235.

Worden, J.W. (2009) *Grief Counseling and Grief Therapy: A Handbook for the Mental Health Practitioner* (4th edn). Hove: Brunner-Routledge.

World Health Organization (2016) *Definition of Palliative Care*. Available at: http://www.who.int/cancer/palliative/definition/en/ (accessed 22 August 2016).

Yoo, M.S. and Park H.R. (2015) Effects of case-based learning on communication skills, problem-solving ability, and learning motivation in nursing students. *Nursing and Health Sciences*, 17: 166–72.

Physical symptom management, with a focus on nursing interventions for complex symptoms

Anna-Marie Stevens and Diane Laverty

Introduction

This chapter offers insight into the pivotal role that nurses can play in supporting patients with complex symptoms who require palliative care. The remit of palliative nursing, it has been suggested, is in considering a whole person philosophy of care that can be offered to patients irrespective of disease, prognosis or in which setting they are being cared for (Coyle 2015). When caring for the patient, palliative care nursing also includes the care of those closest to the patient and recognising the impact that the patient's disease and symptoms caused by the disease is having on the family, carers or those closest to the patient.

Alleviating suffering and improving the quality of life through symptom management cannot be underestimated within palliative care nursing. While the assessment and management of symptoms are not undertaken by the palliative care nurse in isolation, it is often the nursing team who are with patients throughout the clinical episodes of care and are therefore instrumental in bringing issues to the fore for the wider multi-professional teams. Symptoms addressed in this chapter include pain, constipation, fatigue, breathlessness, nausea and vomiting. It could be argued that the principles of palliative care nursing are applicable to all areas of nursing in the delivery of care through an ethos of dignity and compassion, however, palliative care nurses care for patients at a critical time in their lives and building a relationship with the patient should not be underestimated. This is of particular value in relation to the ability to assess and follow through a management plan to aid symptom control and the impact that a healing relationship can have on the patient and family.

Pain

Prevalence of pain

Pain is viewed as one of the most common and distressing symptoms in patients with cancer, affecting between 56–75 per cent of patients with an advanced disease (Hui and Bruera 2014). For nursing staff, pain at the end of life for patients remains of concern, whether this is in the context of pain being unrecognised, or if even when recognised, there is an inadequate or limited approach to the management of pain (Reynolds et al. 2013).

Box 8.1 Definitions of pain

Pain is a multifactorial experience for patients that is often influenced by physiological, psychological and social factors that influence the individual patient experience. The concept of total pain, originally coined by Dame Cicely Saunders, has been well accepted in the palliative care community, which relates to the impact of pain on other components of human functioning, including personality, mood, behaviour, and social relations (IASP 2009). Pain is defined as 'an unpleasant sensory and emotional experience associated with actual or potential tissue damage, or described in terms of such damage' (RCN 2015).

Chronic pain

Chronic pain is commonly referred to as pain that exists for more than 3 months, lasting beyond the usual course of the acute disease or expected time of healing (IASP 1996). The effects of chronic pain are often linked to an alteration in the patient's temperament and behaviour, as well as having an impact on their activities of daily living, which can in turn impact on social interaction with those closest to them (Orenius et al. 2013). In addition, neuropathic pain has been described as pain related to irregularity within the nervous system (Mann 2008). A failure of the nerves to function normally can be caused by a variety of problems such as surgery, infection, cancer and its treatments and injury such as trauma (Mann 2008).

Cancer pain

Cancer pain can be influenced by a plethora of elements. These include factors such as the cancer itself, treatments for cancer or in situations where the cancer itself is destroying nerves resulting in abnormal function. As in Case Study 8.1, this young woman was unable to wash herself, stand or walk any distance, which was having a huge impact on her quality of life. For some patients, pain reminds them that they have a cancer diagnosis which can impact emotionally on them, although not all pain is a sign that the cancer has returned or is advancing.

Case Study 8.1: Types of pain

A patient with metastatic cancer of the cervix, aged 35, had completed all lines of possible anti-cancer therapy. She was confirmed as having disease in her right pelvic side wall, resulting in pain in the right leg and groin. The pain she described as burning or shooting down her leg with altered sensations of her skin. The pain had been increasing over a period of 3 months. She was limited in movement which was having a significant impact on washing and sleeping, and her overall quality of life was affected by pain. She was experiencing chronic pain and on further assessment was found to be experiencing neuropathic pain.

Pain assessment: considerations of pain assessment

One of the fundamental attributes of the role of the nurse in pain is in ensuring detailed assessments are central in being able to provide individualised care. Assessment of all aspects, both physical and non-physical, is important in order to best know and understand the patient's perception of the pain and how best to aid and approach pain relief. The importance of pain assessment can never be underestimated, and as nurses are with patients more than any other clinician, they are best placed to guide this.

Assessment tools

The three most commonly used pain scales are: (1) the numeric rating scale; (2) the visual analogue scale; and (3) the categorical scale (Swarm et al. 2010). The patient in Case Study 8.1 described her pain as 7/10 at worst, using the numerical rating scale. Pain assessments should be seen as assessments that occur throughout routine episodes of clinical care (Hui and Bruera 2014). Additional assessment tools are available for those patients who may have specific needs, such as dementia or learning disabilities, which can guide the nurse in how best to approach an holistic pain assessment. A variety of acronyms/mnemonics currently exist to support professionals in identifying important elements for patients in assessing their pain. There are many ways of undertaking a detailed assessment of pain. One guide to help professionals remember the key questions in pain assessment involves SOCRATES, which determines the severity, the onset, the characteristic, the radiation of the pain, and anything that helps or makes the pain worse, and the actual site of the pain (Clayton et al. 2000).

Pain management

While the focus of pain management may be linked to a combination of pharmacological and non-pharmacological interventions, both these methods invariably require a multi-professional approach to care. Some patients' attitudes and concerns over commencing strong painkillers can be a limiting factor with concordance, which subsequently affects overall response to pain. Patients may also be concerned regarding side effects, and may equate this with a sign that their disease is advancing.

Persistent chronic cancer pain

The control of pain continues to be driven by the 'analgesic ladder', which was presented by the World Health Organization (WHO) in 1996 as a guide to the management of persistent cancer pain. It is also often used to guide the management of chronic persistent pain. It involves a stepwise approach to the use of analgesics, including non-opioids (step 1), opioids for mild-to-moderate pain (step 2), and opioids for moderate-to-severe pain (step 3). Adjuvant drugs are those that contribute to pain relief but are not primarily indicated for pain management. They can be used at all steps of the ladder. Examples include anti-depressant and anti-convulsant medications, corticosteroids, benzodiazepines, anti-spasmodics and bisphosphonates. The patient in Case Study 8.1 was previously taking medication orally consistent with a step 2 analgesic. As her pain was inadequately controlled, this was increased to a step 3. The introduction of medication on a regular basis allowed her pain to be better controlled following regular review of the response to the changes in medications.

All applications of medications run parallel with an holistic assessment of the emotional and psychological well-being of the patient and the impact that the pain may be having on these areas. Medications can be given via the oral route or the parenteral route, depending on the needs of the patient and other symptoms such as nausea, which may indicate the pain should be managed via an alternative route, such as the use of a subcutaneous syringe pump, which will ensure that the medication being delivered to the patient is being absorbed (see Chapter 16 in this volume). For the palliative care nurse, the attention to detail in terms of reviewing the response to any intervention must not be underplayed.

Step 1: non-opioid drugs

Paracetamol and non-steroidal anti-inflammatory drugs (NSAIDs) are recognised as types of non-opioid medications. These medications, while not exhaustive within this group, are of particular benefit to those patients who experience bone and visceral pain (Twycross et al. 2014). Aspirin, paracetamol and non-steroidal anti-inflammatory drugs (NSAIDs) are examples of non-opioid drugs that are effective for mild-to-moderate pain. It should be noted that these drugs are especially effective for musculoskeletal and visceral pain (Twycross et al. 2014).

Step 2: Adjuvant drugs

Adjuvant drugs are a miscellaneous group of drugs, whose primary indication is for conditions other than pain, which may, however, relieve pain in specific circumstances

(Twycross et al. 2014). Examples of this category of drugs include NSAIDs used for bone and visceral pain, steroids for pressure, bone pain and raised intracranial pressure, anti-depressants, and anti-epileptics for neuropathic pain.

Step 3: Opioids

Step 2 and Step 3 medications include those stronger pain killers (opioids) used for both mild-to-moderate pain (step 2) and those for moderate-to-severe pain (step 3). For those medications required at step 2, codeine-based medications are often prescribed. The latter occurs when pain relief with medications used in step 1 are not controlling the pain alone. Medications prescribed at step 3 include drugs such as morphine, oxycodone and fentanyl. Again this list is by no means exhaustive and further information can be sourced from local guidelines or from the British Pain Society and the Palliative Care Formulary.

Considerations for the nurse when a patient is being started on opioid medication

To support the commencement of opioids, both verbal and written information should be offered which should include information regarding when and why strong opioids are used to treat pain and how effective they are likely to be (NICE 2012). In addition to this, how to store medications and who to contact for further advice are also important.

The National Institute for Health and Care Excellence (NICE) in the UK in a guideline in 2012 suggested that when starting treatment with strong opioids, nurses should offer patients with advanced and progressive disease regular oral sustained-release or oral immediate-release morphine (depending on patient preference), with rescue doses of oral immediate-release morphine for breakthrough pain. The most common side effects of opioids are listed in Table 8.1. On-going nursing assessment is integral to the early recognition of the side effects of opioids. Considerations in changing to a different type of opioid may need to be discussed to ensure the medication is tolerated, of benefit to the patient and is not causing more harm than benefit (Walsh et al. 2001).

Table 8.1 Side effects of opioids

Common	Less common
Constipation	Hyperalgesia
Nausea/vomiting	Allodynia
Drowsiness	Myoclonus
Unsteadiness	Hallucinations
Delirium	Sweating
Dry mouth	Itching
	Urinary retention

Adjuvant drugs (co-analgesics)

Most chronic pain contains elements of nerve pain. Patients with nociceptive pain, that is, pain resulting 'from activity in neural pathways secondary to actual tissue damage or potentially tissue-damaging stimuli' (Nicholson 2006), are likely to gain some benefit from standard medications such as NSAIDs, but these drugs come with a strong side effect profile. It is probable that those patients who experience a form of neuropathic pain will be expected to achieve some benefit from co-analgesics, including drugs such as tricyclic anti-depressants (e.g. amitriptyline and nortriptyline) and anti-convulsant drugs (e.g. gabapentin and pregabalin) (Mackintosh and Elson 2008). The WHO analgesic ladder endorses the use of these drugs in combination with non-opioids, opioids for mild-to-moderate pain and opioids for moderate-to-severe pain. Further information on medications and recommended dose conversions can be accessed through the Palliative Care Formulary (PCF) (Twycross et al. 2014) or palliativedrugs.com. Additional medications such as the use of nitrous oxide (Entonox) can be helpful for those individuals who experience pain that is temporary and related to a specific activity, such as a dressing change. The use of local anaesthetic patches such as Lidocaine can also be helpful to manage neuropathic pain. An example of this might be a patient with neuropathic pain in the leg from a spinal cord compression. The use of epidurals/intrathecal can also be considered for complex pain but will obviously depend on access to resources.

The patient in Case Study 8.1 required an intrathecal catheter to be inserted into her back, which helped alleviate the pain. These interventions can be useful but careful consideration and assessment must take place to ensure that any potential side effects are discussed with the patient, as anaesthetic interventions may severely limit the patient's activities and impact on the patient's place of care.

Non-pharmacological methods of managing pain

Therapies other than pharmacology can serve as adjuncts, including talking therapies. Often these therapies run alongside medication therapy. These therapies can often aid relaxation and provide distraction for the patient (Coyle 2015).

Creating trusting therapeutic relationships

By creating trusting relationships with patients, nurses are instrumental in reducing anxiety and helping patients to cope with pain. Nurses may underestimate the benefits and comfort they bring by staying with a patient who is experiencing pain, as well as appreciating how they can help to alleviate barriers to pain control by exploring issues of fear regarding taking medications. For some patients, the fear is that pain may be associated with disease progression of cancer (Chapman 2012).

Relaxation

Evidence suggests that relaxation not only can make a patient feel better but can diminish the emotional components of pain and increase coping abilities to be able to deal with pain (Schaffer and Yucha 2004).

Music

The use of music in the healthcare setting can also provide relaxation and distraction from pain and has been recognised as having a positive impact on chronic pain (Persson 2014). Vaajoki et al. (2012) recognised lower pain intensity and pain distress in bed rest on the second post-operative day in a music group compared with a control group after elective abdominal surgery.

Art

The literature suggests that art therapy could be used to alleviate physical symptoms in some patients with chronic pain (Angheluta 2011). The skills of an art therapist are required to ensure the successful use of this intervention; this is to ensure the safety of the patient.

Mindfulness

In mindfulness meditation patients are encouraged to become more aware of their breathing, thoughts and physical sensations in the present moment and to review them without judgement (Tang and Leve 2016). Evidence has recently suggested that mindfulness meditation can help with the reduction of pain relating to chronic back pain (Cherkin et al. 2016) but researchers have recognised that further research into this area is necessary before clinicians may add this therapy to everyday clinical practice (Jacob 2016).

Learning exercise 8.1

- What influences a patient's perception of pain?
- How would you as a nurse empower patients to be involved in their pain control and what skills would you use to help them self-manage their pain?
- As a nurse what would you draw on to be able to guide and better support patients who are experiencing pain?

Constipation

Constipation is one of the most prevalent issues experienced by patients in palliative care (Larkin et al. 2008). The incidence of constipation diverges in different literature, however, the overall occurrence is between 32–87 per cent (Fallon and O'Neill 1997; Sykes 1998; Potter et al. 2003; Clark et al. 2010). There is no universally agreed definition of constipation (Clark et al. 2010) and for the nurse in palliative care, this is significant as what is constipation to one patient will not be constipation to another, signifying the importance of individualised care planning and assessment. There is limited evidence guiding the management of constipation or the use of laxatives in those patients with palliative care needs.

Constipation assessment

An accurate history is critical for the diagnosis and effective management of constipation and should incorporate questions about stool frequency (number of times per week), whether the patient feels they are constipated and any associated symptoms such as abdominal pain, nausea and vomiting or bloating. In considering stool consistency, the Bristol Stool Chart provides a visual description (Lewis and Heaton 1997).

Constipation can be debilitating for patients and, where possible, you should treat or prevent the symptom. It is important to review drugs that may cause constipation as well as monitor change in activities of daily living and fluid intake.

Constipation management

It is likely that most patients with advanced disease will require some drug management of constipation, however, it is also important to consider non-pharmacological interventions, such as encouraging oral fluids, where possible, increasing mobility and above all ensuring the person has privacy and can sit on a toilet/commode. The pharmacological management of constipation involves both oral and rectal laxatives as well as non-laxative medications, including peripherally restricted opioid receptor antagonists. As with all issues relating to optimal symptom control, laxatives should be prescribed, reviewed and titrated according to individual patient need and symptoms.

Laxatives may be organised according to their mode of action and whether they are predominately softening or stimulating. It is important to be aware of the adverse effects of laxatives to ensure the most appropriate medication is selected, depending on the assessment that has been undertaken. In some circumstances, rectal laxatives may be useful in patients who cannot tolerate oral laxatives or who have distal faecal impaction. Rectal laxatives include suppositories and enemas. There are occasions when non-laxative medications such as the use of prokinetics, which are medications to enhance gastrointestinal activity, are implemented to stimulate the bowel, and medications that affect constipation induced by opioids can be considered, but this is usually with the support of specialist teams such as specialist palliative care. Further information on laxatives can be sourced from palliativedrugs.com and information from the National Clinical Effectiveness Committee (DH Dublin National Clinical Effectiveness Committee 2015).

Considerations for the nurse

Ensuring privacy and dignity (NMC 2015) for the patient is paramount at this time. Environmental factors such as ease of getting to the toilet, shared bathroom facilities, or being physically comfortable to sit on the toilet in the correct position can all have an impact on constipation being relieved. Nurses are also ideally placed to anticipate those patients who may be prone to becoming constipated and to evaluate interventions for constipation, as well as being able to initiate conversations about such sensitive and, for some people, embarrassing symptoms.

Nausea and vomiting

Nausea and vomiting are unpleasant symptoms, which may be experienced by people with advanced illness. The causes are multi-factorial and management is based on the emetic pathway (Figure 8.1) or prescribing experience of the practitioner (Harris 2010; Glare et al. 2012).

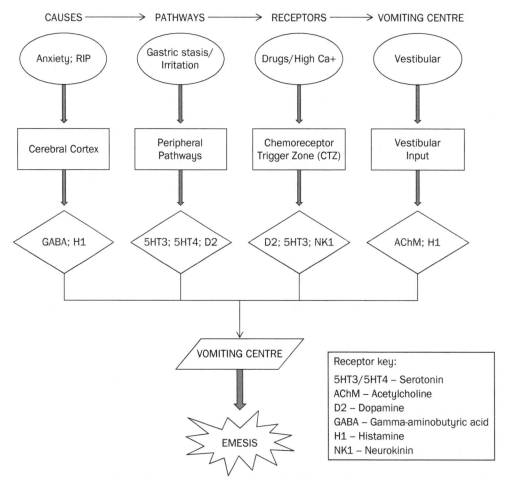

Figure 8.1 The emetic pathway
Source: Adapted from Harris (2010).

Box 8.2   Definitions of nausea and vomiting

- Nausea is 'an unpleasant feeling of the need to vomit, often accompanied by autonomic symptoms such as pallor, cold sweat, salivation, tachycardia and diarrhoea'.
- Vomiting is 'the forceful expulsion of gastric contents through the mouth through a complex reflex involving coordinated activities of the gastrointestinal tract, diaphragm and abdominal muscles' (Harris 2010).

Brief physiology of vomiting

Harmful substances ingested or an increase in the body chemicals are detected by receptors within the gastrointestinal tract and the chemoreceptor trigger zone (CTZ), which prepare the body for expulsion of the unwanted harmful substances. The CTZ is a complex neural network containing receptors, which relay messages. It is situated outside the blood-brain barrier and is therefore able to detect any circulating toxins in the blood (Harris 2010).

Vomiting assessment

Nurses are ideally situated to do a thorough and on-going assessment of nausea and vomiting. Frequently the cause is multi-factorial and the treatment should reflect this (see Table 8.2), however, in some cases, there may be no clearly identifiable cause (NICE 2016). The consequences of persistent nausea and vomiting might require correction to improve symptom control, e.g. dehydration and loss of essential electrolytes.

Interventions: pharmacological

The pharmacological management is concerned with anti-emetic drugs, which block the neurotransmitters (see Table 8.3).

Any reversible conditions, e.g. hypercalcaemia, should be treated (Harris 2010). The subcutaneous route should be considered (NICE 2016) and other anti-emetics added if required (Cox et al. 2015; Murray-Brown and Dorman 2015).

Non-pharmacological interventions

Non-pharmacological management enables control and self-management techniques. Some research has looked at acupuncture and acupressure in chemotherapy-induced nausea and vomiting. The acupressure point is stimulated by wearing a 'sea band' that is cheap, acceptable to the patient and can be married up with anti-emetics (Ezzo et al. 2006).

Table 8.2 Common anti-emetic drugs and their use

Syndrome	Causes	Emetic pathway/receptors	Drugs and dosage
Anxiety	Anticipatory Anxiety	Cerebral cortex GABA; Histamine	Lorazepam 0.5–1 mg PRN
Gastric stasis	Gastric outlet obstruction Cancer Ascites Opioids Constipation	Peripheral Serotonin Dopamine	Metoclopramide 10–20 mg TDS OR Domperidone 10–20 mg TDS + Levomepromazine 6.25–25 mg**
Gastric irritation	Bowel obstruction	Peripheral Serotonin Dopamine	Cyclizine 50 mg TDS OR Haloperidol** 1.5–3 mg BD OR Hyoscine Butylbromide 80–120 mg OD SC + Levomepromazine 6.25–25 mg OD** + Dexamethasone 8–16 mg OD AND/OR Octreotide 300–600 mcg OD SC
Biochemical	Hypercalcaemia Liver disease Bowel obstruction Opioids Chemotherapy Antibiotics	CTZ Dopamine Serotonin Neurokinin	Haloperidol** 1.5–3 mg BD OR/AND Levomepromazine** 6.25–12.5 mg OD OR Ondansetron 4–8 mg BD
Raised intracranial pressure	Cancer: – brain primary – cerebral secondary Meningeal disease Bleeding	Cerebral cortex GABA Histamine	Dexamethasone 8–12 mg OD AND Cyclizine 50 mg TDS
Vestibular	Cancer – brain primary – cerebral secondary	Vestibular input Acetylcholine Histamine	Cyclizine 50 mg TDS OR Prochloperazine 5 mg TDS

** Doses can differ by subcutaneous route.

Table 8.3 Less common anti-emetic drugs

Drug	Use
Olanzapine	Some evidence in refractory nausea and vomiting (Glare et al. 2012)
Nabilone*	Little evidence to support this and not superior to conventional anti-emetics (Peat 2010)
Erythromycin	Some prokinetic activity (Glare et al. 2012)
Aprepitant	Nausea and vomiting associated with chemotherapy (Aapro et al. 2015)

* Heavy burden of side effects.

Guided imagery or distraction can be useful for behaviour and relaxation in anticipatory nausea and vomiting (Mundy et al. 2003).

Non-surgical interventions

Alternative means of symptom management can enhance the quality of life; for example, a venting gastrostomy (if patient wants to continue eating), a percutaneous endoscopic gastrostomy (PEG) (bypasses the oesophagus/stomach) and stents (dilates oesophagus and passes any obstruction) (Glare et al. 2012).

The nursing role

Regular assessment by the nurse will determine and treat the cause or effect. Administration of drugs and consideration of all non-drug options are ideally suited to the nurse's role, followed by timely evaluation and appropriate education. Attention to the current condition is essential to address if treatment is justified. Adverse consequences of persistent nausea and vomiting must be identified and treated if necessary or appropriate, for example, dehydration. Personal individualised care of the patient is a key nursing role, alongside reassurance, care and comfort, for example, good mouth care and sipping ice cubes.

Dyspnoea (shortness of breath)

Box 8.3   Definition of dyspnoea

Dyspnoea is 'a subjective experience of breathing discomfort that consists of qualitatively distinct sensations that vary in intensity. The experience derives from interactions among multiple physiological, psychological, social and environmental factors and may induce secondary physiological and behavioral responses' (ATS 1999, p. 322).

Case Study 8.2: Danny

Danny is a 56-year-old man with colorectal cancer. He has had surgery and several courses of chemotherapy. Recently he reported feeling breathless while walking up stairs. A CT scan revealed a grossly enlarged liver pressing on his diaphragm due to metastases.

Danny had always valued his independence. Before the cancer diagnosis he had enjoyed good health, been a regular member of the gym and had participated in local sports; now the breathlessness was increasing, culminating in fatigue and weakness. This combination of symptoms significantly limited what he could manage. He felt frustrated with his lack of activity and needing to ask for help with everyday things.

Dyspnoea (shortness of breath) is an extremely debilitating symptom which can significantly affect a person's quality of life and cause notable suffering. It can be due to a malignant or non-malignant condition. There is a distinct similarity in symptoms (physical and psychosocial) and the care required but the prognosis may be different, with non-malignant conditions being slower progressing in comparison to a malignancy (Edmonds et al. 2001).

Brief physiology of dyspnoea

There are numerous stimuli that could result in dyspnoea, for example, increased cardiac/respiratory workload, resistance in the airways, weakened ventilator muscles and changes in internal gases. Dyspnoea is also believed to be influenced by signals from the motor cortex that send messages to the sensory cortex, alongside commands to the ventilator muscles (Manning and Schwartzstein 1995).

Assessment

It is important to determine whether the dyspnoea is potentially reversible (e.g. infection, anaemia, pulmonary embolism, superior vena cava obstruction, lymphangitis) or whether it is due to general deterioration.

The most commonly adopted assessment tools are the visual analogue scale (VAS) or the numerical rating scale (NRS) with points that range from 'no breathlessness' to the 'worst intensity/unpleasant breathlessness'. Other outcome measures such as the Integrated Palliative Outcome Score (IPOS) are also useful (www.pos-pal.org).

Case Study 8.2 continued: Danny's breathlessness

The enlarged liver and pressure on the diaphragm will reduce lung volume and cause breathlessness. This will result in Danny being less active and increasingly dependent on others to help him with everyday activities.

Table 8.4 Common treatments used in the management of dyspnoea

Treatment	Use
Oxygen	Reduce risk of hypoxia
Salbutamol/Terbutaline	Short-acting bronchodilators
Furosemide	Bronchodilator/diuretic
Tiotropium/Ipratropium Bromide	Long-acting bronchodilators
Carbocisteine	Mucolytic – loosens secretions
Theophylline	Bronchodilator – added if not getting benefit from optimum doses of inhaled bronchodilators
Salmeterol	Long-acting bronchodilator – may be used in combination with inhaled steroids
Opioids	Reduce sensation of breathlessness
Steroids	Reduce inflammation
Lorazepam	Relaxant
Saline	Loosen secretions

Management

Any reversible causes should be treated initially but if symptomatic relief is the aim of treatment, combining both pharmacological and non-pharmacological interventions will improve symptom burden and quality of life (Currow et al. 2013) (Table 8.4).

Pharmacological interventions

A Cochrane Review showed some evidence of clinical effect with *oral opioids* but not for the nebulised route (Barnes et al. 2015). Dosing tends to be small, for example, 5 mg sustained released morphine twice daily can be sufficient in people who respond to opioids (Currow et al. 2011). *Benzodiazepines* have been linked to the management of anxiety, though a Cochrane Review showed no evidence of beneficial effect (Simon et al. 2010).

Patients may be unable to coordinate a good *inhalation delivery* and not gain adequate benefit from the drugs. Spacers to aid inhalation or nebulised preparations of the drugs can also be used. *Steroids* can be inhaled or used as an oral preparation. They reduce local inflammation but must be reduced or stopped as soon as possible (NICE 2010). *Mucolytics* loosen secretions if patients experience chronic cough and difficulty in expectorating (NICE 2010). Similarly, *nebulised saline* is used to clear secretions and moisten the airway.

Pleural effusion (an abnormal collection of fluid in the pleural cavity) *drains* can be indwelling to prevent exposure to infection from repeated insertions There is evidence to suggest that the indwelling drains may improve breathlessness but do not necessarily prevent the accumulation of fluid (Clive et al. 2016). *Oxygen* will only be useful in patients who have hypoxia. Education regarding accumulation and retention of carbon dioxide is essential. Finally, *nebulised furosemide* limits bronchospasm and can promote mild bronchodilation (Newton et al. 2008).

Case Study 8.2 continued: Danny's drug treatment

It is likely that Danny will gain some benefit from steroids (to reduce inflammation relating to the liver metastases), opioids (to reduce the sensation of breathlessness) and benzodiazepines (to reduce any associated anxiety). Each pharmacological intervention should be introduced with support, information and adequate monitoring by the nurses.

Non-pharmacological interventions

Non-pharmacological interventions give patients control and independence. There is an armoury of techniques available, which nurses can instigate. *Fan therapy* creates a flow across the face, stimulating the skin and mucosa and causing activation of the second and third branches of the trigeminal nerve (Booth et al. 2016). *Patient-taught programmes* of breathing training, managing anxiety and panic, pacing activities and energy conservation have been shown to be advantageous for patient control and self-management techniques (Booth et al. 2012; Currow et al. 2013). Correct *body positioning* can increase lung ventilation.

Systematic reviews show limited evidence that *acupuncture or acupressure* are beneficial in dyspnoea (Towler et al. 2013), however, there has been some positive evaluation of semi-permanent indwelling studs which can be massaged by the patient (Filshie et al. 1996; Vickers et al. 2005). There is minimal evidence to show *relaxation* is effective (Bausewein et al. 2008) but it promotes positive well-being.

Non-invasive ventilation (NIV) provides additional support during recovery from exacerbations, progressive respiratory disease or repeated episodes of hypoxia and hypercapnia (carbon dioxide retention), despite optimum oxygen therapy (NICE 2010). For some patients, NIV cannot be tolerated or is not effective. As this is often the ceiling of treatment for advanced respiratory disease, this needs sensitive and careful exploration. Nurses are well placed to incorporate this into advance care planning discussions.

> ## Case Study 8.2 continued: Danny's non-pharmacological interventions
>
> Additional interventions may also benefit Danny. Positioning to ensure maximum lung ventilation and complementary therapies will encourage self-management of pacing activities that may lessen frustration by promoting enablement, resilience and independence.

The nursing role

Nurses have conducted research and been influential in many areas including assessing, monitoring and evaluating interventions, promotion of self-management programmes and maximising functionality by setting realistic goals (Bredin et al. 1999; Booth et al. 2012). They also promote timely advance care planning discussions, good inhaler technique, observe for side effects of treatment, for example, steroids (NICE 2010) and explore the patient's home circumstances and what support they require (Boland et al. 2013). Finally, nurse-led clinics embrace a holistic approach and have proved to be cost-effective, safe and improve satisfaction with follow-up in lung cancer patients (Moore et al. 2002).

> ## Case Study 8.2 continued: Danny's symptom management
>
> Danny's disease progression means he requires timely symptom management, explanation, information and support. Nurse-led care will be key to his ongoing sustainability by setting realistic goals and helping him adapt to his altered life.

The subjectivity of the symptom lends itself well to patient self-management programmes and nurse-led care. Collaborative working with the multi-professional team ensures a bespoke care plan is devised alongside the patient and their carers/family.

> ## Learning exercise 8.2
>
> Think about a patient you cared for recently who was extremely short of breath.
>
> - How did you feel, as a nurse, you were able to respond to their care needs?
> - What specific care did you deliver?
> - On reflection, how did it make you feel being with a patient when they suffered an attack of breathlessness?

Fatigue

Fatigue is one of the most common symptoms of advanced illness and can have a major impact on the patient's physical, psychological and social well-being (Radbruch et al. 2008).

Box 8.4   Definition of fatigue

Fatigue is 'a subjective feeling of tiredness, weakness or lack of energy' (Radbruch et al. 2008).

Brief physiology

The causes of fatigue are often multi-factorial and are an expected consequence of advanced illness/treatment. The most common identified factors are:

- anaemia
- electrolyte imbalance
- deconditioning – prolonged bed rest, weakness
- hypercalcaemia
- co-morbidities, e.g. diabetes, heart/lung disease
- symptoms, e.g. pain, dyspnoea, insomnia, depression
- drugs, e.g. opioids, benzodiazepines
- infection
- side effects of treatment
- poor appetite/weight loss.

Assessment

Fatigue is a subjective measure, which should be self-assessed to ascertain if it is the primary symptom (disease-related) or the secondary symptom (treatment-related). Assessment tools can measure performance status or functional capacity, including fatigue severity, level of interference in normal daily activities, onset and length of time the fatigue is experienced and underlying causes and associated problems or concerns.

If death is approaching, it may be futile to treat fatigue when this may be of benefit in sheltering the patient from unnecessary emotional distress or awareness of the dying process (Radbruch et al. 2008).

Case Study 8.2 continued: Danny's fatigue

Danny's level of fatigue should be assessed, focusing on his functionality and ability to perform activities of daily living. His fatigue may originate from a number of causes, such as possible anaemia, drug therapy, anxiety, weakness and poor appetite.

Interventions

There are few robust studies determining the value of conventional treatment for managing fatigue in advanced progressive illness but there is some evidence, both empirical and anecdotal, to support some pharmacological and non-pharmacological interventions (Payne, Wiffen and Martin 2012).

Pharmacological interventions

Trials in the use of *erythropoietin agents* have persistently shown a response to treating anaemia and reducing levels of fatigue. The limitation is that it may take up to 12 weeks to have an effect (Radbruch et al. 2008). Routine *blood transfusions* can be expensive, may require an overnight stay, can be an unnecessary burden for patients and have minimal effect, which is short-lived (Preston et al. 2012). Careful thought and discussion are necessary before embarking on this treatment.

There are limited good quality trials to support the use of *corticosteroids* but substantial anecdotal evidence reports benefits if prescribed for the shortest possible time to allow for a longed-for event, for example. a wedding, birth of a child (Radbruch et al. 2008; Begley et al. 2016).

Studies of psychostimulant drugs in the management of fatigue have shown some positive evidence (Radbruch et al. 2008). Methylphenidate is used for depression due to its fast action onset, which is particularly advantageous in this population of patients. Modafinil has shown some benefit in patients with advanced neurological diseases, for example, multiple sclerosis.

There is some evidence that Megestrol Acetate can show a rapid improvement in appetite and fatigue (Bruera et al. 1993). Vitamin D insufficiency could be significant in causing fatigue. Vitamin D supplementation should be considered in patients with advanced cancer who have low serum levels of vitamin D (Martinez-Alonso et al. 2016). Reviewing medication can be beneficial by considering the effects of polypharmacy.

Case Study 8.2 continued: Danny's therapeutic interventions

Danny may benefit from some therapeutic interactions. A course of steroids will be useful for improving his appetite and energy levels. If he is anaemic, a blood transfusion could be tried and evaluated regarding its benefits. If his fatigue was particularly troublesome for Danny, a trial of psychostimulants would be worthwhile.

Non-pharmacological interventions

Fatigue lends itself well to nurse-led self-management techniques and management. Regular and aerobic *exercise* and pacing can improve mental well-being and motivation

(Payne, Wiffen and Martin 2012). Some studies on *acupuncture* have shown promising results (Towler et al. 2013) and a multitude of *complementary therapies*, such as massage, reflexology and mindfulness, promote a sense of well-being and quality of life (Frenkel and Shah 2008).

Fatigue is frequently associated with low mood, either as a primary cause or as a result. Providing *counselling*, support and adequate and timely information regarding side effects of treatment can prepare patients for what might be expected.

Nursing care

Nurses should focus on empowering the person to become independent and pacing themselves to suit their energy levels. Encouragement and motivation are fundamental elements when exploring their goals for the future. They can play a key role in exploring expectations, creating achievable goals, providing information to understand the reasons behind fatigue, and recommending management techniques. Of equal importance is acknowledging the severity of this symptom for patients. As a previous study demonstrates, fatigue affects more patients than any other symptom and patients identify it as more important than pain or nausea/vomiting (Stone et al. 2000). Nurses have a key role in identifying and managing this symptom.

Fatigue remains an unexplored and under-researched symptom in palliative care. We have gained some knowledge and treatment options from work done in cancer but this area of care remains ripe for further nursing study.

Conclusion

This chapter has explored the most commonly experienced symptoms of pain, constipation, nausea and vomiting, dyspnoea and fatigue. Key elements of symptom management are assessment, planning and implementation of care. There should be a balance between drug therapy and non-pharmacological interventions, which will provide optimum symptom control and a tailored approach to the patient's individual needs.

The nurse's role in symptom management is key and indisputable. Nurses spend a great deal of time with patients and are well placed to observe the changes in patients as they present and to offer on-going support and interventions. They have numerous skills which complement and work in parallel with other disciplines and these should always be explored. Collaborative working ensures a holistic approach to the patient's care and avoids isolated working streams. This is governed by adequate, continuous and timely assessments which feed valuable knowledge into care planning.

Nurses have high-level communication skills which are of great benefit when considering all aspects of care. These essential qualities bring the nurse and patient closer and aid partnership working. They also allow effective patient education and information.

Nurses have started to take a lead in identifying difficult symptoms which nurses can help manage, with dyspnoea being an obvious example. The role of nurses here could be expanded to start to develop symptom research. Finally, the therapeutic relationship between nurses and patients must never be underestimated in the journey towards end of life. Forming a trusting, empathetic and responsive connection results in the achievement of goals, wishes and preferences.

References

Aapro, M., Carides, A., Rapoport, B.L. et al. (2015) Aprepitant and Fosaprepitant: a 10 year review of efficacy and safety. *The Oncologist.* doi: 10.1634/theoncologist.2014-0229 (accessed 12 July 2016).

Angheluta, A. (2011) Art therapy for chronic pain. *Canadian Journal of Counselling and Psychotherapy*, 45(2): 112–31.

ATS (American Thoracic Society) (1999) Dyspnoea – mechanisms, assessment and management: a consensus statement. *American Journal of Respiratory and Critical Care Medicine*, 159: 321–40.

Barnes, H., McDonald, J., Smallwood, N. and Manser, R. (2015) Opioids for the palliation of refractory breathlessness in adults with advanced disease and terminal illness. *Cochrane Database Systematic Review*, 3. CD011008.

Bausewein, C., Booth, S., Gysel, M. and Higginson, I. (2008) Non-pharmacological interventions for breathlessness in advanced stages of malignant and non-malignant diseases. *Cochrane Database of Systematic Review*, 2: CD005623.

Begley, S., Rose, K. and O'Connor, M. (2016) The use of corticosteroids in reducing cancer-related fatigue: assessing the evidence for clinical practice. *International Journal of Palliative Nursing*, 22(1): 5–9.

Boland, J., Martin, J., Wells, A.U. and Ross, J.R. (2013) Palliative care for people with non-malignant lung disease: summary of current evidence and future direction. *Palliative Medicine*, 27(9): 811–16.

Booth, S., Galbraith, S., Ryan, R. et al. (2016) The importance of the feasibility study: lessons from a study of the hand-held fan used to relieve dyspnoea in people who are breathless at rest. *Palliative Medicine*, 30(5): 504–9.

Booth, S., Moffat, C. and Burkin, J. (2012) *Cambridge Breathlessness Intervention Service Manual.* Addenbrookes: BIS Press. Available at: http://www.cuh.org.uk/breath lessness

Bredin, M., Corner, J., Krishnasamy, M. et al. (1999) Multicentre randomised controlled trial of nursing intervention for breathlessness in patients with lung cancer. *BMJ*, 318: 901–4. Available at: www.bmj.com/cgi/content/full/318/7188/901

Bruera, E., Ernst, S., Hagen, N. et al. (1993) Effectiveness of megestrol acetate in patients with advanced cancer: a randomised, double-blind, crossover study. *Cancer Prevention and Control*, 2(2): 74–8.

Chapman, S. (2012) Cancer pain part 2: assessment and management. *Nursing Standard*, 26(48): 44–9.

Cherkin, D.C., Sherman, K.J., Balderson, B.H. et al. (2016) Effect of mindfulness-based stress reduction vs cognitive behavioral therapy or usual care on back pain and functional limitations in adults with chronic low back pain: a randomized clinical trial. *JAMA*, 315(12): 1240–9. doi: 10.1001/jama.2016.2323.

Clark, K., Urban, K. and Currow, D.C. (2010) Current approaches to diagnosing and managing constipation in advanced cancer and palliative care. *Journal of Palliative Medicine*, 13(4): 473–6.

Clayton, H.A., Reschak, G.L., Gaynor, S.E. and Creamer, J.L. (2000) A novel program to assess and manage pain. *Medical-Surgical Nurses*, 9(6): 318–21.

Clive, A.O., Jones, H.E., Bhatnagar, R. et al. (2016) Interventions for the management of malignant pleural effusions: a network meta-analysis. *Cochrane Database of Systematic Reviews*, 5: CD010529. doi: 10.1002/14651858.CD010529.pub2.

Cox, L., Darvill, E. and Dorman, S. (2015) Levomepromazine for nausea and vomiting in palliative care. *Cochrane Database of Systematic Reviews*, 11: CD009420. doi: 10.1002/14651858.CD009420.pub

Coyle, N. (2015) Introduction to palliative care nursing. In Ferrell, B.R., Coyle, N. and Paice, J. (eds) *Oxford Textbook of Palliative Nursing* (4th edn). Oxford: Oxford University Press.

Currow, D., Higginson, I.J. and Johnson, M.J. (2013) Breathlessness – current and emerging mechanisms, measurement and management: a discussion from a European Association of Palliative Care workshop. *Palliative Medicine*, 27(10): 932–8.

Currow, D., McDonald, C., Oaten, S. et al. (2011) Once daily opioids for chronic dyspnoea: a dose increment and pharmacovigilance study. *Journal of Pain and Symptom Management*, 42(3): 388–99.

DH Dublin National Clinical Effectiveness Committee (2015) *Management of Constipation in Adult Patients Receiving Palliative Care*. National Clinical Guideline No. 10. Dublin: DH.

Edmonds, P., Karlsen, S., Khan, S. and Addington-Hall, J. (2001) A comparison of the PC needs of patients dying from chronic respiratory diseases and lung cancer. *Palliative Medicine*, 15: 287–95.

Ezzo, J., Streitberger, K. and Schneider, A. (2006) Cochrane systematic reviews examine P6 acupuncture-point stimulation for nausea and vomiting. *Journal of Alternative and Complementary Medicine*, 12(5): 489–95.

Fallon, M. and O'Neill, B. (1997) ABC of palliative care: constipation and diarrhoea. *BMJ*, 315: 1293–6.

Filshie, J., Penn, K., Ashley, S. and Davis, C.L. (1996) Acupuncture for the relief of cancer-related breathlessness. *Palliative Medicine*, 10(2): 145–50.

Frenkel, M. and Shah, V. (2008) Complementary medicine can benefit palliative care – part 1. *European Journal of Palliative Care*, 15(5): 238–43.

Glare, P., Nikolova, T., Tickoo, R. et al. (2012) An overview of anti-emetic medications for their use in palliative care. *European Journal of Palliative Care*, 19(4): 162–7.

Harris, D.G. (2010) Nausea and vomiting in advanced cancer. *British Medical Bulletin*. doi: 10.1093/bmb/ldq031 (accessed 23 August 2016).

Hui, D. and Bruera, E. (2014) A personalized approach to assessing and managing patients with cancer. *Journal of Clinical Oncology*, 32(16): 1640–6.

IASP (International Association for the Study of Pain) (1996) Classification of chronic pain. *Pain*, 3(Suppl.).

IASP (International Association for the Study of Pain) (2009) *Global Year against Cancer Pain.* Washington, DC: IASP.

Jacob, J.A. (2016) As opioid prescribing guidelines tighten, mindfulness meditation holds promise for pain relief. *JAMA*, 315(22): 2385–7.

Larkin, P. J., Sykes, N. P., Centeno, C. et al. (2008) The management of constipation in palliative care: clinical practice recommendations. *Palliative Medicine*, 22: 796–807.

Lewis, S. and Heaton, K. (1997) Stool form scale as a useful guide to intestinal transit time. *Scandinavian Journal of Gastroenterology*, 32(9): 920–4.

Mackintosh, C.L. and Elson, S. (2008) Chronic pain: clinical features, assessment and treatment. *Nursing Standard*, 23(5): 48–56.

Mann, E. (2008) Neuropathic pain: could nurses become more involved? *British Journal of Nursing*, 17(19): 1208–13.

Manning, H.L. and Schwartzstein, R.M. (1995). Pathophysiology of dyspnoea: mechanisms of disease. *New England Journal of Medicine*, 333(23): 1547–53.

Martinez-Alonso, M., Dusso, A., Ariza, G. and Nabal, M. (2016) Vitamin D deficiency and its association with fatigue and quality of life in advanced cancer patients under palliative care: a cross-sectional study. *Palliative Medicine*, 30(1): 89–96.

Moore, S., Corner, J., Haviland, J. et al. (2002) Nurse led follow up and conventional medical follow up in management of patients with lung cancer: randomised trial. *British Medical Journal*, 325: 1145–55.

Mundy, E.A., DuHamel, K.N. and Montgomery, G.H. (2003) The efficacy of behavioural interventions for cancer treatment-related side effects. *Seminars in Clinical Neuropsychiatry*, 8(4): 253–75.

Murray-Brown, F. and Dorman, S. (2015) Haloperidol for the treatment of nausea and vomiting in palliative care patients. *Cochrane Database of Systematic Reviews*, 11: CD006271. doi: 10.1002/14651858.CD006271.pub3.

Newton, P., Davidson, P.M., Macdonald, P. et al. (2008) Nebulised furosemide for the management of dyspnoea: does the evidence support its use? *Journal of Pain and Symptom Management*, 36(4): 424–41.

NICE (National Institute for Clinical Excellence) (2010) *COPD: Management of COPD in Adults in Primary and Secondary Care.* Clinical Guideline No. 101. London. NICE.

NICE (National Institute for Health and Care Excellence) (2012) *Opioids in Palliative Care: Safe and Effective Prescribing of Strong Opioids for Pain in Palliative Care of Adults*, CG140. London: NICE. Available at: www.nice.org.uk/guidance/CG140

NICE (National Institute for Health and Care Excellence) (2016) *Palliative Care – Nausea and Vomiting*: Clinical Knowledge Summary. London: NICE.

Nicholson, B. (2006) Differential diagnosis: nociceptive and neuropathic pain. *American Journal of Managed Care*, 12(9 Suppl.): 256–62.

Nursing and Midwifery Council (2015) *The Code: Standards of Conduct, Performance and Ethics for Nurses and Midwives.* London: Nursing and Midwifery Council.

Orenius, T., Koskela, T., Koho, P. et al. (2013) Anxiety and depression are independent predictors of quality of life of patients with chronic musculoskeletal pain. *Journal of Health Psychology*, 18(2): 167–75.

Payne, C., Wiffen, P.J. and Martin, S. (2012) Interventions for fatigue and weight loss in adults with advanced progressive illness. *Cochrane Database of Systematic Reviews*, 1: CD008427. doi: 10.1002/14651858.CD008427.pub2.

Peat, S. (2010) Using cannabinoids in pain and palliative care. *International Journal of Palliative Nursing*, 16(10): 481–5.

Persson, C. (2014) Music can relieve chronic pain. *Science Nordic*, Available at: http://sciencenordic.com/music-can-relieve-chronic-pain

Potter, J., Hami, F., Bryan, T. and Quigley, C. (2003). Symptoms in 400 patients referred to palliative care services: prevalence and patterns. *Palliative Medicine*, 17: 310–14.

Preston, N.J., Hurlow, A., Brine, J. and Bennett, M.I. (2012) Blood transfusions for anaemia in patients with advanced cancer. *Cochrane Database of Systematic Reviews*, 2: CD009007. doi: 10.1002/14651858.CD009007.pub2.

Radbruch, L., Strasser, F., Elsner, F. et al. for the Research Steering Committee of the European Association for Palliative Care (EAPC) (2008) Fatigue in palliative care patients: an EAPC approach. *Palliative Medicine*, 22: 13–32.

Reynolds, J., Drew, D. and Dunwoody, C. (2013) American Society for Pain Management Nursing position statement: pain management at the end of life. *Pain Management Nursing*, 14(3): 172–5. doi: 10.1016/j.pmn.2013.07.002.

Royal College of Nursing (2015) *Pain Knowledge and Skills Framework for the Nursing Team*. London: RCN.

Schaffer, S. and Yucha, C. (2004) Relaxation and pain management: the relaxation response can play a role in managing chronic and acute pain. *American Journal of Nursing*, 104(8): 75–82.

Simon, S., Higginson, I., Booth, S. et al. (2010) Benzodiazepines for the relief of breathlessness in advanced malignant and non-malignant diseases in adults. *Cochrane Database of Systematic Reviews*, 10: CD007354. doi: 10.1002/14651858.CD007354.pub2.

Stone, P., Richardson, A., Ream, E. et al. (2000) Cancer related fatigue: inevitable, unimportant and untreatable? Results of a multi-centre patient survey. Cancer Fatigue Forum. *Annals of Oncology*, 11(8): 971–5.

Swarm, R., Abernethy, A.P., Anghelescu, D.L. et al. (2010) Adult cancer pain. *Journal of the National Comprehensive Cancer Network*, 8: 1046–86.

Sykes, N. (1998) The relationship between opioid use and laxative use in terminally ill cancer patients. *Palliative Medicine*, 12: 375–82.

Tang, Y.Y. and Leve, L.D. (2016) A translational neuroscience perspective on mindfulness meditation: a prevention strategy. *Translational Behavioural Medicine*, 6(1): 63–72.

Towler, P., Molassiotis, A. and Brearley, S.G. (2013) What is the evidence for the use of acupuncture as an intervention for symptom management in cancer supportive and palliative care? An integrative overview of reviews. *Supportive Care Cancer*, 21: 2913–23.

Twycross, R., Wilcock, A. and Howard, P. (2014) *Palliative Care Formulary*. Available at: www.Palliative Drugs.com

Vaajoki, A., Pietilä, A.M., Kankkunen, P. and Vehviläinen-Julkunen, K. (2012) Effects of listening to music on pain intensity and pain distress after surgery: an intervention. *Journal of Clinical Nursing*, 21(5–6): 708–17.

Vickers, A.J., Feinstein, M.B., Deng, G.E. and Cassileth, B.R. (2005) Acupuncture for dyspnoea in advanced cancer: a randomised, placebo-controlled pilot trial. *BMC Palliative Care*, 4: 5. doi: 10.1186/1472-684X-4-5.

Walsh, D., Mahmoud, F.A. and Sarhill, N. (2001) Parenteral opioid rotation in advanced cancer: a prospective study. *Supportive Care in Cancer*, 9(307): 14–15.

World Health Organization (1996) *Cancer Pain Relief* (2nd edn) (with a guide to opioid availability). Geneva: World Health Organization.

Psychological symptoms and the promotion of psychological well-being

Craig A. White

Introduction

This chapter will outline a broad definition of psychological distress that can be used to consider nursing assessment and intervention in palliative care. It will include some of the issues to be considered during assessment and summarise some of the psychological processes known to influence effective care and support planning. It is important that nurses working in palliative care, who have a key role to play in conducting an assessment of the patient's state of mind, are confident and have a comprehensive understanding of the range of ways in which psychological factors can influence adjustment to the sorts of conditions that often require the provision of palliative care. The wide range of psychological processes and issues raised by individual experience of progressive life-limiting disease can mean that psychological issues are less well represented in planning care. Coordination and communication about the physical dimensions of people's experiences and care planning are often easier for nurses as there is a widespread commonly accepted understanding of terminology, concepts and interventions.

Understanding distress

Increasing medical advances have meant that more people than ever before are living longer with a range of medical conditions (Roser 2017). Almost everyone who is told that they have a condition that will be life-limiting or life-shortening will experience a period of shock and psychological distress. For the majority of people, this will be a self-limiting experience, which does not cause any lasting psychological symptoms or problems and which can be understood as part of a so-called 'normal' adjustment reaction. However, some people will experience more severe psychological distress, requiring specific help to understand how to manage the distress.

Psychological distress is a well-recognised feature of people's response to the diagnosis of a progressive incurable physical disease. Although there has been some debate in the literature about the conceptual basis for distress, the definition of the National Comprehensive Cancer Network is still very helpful as a basis for considering care delivery across a wide range of clinical conditions and presentations:

> A multifactorial unpleasant emotional experience of a psychological (cognitive, behavioral, emotional), social and/or spiritual nature that may interfere with the ability to cope effectively with cancer, its physical symptoms, and its treatments. Distress extends along a continuum, ranging from common normal feelings of vulnerability, sadness, and fears to problems that can become disabling, such as depression, anxiety, panic, social isolation, and existential and spiritual crisis.
>
> (Holland et al. 2010, p. 450)

This definition has general application across a range of conditions, reflecting as it does the holistic nature of palliative care nursing and taking account of the need to consider emotional responses to life events, guarding against the tendency to consider everything through a biomedical lens. Currently available estimates suggest that around 1 in 4 people will experience these more severe levels of distress (Snowden et al. 2011). White (2016a) has outlined that distress is more common among the following groups of people:

- those of a younger age;
- people who are single and live alone;
- patients with children still living at home.

Other factors that can increase distress are:

- when illness co-occurs with economic adversity;
- there is perceived lack of social support;
- poor marital or family functioning;
- among people who have a prior history of psychiatric problems, several previously stressful life events and a history of alcohol or other substance abuse.

This has also been confirmed recently by Costantini et al. (2015).

Clinically significant psychological problems usually occur as part of an adjustment disorder, a major depressive disorder, or one of the anxiety disorders such as Post Traumatic Stress Disorder (White and Macleod 2002).

As White (2016a) has outlined:

Many people have to face treatment regimes that are difficult to tolerate, that require frequent hospital visits and levels of motivation that can be difficult to generate or sustain. Non-physical treatment side effects such as anger, anxiety or apprehension are often rated by patients as being more severe than physical side effects.

However, advances in drug therapies have resulted in a reduction in the incidence of side effects for many of the medications used in palliative care settings. Neuropsychological symptoms may need to be considered and specific consideration of detailed assessment of areas such as sexual functioning should be included in comprehensive nursing assessments. Physical symptoms such as fatigue are commonly linked to related problems with sleep and both need to be understood in terms of emotional, social and practical dimensions of quality of life (Wagland et al. 2016).

Psychologically sensitive assessments

Part of the nursing role can be to provide a psychologically sensitive assessment. The process of including psychological factors and impact within a nursing assessment can be therapeutic itself, particularly for a patient who has not had an opportunity to talk about their experiences. Nurses should not underestimate the therapeutic value that can be gained from an assessment that has been sensitively conducted. The timing and arrangements made for assessment need to be taken into account, for example, nurses should consider the impact of assessment activity that takes place in the presence of a relative, as it is common for the patient to 'censor' what they disclose for fear of causing further distress to their relative, whom they know is already distressed by what they have been experiencing (Applebaum et al. 2016).

Assessments should therefore always include the offer of a time when the person would be able to speak with the nurse in private. Nursing assessment should aim to focus on what matters most to the people who are receiving care (as opposed to the regrettably still too common 'What's wrong with you?' emphasis that still dominates many of the care systems and processes). This is of course not to ignore that fact that a nursing assessment needs to be informed and influenced by what is known clinically about the conditions being experienced by someone – emphasis on what matters and who matters to people will ultimately lead to a more sensitive psychological assessment.

It has been suggested that there are too many instances where assessment and care planning for psychological care and symptoms in nursing and medicine are approached with no rationale, frame of reference or model to guide what is considered. Perhaps more importantly when it comes to making sense of information and synthesising for care planning, what happens with the information that is used is often unclear. In some circumstances the application of clinical tools can enhance assessment and care planning. Screening assessments and patient-reported outcome measures can be effective in identifying unmet need, facilitating communication and supporting the monitoring of outcomes over time.

Hudson et al. (2016) have reviewed what is available and recommend clinical tools that assist with assessment and care planning of specialist palliative care provision (Table 9.1). They highlighted the benefits of supporting delivery of a consistent

Table 9.1 Overview of clinical tools recommended for widespread use

Domain of Palliative Care	Clinical Tool	Initial/Screening Assessment	Comprehensive Assessment	Follow-Up	Special Situation	Reference
Multidomain assessment/needs assessment	Problem Severity Score	✓		✓		Palliative Care Outcomes Collaboration (2011) (www.pcoc.org.au)
	Distress Thermometer	✓		✓		National Comprehensive Cancer Network (2015) (www.nccn.org)
Pain	Initial Pain Assessment Tool		✓			McCaffery and Pasero (1999)
Family/caregiver	Carer Support Needs Assessment Tool		✓			Ewing and Grande (2012)
Emotional distress	GHQ12		✓			Goldberg (1978)
Spirituality	FICA Spiritual History Tool		✓			George Washington Institute for Spirituality and Health (2015)
Symptoms	Symptom Assessment Scale	✓		✓		Palliative Care Outcomes Collaboration (2010) (www.pcoc.org.au)
Performance/function	Australian-modified KPS	✓				Abernethy (2005)
Quality of life	FACIT-PAL	✓				FACIT.org (2015) (www.facit.org)
Prognosis	PaP				✓	Glare et al. (2003)
	PPI				✓	Stone et al. (2008)
Care of dying patient	Liverpool Care Pathway				✓	Marie Curie Palliative Care Institute (2015)

Reprinted with permission from Hudson et al. (2016).

approach to care. Nurses in palliative care could consider how the testing of the implementation of such tools might influence the delivery of clinical excellence, particularly through supporting the consistent and reliable delivery of comprehensive assessments that minimise the sort of variation that can exist through individual differences in knowledge level, confidence and the wide range of human factors that influence what people include in their assessments.

Learning exercise 9.1

Take some time to think about the way that you assess distress, pain and carer support needs currently. Consider how you might locate a copy of one of the clinical tools that Hudson et al. (2016) recommend and set aside some time to review one improvement you could make to your approach to assessment. For example, you might seek to add in a new question you ask the next patient about their coping with distressing symptoms.

Moving beyond symptom presence

Nursing assessments often stop at the point where psychological symptoms or distress are identified, missing out on the opportunity to explore their expression. Symptoms fluctuate in intensity from moment to moment and hour to hour and it is helpful to measure this variation. Nurses need to be able to consider and then account for the factors that seem to influence the changes in symptom frequency and intensity. This can also provide a good opportunity to determine tolerance thresholds for the experience of key symptoms (such as times when the same symptom is experienced differently from a psychological perspective). Using descriptive examples from different times can engage people in understanding the importance of cross-situational factors that will influence their overall response to illness. Patients who have become preoccupied by illness and its impact often report that their lives are 'ruled' by it (Hundt et al. 2015). This can then lead to the establishment of links with prior beliefs or thoughts that determine current behaviours. Prospective monitoring over a range of situations can begin to unpack the basis for beliefs with the potential for pervasive impact.

Illness perceptions are key determinants of interactions with care delivery systems (Rutter and Rutter 2002; Ashley et al. 2013; Baines and Wittkowski 2013). White (2016b) has emphasised how the core of most adjustment, anxiety and mood disorders relates to personal threat, danger, loss and an inability to cope with such threatening or dangerous situations. Assessments should feature everything that is spontaneously offered by the patient as a concern. Other elements not disclosed should be screened, taking account of illness-specific factors.

Interpersonal factors that relate to interactions with and relationships to professional caregivers should be considered. Family functioning should be assessed by examining the issues of cohesion, team work, openness of communication and conflict resolution (Merz and Consedine 2009). This is important because family interactions are often increased during episodes of physical ill health and may therefore buffer or precipitate crises (Rosland and Piette 2010). Family members are often vital as support during the care provided in acute hospital settings. Lack of social support is a well-established risk factor for negative health outcomes (including mortality) and vulnerability to psychological distress (Cohen and Wills 1985).

Care and support planning should consider whether psychological symptoms might be primarily the result of a medical factor. For example, someone who has a biochemically mediated anxiety reaction is unlikely to benefit from strategies designed to reduce autonomic arousal or challenge thoughts relating to panic. Conversely, the same applies to psychological symptoms that are conceptualised solely from a biological or biomedical viewpoint. For instance, prescribing anxiolytic medication or ignoring the individual style of thinking, way of coping or relationship support will most likely result in only a partial reduction in the severity of anxiety (Watts et al. 2015).

Meaning is a concept that is often mentioned in respect of psychological adjustment in palliative care settings, though its practical integration into assessment protocols and care planning is often difficult. Illness challenges people's views of the world. 'What it all means' is a common focus of thinking. The nurse should find ways of engaging with what matters most to people as this is often the route to enabling them to make sense of what is most personally meaningful in their illness experience (Haugan 2014).

A revision of priorities in life and the establishment of new motivational structures may have taken place. Coward (1997) has referred to a process of 'severe spiritual disequilibrium' and suggests that the process of searching for meaning is a response to this state. It has been proposed that psychological adjustment is more likely when there can be an integration of illness experiences into what is sometimes referred to as a 'pre-existing mental model' (Lepore and Helgeson 2011). O'Connor, Wicker and Germino (1990) helpfully describe the process of searching for meaning as reflective of there being questions posed 'in order to give the experience purpose and to place it in the context of a total life pattern'. While there are some people who are able to retain feelings of self-control and worth throughout their experience of progressive incurable physical disease, there are a substantial minority for whom loss of control can become a significant issue influencing adjustment. Nursing assessments and interventions can provide a useful way of empowering people to take control of the areas of their life that illness has negatively influenced.

Social and family support can act as a significant personal resource for many patients, yet for others the lack of such support leads to feelings of isolation and loneliness (Mushtaq et al. 2014). It is important that nurses, therefore, identify what if any social support patients have. Nursing care and support interventions may need to ensure that the negative impact of loneliness is considered an important part of planning care. Useful questions to explore these issues and incorporate into nursing assessment and care include: 'Has your illness had an effect on your relationships with other people?' or 'How have your relationships with other people affected how you have been feeling emotionally?' Some relatives of patients are more distressed than the person they are caring for, something that should be borne in mind when conducting an initial assessment. The way in which other clinical and care staff have interacted with the person will often be significant and should be assessed. This can become very significant in terms of beliefs about staff sensitivity and support (crucial when it comes to later efforts to access supportive care) and the fact that distress in the early months after a diagnosis is predictive of later levels of distress.

Most patients want to be fully informed about their care and treatment (Jenkins, Fallowfield and Saul 2001). Satisfaction with the information provided also is a very significant determinant of overall psychosocial adjustment. It is important that nurses ensure that people are asked about their current level of understanding of their illness and treatment. This can reveal misconceptions and information needs that then become a key factor in subsequent intervention. Experience of physical ill health can result in the recall of a number of memories of physical illness within families, and thus the following questions may be helpful: 'Do you find that you get unwanted thoughts about illness? Have you experienced more memories of times that you or your loved ones have been ill?' (Brewin et al. 1998). Images often have their origins in life events such as a relative who was unwell, witnessing another person in a care setting with the same illness or re-experiencing events from earlier care experiences, such as the recall of statements that have been made by medical or nursing staff. The occurrence and frequency of intrusive memories and thoughts about illness experiences should be assessed. It is crucial to take time to explore any images and in particular to consider any personally salient fears or concerns reflected within them.

Some people survive by developing a global avoidance strategy. This can make assessment difficult (as this involves reversal of avoidance). Avoidance is often a key maintaining factor for problems associated with anxiety and depression. This should be distinguished from denial, as the concepts used in formulation and the strategies which are used to manage each are different. Avoidant patients differ from those in denial, as they know that they have cancer and choose not to think about this. This can usually easily be determined by asking patients, 'What is your understanding of what disease you have?', or in some cases the more direct, 'Do you think you have an incurable illness?'

Learning exercise 9.2

Think about one of your recent patients that you have provided care to, and reviewing the information in the section 'Moving beyond symptom presence', list some of the ways in which you can integrate an expanded range of issues into nursing assessment process, care and support planning.

Significant numbers of people will have experienced anxiety and depressive symptoms prior to their diagnosis. Katz, Rodin and Devins (1995) state: 'The integration of the illness into the self-concept without undue loss of self-esteem may protect those with serious medical illnesses from clinical depression.' White (2016a) outlined how information on someone's self-esteem is often key and should inform screening questions such as 'How do you feel about yourself compared to other people?' or 'Do you ever feel worthless?'

White (2016a) has previously emphasised how the following factors need to be borne in mind when considering clinical assessment and care management:

- positive contributions in providing emotional support;
- family composition outlined in a 'family tree' diagram (taking account of age and developmental life stage);
- levels of knowledge, support and involvement (taking account of frequency of contact, practical support and confiding relationships);
- family myths or views of the world (in terms of constructs such as fair, safe, predictable);
- lifelong copying styles;
- exposure to physical ill health and nursing care delivery.

People often have to manage uncertainty about their future, search for meaning, deal with loss of control, and address the need for openness about illness and vulnerability. Some people have unrealistic perceptions, for example, overly optimistic or inappropriately pessimistic views regarding their illness and its treatment. This can lead to problems, particularly when it becomes clear that their perception of their illness is at odds with information from other sources. Expectations tend to influence emotional reactions in response to new events. When symptoms recur, patients who did not expect recurrence tend to be more distressed than those who at some level did expect it. When patient expectations and perceptions are included within a formulation, it is important to outline the hypothesised contributors to the perception (e.g. a long-standing avoidant coping style, the presence of severe distress at the time of information provision). White (2016b) described how information on the range of triggering factors, both internal (e.g. physical symptoms, memory of prior illness) and external (e.g. hospital attendance, comment by family member) should be considered for each of the presenting problems within a formulation.

Generally speaking, people who engage in greater levels of avoidance of memories experience greater levels of anxiety. Sometimes people have had previous psychological problems or are still experiencing these at the point when they encounter physical health problems. Events within people's earlier personal histories can resurface during illness experiences and related care and support planning. Issues relating to separation, abandonment or mistrust can influence the psychological experiences of some patients.

Given the pivotal role of social, partner and family support in coping with adjustment to illness, nurses need to include this in assessments and the linked care and support planning work they undertake. Feelings of helplessness, hopelessness, procrastination or a lack of opportunity to socialise, or sometimes anxiety can all contribute to isolation and loneliness. Sometimes friends and relatives may avoid people because of their own difficulties in making sense of the events. When relatives are uncertain about how best to help the patient, nurses may need to arrange to provide advice on practical strategies and on how to overcome some of the obstacles to providing support.

What to do with the psychosocial information?

Although first presented for psychologists and psychiatrists wishing to improve the way they conceptualised psychological problems occurring in the context of physical health problems, the following checklist by White (2016b) can also be applied to nursing assessment (and has been adapted here for this purpose):

- Determine a list that covers all of the presenting physical, psychological, social and interpersonal problems, issues or concerns reported.
- Use this to identify which ones require more detailed exploration and consideration as part of a nursing assessment. This could form part of the way in which nurses would identify areas where they have a specific professional responsibility to conduct further nursing assessment or where they need to highlight the need to another appropriately qualified person.
- Consider all of the information that is available and, then, through consideration of what matters most to the person concerned, begin to look at the ways in which the various areas are linked and what support they might wish in respect of each.

Some families have difficulty modifying their initial response to the illness when the acute phase has passed (Kreutzer et al. 2002). It is important to keep this in mind, with particular emphasis on the extent to which these responses seem to take account of changes in illness course, treatment or prognosis.

Integrating psychological care into care and support planning

Psychodynamic psychotherapy can help people understand the links between unresolved childhood conflicts and current relationships. Physical ill-health can often foster feelings of dependency that have been felt at other times in their lives. Sometimes people idealise caregivers or may become extremely angry when the nurturance they seek is not experienced. Nurses working in palliative care need to ensure that they consider the ways in which attachment and experience of relationships throughout a person's life might influence the way in which they expect to experience caregiver relationships in illness.

Nurses may develop what are referred to as counter-transference feelings, that is, emotional responses to the patient that may be rooted in their own needs and conflicts. Nursing staff may feel out of control and helpless to impact positively on the people they are caring for. White (2016a) has proposed that it can be helpful to stop and think about what the person being cared for's deepest unexpressed feelings could be and discuss within the wider team how it might be possible to help them understand and process those feelings. When someone does not need to expend emotional energy defending against feelings, they are better able to cope with illness-related distress. Nurses should consider whether conflict and the expression of these within current relationships may need to be a central element of care planning.

Care and support planning may need to seek to enhance communication and facilitate interpersonal relationships that are sensitive to the emotional and psychological dimensions of the family member who is unwell. The focus in care and support planning often needs to be on enabling people to tackle avoidance of communication, particularly on emotionally charged topics such as death. Families may need support to ensure that illness does not become a dominant feature in influencing all relationships and responses to everyday events. It could help with care planning to focus on the identification of shared assets and to engage in a process whereby people can begin to prioritise the problems that face them or consider how they might have untapped resources that could be used to address problems.

Nurses need to consider how to support people to maintain a degree of stability, ensuring that the non-medical needs are met throughout care. However, clinical and care staff may need to devote time too to reinforcing the non-medical needs of the person being cared for (and possibly those of key family members, especially those of young children).

Conclusion

Nurses working in palliative care are uniquely placed to identify the very personal aspects of experience of a progressive incurable disease, supporting the patient through their assessment and discovering what matters most to the person being cared for, and moving beyond descriptions of psychological symptoms of distress to truly appreciating the ways in which a wider range of psychosocial factors influence coping, adjustment and quality of life. This knowledge can then be used in caring for people in a person-centred way, ensuring that psychological care and support plans empower the patients to live their lives in the way they wish for as long as they are able to.

References

Applebaum, A.J., Kryza-Lacombe, M., Buthorn, J. et al. (2016) Existential distress among caregivers of patients with brain tumors: a review of the literature. *Neuro-Oncology Practice*, 3(4): 232–44.

Ashley, L., Smith, A.B., Keding, A. et al. (2013) Psychometric evaluation of the revised Illness Perception Questionnaire (IPQ-R) in cancer patients: confirmatory factor analysis and Rasch analysis. *Journal of Psychosomatic Research*, 75(6): 556–62.

Baines, T. and Wittkowski, A. (2013) A systematic review of the literature exploring illness perceptions in mental health utilising the self-regulation model. *Journal of Clinical Psychology in Medical Settings*, 20(3): 263–74.

Brewin, C.R., Watson, M., McCarthy, S. et al. (1998) Intrusive memories and depression in cancer patients. *Behaviour Research and Therapy*, 36(12): 1131–42.

Cohen, S. and Wills, T.A. (1985) Stress, social support, and the buffering hypothesis. *Psychological Bulletin*, 98(2): 310–57.

Costantini, A., Grassi, L., Picardi, A. et al. (2015) Awareness of cancer, satisfaction with care, emotional distress, and adjustment to illness: an Italian multicenter study. *Psycho-Oncology*, 24(9): 1088–96.

Coward, D.D. (1997) Constructing meaning from the experience of cancer. *Seminars in Oncology Nursing*, 13(4): 248–51.

Haugan, G. (2014) Meaning-in-life in nursing-home patients: a valuable approach for enhancing psychological and physical well-being? *Journal of Clinical Nursing*, 23(13–14): 1830–44.

Holland, J.C., Andersen, B., Breitbart, W.S. et al. (2010) Distress management: clinical practice guidelines in oncology™. *Journal of the National Comprehensive Cancer Network*, 8(4): 448–85.

Hudson, P., Collins, A., Bostanci, A. et al. (2016) Toward a systematic approach to assessment and care planning in palliative care: a practical review of clinical tools. *Palliative and Supportive Care*, 14(2): 161–73.

Hundt, N.E., Bensadon, B.A., Stanley, M.A. et al. (2015) Coping mediates the relationship between disease severity and illness intrusiveness among chronically ill patients. *Journal of Health Psychology*, 20(9): 1186–95.

Jenkins, V., Fallowfield, L. and Saul, J. (2001) Information needs of patients with cancer: results from a large study in UK cancer centres. *British Journal of Cancer*, 84(1): 48–51.

Katz, M.R., Rodin, G. and Devins, G.M. (1995) Self-esteem and cancer: theory and research. *Canadian Journal of Psychiatry*, 40(10): 608–15.

Kreutzer, J.S., Kolakowsky-Hayner, S.A., Demm, S.R. and Meade, M.A. (2002) A structured approach to family intervention after brain injury. *Journal of Head Trauma Rehabilitation*, 17(4): 349–67.

Lepore, S.J. and Helgeson, V.S. (2011) Social constraints, intrusive thoughts, and mental health after prostate cancer. *Journal of Social and Clinical Psychology*, 17(1): 89–106.

Merz, E.M. and Considine, N.S. (2009) The association of family support and wellbeing in later life depends on adult attachment style. *Attachment & Human Development*, 11(2): 203–21.

Mushtaq, R., Shoib, S., Shah, T. and Mushtaq, S. (2014) Relationship between loneliness, psychiatric disorders and physical health? A review on the psychological aspects of loneliness. *Journal of Clinical and Diagnostic Research*, 8(9): WE01–04.

O'Connor, A.P., Wicker, C.A. and Germino, B.B. (1990) Understanding the cancer patient's search for meaning. *Cancer Nursing*, 13(3): 167–75.

Roser, M. (2017) Life expectancy. Available at: https://ourworldindata.org/life-expectancy/ (accessed 9 May 2017).

Rosland, A.M. and Piette, J.D. (2010) Emerging models for mobilizing family support for chronic disease management: a structured review. *Chronic Illness*, 6(1): 7–21.

Rutter, C.L. and Rutter, D.R. (2002) Illness representation, coping and outcome in irritable bowel syndrome (IBS). *British Journal of Health Psychology*, 7(4): 377–91.

Snowden, A., White, C.A., Christie, Z. et al. (2011) The clinical utility of the distress thermometer: a review. *British Journal of Nursing*, 20(4): 220–7.

Wagland, R., Richardson, A., Ewings, S. et al. (2016) Prevalence of cancer chemotherapy-related problems, their relation to health-related quality of life and associated supportive care: a cross-sectional survey. *Supportive Care in Cancer*, 24(12): 4901–11.

Watts, S.E., Turnell, A., Kladnitski, N. et al. (2015) Treatment-as-usual (TAU) is anything but usual: a meta-analysis of CBT versus TAU for anxiety and depression. *Journal of Affective Disorders*, 175: 152–67.

White, C.A. (2016a) Cancer. In Carr, A. and McNulty, M. (eds) *The Handbook of Adult Clinical Psychology: An Evidence Based Practice Approach*. London: Routledge.

White, C.A. (2016b) Physical health problems. In Tarrier, N. and Johnson, J. (eds) *Case Formulation in Cognitive Behaviour Therapy: The Treatment of Challenging and Complex Cases*. London: Routledge.

White, C.A. and Macleod, U. (2002) ABC of psychological medicine: cancer. *British Medical Journal*, 325(7360): 377–80.

Spirituality, spiritual care and the role of nurses in palliative care

Hamilton Inbadas

Spiritual care has been recognised as an important aspect of palliative care that contributes to the overall well-being of the persons receiving care and their families. It has been widely acknowledged that patients facing death and their loved ones are confronted with spiritual and existential distress. The philosophy of palliative care recognises the criticality of spiritual pain at the end of life and includes it as part of the sum of the experiences that patients undergo. Cicely Saunders, the founder of the modern hospice movement, emphasised this in recognising spiritual pain as a significant part of the suffering patients experienced at the end of life, which she conceived as 'total pain', consisting of physical, psychological, social and spiritual aspects (Saunders 1996; Clark 1999). To explore the place of spiritual care in palliative care, it is necessary to understand the concept of spirituality, its significance at the end of life, as well as available methods and tools for addressing spiritual distress.

This chapter begins with describing the concept of spirituality, particularly in the context of the end of life by exploring how it is defined in academic discourses and by addressing issues pertaining to its relationship with religion. This will be followed by sections on manifestations of spiritual needs and approaches and tools available for dealing with spiritual distress. Following a section on aspects of providing spiritual care at the end of life the chapter will conclude with an analysis of the role of nurses in palliative care.

In order to address the various aspects of total pain that patients experience at the end of life, palliative care offers the framework of 'total care', which has four components: the physical, psychological, social and spiritual (Twycross 2003). However, in practice, several authors have observed a hierarchy of these four, starting from the physical to the spiritual, where spiritual care receives the least attention and remains the least developed component of the total care that palliative care promises to provide (Puchalski 2009; Rajagopal 2010). Larkin rightly observes that spiritual care is often 'subsumed under the concept of psychosocial care' and therefore lacking the attention needed to understand and adequately support complex spiritual issues (2010, p. 336).

Understanding spirituality

The literature on the subject of spirituality in healthcare reveals that defining 'spirituality' is a challenging task. The notion of spirituality either does not seem to neatly fit into any one description or it tends to lose significance when broadened to include the wide range of elements it incorporates (McSherry and Cash 2004; Gunaratnam and Oliviere 2009). Due to the multiplicity of ways in which spirituality is described, there seems to be an increasing awareness that the only point of agreement we can arrive at is to accept the conceptual ambiguity of spirituality (Sinclair et al. 2006). However, several authors have stressed the need for a definition, in order to promote the understanding of spirituality among healthcare professionals and to help recognise and appropriately care for patients (Vachon et al. 2009).

Several definitions of spirituality can be found and they all represent a multifaceted understanding of spirituality: 'Spirituality is the inner essence of life', 'a dimension of the whole person', that is integral to and interacts with all other aspects of life, both physical and psychosocial (Wright 1998; Dom 1999; Carroll 2001; Narayanasamy 2006b). It is the aspect of life that gives meaning and purpose to life and facilitates self-transcendence (Puchalski 2007; Vachon et al. 2009). Spirituality involves a relationship with God, others, nature and oneself (Dyson et al. 1997; Hermann 2001; Narayanasamy 2010). Spirituality thus offers the possibility of a sense of identity and wholeness in life. A recent consensus conference proposed the following definition of spirituality, which attempts to bring these various dimensions together:

> Spirituality is a dynamic and intrinsic aspect of humanity through which persons seek ultimate meaning, purpose, and transcendence, and experience relationship to self, family, others, community, society, nature, and the significant or sacred. Spirituality is expressed through beliefs, values, traditions, and practices.
>
> (Puchalski et al. 2014, p. 646)

All these definitions seem to suggest that 'relationship' (to self, others and the significant/sacred other) is at the heart of spirituality. Dean Ornish's definition of spirituality amply captures this thought: 'When I use the word spirituality, . . . I mean whatever it is that helps you feel connected to something that is larger than yourself' (cited in Dunklee 2011, p. 62). Definitions of spirituality, therefore, suggest that spirituality is this 'feeling of connectedness' or 'experiencing a relationship' with something or someone that provides meaning and purpose to life and forms the essence of human life.

Religion and spirituality

The relationship between religion and spirituality is an often-debated question in the study of spirituality. While some scholars argue that a belief in God and participation in religious rituals positively contribute to the well-being and coping of patients, others have cautioned that religion could cause negative consequences in the context of spiritual care at the end of life (Dein and Stygall 1997; Hermsen and ten Have 2004). Some argue that attention to the spiritual dimension adds to the suffering of the patients, particularly those at the end of life. Those who advocate this idea claim that focusing on the spiritual aspect during a period of illness or the prospect of death increases anxiety and a sense of loneliness and thus accounts for a reduced sense of well-being (Fitzgerald Miller 1985; Kaczorowski 1989). Similarly, some authors also argue against the very notion of spirituality and spiritual care (Sloan et al. 1999; Paley 2008). Swinton and Pattison articulately summarise these arguments as follows:

> First, it is argued that terms like these are used in endlessly different and loose ways. Second, this is then taken to be the evidence that, they cannot, and do not, refer to constant essences or objects within people or in the world. Third, from which it is then deduced, that because the usages of spirituality are emergent, changing, pluriform, diffuse, and non-referential, they really have no legitimate use or value; spirituality does not exist.
>
> (Swinton and Pattison 2010, p. 227)

With the increasing secularisation of Western societies, there are many who articulate their spiritual identity as 'spiritual but not religious' (Sperry 2016). While steering clear of religious and dogmatic orientations, spirituality outside the boundaries of religion is often framed as 'secular spirituality' (Watson 2016). The relationship between religion and spirituality is thus multifaceted. For some, their spirituality is exclusively shaped by their religious beliefs. Others see them as overlapping concepts. There are also other approaches that view them separately.

There is, however, overwhelming consensus and evidence that spirituality is a crucial aspect of the human person and there is great need for attention to spiritual needs, particularly when people are faced with serious illness or death (Cobb 2001; Swinton and Narayanasamy 2002; Swinton 2010; Swinton and Pattison 2010). Most authors also acknowledge the overlap of spirituality with religiosity for some people and emphasise that spirituality and good spiritual care practice should move beyond the limits of religiosity (Hermann 2001; Gunaratnam and Oliviere 2009). Spirituality and spiritual care are therefore contested topics in healthcare. However, as illustrated earlier, there is a strong body of evidence that confirms that most authors and clinicians consider spirituality as a valuable aspect of person-centred care, and that addressing the spiritual issues of the patient leads to well-being and healing (Swinton 2010).

The conceptual overlap between religion and spirituality and their differences continue to inspire fierce discussions on the topic. Yet, the common beliefs of all converge on the understanding that we are all spiritual beings and that, whether shaped by religious beliefs or otherwise, our spirituality remains an important core factor of what makes us human persons.

Manifestations of spiritual distress

Spiritual distress refers to 'a state of suffering related to the impaired ability to experience meaning in life through connectedness with self, others, world or a Superior Being' (Caldeira et al. 2013, p. 82). In the palliative care context, spiritual distress is often caused by the realisation of the ensuing or imminent death, the implications of this prospect for themselves and for their loved ones, and the demands on one's inner strength to withstand the physical pain and suffering caused by disease and/or treatment. Spiritual distress can manifest in different ways. An extensive review of the literature identified several forms in which spiritual distress is expressed: fear; feeling hopeless, helpless, empty, down, depressed and in despair; feeling angry, cynical and bitter; not being able to find peace, feeling impatient, irritable and restless, with a sense of frustration and unjustness; feeling guilty, blaming themselves; feeling punished or judged by God, and blaming others and finding fault with everybody (Edwards et al. 2010).

Besides these psychological manifestations, spiritual distress can also manifest through intractable physical pain and other symptoms or through more social expressions, such as withdrawal from activities and social engagements and wanting to be alone. Such varied expressions of spiritual distress demand a high level of sensitivity from the palliative care team. While dealing with particular symptoms, even physical ones, it is important to bear in mind that what the treating team are presented with could be indications of spiritual distress, which requires additional attention from a spiritual care perspective, often, in addition to treatment of the presenting physical problem. Recognition of manifestations of spiritual distress should lead to a systematic assessment towards identifying appropriate ways of addressing them.

Spiritual need assessment

Identifying specific engagements that can help in a situation of spiritual distress to patients, often denoted as 'spiritual need' is key to providing spiritual support. This involves getting the person: (1) to face their own spiritual distress and acknowledge their need for support; and (2) to search for sources that give them strength in times of distress. These are very personal and individual. The process of identifying helpful spiritual tools thus can be a very intense reflective process.

Several studies have shown the range of spiritual needs which patients and families identified. Figure 10.1 illustrates the findings of a qualitative study on spiritual need assessment (Hermann 2001). The themes that emerged from the study present a range of specific needs ranging from needs for self – to have a positive outlook, to have control and to accomplish specific goals; for others – to have companionship and meaningful relationships; and to engage with activities within the realms of religious traditions.

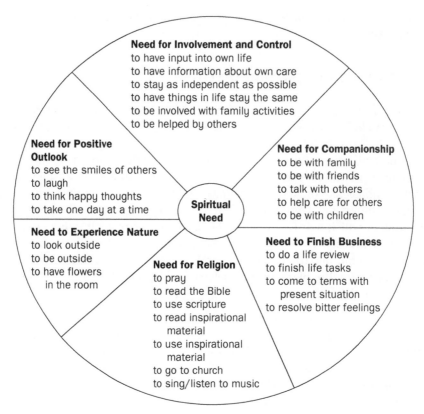

Figure 10.1 Spiritual needs
Source: Hermann (2001).

These needs predominantly arise from the individual's existing spiritual formation and orientation. Kellehear, in his work on spiritual needs, classifies spiritual needs arising from three dimensions, namely: (1) situational transcendence; (2) moral and biographical transcendence; and (3) religious transcendence (Kellehear 2000). Figure 10.2 represents Kellehear's 'model of needs', which is based on the idea that human beings have an innate desire to transcend pain and suffering, and suggests the reality that many of these needs can present at the same time and can have considerable mutual influences among them.

Knowledge of the wide range of spiritual needs that patients and their loved ones can have can function only as a guide that helps explore their actual spiritual needs. The various elements identified on the list of spiritual needs clearly suggest that spiritual needs are not limited to religious rituals and activities or deep searching existential questions, although they comprise a significant part of the spiritual experience of the patients in a palliative care context. It is also important to recognise that some of the elements of spiritual needs can be perceived as social or relational matters without the realisation that these can have deep personal meanings and can contribute to spiritual fulfilment. Spiritual needs assessment, therefore, requires much sensitivity and care to

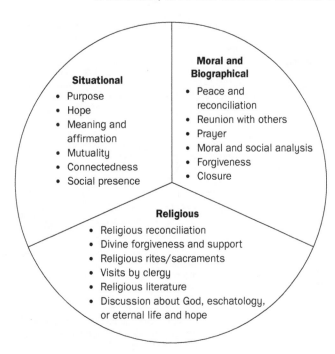

Figure 10.2 Dimensions of spiritual need
Source: Kellehear (2000).

enable nurses to identify specific activities that have the potential to help individuals transcend their spiritual distress in the situation of being faced with death.

Several tools are available that can assist nurses in the process of spiritual care assessment and provision. A few of the most popular ones are as follows:

1   Puchalski introduced the FICA model as a guide which can be used to help the spiritual care provider open a conversation on spiritual matters and initiate a process of understanding the patient's values, beliefs, and hopes. This model includes questions about faith and belief, importance, community, and how the patient wants to address these issues in the care process (Puchalski 2001, 2002).

2   Maugans introduced the SPIRIT model where **S**piritual belief system, **P**ersonal spirituality, **I**ntegration with a spiritual community, **R**itualised practices and restrictions, **I**mplications for medical care, and **T**erminal events planning are presented as the core components of assessing and assisting in spiritual care (Maugans 1996).

3   Gowri Anandarajah proposed the HOPE model where sources of Hope – strength, comfort, meaning, peace, love, and connection, the role of organised religion for the patient, personal spirituality and practices, and effects of medical care and end of life decisions are presented as tools to facilitate spiritual care provision (Anandarajah and Hight 2002).

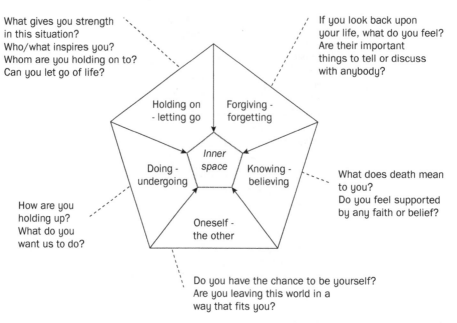

Ars Moriendi Model

Figure 10.3 *Ars Moriendi* model
Source: Vermandere et al. (2013).

Other models have been developed drawing insights from historical traditions. For instance, retrieving the *Ars Moriendi* tradition of medieval Europe, a framework for spiritual history taking has been developed (Leget 2007; Vermandere et al. 2013; Vermandere et al. 2015). Evaluations of this model demonstrated that it was a useful instrument for nurses to use to gain insight into the spirituality of patients. They also showed that the *Ars Moriendi* model of spiritual history taking enhanced patients' spiritual well-being, quality of life and personal relationships. Figure 10.3 illustrates the *Ars Moriendi* model of spiritual history taking.

Besides these, other guidelines have been developed as part of palliative care toolkits for use in various contexts (Bond et al. 2008; Lavy 2009). These are examples of frameworks developed to identify spiritual issues among palliative care patients and can be of great help for nurses involved in such care. They are helpful guides to inform nurses of potential areas of interactions that could lead to identification of spiritual distress as well as indications of directions for opportunities of spiritual healing.

The development of such frameworks and tools has helped make opening a conversation and entering into the spiritual realm of the patient conceivable. They offer a useful set of pointers to keep as a reference while engaging with patients dealing with spiritual issues. However, it has also been noted that spiritual care does not always fit into such set questions and forms of assessment, reiterating the need for an individually focused approach to patients that is culturally sensitive and patient context-specific (Gordon and Mitchell 2004; Alcorn et al. 2010).

Spiritual care

Spiritual care can be broadly described as the entire process of recognising spiritual distress, assessing spiritual needs and taking actions to facilitate and provide spiritual support. What constitutes spiritual care is a critical question. Several approaches to spiritual care have been suggested. In what follows, three dominant paradigms of spiritual care discourse are discussed.

Be present and listen

Nurses being present with the patient and family and actively listening to them provides the safe and protected time and space they often need to explore and express spiritual distress and needs and to consider potential ways of addressing them. Spiritual care is not about the nurse making an intervention and expecting an outcome as a result. It is rather about the way of caring which starts with building trusting relationships (Edwards et al. 2010). Much more than a 'doer' or 'provider' image, offering spiritual care often involves taking the position of a helper who 'assists' patients in finding a source of refuge for themselves (Vasudevan 2003; Lunn 2004).

> The spiritual care provider must ultimately be a presence who respectfully enters into the dying person's experience, affirming and accepting her or his identity, encouraging her or his search for meaning, and allowing for a discussion of fears and hopes concerning existence beyond this life.
>
> (Kaut 2002)

Spiritual care in this sense refers to the ways in which care providers assess and respond to patients' and their families' spiritual needs by being available to them for explorations of their spiritual journeys. This may involve 'being with' and assisting the person in their journey towards spiritual healing as well as facilitating those things or practices that will help the process (Lunn 2004; Greenstreet 2006). It is about providing a safe space and building a trusting relationship where patients are encouraged to ask deep and disturbing questions they may have and explore ways of finding meaning of their experiences.

Religious care

For many people, the process of finding the source of spiritual strength involves a renewed faith in God, which is practically expressed in rituals and practices such as prayer and meditation and a subjective experience of God's presence, love, and care (Narayanasamy 2007). In this aspect of spiritual care involving a relationship with God, religious means and methods are usually found helpful.

In the multi-cultural and religious context of contemporary societies, it is essential that palliative care professionals are appreciative of and sensitive to different religious and cultural traditions, particularly looking for the unique spiritual needs of patients and families, which will, on the one hand, help improve their skills as culturally sensitive spiritual care providers, and, on the other, offer an opportunity for growth by challenging one's own perception of a good death and healthy grieving (Bauer-Wu et al. 2007).

Questions often arise about the appropriateness of nurses offering spiritual support to a patient whose religious affiliation is different from theirs. The core of spiritual care is neither doctrinal nor dogmatic religion, but rather the ability that 'involves touching another at the level that is deeper than ideological and doctrinal differences' (Dom 1999). Therefore, those committed to providing spiritual care should be able to move beyond such differences and support ways that are meaningful and strengthening for the patient.

Providing spiritual care requires immense sensitivity and care. Murray and colleagues (2004) warn that attempts to provide spiritual care without adequate attention to the patients' sense of identity and self-worth can instead cause spiritual distress.

Life review

Life review plays a crucial role in terms of the content of spiritual care, with its scope including issues around the meaning of life, of relationships, and of values. This aspect of spiritual care would involve recontextualising the life of the patient in the circumstances of the present situation, matters of relationships such as forgiveness and love and the continuing search for the meaning and purpose of life (Jenko et al. 2010). The image of the spiritual care provider in this aspect of care is one of an understanding co-traveller, as the patient is trying to unpack the meaning of life as it comes to them at the time of the review in the light of what has gone before. Being truly present with the patient, doing deep listening, and being open to possibilities as directed by the patient are the most fundamental characteristics that are emphasised as necessary (Hegarty 2007). Daaleman (2008) describes this process in three steps: (1) being present; (2) opening eyes; (3) and co-creating. Similar to questions about God and religion, the life review approach also presents a set of questions which are deemed useful to keep in mind in engaging in the process of care. These questions may include, 'What has your life meant? How will you spend the rest of your life? How will you die? What do you need to do to live and die as you wish? What gives you hope in this situation?' (Hegarty 2007). Finding answers to these questions can involve reviewing the past life, trying to grasp the present, and looking ahead at the future within the constraints of the present situation.

Being present and listening attentively, offering religious practices and rituals and creating opportunities for life review thus are broadly understood to constitute the essential forms of spiritual care. Some of these elements take higher significance than others for different individuals depending on their own personal spiritual orientation. While the first two have relevance for all care settings, 'life review' has particular importance to palliative care.

Providing spiritual care

What is the best way to provide spiritual care to palliative care patients and their loved ones? Identifying a reasonable and sensitive approach to enable nurses to enter into such trusting relationships is important to allow them to explore and deal with deep spiritual matters and at the same time remain within the professional frame of being a nurse. Two fundamental issues surface: the first is the question of the content of spiritual care focusing on what is involved in providing spiritual care, and the second pertains to the area of the method in which such care is provided.

Acknowledging the complexity of the subject of spirituality and sensitivities around providing spiritual care, cultivation and expression of a good quality of spirituality and spiritual care is regarded as one of the most challenging tasks for humankind (Dom 1999).

For those whose spiritual orientation is framed in religious rituals and practices, performing or participating in such practices offers access to that layer of meaning and fulfilment. When the patient's source of spiritual strength is based on a belief in God, it is reasonable to support that aspect of the patient's spirituality, irrespective of the caregiver's religious affiliations. A spiritual assessment that includes discussions on the religious beliefs of the patient, the effect of the current life circumstances on their belief, the role such belief plays in coping, and the importance of rituals and prayers can open the way for spiritual care in this direction (Mishra et al. 2010).

The recognition of the importance of religious coping led to exploring the understanding of suffering, death, dying, coping, and associated rituals within major religious traditions (Bauer-Wu et al. 2007). There are others who have tried to develop a religion-neutral or secular understanding of spiritual care (Kaut 2002). While both these approaches are important, their usefulness and appropriateness have been questioned. Studies have shown that even among those who believe in God, coping varied in relation to the images of God that patients held (van Laarhoven 2010). While the formulaic religious approach to spirituality, with its attempt to make direct associations of the meanings of beliefs and rituals as prescribed by religions at the level of the individual's spirituality has been seen as of little help in the pluralistic world in which we live, to replace religious ways of expressing spirituality with a secularised spirituality has also attracted criticism (Pesut and Reimer-Kirkham 2010).

The question of how to provide spiritual care is also about possible methods of offering spiritual care within professional disciplines. Chaplains, in their approach to spiritual care, have traditionally used the tools developed through pastoral theology and pastoral counselling (Brittain 1986). While the applicability of pastoral theology can be questioned in a religiously plural context, how spiritual care is done through professionals of other disciplines is often not clearly laid out (Sinclair et al. 2006). Nevertheless, emphasis on the collective responsibility of spiritual care to patients by all care professionals in palliative care encourages nurses to engage in providing spiritual care at levels feasible to them.

The tools of spiritual needs assessment discussed earlier – for example, FICA, SPIRIT and HOPE – also offer guidance and frameworks for providing spiritual care. The European Association of Palliative Care has set up a task force on spiritual care with the objective of developing spiritual care for palliative care in the European context. Their work includes continued research, education and training in spiritual care and implementation of spiritual care provision in palliative care services (European

Association for Palliative Care 2011). Such continued efforts further sharpen our understanding of the best ways in which nurses can provide spiritual care for patients and their families.

As has been discussed, the use of such frameworks and tools can help nurses open a conversation and enter the spiritual realm of the patient. It is therefore critically important that besides using assessment and care delivery tools, nurses need to be extremely sensitive to the person in front of them, seeking to understand the individuality of the person's spirituality and opportunities of spiritual support with an open-minded and non-judgemental approach.

Learning exercise 10.1

Spiritual care and nursing

Using one of the tools described in the chapter on two patients (one religious and one non-religious), compare how you would behave with each.

What is the role of nurses in spiritual care provision? There are situations where nurses are well aware of the need for spiritual care in their own care setting and have a desire to engage in spiritual care provision, but are unable to do so due to lack of a knowledge base, often owing to curricular deficiencies in nursing education and lack of competence, since many do not receive any training and support on this aspect of patient care (Narayanasamy 2006a; Austin et al. 2016). Over the years 'who should provide spiritual care' has become a much contested question. Some studies evidenced that patients want their religious and spiritual needs to be recognised and addressed by their physicians (Chattopadhyay 2007). There are those who move spiritual care into the realm of the professional and ethical responsibility of nurses (Wright 1998; Rodin et al. 2015). Palliative care in general emphasises an interdisciplinary team approach to care, where the role of a chaplain or spiritual care provider is included (Crawford 2003). Spiritual care is rather understood as a fundamental aspect of care where the skills of spiritual support are embedded in the daily clinical practice of all the members of the team (Chattopadhyay 2007).

It is well known that nurses do spend more time with patients than other members of the treating team and are often placed in the best position to recognise spiritual distress and to engage in a conversation which may lead to exploring measures of spiritual strength (Keall et al. 2014). Therefore, it is essential that nurses receive opportunities to gain and expand their knowledge and skills on spirituality and spiritual care. Nurses who have received training and education in spiritual care have demonstrated a higher level of confidence and expertise in addressing the existential and spiritual concerns of their patients (Attard et al. 2014).

Some trace the importance of nurses' role in providing spiritual care in the historical roots of nursing as a vocation. Bradshaw (1994) suggests that the principles of nursing, emerging from Christian theology, considerably influenced the history of caring for the dying and was part of the history, culture and tradition of Britain. This approach suggests that the requirement to provide spiritual care is part of the foundations of nursing care.

Such viewpoints about the nursing profession and its relationship to spirituality reinforce that nurses have an important responsibility for the spiritual care of their patients. However, there are practical challenges. In exploring barriers to providing spiritual care, Daaleman and colleagues (2008) reported lack of sufficient time as the most important barrier to providing spiritual care. In addition, they also have identified social, religious, or cultural differences between caregiver and patients, which are sometimes a source of mistrust, and institutional obstacles such as the absence of privacy and lack of continuity. The issue of trust due to different religious backgrounds remains for a chaplain or spiritual care provider as well; but time, space, and continuity seem to pose the primary challenge. One of the most important aspects of spiritual care provision is the possibility of ample and unrestrained quality time to listen to the patient (Edwards et al. 2010). Given the pressure on time nurses already have with their routine clinical work, having sufficient time for in-depth discussions on spiritual issues without having to compromise on competing clinical demands becomes impossible.

Recognising the limitations within clinical settings for nurses to provide spiritual care offers the possibility of finding feasible opportunities. There is no doubt that every occasion of contact with the patient and their loved ones can be an opportunity for supporting their spirituality. Adequately assessed and used, such encounters can bring opportunities for healing and spiritual well-being for the patient and for their loved ones.

While it is important to give as much attention as possible to patients' spiritual care needs, it is also important for nurses to make appropriate referrals for further spiritual support. Making referrals to chaplaincy services or other relevant spiritual leaders is part of the function of spiritual care (Epstein-Peterson et al. 2015). It is often useful to be aware of available spiritual care resources available in individual care settings so that potential spiritual caregivers can be identified and patients can be directed to their care. These may include chaplains or other pastoral care providers. It is also important for nurses involved in spiritual care to receive adequate supervision (Zollfrank et al. 2015).

Nurses, therefore, have an important role to play in the spiritual domain of patient care. Despite challenges and limitations, nurses have many opportunities to engage in identifying and responding to the spiritual distress of patients. Such engagements need to be undertaken in an organised and co-ordinated manner in consultation with chaplaincy teams or spiritual care specialists. Team spirit and collaborative work, which are well-known concepts in palliative care, are essential for spiritual care.

Conclusion

Spirituality is continuing to emerge as a significant field in palliative care. Much of the current understanding of spirituality centres around the meaning and purpose of life for individuals. There is much more to be understood about spirituality, particularly how philosophical and theological contexts and tenets of history, cultures and traditions of particular contexts contribute to the construction of the notion of spirituality (Inbadas 2016). While it is extremely important to continue to explore what the experience of facing death means for individuals and their loved ones, it is also critical to recognise the relationship between personal constructions and the contextual constructions of the meanings of life, death and dying.

Palliative care has contributed much to the inclusion of spiritual care as part of the holistic approach of care provided in a modern healthcare context. Assessing spiritual needs and facilitating spiritual support must be done with the utmost care and sensitivity. Spiritual care may still be far from becoming an integral part of mainstream healthcare in many settings. But it is encouraging that its importance has been well recognised in palliative care and its recognition is gradually growing across other fields of medicine. The process of spiritual care can be time-consuming and demanding. Such spiritual care diligently provided can offer a meaningful experience of facing death with hope and dignity for palliative care patients and their loved ones.

Learning exercise 10.2

Take time to understand your own spirituality. Develop your self-care plan and create space for spiritual nourishment in your regular schedule.

References

Alcorn, M., Prigerson, H., Reynolds, A. et al. (2010) 'If God wanted me yesterday, I wouldn't be here today': religious and spiritual themes in patients' experiences of advanced cancer. *Journal of Palliative Medicine*, 13: 581–8.

Anandarajah, G. and Hight, E. (2002) Spirituality and medical practice. *American Family Physician*, 63: 1–6.

Attard, J., Baldacchino, D.R. and Camilleri, L. (2014) Nurses' and midwives' acquisition of competency in spiritual care: a focus on education. *Nurse Education Today*, 34: 1460–6.

Austin, P.D., Macleod, R., Siddall, P.J. et al. (2016) The ability of hospital staff to recognise and meet patients' spiritual needs: a pilot study. *Journal for the Study of Spirituality*, 6: 20–37.

Bauer-Wu, S., Barrett, R. and Yeager, K. (2007) Spiritual perspectives and practices at the end-of-life: a review of the major world religions and application to palliative care. *Indian Journal of Palliative Care*, 13: 53–8.

Bond, C., Lavy, V. and Wooldridge, R. (2008) *Palliative Care Tool Kit: Improving Care from the Roots Up in Resource Limited Settings*. London: Help the Hospices.

Bradshaw, A. (1994) *Lighting the Lamp: The Spiritual Dimension of Nursing Care*. London: Scutari Press.

Brittain, J.N. (1986) Theological foundations for spiritual care. *Journal of Religion and Health*, 25: 107–21.

Caldeira, S., Carvalho, E.C. and Vieira, M. (2013) Spiritual distress: proposing a new definition and defining characteristics. *International Journal of Nursing Knowledge*, 24: 77–84.

Carroll, B. (2001) A phenomenological exploration of the nature of spirituality and spiritual care. *Mortality*, 6: 81–98.

Chattopadhyay, S. (2007) Religion, spirituality, health and medicine: why should Indian physicians care? *Journal of Postgraduate Medicine*, 53: 262–6.

Clark, D. (1999) Total pain, disciplinary power and the body in the work of Cicely Saunders, 1958–1967. *Social Science and Medicine*, 49: 727–36.

Cobb, M. (2001) *The Dying Soul: Spiritual Care at the End of Life*. Buckingham: Open University Press.

Crawford, G.B. (2003) Team working: palliative care as a model of interdisciplinary practice. *Medical Journal of Australia*, 179: 32–4.

Daaleman, T.P., Usher, B.M., Williams, S.W. et al. (2008) An exploratory study of spiritual care at the end of life. *Annals of Family Medicine*, 6: 406–11.

Dein, S. and Stygall, J. (1997) Does being religious help or hinder coping with chronic illness? A critical literature review. *Palliative Medicine*, 11: 291–8.

Dom, H. (1999) Spiritual care, need and pain-recognition and response. *European Journal of Palliative Care*, 6: 87–90.

Dunklee, L.G. (2011) Religion, spirituality and the search for common ground. *Health Progress: St Louis*, 92: 62–4.

Dyson, J., Cobb, M. and Forman, D. (1997) The meaning of spirituality: a literature review. *Journal of Advanced Nursing*, 26: 1183–8.

Edwards, A., Pang, N., Shiu, V. and Chan, C.L.W. (2010) The understanding of spirituality and the potential role of spiritual care in end-of-life and palliative care: a meta-study of qualitative research. *Palliative Medicine*, 24: 753–70.

Epstein-Peterson, Z.D., Sullivan, A.J., Enzinger, A.C. et al. (2015) Examining forms of spiritual care provided in the advanced cancer setting. *American Journal of Hospice and Palliative Medicine*, 32: 750–7.

European Association for Palliative Care (2011) *EAPC Taskforce on Spiritual Care in Palliative Care*. Available at: www.eapcnet.eu/Themes/ClinicalCare/SpiritualCarein PalliativeCare.aspx (accessed 21 March 2017).

Fitzgerald Miller, J. (1985) Assessment of loneliness and spiritual well-being in chronically ill and healthy adults. *Journal of Professional Nursing*, 1: 79–85.

Gordon, T. and Mitchell, D. (2004) A competency model for the assessment and delivery of spiritual care. *Palliative Medicine*, 18: 646–51.

Greenstreet, W. (2006) *Integrating Spirituality in Health and Social Care: Perspectives and Practical Approaches*. Oxford: Radcliffe Publishing.

Gunaratnam, Y. and Oliviere, D. (2009) *Narrative and Stories in Health Care: Illness, Dying and Bereavement*. Oxford: Oxford University Press.

Hegarty, M. (2007) Care of the spirit that transcends religious, ideological and philosophical boundaries. *Indian Journal of Palliative Care*, 13: 42–7.

Hermann, C.P. (2001) Spiritual needs of dying patients: a qualitative study. *Oncology Nursing Forum*, 28: 67–72.

Hermsen, M.A. and Ten Have, H.A. (2004) Pastoral care, spirituality, and religion in palliative care journals. *American Journal of Hospice and Palliative Medicine*, 21: 353–6.

Inbadas, H. (2016) History, culture and traditions: the silent spaces in the study of spirituality at the end of life. *Religions*, 7(5): 53.

Jenko, L., Alley, P.M. and Gonzalez, P. (2010) Life review in critical care: possibilities at the end of life. *Critical Care Nurse*, 30: 17–28.

Kaczorowski, J.M. (1989) Spiritual well-being and anxiety in adults diagnosed with cancer. *Hospice Journal*, 5: 105–16.

Kaut, K.P. (2002) Religion, spirituality, and existentialism near the end of life. *American Behavioral Scientist*, 46: 220–34.

Keall, R., Clayton, J.M. and Butow, P. (2014) How do Australian palliative care nurses address existential and spiritual concerns? Facilitators, barriers and strategies. *Journal of Clinical Nursing*, 23: 3197–205.

Kellehear, A. (2000) Spirituality and palliative care: a model of needs. *Palliative Medicine*, 14: 149–55.

Larkin, P.J. (2010) Listening to the still small voice: the role of palliative care nurses in addressing psychosocial issues at end of life. *Progress in Palliative Care*, 18: 335–40.

Lavy, V. (2009) *Palliative Care Toolkit Training Manual*. London: Help the Hospices.

Leget, C. (2007) Retrieving the *ars moriendi* tradition. *Medicine, Health Care and Philosophy*, 10: 313–19.

Lunn, J.S. (2004) Spiritual care in a multi-religious context. *Journal of Pain and Palliative Care Pharmacotherapy*, 17: 153–66.

Maugans, T.A. (1996) The spiritual history. *Archives of Family Medicine*, 5: 11–16.

Mcsherry, W. and Cash, K. (2004) The language of spirituality: an emerging taxonomy. *International Journal of Nursing Studies*, 41: 151–61.

Mishra, S., Bhatnagar, S., Philip, F.A. et al. (2010) Psychosocial concerns in patients with advanced cancer: an observational study at regional cancer centre, India. *American Journal of Hospice and Palliative Medicine*, 27: 316–19.

Murray, S.A., Kendall, M., Boyd, K. et al. (2004) Exploring the spiritual needs of people dying of lung cancer or heart failure: a prospective qualitative interview study of patients and their carers. *Palliative Medicine*, 18: 39–45.

Narayanasamy, A. (2006a) The impact of empirical studies of spirituality and culture on nurse education. *Journal of Clinical Nursing*, 15: 840–51.

Narayanasamy, A. (2006b) *Spiritual Care and Transcultural Care Research*. London: Quay Books.

Narayanasamy, A. (2007) Palliative care and spirituality. *Indian Journal of Palliative Care*, 13: 32–41.

Narayanasamy, A. (2010) Recognising spiritual needs. In Mcsherry, W. and Ross, L. (eds) *Spiritual Assessment in Healthcare Practice*. Keswick: M&K Update Ltd.

Paley, J. (2008) Spirituality and nursing: a reductionist approach. *Nursing Philosophy*, 9: 3–18.

Pesut, B. and Reimer-Kirkham, S. (2010) Situated clinical encounters in the negotiation of religious and spiritual plurality: a critical ethnography. *International Journal of Nursing Studies*, 47: 815–25.

Puchalski, C.M. (2001) Spirituality and health: the art of compassionate medicine. *Hospital Physician*, 37: 30–6.

Puchalski, C.M. (2002) Spirituality and end-of-life care: a time for listening and caring. *Journal of Palliative Medicine*, 5: 289–94.

Puchalski, C.M. (2007) Spirituality and the care of patients at the end-of-life: an essential component of care. *OMEGA: Journal of Death and Dying*, 56: 33–46.

Puchalski, C.M. (2009) Spiritual issues in palliative care. In Chochinov, H.M. and Breitbart, W. (eds) *Handbook of Psychiatry in Palliative Medicine*. New York: Oxford University Press.

Puchalski, C.M., Vitillo, R., Hull, S.K. and Reller, N. (2014) Improving the spiritual dimension of whole person care: reaching national and international consensus. *Journal of Palliative Medicine*, 17: 642–56.

Rajagopal, M.R. (2010) Disease, dignity and palliative care. *Indian Journal of Palliative Care*, 16: 59–60.

Rodin, D., Balboni, M., Mitchell, C. et al. (2015) Whose role? Oncology practitioners' perceptions of their role in providing spiritual care to advanced cancer patients. *Supportive Care in Cancer*, 23: 2543–50.

Saunders, C. (1996) Into the valley of the shadow of death: a personal therapeutic journey. *British Medical Journal*, 313: 1599–601.

Sinclair, S., Pereira, J. and Raffin, S. (2006) A thematic review of the spirituality literature within palliative care. *Journal of Palliative Medicine*, 9: 464–79.

Sloan, R.P., Bagiella, E. and Powell, T. (1999) Religion, spirituality, and medicine. *The Lancet*, 353: 664–7.

Sperry, L. (2016) Secular spirituality and spiritually sensitive clinical practice. *Spirituality in Clinical Practice*, 3: 221–3.

Swinton, J. (2010) The meaning of spirituality: a multi-perspective approach to 'the spiritual'. In Mcsherry, W. and Ross, L.A. (eds) *Spiritual Assessment in Healthcare Practice*. Keswick: M&K Update Ltd.

Swinton, J. and Narayanasamy, A. (2002) Response to:'A critical view of spirituality and spiritual assessment' by P. Draper and W. McSherry (2002) *Journal of Advanced Nursing* 39, 1–2. *Journal of Advanced Nursing*, 40: 158–60.

Swinton, J. and Pattison, S. (2010) Moving beyond clarity: towards a thin, vague, and useful understanding of spirituality in nursing care. *Nursing Philosophy*, 11: 226–37.

Twycross, R.G. (2003) *Introducing Palliative Care*. Oxford: Radcliffe Publishing.

Vachon, M., Fillion, L. and Achille, M. (2009) A conceptual analysis of spirituality at the end of life. *Journal of Palliative Medicine*, 12: 53–9.

van Laarhoven, H.W.M. (2010) Images of God in relation to coping strategies of palliative cancer patients. *Journal of Pain and Symptom Management*, 40: 495–501.

Vasudevan, S. (2003) Coping with terminal illness: a spiritual perspective. *Indian Journal of Palliative Care*, 9: 19–24.

Vermandere, M., Bertheloot, K., Buyse, H. et al. (2013) Implementation of the ars moriendi model in palliative home care: a pilot study. *Progress in Palliative Care*, 21: 278–85.

Vermandere, M., Warmenhoven, F., Van Severen, E. et al. (2015) The ars moriendi model for spiritual assessment: a mixed-methods evaluation. *Oncology Nursing Forum*, 42: 294–301.

Watson, J. (2016) Secular spirituality: the next step towards enlightenment. *Journal for the Study of Spirituality*, 6: 121–4.

Wright, K.B. (1998) Professional, ethical, and legal implications for spiritual care in nursing. *Journal of Nursing Scholarship*, 30: 81–3.

Zollfrank, A.A., Trevino, K.M., Cadge, W. et al. (2015) Teaching health care providers to provide spiritual care: a pilot study. *Journal of Palliative Medicine*, 18: 408–14.

Identity, the dignified self and person-centred approaches in palliative care

Susan McClement and Genevieve Thompson

The relief of suffering is a fundamental aspect of all nursing practice (Ferrell and Coyle 2008). However, when individuals are confronted with a life-limiting illness, attention to their suffering becomes even more pronounced. The central work of nursing at this stage becomes the ability to recognise and respond to distress. In particular, nurses must realise that suffering arises not only out of physical distress but rather can occur when an individual feels voiceless, invisible, or they believe their dignity is fractured (Chochinov et al. 2002; Hack et al. 2004; Ferrell and Coyle 2008). Research examining what constitutes a 'good death' consistently underscores the importance of not only meticulous attention to pain and symptom management, but also to the affirmation of the entire person, including respecting their needs in regards to psychological, social and spiritual wholeness (Steinhauser et al. 2000; Oechsle et al. 2014). Implicit in this is an understanding that those we care for are complete persons beyond their illness.

This chapter will explore the idea that to alleviate suffering in patients receiving palliative care, we as nurses need to consider how identity and sense of self are supported and ultimately, how we can ensure that individuals feel whole and that their dignity is bolstered or remains intact as they near the end of life.

Identity, dignity, and suffering

Early work exploring the patient experience of chronic illness has underscored that illness can have a profound impact on how individuals view themselves and are viewed by others. The concept 'loss of self' (Charmaz 1983) describes the process of the gradually increasing impact of an illness on every aspect of one's life. Illness, and in particular advanced life-limiting illness, threaten the potential to maintain a coherent sense of self and identity (Reeve et al. 2009). Social roles may become diminished, physical abilities decline, and one's personal identity may become eroded as the 'patient' identity begins to predominate (Nanton et al. 2016).

Indeed, over time, as a life-limiting illness begins to permeate every aspect of life and death becomes closer to a reality, individuals begin to reassess who they are and what constitutes self. This is particularly poignant as one begins to realise that one's body may not function as it once did and previously taken for granted abilities such as bathing, getting dressed, eating, or going for a walk become difficult, if not impossible. When experiencing this altered body, people begin to compare their present body with their past body, and often these bodily changes are viewed with a sense of betrayal (Charmaz 1995). Feelings of guilt, anger, and shame at the inability to care for oneself, feeling a burden to others, for potentially a changed physical appearance, or the realisation that a future no longer exists as a 'well' person, are sources of potential suffering that nurses providing care to those with life-limiting illness need to understand. Part of the responsibility of nurses in the dying process is to provide opportunities for the possibility of retaining as much of a person's identity or self as possible until the moment of death (Ternestedt 2009).

One's sense of self or personal identity is derived from many factors. Central to identity is a multi-dimensional understanding of 'who I am'; a person with a life story, roles, personality, and values that encompass all aspects of life (e.g. spirituality, physical, sexuality, political, ideological, existential, and social) (Jeppsson and Thomé 2015). The self is situated in the person and develops through the interaction between biological, psychological, social, and cultural processes (Ternestedt 2009). Identity can help serve an integrative function in a human life as we continuously reassess ourselves in regard to previous experiences and ideas of the future (Erikson 1998). Our identity is constructed through life-long evolving self-narratives, including the end of life, and helps people make sense of their reality and to find meaning and purpose (Carlander et al. 2011). Through storytelling, people 'discover themselves and at the same time reveal and construct their identity and self-image' (Carlander et al. 2011, p. 5932). Therefore, our identity is also comprised by how we wish to define ourselves (Charmaz 1995). In this regard, we may hold different notions of self that are expressed publicly versus those regarded as more private. A life-limiting illness may, therefore, alter what people choose to express of themselves or wish to be defined by as a means of maintaining their sense of self, for example, a person with advanced lung disease who values their physical strength and defines themselves as a gardener, may try to mitigate the physical difficulties they experience in getting outdoors to continue such a role. Tensions arise when the ability to continue with previously held identities become difficult, and fulfilling the expectations of others (or of one's self) based on these identities is challenged (Charmaz 1983). This might arise also in those experiencing some degree of cognitive impairment whereby the ability to fulfil past roles, meet previous expectations, and changes in ability to express oneself verbally become increasingly difficult. In this regard, we need to look beyond the ability of what a person can 'do' as a defining feature of identity, to notions of the inherent dignity of people.

While identity or self is shaped by our lived experience and may be intimately tied to notions of autonomy, rationality, self-consciousness, and control (Kitwood 1997), the idea of dignity helps us to move beyond these conceptions. Dignity is defined as 'the quality or state of being worthy, honored, or esteemed' *(Merriam-Webster Dictionary* 2017). For patients living with life-threatening or life-limiting illness, a sense of dignity is intimately connected to the feeling that they are respected and deserving of respect, despite the physical deterioration of their bodies and the psychological distress their illness may bring. Dignity includes notions of being able to maintain feelings of physical comfort, autonomy, meaning, spiritual comfort, interpersonal connectedness, belonging, and hopefulness (Proulx and Jacelon 2004; Chochinov and Cann 2005; Rodríguez-Prat et al. 2016). The transgression of personal boundaries, coupled with an acute sense of vulnerability, can impact a patient's sense of self (Lomborg et al. 2005; Ahlstrom 2007).

Palliative care researchers have identified a significant association between functional dependency and loss of dignity among terminally ill patients (Chochinov et al. 2002; Hack et al. 2004). Chochinov and colleagues (2002) found that loss of functional capacity altered patients' sense of self, resulting in a profound loss of dignity. In response to this finding, Hack et al. (2004) proposed the concept of intimate dependency to describe a patient's level of dependency for the most personal aspects of their care such as assistance with bathing, toileting, dressing and continence care. Using factor analysis and regression methods on survey data with 213 palliative care patients, their study found that intimate dependency was significantly associated with loss of dignity. With this understanding, it is critical that nurses realise the psychological impact that being dependent for basic care needs, can have on individuals. Therefore, as nurses, we need to change how we view providing this care; that it is not simply a task to perform but rather requires a delicate negotiation and a deep awareness of the potential suffering of the other. It also requires that when this care has been delegated to others, such as healthcare assistants, that we are role modelling and educating them about the delicacy this care requires to preserve dignity.

Just as identity is developed and maintained through social relations (Charmaz 1983; Jeppsson and Thomé 2015), dignity can be profoundly shaped by our relationships with others (Pullman 2004; McClement and Chochinov 2006). Most people describe feeling connected to others and belonging to a group, whether that is family, a social group, or care providers, as critical to their sense of self (Ternestedt 2009). Dignity can be nurtured and supported by personal relationships that are empowering throughout life (Street and Kissane 2001). In this sense, dignity may be a function of the attitudes and behaviours communicated by others (Chochinov 2007). Negative attitudes, such as anger or blame, can undermine empathy and the helping behaviours of caregiving families towards their dying loved one (Lobchuk et al. 2008). Expressions of empathy, the imaginative ability of being able to step inside another person's shoes to understand and validate their emotional pain, can mitigate suffering and enhance the quality of life for patients nearing death (Davis 1994; Devoldre et al. 2010).

In healthcare, this relational approach is central to work on identity and suffering (Kitwood 1997; Cassell 2004) as well as earlier research on the preservation of patient dignity at end of life (Chochinov 2002; Chochinov et al. 2002; Pleschberger 2007; Lin et al. 2011; Jacelon 2014). Cassel (2004) described the critical relationship between suffering and perceived threats to, or diminished sense of, self. When self is threatened or diminished, patients suffer. In our studies, nearly 75 per cent of patients nearing death report that 'no longer feeling like the person they once were' would undermine their sense of dignity (Chochinov et al. 2006); with 36 per cent indicating this is a current and significant problem (Chochinov et al. 2009). In a study of non-malignant life-limiting conditions, we reported that being significantly troubled by 'no longer feeling like the person they once were' ranged from 14 per cent in the frail institutionalised elderly to as high as 42 per cent in those with amyotrophic lateral sclerosis (ALS) (Chochinov et al. 2016). Hence, for nurses to effectively address suffering, they must understand who patients are as persons beyond individualistic ideas or abilities, and appreciate key facets of their core identity or self.

Learning exercise 11.1

- What do you think are the things that matter to you as a person?
- What would be important to you if you were in hospital and dependent on others?
- Do you ask patients 'What matters to you?'?
- Consider using this question in your everyday practice.

Models of care: person-centred and dignity-conserving care

The basic tenets of palliative care, including symptom control, psychological and spiritual well-being, and care of the family, align themselves with the philosophical underpinnings of the person-centred care model being widely embraced in healthcare. At their core, both models are focused on providing care that meets and responds to the unique needs of persons and their families. In order to achieve this goal, person-centredness requires intimate knowledge of a person's needs, hopes, and preferences in order to promote a continuation of self and normality despite a life-limiting illness, to enable shared decision-making, and to facilitate experiences of comfort, empathetic awareness, respect, and meaningful experiences of life (McCormack and McCance 2006; Edvardsson and Innes 2010). Person-centred care, like palliative care, requires nurses to shift their focus from the task to the person (Edvardsson et al. 2014) and engage in conversations with individuals that elicit the essence of who that person is. While difficult in those with diminishing cognitive capacity, either as the result of advancing disease process (e.g. dementia, brain metastases) or the proximity to death, a person-centred approach demands that nurses find ways to ensure the self or dignity is maintained (Thompson et al. 2016).

Person-centred care can improve patient satisfaction, patient treatment adherence, the quality of healthcare, the perceived health outcomes, and symptom management

(Morgan and Yoder 2012; Lusk and Fater 2013; Jakimowicz and Perry 2015). It can also decrease implicit healthcare provider prejudice; increase healthcare provider work satisfaction; is related to better healthcare provider retention; and can even yield economic benefits (Hall et al. 2015; Jakimowicz and Perry 2015; Sharma et al. 2015). While person-centred care is guided by core concepts such as patient engagement and empowerment, mutual respect and dignity, effective communication, collaborative decision-making, and healthcare provider self-awareness (Jakimowicz and Perry 2015), putting these concepts into practice requires a relational approach. This approach organises care around the health needs and expectations of people rather than illnesses (World Health Organization 2017), and addresses the whole person, with nurses extending themselves as relational beings to those for whom they care. Being seen as a person with a past and life experiences, and being remembered as someone, is critical near the end of life (Ternestedt 2009). By deepening the relationships between patients and nurses, joint understandings can lead to patient empowerment, helping them fulfil their personal aspirations and ultimately increasing the potential for a good death.

Dignity-conserving care actions

While nurses may be clear about the importance of providing care to patients that supports identity and dignity, they may feel less sure about what actions they can take to accomplish that goal. The model of dignity-conserving care developed by Chochinov and colleagues is instructive in this regard (Chochinov 2002; Chochinov et al. 2002; McClement et al. 2004). Empirically derived from interviews with Canadian and Australian patients with cancer with palliative care needs, validated, and supported by factor analysis (Hack et al. 2004), the model helps nurses understand the three main issues that affect a patient's sense of dignity. These include: (1) illness-related issues; (2) the patient's dignity-conserving repertoire; and (3) the nature and quality of interactions with others (i.e. the social dignity inventory) (Figure 11.1). Illness-related concerns alert clinicians to the importance of attending to patients' physical and psychosocial symptom distress, as well as challenges that can arise with cognitive acuity and functional independence in activities of daily living.

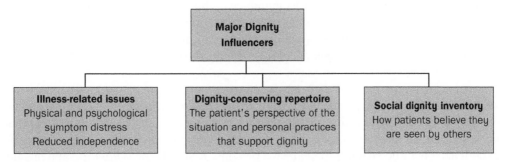

Figure 11.1 The main components of dignity

Understanding of the patients' dignity-conserving repertoire requires an appreciation of the patient's perspective about such things as sense of self, pride, hope, generativity, and ability to fulfil roles; all of which can impact patient dignity. It also requires that nurses understand that patients employ personal approaches and techniques to bring dignity to their lives when they are ill. These dignity-conserving practices include such things as living in the moment instead of worrying about the future; maintaining routines that help in the management of day-to-day challenges; and finding comfort in spiritual practices that are meaningful to them. Taking the time to discover these unique approaches and techniques is important. It helps the nurse to see the patient not as someone with illness-induced deficits, but as an individual with inherent strengths and resources that can be supported and optimised. The assumed benefits of a strengths-based approach to nursing care include empowerment, self-efficacy and hope – outcomes that are clearly related to supporting patient dignity (Gottlieb 2014).

Learning exercise 11.2

- Do you consider your own approach, attitudes and behaviour when caring for patients?
- Write a reflection on the last patient you cared for with palliative care needs; did anything about your approach, attitudes or behaviour change the way you cared? Consider whether you felt anxious, busy or distracted by something else in your work or in your own life. All of these will reflect on the care we give.

The nature and quality of interactions that patients have with others – the Social Dignity Inventory component of the model – remind nurses to be respectful of patient privacy and recognise the importance of patient social support systems. Nurses must also remember that patients can become distressed if they are made to feel a burden to caregivers, and may harbour concerns about how their death will affect those left behind. The Social Dignity Inventory also requires that nurses pay attention to the tone of care they deliver. This 'care tenor' requires vigilance on the part of nurses to ensure that the care they provide embodies the values of kindness, humanity and respect. These values are espoused in the ABCD of dignity-conserving care, an acronym that serves as a guide for putting the principles of dignity in care into action by Chochinov (2007) (Figure 11.2).

The *A* of the ABCD of dignity-conserving care stands for *attitudes* and reminds us that our beliefs about others influence the way we respond to them. Thus, it is critical that nurses reflect on their attitudes and the extent to which personal beliefs, values and life experiences may be shaping the care we provide. *B* stands for *behaviour* and speaks to the importance of ensuring that care provided is based on respect and kindness.

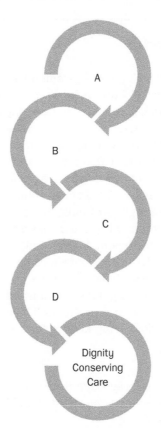

Figure 11.2 The ABCD of dignity-conserving care

Compassion, the *C* in the ABCD acronym, refers to what Sinclair and colleagues have defined as 'a virtuous response that seeks to address the suffering of a person through relational understanding and action' (Sinclair et al. 2016a, 2016b). A compassionate response requires a basic interest in humanity, and requires that nurses find ways to identify with those who are suffering. *Dialogue*, the *D* in the ABCD of dignity-conserving care, is more than just taking a medical history and providing information about tests and procedures, though such interactions are clearly important. Dialogue pushes us to ask questions that allow us to learn who the patient is as a person, and the emotional impact that is part of the illness experience.

An integrative review conducted by Johnston and colleagues (Johnston et al. 2015b) that examined dignity-conserving care actions in palliative care settings supports the use of the dignity-conserving care model as a useful heuristic device for nurses to help think about how to provide care that supports dignity. Their review identified that although there were less reported care actions related to the level of independence and aftermath concerns, the majority of care actions could be classified under the themes of the dignity-conserving care model. To help you consider how you might use the model in practice, consider the following clinical scenario in Case Study 11.1.

Case Study 11.1: Marietta

Mrs. Marietta Kowalchuk is a 45-year-old woman who experienced her first diagnosis of breast cancer at age 30. Until the past year, she has been doing well, running the family business with her husband and keeping busy with her two children, ages 8 and 10. Over the past year, her breast cancer has recurred with metastases to her liver, left femur, and spine. Her care has been managed in the community, with regular visits from the palliative care team. You have been Marietta's primary nurse for several months and have noticed small changes in her physical abilities, especially in the past week. She has started having trouble with mobility and is requiring much more assistance with activities of daily living such as bathing. She indicates that her back hurts constantly and it is particularly painful to walk. Marietta also indicates to you that lately she has had several nights of 'terrifying dreams' that have caused her to have restless sleep and she is having difficulty staying awake during the day. Overall, she seems to have less energy and her appetite has become poor. When you arrive this morning, you find Marietta lying in bed, clutching her left leg, and sobbing. She looks at you and says: 'I have to get well . . . I have to get well. I don't want to be a burden on my kids. How can I die now?'

Consider the following:

* What potential threats to self/dignity do you see in this case?
* What nursing assessments/questions would you suggest be used to explore these threats?
* Looking at the dignity-conserving care model, what interventions can you as a nurse use to address or support the following?:

  ○ illness-related concerns
  ○ dignity-conserving repertoire
  ○ dignity-conserving practices
  ○ the social dignity inventory

Response

Marietta has several potential threats to her sense of self and dignity we need to think about. She is a mother, wife, and business owner; each of these may profoundly shape how she sees herself and what is important to her. Other threats including advancing physical symptoms (e.g. illness-related concerns including pain, fatigue/difficulty sleeping, mobility, poor appetite, disease progression); feeling a sense of burden; increasing dependency for activities of daily living; and worries about the future care of her children.

In speaking with Marietta, a helpful starting point may be to start the conversation by saying: 'I can sense that there are things that have happened that are bothering you. Why don't you start by telling me what you are concerned about.' This open type of question not only conveys our concern about her, but will also elicit the issues that are her priority. We may need to probe further by asking things such as 'Can you tell me more about why that is bothering you?' or 'What is the one wish you have for today that I might help you achieve?' Once we establish what needs are her priority, we can then begin to delve deeper by applying the model of dignity-conserving care.

When applying the dignity-conserving care model to this case, think about the assessments and interventions in Table 11.1.

Table 11.1 Assessments and interventions divided into categories related to the dignity-conserving care model

Dignity-conserving care categories	Case-specific relevant theme or subtheme	Case-specific indicator	Interventions (McClement et al. 2004; Thompson and Chochinov 2008; Östlund et al. 2012)
Illness- related concerns			
Symptom distress	Physical distress	Pain Fatigue	On-going assessment and management of physical symptoms, such as pain control, energy conservation strategies
		Poor appetite	Discuss the role of food and fluid near the end of life; explore options for smaller meals if desired
		Dreams	Explore meaning of dreams; encourage discussion of the dreams
	Psychological distress	Death anxiety	Explore concerns related to illness progression; reassurance that care will continue into the future; explore realistic goals
Level of independence	Functional capacity of daily living	Decreasing mobility	Support independence through provision of supports (e.g. walker); teach her what is normal as her illness progresses
		Changes in activities of daily living (e.g. bathing)	Promote self-care where appropriate; ensure proper equipment is available; protect privacy
Dignity-conserving repertoire			
Dignity-conserving perspectives	Role preservation	Concerns about her continued abilities to act in her various roles	Explore ways that she can still enact important roles and how that might be supported

(Continued)

Table 11.1 (Continued)

Dignity-conserving care categories	Case-specific relevant theme or subtheme	Case-specific indicator	Interventions (McClement et al. 2004; Thompson and Chochinov 2008; Östlund et al. 2012)
	Hopefulness	Desire to 'beat this'	Encourage discussion around changing what is hoped for. Rather than hoping for a cure, may look at short-term goals such as hoping for a pain-free day, hoping for more restful sleep or hope to watch a movie with her children
	Generativity/ legacy		Facilitate the sharing of memories that are meaningful for her; explore idea of memory-making activities for her children
Dignity-conserving practices	Maintaining normalcy	Carrying on usual routines	Talk with her about things beyond her illness; find ways to remain connected to the larger community and stay engaged in her children's activities/school work
	Living 'in the moment'	Focusing on the present and not worrying about the future	
Social dignity inventory	Burden to others	Worried about feeling a burden to her children	Explore why she feels this way
	Aftermath concerns	Worried about the impact her death may have on those left behind, particularly her children but also the business	Encourage reflection on the perceived challenges and difficulties that may be experienced because of her death

The previously described model of dignity-conserving care spawned the development of a question that nurses can ask in the service of inquiring about identity and supporting patient dignity. The Patient Dignity Question (PDQ) asks, 'What do I need to know about you as a person to give you the best care possible?' (Chochinov et al. 2015). This brief yet important question speaks to the association between sense of dignity and patients feeling known for who they are and what is important to them – not for the malady they have. Because the answers elicited from the PDQ contain salient information about identity and self, nurses' awareness and perspective about who the patient is as a person are also enhanced, and perhaps changed.

The impact of the PDQ on patients with palliative care needs, their families, and healthcare providers has been empirically evaluated in several studies (Chochinov et al. 2015; Johnston et al. 2015a; Johnston et al. 2015c), including a recent systematic review (Arantzamendi et al. 2016). In the study by Chochinov and colleagues (2015), in-patients with palliative care needs or their family members were invited to respond to the PDQ. Responses were summarised, vetted by participants to ensure their accuracy, and then placed on patients' charts where they were accessible to clinicians. The majority of patients (93 per cent) felt that the information elicited by the PDQ was important for clinicians to know. Ninety per cent of clinicians reported that they learned something new from reading responses to the PDQ, 64 per cent were emotionally affected by what they read, 59 per cent indicated that it influenced their sense of empathy, and 44 per cent endorsed that it influenced their care. The PDQ does not obviate the need for on-going more in-depth discussion about matters of identity and self, but evidence indicates that it is a place from which to being to ensure that sense of self does not get short shrift in the clinical encounter.

Research supports the use of the PDQ in environments beyond palliative care. Johnston and colleagues confirmed the feasibility and acceptability of asking this question in acute care settings in Scotland (Johnston et al. 2015a). Their mixed methods study used a before and after study design to evaluate the PDQ as an intervention to promote a person-centred climate of care by fostering a therapeutic relationship between patients and healthcare providers. Thirty acute care patients who did have palliative care needs, 4 family members, and 17 healthcare providers participated. Main outcome measures included the Consultation and Relational Empathy (CARE) measure, the Person-Centred Climate Questionnaire (PCQ-P), and the Patient Dignity Question feedback questionnaire. Findings indicated that asking the PDQ can foster the creation of a person-centred environment, and enhance the levels of empathy patients perceive they receive from care providers. Patients and healthcare providers positively endorsed the PDQ. Patients wanted health- care providers to know them as a person, and provide care that allowed for patient individuality. Healthcare providers learned new information about the patients for whom they were caring; information that ostensibly could help them better appreciate such individuality and consider it when planning and providing. Having this simple phrase in our lexicon can significantly change how patients are viewed not only by nurses but other members of the healthcare team, thereby promoting and enhancing a person-centred approach to palliative care.

Conclusion

Enriching a sense of self, identity and ultimately patient dignity is a key issue for nurses working with those experiencing life-limiting illness across settings of care. When dignity is undermined, patients feel that their life may no longer have meaning and purpose, they feel they are suffering, and they may be more apt to make requests for a hastened death (Wilson et al. 2007). By having tools such as the dignity-conserving care model and the patient dignity question (PDQ) in our toolbox, nurses can strive to uncover what it is about the person they are caring for that is important to that person's well-being. By supporting the core identity and sense of self of the individual in our care, person-centred care is promoted and the potential for a good death is increased.

References

Ahlstrom, G. (2007) Experiences of loss and chronic sorrow in persons with severe chronic illness. *Journal of Clinical Nursing*, 16(3A): 76–83.

Arantzamendi, M., Belar, A. and Martínez, M. (2016) Promoting patient-centred palliative care: a scoping review of the patient dignity question. *Current Opinion in Supportive and Palliative Care*, 10(4): 324–9.

Carlander, I., Ternestedt, B., Sahlberg-Blom, E. et al. (2011) Four aspects of self-image close to death at home. *International Journal of Qualitative Studies on Health and Well-being*, 6(2).

Cassell, E.J. (2004) *The Nature of Suffering and the Goals of Medicine*. Oxford: Oxford University Press.

Charmaz, K. (1983) Loss of self: a fundamental form of suffering in the chronically ill. *Sociology of Health & Illness*, 5(2): 168–95.

Charmaz, K. (1995) The body, identity, and self: adapting to impairment. *Sociological Quarterly*, 36(4): 657–80.

Chochinov, H.M. (2002) Dignity-conserving care – a new model for palliative care: helping the patient feel valued. *Journal of the American Medical Association*, 287(17): 2253–60.

Chochinov, H.M. (2007) Dignity and the essence of medicine: the A, B, C, and D of dignity conserving care. *BMJ (Clinical Research Ed.)*, 335(7612): 184–7.

Chochinov, H.M. and Cann, B.J. (2005) Interventions to enhance the spiritual aspects of dying. *Journal of Palliative Medicine*, 8 (Suppl. 1): s103–15.

Chochinov, H.M., Hack, T., McClement, S. et al. (2002) Dignity in the terminally ill: a developing empirical model. *Social Science & Medicine (1982)*, 54(3): 433–43.

Chochinov, H.M., Krisjanson, L.J., Hack, T.F. et al. (2006) Dignity in the terminally ill: revisited. *Journal of Palliative Medicine*, 9(3): 666–72.

Chochinov, H.M., Hack, T., Hassard, T. et al. (2002) Dignity in the terminally ill: a cross-sectional, cohort study. *Lancet*, 360(9350): 2026–30.

Chochinov, H.M., Hassard, T., McClement, S. et al. (2009) The landscape of distress in the terminally ill. *Journal of Pain and Symptom Management*, 38(5): 641–9.

Chochinov, H.M., Johnston, W., McClement, S.E. et al. (2016) Dignity and distress towards the end of life across four non-cancer populations. *PLoS One*, 11(1): e0147607.

Chochinov, H.M., McClement, S., Hack, T. et al. (2015) Eliciting personhood within clinical practice: effects on patients, families and health care providers. *Journal of Pain and Symptom Management*, 49(6): 974–80.

Davis, M.H. (1994) *Empathy: A Social Psychological Approach*. Madison, WI: Westview Press.

Devoldre, I., Davis, M.H., Verhofstadt, L.L. and Buysse, A. (2010) Empathy and social support provision in couples: social support and the need to study the underlying processes. *Journal of Psychology*, 144(3): 259–84.

Edvardsson, D. and Innes, A. (2010) Measuring person-centred care: a critical comparative review of published tools. *Gerontologist*, 50(6): 834–46.

Edvardsson, D., Varrailhon, P. and Edvardsson, K. (2014) Promoting person-centeredness in long-term care: an exploratory study. *Journal of Gerontological Nursing*, 40(4): 46–53.

Erikson, H.E. (1998) *The Life Cycle Completed: Extended Version with New Chapters on the Ninth Stage of Development by Joan M. Erikson*. New York: W.W. Norton & Company, Inc.

Ferrell, B.R. and Coyle, N. (2008) *The Nature of Suffering and the Goals of Nursing*. New York: Oxford University Press.

Gottlieb, L.N. (2014) Strengths-based nursing. *American Journal of Nursing*, 114(8): 24–32.

Hack, T.F., Chochinov, H.M., Hassard, T. et al. (2004) Defining dignity in terminally ill cancer patients: a factor-analytic approach. *Psycho-Oncology*, 13(10): 700–8.

Hall, W.J., Chapman, M.V., Lee, K.M. et al. (2015) Implicit racial/ethnic bias among health care professionals and its influence on health care outcomes: a systematic review. *American Journal of Public Health*, 105(12): e60–76.

Jacelon, C.S. (2014) Strategies used by older adults to maintain or restore attributed dignity. *Research in Gerontological Nursing*, 7(6): 273–83.

Jakimowicz, S. and Perry, L. (2015) A concept analysis of patient-centred nursing in the intensive care unit. *Journal of Advanced Nursing*, 71(7): 1499–517.

Jeppsson, M. and Thomé, B. (2015) How do nurses in palliative care perceive the concept of self-image? *Scandinavian Journal of Caring Sciences*, 29(3): 454–61.

Johnston, B., Gaffney, M., Pringle, J. and Buchanan, D. (2015a) The person behind the patient: a feasibility study using the Patient Dignity Question for patients with palliative care needs in hospital. *International Journal of Palliative Nursing*, 21(2): 71–7.

Johnston, B., Larkin, P., Connolly, M. et al. (2015b) Dignity-conserving care in palliative care settings: an integrative review. *Journal of Clinical Nursing*, 24(13–14): 1743–72.

Johnston, B., Pringle, J., Gaffney, M. et al. (2015c) The dignified approach to care: a pilot study using the patient dignity question as an intervention to enhance dignity and person-centred care for people with palliative care needs in the acute hospital setting. *BMC Palliative Care*, 14: 9.

Kitwood, T. (1997) *Dementia Reconsidered: The Person Comes First*. Maidenhead: McGraw-Hill Education.

Lin, Y.P., Tsai, Y.F. and Cheng, S.F. (2011) Patient dignity in the hospital setting from patients' perspectives. *Journal of Clinical Nursing*, 5–6: 794–801.

Lobchuk, M.M., McClement, S.E., McPherson, C. and Cheang, M. (2008) Does blaming the patient with lung cancer affect the helping behaviour of primary caregivers? *Oncology Nursing Forum*, 35(4): 681–9.

Lomborg, K., Bjorn, A., Dahl, R. and Kirkevold, M. (2005) Body care experienced by people hospitalized with severe respiratory disease. *Journal of Advanced Nursing*, 50(3): 262–71.

Lusk, J.M. and Fater, K. (2013) A concept analysis of patient-centred care. *Nursing Forum*, 48(2): 89–98.

McClement, S.E. and Chochinov, H.M. (2006) Dignity in palliative care. In Bruera, E., Higginson, I., von Gunten, C. and Ripamonti, C. (eds) *Textbook of Palliative Medicine*. New York: Edward Arnold, pp. 100–7.

McClement, S.E., Chochinov, H.M., Hack, T.F. et al. (2004) Dignity-conserving care: application of research findings to practice. *International Journal of Palliative Nursing*, 10(4): 173–9.

McCormack, B. and McCance, T.V. (2006) Development of a framework for person-centred nursing. *Journal of Advanced Nursing*, 56(5): 472–9.

Merriam-Webster Dictionary (2017) Dignity. Available at: http://www.merriam-webster. com

Morgan, S. and Yoder, L.H. (2012) A concept analysis of person-centred care. *Journal of Holistic Nursing: Official Journal of the American Holistic Nurses' Association*, 30(1): 6–15.

Nanton, V., Munday, D., Dale, J. et al. (2016) The threatened self: considerations of time, place, and uncertainty in advanced illness. *British Journal of Health Psychology*, 21(2): 351–73.

Oechsle, K., Wais, M.C., Vehling, S. et al. (2014) Relationship between symptom burden, distress, and sense of dignity in terminally ill cancer patients. *Journal of Pain and Symptom Management*, 48(3): 313–21.

Östlund, U., Brown, H. and Johnston, B. (2012) Dignity conserving care at end-of-life: a narrative review. *European Journal of Oncology Nursing*, 16(4): 353–67.

Pleschberger, S. (2007) Dignity and the challenge of dying in nursing homes: the residents' view. *Age and Ageing*, 36(2): 197–202.

Proulx, K. and Jacelon, C. (2004) Dying with dignity: the good patient versus the good death. *American Journal of Hospice & Palliative Care*, 21(2): 116–20.

Pullman, D. (2004) Death, dignity, and moral nonsense. *Journal of Palliative Care*, 20(3): 171–8.

Reeve, J., Lloyd-Williams, M., Payne, S. and Dowrick, C. (2009) Towards a reconceptualisation of the management of distress in palliative care patients: the self-integrity model. *Progress in Palliative Care*, 17(2): 51–60.

Rodríguez-Prat, A., Monforte-Royo, C., Porta-Sales, J. et al. (2016) Patient perspectives of dignity, autonomy and control at the end of life: systematic review and meta-ethnography. *PLoS One*, 11(3): e0151435.

Sharma, T., Bamford, M. and Dodman, D. (2015) Person-centred care: an overview of reviews. *Contemporary Nurse*, 51(2–3): 107–20.

Sinclair, S., McClement, S., Raffin-Bouchal, S. et al. (2016b) Compassion in health care: an empirical model. *Journal of Pain and Symptom Management*, 51(2): 193–203.

Sinclair, S., Torres, M.B., Raffin-Bouchal, S. et al. (2016a) Compassion training in healthcare: what are patients' perspectives on training healthcare providers? *BMC Medical Education*, 16: 169.

Steinhauser, K.E., Christakis, N.A., Clipp, E.C. et al. (2000) Factors considered important at the end of life by patients, family, physicians, and other care providers. *Journal of the American Medical Association*, 284(19): 2476–82.

Street, A.F. and Kissane, D.W. (2001) Constructions of dignity in end-of-life care. *Journal of Palliative Care*, 17(2): 93–101.

Ternestedt, B. (2009) A dignified death and identity-promoting care. In Nordenfelt, L. (ed.) *Dignity in Care for Older People.* Oxford: Blackwell, pp. 146–67.

Thompson, G.N. and Chochinov, H.M. (2008) Dignity-based approaches in the care of terminally ill patients. *Current Opinion in Supportive and Palliative Care,* 2(1): 49–53.

Thompson, G.N., McArthur, J. and Doupe, M. (2016) Identifying markers of dignity-conserving care in long-term care: a modified Delphi study. *PLoS One,* 11(6): e0156816.

Wilson, K.G., Chochinov, H.M., McPherson, C.J. et al. (2007) Desire for euthanasia or physician-assisted suicide in palliative cancer care. *Health Psychology: Official Journal of the Division of Health Psychology, American Psychological Association,* 26(3): 314–23.

World Health Organization (2017) *Framework on Integrated People-Centred Health Services.* Available at: http://www.who.int.uml.idm.oclc.org/servicedeliverysafety/areas/people-centred-care/framework/en/

Caring for informal carers

Samar M. Aoun and Gail Ewing

Introduction

The fundamental goal of palliative care is to attain the best possible quality of life and support for terminally ill people and their families (National Institute for Health and Clinical Excellence 2004; Palliative Care Australia 2005; World Health Organization 2007; National Hospice and Palliative Care Organization 2008). The ethos of palliative care embraces not just the patient, but also family members or friends who are their informal carers. Without the involvement of family or informal carers, the well-being of most terminally ill people would be disadvantaged (Hudson 2003; Aoun et al. 2005b). Several reports have argued that the changing demographics at the end of life, including the reduction in numbers of potential family carers, have considerable outcomes for service delivery (Hudson 2003; Rolls et al. 2011).

Recognition of the impacts of caregiving has resulted in health policy recommendations on the need to support carers in several countries, such as Australia (Palliative Care Australia 2005; Commonwealth of Australia 2010), Canada (Carstairs and Keon 2009; Canadian Hospice Palliative Care Association 2013) and the UK, where the National Institute for Clinical Excellence (2004, p. 157) stressed that carers' needs should be 'assessed, acknowledged and addressed'. The subsequent UK End of Life Care Strategy (Department of Health 2008) further acknowledged the central role of carers in care provision as 'co-workers' but also identified that they have their own needs separate from those of patients. More recently, Actions for End of Life Care (NHS England 2014) refreshed the End of Life Care Strategy (Department of Health 2008) and set out the commitments of NHS England for support to carers (as well as patients), indicating that they are to be offered comprehensive holistic assessments and holistic support, following a person-centred model of care.

Thus, a key aspect of palliative care nursing is not just caring for patients, but also supporting their carers. This chapter provides an overview of caring for informal carers in three sections:

1   Carers in palliative care: their key role and the impact that caring has on them.
2   Assessing carers: carer support needs, assessment tools and person-centred care.
3   Supportive interventions for carers in palliative care.

Carers in palliative care

Definitions

In this chapter, the term 'carer' refers to people who provide *unpaid* support to a family member/friend (as opposed to those who provide caring support in a paid capacity in health or social services and may also be referred to as 'carers'). However, it is important to be aware that other terms may also be used to refer to those in an unpaid caring role such as caregivers, family carers, informal carers or lay carers, as these terms tend to be used interchangeably.

Just as there are different names for carers, so too are there many different definitions of a 'carer'. The UK charity Carers Trust, whose remit is supporting carers more broadly than palliative care, defines a carer as 'anyone who cares, unpaid, for a friend or family member who due to illness, disability, a mental health problem or an addiction cannot cope without their support' (Carers Trust 2015). In palliative care, a useful definition is 'lay people in a close supportive role who share in the illness experience of the patient and who undertake vital care work and emotion management' (National Institute for Health and Clinical Excellence 2004). This definition is used here because it includes the important work of emotional support many carers provide within a palliative care context.

While most reports state the number of people with a caring role in general, there are only estimates of the numbers of those caring in palliative and end of life care, for example, in the UK it is estimated to be at least half a million (based on UK number of deaths per year), and this figure may be an underestimate as often there is more than one carer involved (The National Council for Palliative Care 2013). In Australia, there are 159,000 deaths per year (Australian Bureau of Statistics, 2015), and the proportion of expected deaths varies between 25–50 per cent (Commonwealth of Australia 2010).

Profile and role of carers

Caring is related to gender, as more women than men provide care, and with differing life expectancies between the two genders, it is expected that the majority of older carers in palliative care are women (Payne and EAPC Task Force on Family Carers 2010). In a more recent Australian study on family carers at end of life, 71 per cent were women, average age was 64 years, 68 per cent were spouses and 20 per cent were adult children of care recipients (Aoun et al. 2015b). The profile of this study was similar to that of many studies where family carers were predominantly women, spouses, retirees, and caring for older family members with mainly a malignant disease, and in particular comparable to a similar study conducted in the UK (Ewing et al. 2013).

The important role carers play in home-based palliative care involves a range of tasks such as managing symptoms and administering medications, providing personal care such as washing and dressing, different aspects of practical support such as assisting with walking and positioning and sourcing or managing equipment needed for patient care, providing emotional support and coordinating appointments and input from care providers (Aoun et al. 2005a; Bee et al. 2009; Funk et al. 2010; Stajduhar et al. 2010). Estimates of the time spent on caring vary, from 20 or more hours per week (The National Council for Palliative Care 2013) to over 69 hours per week reported in a new national post bereavement census survey (Rowland et al. 2017). In so doing, they provide much of the support needed by the patient as well as reducing the costs of formal care (Aoun et al. 2005a; Stajduhar et al. 2010; Haines 2011).

Carer influence on place of care and place of death

As seen previously in Chapter 3, most people express a preference to die at home (Gomes et al. 2013). In Australia, up to 90 per cent of terminally ill patients spend the majority of their last year of life at home, and approximately one-third of all Australian patients receiving palliative care services die at home (Australian Institute of Health and Welfare 2012). In England, the percentage of patients cared for at home in the last year of life is not clear, although many remain under the care of the primary care team. We do know that although 22 per cent of deaths in England take place at home (Public Health England 2015), nearly 90 per cent of patients attend hospital in some form in their last year (Georghiou et al. 2012). In a systematic review of variables affecting place of death for terminally ill cancer patients in the UK, living with relatives was identified as strongly associated with dying at home (Gomes and Higginson 2006). An Australian study reported that, compared to terminally ill patients with a carer, those without a carer were less likely to die at home (35 per cent compared to 57 per cent), 2.5 times more likely to die in a hospital and twice as likely to die in a hospice (Aoun et al. 2007). In this context, carers play an essential role in enabling patients to be cared for at home and die there if that is their choice.

Impact of caring

Providing home-based caregiving for the terminally ill is not without a cost to carers: the impact of taking on this role is well documented, with an extensive literature reporting adverse effects of caregiving. Negative impacts are reported on physical and emotional health, social isolation and pressures on work and finances (Aoun et al. 2005a; Grande et al. 2009; Stajduhar et al. 2010; Aoun et al. 2017), and there is evidence of increased mortality (Schulz and Beach 1999). However, not all aspects of caregiving are negative. Despite difficult circumstances, carers report positive experiences about their caregiving role, gaining a sense of reward and self-fulfilment (Hudson 2004; Wong and

Ussher 2009). These positive aspects may have some buffering effect on the challenges carers can also face.

There is also evidence that provision of adequate support by services during care-giving improves family carers' psychological outcomes (Ferrario et al. 2004; Grande et al. 2004; Kissane et al. 2006), while identifying and addressing concerns early leads to better carer health outcomes (Grande et al. 2004; Aoun et al. 2015b). Therefore, in order to ameliorate the negative effects of caregiving, family carers need to be supported in their central role of caring.

Barriers to supporting carers

There are a number of barriers that can hinder carers in being supported as needed (Austin et al. 2017). While the ethos of palliative care is to support not only the patient but also family members/friends who are carers, the primary focus of services is on patients as they are clients of the service. As a consequence, identification of carers' needs, where it does take place, tends to be informal and without any guiding frame-work and can often go undocumented (Ewing et al. 2013; Aoun et al. 2015c). Moreover, there is often reluctance by family carers to express their own needs (Grande et al. 2009) either because they prefer the focus of service providers to be the patient (Ewing and Grande 2013) or because they do not identify themselves as being 'carers', but rather see themselves as husband/wife, son/daughter, friend, etc. (Corden and Hirst 2011; Burns et al. 2013; Carduff et al. 2014). Carers tend to be overlooked and often referred to as 'hidden patients' (Kristjanson and Aoun 2004).

Learning exercise 12.1 Examining existing practice with carers

This is a useful stage to review your own practice in identifying carers' needs. You may wish to reflect on these questions as you complete this exercise:

- How often do you find yourself asking a carer 'How are you?' on the door-step or in a ward corridor?
- Do you use any kind of assessment tool to help identify needs?
- How much do you rely on picking up cues?
- Carers are often included in the joint assessment with the patient: but whose needs are the focus?

Reflect on your current practice working with carers and make some short notes on the following areas:

- How do you currently become aware of carers' support needs?
- What limitations do these methods have?
- What are the positives that you would wish to retain?

Assessing carers

Carer support needs

There is an extensive literature on carers' support needs in end of life care and we refer readers to reviews such as Stajduhar et al. (2010) and Payne et al. (2010) for a full discussion. However, in terms of delivering nursing support to carers, the study by Ewing and Grande (2013), which focused directly on carers' support needs, provides a useful, practical framework of 14 support domains (each a broad area of support needs) that encompass physical, practical, social, financial, psychological and spiritual support that current policy guidance indicates should be delivered to carers during end of life care. What is important to note is that these domains fall into two distinct groupings (Box 12.1):

1   Support that carers need to enable them to care for their relative/friend, for example, with managing symptoms or medicines or knowing what to expect in the future. These are areas of support for the 'co-worker' role taken on by carers in end of life care. Carers often feel a great responsibility in ensuring appropriate care for their relative/friend and frequently have great expertise in this role which needs to be recognised.
2   More direct support for carers themselves in terms of their own health and well-being, for example, with dealing with their feelings and worries or having time for themselves in the day. These support domains reflect that carers also have the role of 'client' in palliative and end of life care where the remit of services is to care not just for the patient but to support the carer and family.

Box 12.1 Carer support needs

Seven domains of support enabling the carer to care (the 'co-worker' role)

1   Understanding their relative's illness.
2   Managing their relative's symptoms, including giving medicines.
3   Providing personal care (e.g. dressing, washing, toileting).
4   Knowing whom to contact when concerned.
5   Equipment to help care for their relative.
6   Talking with their relative about his/her illness.
7   Knowing what to expect in the future when caring for their relative.

Seven domains of support in relation to their own health and well-being (the 'client' role)

1   Looking after their own physical health.
2   Having time for self in the day.
3   Any financial, legal, or work issues.

4   Dealing with feelings and worries.
5   Beliefs or spiritual concerns.
6   Practical help in the home.
7   Getting a break from caring overnight.

Despite an evidence base of the impact of caregiving on carers and recognition of their support needs, carers are not always well supported. Figure 12.1 demonstrates the extent of unmet support needs of carers from two recent studies in the UK and Australia (Ewing et al. 2013; Aoun et al. 2015b). The four domains in which most carers needed more support were similar in both countries: knowing what to expect in the future, having time for yourself in the day, dealing with your feelings and worries and understanding your relative's illness. What is important to note here is that clearly carers have support needs in both aspects of their role, as 'co-workers' as well as 'clients'.

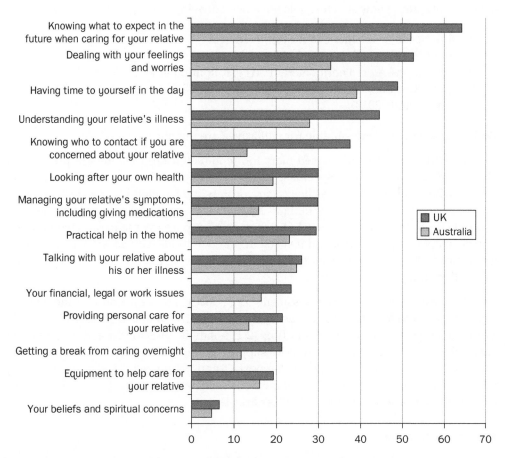

Figure 12.1 Unmet carer support needs in the UK (n = 216–222) and Australia (n = 215)
Source: Adapted from Aoun et al. (2015b) and Ewing et al. (2013).

Carer assessment tools in palliative care

Many carer assessment tools have been developed for long-term caregiving, particularly for carers of people with dementia and Alzheimer's disease (Deeken et al. 2003) or developed for the field of gerontology such as the COAT (Hanson et al. 2006) or CARE (Keefe et al. 2008) tools, but these have not been widely implemented in palliative care. A review by Hudson et al. (2010b) identified 62 measures for use with family caregivers of palliative care patients. Although a large number of tools were reviewed, most did not measure 'needs' directly, rather, they were indirect measures, including carer burden, distress, preparedness, anxiety and depression. As such, these tools are *indicators* of caregiving difficulties and the need for carers to be supported, but they do not assess what the carers' needs are (Stajduhar et al. 2010; Ewing and Grande 2013).

There are some well-tested research tools to measure carers' needs directly such as the Home Caregiver Needs Survey (Hileman et al. 1992), the Caregiving at Life's End Questionnaire (Salmon et al. 2005) and the Problems and Needs in Palliative Care (Osse et al. 2006) but they are very lengthy and not suitable for use in routine practice. However, recently three new shorter tools have been developed for practice. These are:

1 the Needs Assessment Tool-Caregivers (NAT-C) developed in Australia (Mitchell et al. 2010), which is intended for use by GPs;
2 the Carers' Alert Thermometer (CAT) (Knighting et al. 2015);
3 the Carer Support Needs Assessment Tool (CSNAT) (Ewing et al. 2013; Ewing and Grande 2013).

Both CAT and CSNAT are suitable for palliative care nursing.

The CAT is an evidence-based alert tool completed by a healthcare professional and intended for use by non-specialist palliative care providers. It has ten questions to discuss with carers to enable the healthcare professional to identify any alerts requiring action. Each question has a traffic light system of green (Low), amber (Intermediate) and red (High) to identify the level of risk each alert poses to the caregiving situation. The developers report that it can be used in practice to identify carers who are at risk and in need of a formal needs assessment. The CAT has not yet been implemented fully in practice (Knighting et al. 2015).

The Carer Support Needs Assessment Tool (CSNAT) takes account of the dual role of carers, as both 'co-workers' and as 'clients' themselves and is structured around the 14 broad support domains shown in Box 12.1. A simple question format is used to ask carers directly whether they need more support in the 14 areas and carers themselves are able to indicate how much more support, if any, they need. This screening design allows the tool to be brief but also comprehensive. Thus, unlike the CAT, which is a professionally led assessment, the CSNAT is carer-led.

Person-centred care

Person-centred care is widely promoted in healthcare, where collaboration between service providers and service users can be a marker of quality of care (Collins 2014; Health Foundation 2014). 'It is about working "with" people rather than doing "to" them'

(Ewing et al. 2015, p. 580). Person-centred care is central to NHS England's (2014) vision for end of life care for 2015 and beyond, for both carers as well as patients. However, while the term 'person-centred care' is widely used, it is not always clear how this can be delivered in healthcare practice. To help address this issue for carer assessment and support, the CSNAT research team has defined a five-stage person-centred process, the CSNAT Approach, to be used with the CSNAT itself, to enable a holistic and systematic process of assessment and support that is carer-led and tailored to their individual support needs (Ewing et al. 2015) (Figure 12.2).

Figure 12.2 provides an illustration of the CSNAT Approach which can be a useful reminder of the stages of this person-centred process:

- Stage 1: the CSNAT (the tool itself) is introduced to the carer as an opportunity to discuss their situation and any support they may need, not as a questionnaire to fill in.
- Stage 2: the carer needs time to consider the domains where they may need more support and prioritise those most important to them.
- Stage 3: the carer and practitioner can discuss the carer's specific support needs during an 'assessment conversation'.
- Stage 4: the carer and practitioner agree on what further supportive input the carer feels would be valuable and create a shared action plan tailored to the carer's individual needs.
- Stage 5: review of the carer's support needs is ongoing, initiated by either the carer or the practitioner.

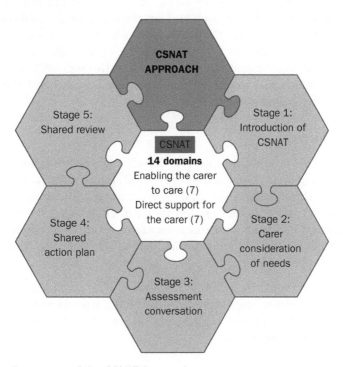

Figure 12.2 The five stages of the CSNAT Approach

Using the CSNAT Approach in practice entails a shift from the informal health professional-led methods of identifying carers' support needs to a carer-led approach facilitated by the health professional. Case Study 12.1 provides an illustration of use of the CSNAT Approach in hospice home care. In this organisation, experienced healthcare assistants as well as nursing staff received training in the CSNAT Approach and one of the team provided an exemplar of its use in practice.

Case Study 12.1: Using the CSNAT Approach in practice

Exemplar from a Health Care Assistant (HCA)

Context

Sarah, the Health Care Assistant (HCA), was part of a team of practitioners who were supporting the family in their home. Sarah had attended a short training session on using the CSNAT Approach in practice.

Stage 1: Introduction

Sarah was visiting the patient to help with his morning care needs. The patient had deteriorated over the previous week and when she arrived she found the carer in tears. The CSNAT Approach had just been introduced into the service so Sarah decided to take the opportunity to use it with this distressed carer. Sarah's approach was simple: she sat down with the carer, introduced the CSNAT and explained what it was for and asked her to read it through while she went off to attend to the patient. She explained that when she had finished, they would sit together and have a chat about things.

Stage 2: Consideration

The carer had time to read through the CSNAT while Sarah spent time with the patient. Then they looked together at the CSNAT. Sarah asked the carer if it was OK if they went through it together and the carer agreed, so Sarah simply read out the questions and asked the carer to tell her whether she needed more support for each domain and recorded the carer's responses. Both were comfortable doing this. Sarah didn't explore any domains in detail at this time; she first gathered all of the carer's support needs.

Most often carers complete the CSNAT themselves. This particular carer preferred that Sarah recorded her responses. However, what was recorded was what the carer said was needed in terms of more support with the different domains. Sarah did not interpret her responses.

Stage 3: Assessment conversation

Once the domains where more support was needed had been identified, Sarah asked the carer to tell her which areas were most important (her immediate priorities). Sarah then circled the key support domains from those she had highlighted on the CSNAT. What surprised Sarah was that the carer's priorities were not at all what she had expected: 'This is why I think it [the CSNAT Approach] is so good because we go in there day in day out, and we think we know what they need, and we're totally wrong.'

Then they went on to discuss further each of the carer's priority areas, which were: (1) talking with her husband about his illness and understanding it more, and (2) having time for herself in the day: she had grandchildren she wanted to see but they lived at a distance and so they discussed the best type of respite that would allow her to spend some time with them.

Stage 4: Shared action plan

In this instance, Sarah had the assessment conversation with the carer. Sarah therefore fed back this conversation to the nursing team along with the CSNAT which enabled a nurse from the team to continue the conversation with the carer and put an action plan in place. The nursing team arranged for a Macmillan nurse to visit for a discussion about the patient's illness and a respite placement was arranged to enable the carer to visit her grandchildren.

Stage 5: Shared review

As Sarah visited the patient and carer on a regular basis, the carer took the opportunity to let Sarah know that she still felt she would like to understand more about the illness, in addition to the information she had already received. This carer was therefore able to initiate a review of her support needs herself. This prompted another contact by the nursing team to provide further help with this.

Benefit of using the CSNAT Approach

Sarah commented on the beneficial on-going review of this carer's support needs, which she felt came about as a direct result of using the CSNAT Approach:

> The last point I'd like to make is that I believe because of the CSNAT and the trust that we built up with the lady, she has been able to ask us any questions and we've been able to give her much more support than maybe we would have done previously.

Learning exercise 12.2

Now that we have introduced you to the CSNAT Approach, this is a good opportunity to reflect on what you have read about each of the stages and consider how you might use it in your own practice. Work through the five stages in Figure 12.2 and consider the questions asked at each stage.

Stage 1: Introduction

How and when could you first introduce the CSNAT to a carer (to ensure the carer perceives the CSNAT as an *opportunity* to consider their needs, *not an obligation* to 'fill in a form')?

Stage 2: Carer's consideration of needs

How will you ensure that the carer has space and time to consider what their own needs are?

Stage 3: Assessment conversation

The assessment conversation takes place once the carer has had the opportunity to consider their own support needs. When would you be able to complete this conversation (e.g. at the same time as it is introduced, at a follow-up visit, over the phone)?

Stage 4: Shared action plan

Will you be able to produce a short action plan following the assessment conversation?

Where will the plan be recorded?

Stage 5: Shared review

Think about whether you have any opportunities to review the whole process.

For permission to use the CSNAT, please contact Gail Ewing: ge200@cam.ac.uk. Further details about the CSNAT Approach can be accessed from CSNAT.org

Benefits of the CSNAT Approach

The CSNAT Approach has demonstrated benefits for both carers and practitioners. Trials of its use showed a significant reduction in caregiver strain in current carers (Aoun et al. 2015b) and significantly lower levels of early grief and better psychological and physical health in bereavement (Grande et al. 2017).

Feedback from nurses was also very positive: using the CSNAT provided guidance, focus, and a structure to facilitate discussion with family carers, and identified needs and responses that would not otherwise have been undertaken (Aoun et al. 2015c, p. 929).

It also appeared to legitimise support provision for carers, and demonstrate practitioners' interest in supporting them (Aoun et al. 2015c; Ewing et al. 2016).

Carers themselves also reported feelings of validation, reassurance, and empowerment and felt they had timely access to support and that services put in place were responsive to their needs (Aoun et al. 2015a, p. 508). Overall, the experience provided carers with confidence in their ability to cope.

Supportive interventions for carers

While routine use of a carer assessment process in practice can be viewed as a supportive intervention that is available to the wider population of carers in order to address their needs, it is more usual to think of 'one-to-one' or group interventions for carer support. There is a growing palliative care literature on supportive interventions, in particular, a number of reviews of current evidence (Caress et al. 2009; Hudson et al. 2010a; Parker et al. 2010; Candy et al. 2011; Harding et al. 2012; Farquhar et al. 2016).

To help practitioners consider which interventions they might use in practice, Payne and Morbey (2013) provide a useful typology of supportive interventions for carers in three categories according to complexity of therapeutic intent:

- The most basic level, which they consider can be offered to all carers, is information, training and education. This includes information resources on topics such as disease processes and symptom management, accessing advice on benefits or education in different aspects of care provision.
- One level up in complexity are 'supportive activities' which include drop-in centres, activity groups and befriending schemes that hospices are often well placed to deliver.
- Finally, the most complex are 'therapeutic activities' which include interventions such as counselling, mindfulness classes or complementary therapies.

What do we know about the effectiveness of interventions?

While the typology offers practitioners a useful means of categorising interventions, it does not address the question of their effectiveness. Despite the increasing number of intervention studies, clear evidence of their effectiveness is limited. This is for three main reasons (Parker et al. 2010; Candy et al. 2011; Farquhar et al. 2016):

- inadequate description of the intervention itself making it difficult to replicate but also to determine which components may have had an impact;
- limitations in the reporting of study methods;
- a lack of experimental designs to permit evaluation of effectiveness of the intervention.

The one high quality study with a significant treatment effect was an RCT by Hudson et al. (2005), in which a one-to-one psycho-educational intervention was delivered to carers by palliative care nurses. Carers in the intervention group had a significantly more positive experience of caregiving compared to those receiving standard care. However, it has to be noted that the intervention delivered was resource-intensive, which calls into question feasibility in routine practice.

A Cochrane Review (Candy et al. 2011), which assessed the effects of supportive interventions that aimed to improve the psychological and physical health of carers, has a lot of relevance for palliative care nursing. Interventions could be practical, emotional, facilitating coping skills, and included carer support delivered indirectly via patient care. While it was not clear from the review which types of support may be of more benefit, emotional support and providing information on caring for the patient were common features of the interventions that were found to help buffer against psychological distress. The conclusion offered by the authors provides some guidance for practice – that at the very least, healthcare professionals should enquire about the concerns of family and friends caring for someone with a terminal illness and consider that they may benefit from additional support.

On the whole, therefore, there remains much work to be done on developing supportive intervention for carers that show effectiveness. It is also the case that interventions that have been developed have a focus on carers of patients with cancer. There is considerably less information about interventions for carers of people with other life-limiting illnesses. Farquhar et al.'s (2016) review of education interventions for lay carers of patients with any advanced disease, not just cancer, concluded that published evaluations are limited, particularly for non-cancer conditions.

Although this chapter has focused on adult carers of adult people with life-limiting illnesses, other carer groups that also deserve attention in further work on informal carers are young carers and parent-carers of children with life-limiting illnesses. Reviews in developed countries (Day 2015; Stamatopoulos 2016) have called for more research on the extent and nature of informal young caregiving to improve recognition and targeted support for young carers and minimise the adverse impact on their future life opportunities. Addressing the support needs of parent-carers in paediatric palliative care is also under-researched. Despite increasing knowledge that parent-carers experience a variety of unmet physical, emotional, social and spiritual support needs, assessment of these needs is typically performed in an ad-hoc, informal manner, and there is a lack of congruency between parents' needs and the services provided to them (Collins et al. 2016; Coombes et al. 2016). CSNAT is not yet validated for these two groups of informal carers.

Conclusion

In this chapter we have drawn on international contemporary research evidence in the field of palliative care. The caregiving context is set by describing the key role of carers in end of life care. Although the impact of their caring role is well recognised and there is good evidence that provision of support can improve outcomes, carers still are not always well supported. There is now a growing palliative care literature on one-to-one and group interventions for carers and systematic reviews to support nurses in identifying those most effective in practice. However, within palliative care nursing the intervention with the potential to have the greatest 'reach', available to a wide population of carers, is the adoption of a comprehensive, person-centred approach to carer assessment in routine practice, ensuring that carers have the opportunity to consider and express their support needs to enable practitioners to deliver support tailored to their individual circumstances. Learning exercises and the case study serve to promote reflective thinking about the issues that practitioners face in routine practice and provide some initial guidance on using an evidence-based person-centred approach to support carers.

Box 12.2 summarises the key learning points from this chapter.

Box 12.2 Key learning points

- Carers play a crucial role in palliative and end of life care: without their support many patients would not achieve their preferred place of care or place of death.
- The impact of taking on a caregiving role is substantial, affecting carers' physical, social and emotional health and well-being, even affecting their mortality.
- To ameliorate some of the negative effects of caregiving, carers need support in their dual role: support to enable them to care for the patient (their 'co-worker' role) and also direct support for their own health and well-being (their 'client' role).
- Use of an evidence-based tool in palliative and end of life care to assess and support carers provides an intervention to support a wider population of carers in everyday practice.
- The Care Support Needs Assessment Tool (CSNAT) is an evidence-based, comprehensive assessment tool which is integrated into a person-centred process of assessment and support. Together as 'The CSNAT Approach', they enable a holistic and systematic process of assessment and support that is carer-led and tailored to their individual support needs.
- There have been many interventions developed for carers in end of life care, mostly for carers of patients with cancer, but these are delivered to relatively few carers at any time and evidence of their effectiveness is limited.

References

Aoun, S., Deas, K., Kristjanson, L.J. and Kissane, D.W. (2017) Identifying and addressing the support needs of family caregivers of people with motor neurone disease using the Carer Support Needs Assessment Tool. *Palliative and Supportive Care*, 15(1): 32–43.

Aoun, S., Deas, K., Toye, C. et al. (2015a) Supporting family caregivers to identify their own needs in end-of-life care: qualitative findings from a stepped wedge cluster trial. *Palliative Medicine*, 29(6): 508–17.

Aoun, S., Grande, G., Howting, D. et al. (2015b) The impact of the Carer Support Needs Assessment Tool (CSNAT) in community palliative care using a stepped wedge cluster trial. *PLoS One*, 10(4): e0123012.

Aoun, S., Kristjanson, L.J., Currow, D.C. and Hudson, P.L. (2005a) Caregiving for the terminally ill: at what cost? *Palliative Medicine*, 19(7): 551–5.

Aoun, S., Kristjanson, L.J., Currow, D. et al. (2007) Terminally-ill people living alone without a caregiver: an Australian national scoping study of palliative care needs. *Palliative Medicine*, 21(1): 29–34.

Aoun, S., Kristjanson, L.J., Hudson, P.L. et al. (2005b) The experience of supporting a dying relative: reflections of caregivers. *Progress in Palliative Care*, 13(6): 319–25.

Aoun, S., Toye, C., Deas, K. et al. (2015c) Enabling a family caregiver-led assessment of support needs in home-based palliative care: potential translation into practice. *Palliative Medicine*, 29(10): 929–38.

Austin, L., Ewing, G. and Grande, G. (2017) Factors influencing practitioner adoption of carer-led assessment in palliative homecare: a qualitative study of the use of the Carer Support Needs Assessment Tool (CSNAT). *PLoS One*, 12(6): e0179287.

Australian Bureau of Statistics (2015) *Causes of Death Australia.*

Australian Institute of Health and Welfare (2012) *Palliative Care Services in Australia 2012*. (Cat. no. HWI120). Canberra: AIHW.

Bee, P.E., Barnes, P. and Luker, K.A. (2009) A systematic review of informal caregivers' needs in providing home-based end-of-life care to people with cancer. *Journal of Clinical Nursing*, 18(10): 1379–93.

Burns, C.M., Abernethy, A.P., Dal Grande, E. and Currow, D.C. (2013) Uncovering an invisible network of direct caregivers at the end of life: a population study. *Palliative Medicine*, 27(7): 608–15.

Canadian Hospice Palliative Care Association (2013) *A Model to Guide Hospice Palliative Care*. Ottawa, ON: Canadian Hospice Palliative Care Association.

Candy, B., Jones, L., Drake, R. et al. (2011) Interventions for supporting informal caregivers of patients in the terminal phase of a disease. *Cochrane Database of Systematic Reviews*, Issue 6. Art. No.: CD007617. doi: 10.1002/14651858.CD007617.pub2.

Carduff, E., Finucane, A., Kendall, M. et al. (2014) Understanding the barriers to identifying carers of people with advanced illness in primary care: triangulating three data sources. *BMC Family Practice*, 15: 48.

Carers Trust (2015) *What Is a Carer?* Vol. 2017. London: Carers Trust.

Caress, A.L., Chalmers, K. and Luker, K. (2009) A narrative review of interventions to support family carers who provide physical care to family members with cancer. *International Journal of Nursing Studies*, 46(11): 1516–27.

Carstairs, S. and Keon, W. (2009) *Canada's Aging Population: Seizing the Opportunity. Special Senate Committee on Aging – Final Report*. Ottawa, ON: Canadian Government.

Collins, A. (2014) *Measuring What Really Matters: Towards a Coherent Measurement System to Support Person-Centred Care*. London: Health Foundation.

Collins, A., Hennessy-Anderson, N., Hosking, S. et al. (2016) Lived experiences of parents caring for a child with a life-limiting condition in Australia: a qualitative study. *Palliative Medicine*, 30(10): 950–9.

Commonwealth of Australia (2010) *The National Palliative Care Strategy: Supporting Australians to Live Well at the End of Life*. Barton, ACT: Commonwealth of Australia.

Coombes, L.H., Wiseman, T., Lucas, G. et al. (2016) Health-related quality-of-life outcome measures in paediatric palliative care: a systematic review of psychometric properties and feasibility of use. *Palliative Medicine*, 30(10): 935–49.

Corden, A. and Hirst, M. (2011) Partner care at the end-of-life: identity, language and characteristics. *Ageing and Society*, 31(2): 217–42.

Day, C. (2015) Young adult carers: a literature review informing the reconceptualisation of young adult caregiving in Australia. *Journal of Youth Studies*, 18(7): 855–66.

Deeken, J.F., Taylor, K.L., Mangan, P. et al. (2003) Care for the caregivers: a review of self-report instruments developed to measure the burden, needs, and quality of life of informal caregivers. *Journal of Pain and Symptom Management*, 26(4): 922–53.

Department of Health (2008) *End of Life Care Strategy: Promoting High Quality Care for All Adults at the End of Life*. London: Department of Health.

Ewing, G., Austin, L., Diffin, J. and Grande, G. (2015) Developing a person-centred approach to carer assessment and support. *British Journal of Community Nursing*, 20(12): 580–4.

Ewing, G., Austin, L. and Grande, G. (2016) The role of the Carer Support Needs Assessment Tool in palliative home care: a qualitative study of practitioners' perspectives of its impact and mechanisms of action. *Palliative Medicine*, 30(4): 392–400.

Ewing, G., Brundle, C., Payne, S. and Grande, G. (2013) The Carer Support Needs Assessment Tool (CSNAT) for use in palliative and end-of-life care at home: a validation study. *Journal of Pain and Symptom Management*, 46(3): 395–405.

Ewing, G. and Grande, G. (2013) Development of a Carer Support Needs Assessment Tool (CSNAT) for end-of-life care practice at home: a qualitative study. *Palliative Medicine*, 27(3): 244–56.

Farquhar, M., Penfold, C., Walter, F.M. et al. (2016) What are the key elements of educational interventions for lay carers of patients with advanced disease? A systematic literature search and narrative review of structural components, processes and modes of delivery. *Journal of Pain and Symptom Management*, 52(1): 117–30. e27.

Ferrario, S.R., Cardillo, V., Vicario, F. et al. (2004) Advanced cancer at home: caregiving and bereavement. *Palliative Medicine*, 18(2): 129–36.

Funk, L., Stajduhar, K., Toye, C. et al. (2010) Part 2: Home-based family caregiving at the end of life: a comprehensive review of published qualitative research (1998–2008). *Palliative Medicine*, 24(6): 594–607.

Georghiou, T., Davies, S., Davies, A. and Bardsley, M. (2012) *Understanding Patterns of Health and Social Care at the End of Life*. London: Nuffield Trust.

Gomes, B., Calanzani, N., Gysels, M. et al. (2013) Heterogeneity and changes in preferences for dying at home: a systematic review. *BMC Palliative Care*, 12: 7.

Gomes, B. and Higginson, I.J. (2006) Factors influencing death at home in terminally ill patients with cancer: systematic review. *BMJ*, 332(7540): 515–21.

Grande, G., Austin, L., Ewing, G. et al. (2015) Assessing the impact of a Carer Support Needs Assessment Tool (CSNAT) intervention in palliative home care: a stepped wedge cluster trial. *BMJ Supportive and Palliative Care*. Published online first. 30 December 2015.

Grande, G., Farquhar, M.C., Barclay, S.I.G. and Todd, C.J. (2004) Caregiver bereavement outcome: relationship with hospice at home, satisfaction with care, and home death. *Journal of Palliative Care*, 20(2): 69–77.

Grande, G., Stajduhar, K., Aoun, S. et al. (2009) Supporting lay carers in end of life care: current gaps and future priorities. *Palliative Medicine*, 23(4): 339–44.

Haines, I.E. (2011) Managing patients with advanced cancer: the benefits of early referral for palliative care. *Medical Journal of Australia*, 194(3): 107–8.

Hanson, E., Nolan, J., Magnusson, L. et al. (2006) COAT: the Carers Outcome Agreement Tool: a new approach to working with family carers. Getting Research into Practice (GRiP) Report No 1. Project Report. Sheffield: University of Sheffield.

Harding, R., List, S., Epiphaniou, E. and Jones, H. (2012) How can informal caregivers in cancer and palliative care be supported? An updated systematic literature review of interventions and their effectiveness. *Palliative Medicine*, 26(1): 7–22.

Health Foundation (2014) *Person-Centred Care Made Simple: What Everyone Should Know about Person-Centred Care*. London: Health Foundation.

Hileman, J.W., Lackey, N.R. and Hassanein, R.S. (1992) Identifying the needs of home caregivers of patients with cancer. *Oncology Nursing Forum*, 19(5): 771–7.

Hudson, P. (2003) Home-based support for palliative care families: challenges and recommendations. *Medical Journal of Australia*, 179(6): S35–S37.

Hudson, P. (2004) Positive aspects and challenges associated with caring for a dying relative at home. *International Journal of Palliative Nursing*, 10(2): 58–65.

Hudson, P., Aranda, S. and Hayman-White, K. (2005) A psycho-educational intervention for family caregivers of patients receiving palliative care: a randomized controlled trial. *Journal of Pain and Symptom Management*, 30(4): 329–41.

Hudson, P., Remedios, C. and Thomas, K. (2010a) A systematic review of psychosocial interventions for family carers of palliative care patients. *BMC Palliative Care*, 9: 17.

Hudson, P., Trauer, T., Graham, S. et al. (2010b) A systematic review of instruments related to family caregivers of palliative care patients. *Palliative Medicine*, 24(7): 656–68.

Keefe, J., Guberman, N., Fancey, P. et al. (2008) Caregivers' aspirations, realities, and expectations: the CARE Tool. *Journal of Applied Gerontology*, 27(3): 286–308.

Kissane, D.W., McKenzie, M., Bloch, S. et al. (2006) Family focused grief therapy: a randomized, controlled trial in palliative care and bereavement. *American Journal of Psychiatry*, 163(7): 1208–18.

Knighting, K., O'Brien, M.R., Roe, B. et al. (2015) Development of the Carers' Alert Thermometer (CAT) to identify family carers struggling with caring for someone dying at home: a mixed method consensus study. *BMC Palliative Care*, 14: 22.

Kristjanson, L.J. and Aoun, S. (2004) Palliative care for families: remembering the hidden patients. *Canadian Journal of Psychiatry*, 49(6): 359–65.

Mitchell, G., Girgis, A., Jiwa, M. et al. (2010) A GP Caregiver Needs Toolkit versus usual care in the management of the needs of caregivers of patients with advanced cancer: a randomized controlled trial, *Trials*, 11: 115.

National Hospice and Palliative Care Organization (2008) *Guidelines for Bereavement Care in Hospice*. Alexandria, VA: National Hospice and Palliative Care Organization.

National Institute for Clinical Excellence (2004) *Guidance on Cancer Services: Improving Supportive and Palliative Care for Adults with Cancer: The Manual*. London: NICE.

NHS England (2014) *NHS England's Actions for End of Life Care*. Leeds: NHS England.

Osse, B.H., Vernooij-Dassen, M.J., Schade, E. and Grol, R.P. (2006) Problems experienced by the informal caregivers of cancer patients and their needs for support. *Cancer Nursing*, 29(5): 378–88; quiz 389–90.

Palliative Care Australia (2005) *Standards for Providing Quality Palliative Care for All Australians*. Canberra, ACT: Palliative Care Australia.

Parker, G., Arksey, H. and Harden, M. (2010) Meta-review of international evidence on interventions to support carers. Working Paper No. DH 2394. Heslington, York: Social Policy Research Unit, University of York.

Payne, S. and EAPC Task Force on Family Carers (2010) White Paper on improving support for family carers in palliative care: part 1. *European Journal of Palliative Care*, 17(5): 238–45.

Payne, S. and Morbey, H. (2013) *Supporting Family Carers: Report on the Evidence of How to Work with and Support Family Carers to Inform the Work of the Commission into the Future of Hospice Care*. London: Help the Hospices.

Public Health England (2015) *National End of Life Care Intelligence Network: What We Know Now 2014*. London: Public Health England.

Rolls, L., Seymour, J.E., Froggatt, K.A. and Hanratty, B. (2011) Older people living alone at the end of life in the UK: research and policy challenges. *Palliative Medicine*, 25(6): 650–7.

Rowland, C., Hanratty, B., Pilling, M. et al. (2017) The contributions of family care-givers at end of life: a national post-bereavement census survey of cancer carers' hours of care and expenditures. *Palliative Medicine*, 31(4): 346–55.

Salmon, J.R., Kwak, J., Acquaviva, K.D. et al. (2005) Validation of the caregiving at life's end questionnaire. *American Journal of Hospice and Palliative Care*, 22(3): 188–94.

Schulz, R. and Beach, S.R. (1999) Caregiving as a risk factor for mortality: the caregiver health effects study. *JAMA*, 282(23): 2215–19.

Stajduhar, K., Funk, L., Toye, C. et al. (2010) Part 1: Home-based family caregiving at the end of life: a comprehensive review of published quantitative research (1998–2008). *Palliative Medicine*, 24(6): 573–93.

Stamatopoulos, V. (2016) Supporting young carers: a qualitative review of young carer services in Canada. *International Journal of Adolescence and Youth*, 21(2): 178–94.

The National Council for Palliative Care (2013) Who cares? Support for carers of people approaching the end of life: A discussion based on a conference held on 6 November 2012. London: The National Council for Palliative Care.

Wong, W.K. and Ussher, J. (2009) Bereaved informal cancer carers making sense of their palliative care experiences at home. *Health and Social Care in the Community*, 17(3): 274–82.

World Health Organization (2007) *Palliative Care*. (Cancer control: Knowledge into action: WHO guide for effective programmes; module 5). Geneva: WHO.

Palliative care for those in disadvantaged groups

Dorry McLaughlin and Brian Nyatanga

Introduction

The concept of palliative care as a human right is identified by the international palliative care community (Gwyther et al. 2009). A European Association of Palliative Care
White Paper recommended equitable access to the provision of palliative care for everyone as applicable to their individual needs (Radbruch and Payne 2010). This means that
everyone should have access to the holistic care, support and advice they require, from
generalist and specialist palliative care services, across sectors and settings. Equity
of service access in meeting individual needs is applicable to all regardless of class,
gender, religion, sexual orientation or ethnicity, yet it is known that many people lack
adequate end of life care (Gwyther et al. 2009) and thus are disadvantaged. This chapter
looks at palliative care for people within some of the disadvantaged groups in society,
drawing specifically on examples of those with learning disabilities and the homeless.
It also considers challenges which exist in delivering care to these populations and
makes suggestions as to how these challenges can be addressed.

Palliative care and people with learning disability

The World Health Organization (WHO) recognises disability as a global human rights
issue (WHO 2011) and yet many people with disabilities lack access to equitable healthcare, including care at the end of their life. Findings are emerging from research studies
across the world suggesting that people with learning disabilities do not have equitable
access to palliative care and are seldom referred for hospice and specialist palliative
care provision (Stein 2008; Tuffrey-Wijne et al. 2008; Ryan et al. 2010; Cross et al. 2012;
McLaughlin et al. 2015). Reports in the United Kingdom also echo growing concerns

about the quality of end of life care which people with learning disabilities sometimes receive (Michael 2008; Heslop et al. 2013).

Defining learning disability

Across the world a number of different terms are used in the context of learning disability. In a number of countries the term 'intellectual disability' has increasingly been recognised while in the United Kingdom the term 'learning disability' is used. However, both terms can be used interchangeably. Internationally, there is agreement that a learning disability can be identified when the following are present: 'intellectual impairment' (or reduced IQ), social or adaptive dysfunction combined with reduced IQ and this all has early onset (Holland 2011, p. 3). In considering this defining criterion, the implications for someone with a learning disability requiring palliative and end of life care become apparent. In a palliative care context a person may need to process information which is cognitively and emotionally complex and they may be required to learn new skills in relation to coping and adaptation, due to the impact of an advanced, progressive disease. However, people with learning disability can have a wide range of disability and there is evidence that this population can possess skills and ability which enable them to show resilience even in a palliative and end of life care situation (Tuffrey-Wijne 2010).

Prevalence of learning disability

It is estimated that a learning disability exists in 1–3 per cent of the population (Mash and Wolfe 2004) and between 5 million and 15 million citizens of the European Union are affected in this way (Pomona 2008). As people with learning disabilities are living longer, this prevalence is expected to increase over the next number of years (McConkey 2006). This has implications for service provision due to an increased risk of advanced, progressive disease in this population, creating a need for access to palliative and end of life care.

Morbidity, causes of death and place of death for people with learning disabilities

People with learning disabilities are living longer than previously, however, they still have a shorter life expectancy than the general population, a higher level of unmet and complex healthcare needs and different common causes of death (National Health Scotland 2004). Further details of common causes of death can be seen in Table 13.1.

A recent European Association for Palliative Care Taskforce on Intellectual Disabilities highlighted a lack of data on people with learning disabilities across Europe, which creates difficulties in knowing what happens at end of life, including place of death (Tuffrey-Wijne et al. 2016). Other studies have found that deaths recorded in death certificates are disease-specific and it is often not noted if the person had a learning disability (Tyrer and McGrother 2009). This makes it difficult to determine the most

Table 13.1 Causes of death in people with learning disabilities

Cause of death	Associated factors
Respiratory disease (Leading cause of death)	Aspiration pneumonia – high rate of *Helicobacter Pylori* virus causing gastric reflux disorder (Douglas 2010; Thillai 2010). Problems with swallowing, feeding and posture
Cardiovascular disease (Second leading cause of death)	Congenital heart disease has a prevalence rate of 40–60 per cent in people with Down Syndrome (Akker et al. 2006; Dooley 2006)
Dementia (Higher rates than in the general population)	High number of people with Down syndrome develop Alzheimer's disease at an early age (McCarron et al. 2005)
Oesophageal, gastric and gall bladder malignancies	Increased incidence and risk (Cooke 1997; Patja et al. 2001)

common place of death for people with learning disabilities so that increased resources can be targeted to address the needs of this population at end of life.

Key issues in nursing people with learning disabilities at end of life

A number of key issues or challenges can exist when providing palliative nursing care to people with learning disabilities. These normally relate to the following areas of practice:

- communication;
- holistic assessment, care planning and care delivery;
- obtaining consent;
- providing bereavement care and support.

Communication

Always remember that people cannot *not* communicate. This means that people with a range of learning disabilities can communicate although this may involve using non-verbal methods or communicating in ways which are not always apparent to those unfamiliar with the person. When caring for someone with a learning disability, it is vitally important to establish how this person communicates and how receptive and expressive communication can be facilitated to and from the person throughout the assessment, care planning and care delivery processes. This often means working jointly and closely with people who are familiar to and with the person, and who have prior knowledge of the person and their communication methods. People familiar to the person with a learning disability, such as family carers, can often interpret what he or she is communicating such as sounds, facial expressions or changes in behaviour. A recent exploratory study by McLaughlin et al. (2015) found that services should be sensitive to the long-term caring role of family carers who have a family member with a learning disability.

People with learning disabilities may use *alternative communication* – a system alternative to speech or they may use *augmentative communication* in supporting their speech through the use of signs, symbols, pictures or photographs (Ferris-Taylor 2007). Caring for someone with a learning disability at the end of their life means taking time with the person to enable them to process information and for communication to take place effectively. Accessible information tailored to the needs of the person may need to be used which can involve the use of pictures and straightforward language. Some useful websites are available where accessible information for use with people with learning disabilities can be downloaded such as: the Easy Health website, which provides accessible information about health issues, including palliative care, for people with learning disabilities (www.easyhealth.org.uk), or the Palliative Care for People with Learning Disability Network website (www.pcpld.org).

Recent research has developed Breaking Bad News Guidelines and resources for use with people with learning disabilities (Tuffrey-Wijne 2013). Details can be found on the following website (www.breakingbadnews.org). A key point to remember is that breaking bad news to a person with a learning disability often takes place through giving chunks of information over a process of time and this may occur in the person's own place of care rather than a hospital clinic. Warning shots, recognised as good practice in breaking bad news with the general population, may not be understood by a person with a learning disability nor the need to ask questions to receive answers and information from professionals.

Family members or carers may be well meaning in protecting the person from discussions about death and dying and may wish to put pressure on professionals not to talk about the person's diagnosis and prognosis. A number of studies have shown that people with learning disabilities are able to have conversations about a taboo topic such as death and dying and can do so in a natural and insightful way (Tuffrey-Wijne et al. 2007; Todd and Read 2010; McLaughlin et al. 2014). This supports the rationale for people with learning disabilities to have equal access to advance care planning and to be facilitated in this process.

Holistic assessment, care planning and care delivery

It is common for a person with a learning disability to have a late diagnosis of an advanced progressive disease leading to a need for palliative and end of life care. According to Lindsey (2002), this late diagnosis can be due to their lack of awareness to attend screening programmes and an inability to recognise signs and symptoms or to mention them to anyone. This can be compounded by 'diagnostic overshadowing' (Reiss and Syszsko 1983) where carers and professionals misinterpret changes in behaviour as part of the learning disability rather than signs and symptoms of something which needs to be explored.

A diagnosis of an advanced progressive disease can cause equal distress to someone with a learning disability as it can cause to anyone else. There is evidence that people with learning disabilities can experience 'total pain' at the end of life and the multidimensional suffering which this entails (Tuffrey-Wijne 2009). This means that this population should be offered holistic end of life assessment and care delivered by a multidisciplinary team.

People with learning disabilities have the same needs at the end of their lives as anyone else, but they can have additional needs which may go unrecognised by services caring for them, causing challenges in assessment, care planning and care delivery. Services need to have an awareness of the importance of adjusting the care and support that they offer to people with learning disabilities at end of life to meet their additional needs (Tuffrey-Wijne et al. 2016). A mixed methods study by McLaughlin et al. (2014) found that partnership working between learning disability and palliative care services, with the person with learning disability and family carers at the centre, can promote a fusion of knowledge and skills, thus enabling more effective holistic assessment, care planning and care delivery.

Some people with learning disabilities will be able to indicate and locate their pain on a photograph or body chart. In people with more severe learning disabilities, people familiar to them will be able to interpret their sounds, mannerisms, changes in behaviour or facial expressions when they are unable to indicate or self-report pain. Professionals should be mindful that identification of distress is only the beginning of the assessment as distress may be caused by anxiety or other symptoms, apart from physical pain. The Disability Distress Assessment Tool (DisDAT) has been developed to help assess and identify distress cues in people with cognitive impairment (Regnard et al. 2007) and is an assessment tool which can be used with people who are learning disabled.

Obtaining consent

Nurses and other healthcare and social care professionals caring for people with learning disabilities at the end of their life should be familiar with and seek advice from their local Disability Discrimination and Capacity/Incapacity legislation and guidelines in relation to obtaining someone's consent for examination, treatment and care. Key to this is to avoid making assumptions that someone with a learning disability lacks capacity to consent to examination, treatment or care, as this can create lack of access to the treatment and care that they require. A person with a learning disability has a right to equitable treatment, respect for their autonomy and to be a partner in decision-making. The person's capacity to provide consent should be assumed unless proven otherwise. They may need to be facilitated to take part in decision-making by professionals providing end of life care. A Speech and Language Therapy Assessment can help to determine how to best communicate with someone with a learning disability and their ability to take part in decision-making concerning their treatment and care.

It is important to remember that if a person with a learning disability is unable to provide consent, another person cannot provide consent on their behalf. Instead 'best interests' decision-making should occur which needs to be clearly documented and based on what is in the best interests of the person with a learning disability.

Providing bereavement care and support

People with learning disabilities can be at risk of disenfranchised grief (Doka 2002), where they may have experienced loss which has not been acknowledged and no bereavement support has been offered to meet their needs. Research carried out over the years, such as that by Oswin (1991), has shown that a person with a learning disability can experience loss, grief and bereavement. A death in the life of someone with a learning disability, particularly of the main carer, can mean that the person may experience multiple losses as they may have to move home and lose their identity, their friends and much of what is familiar to them (Gates and Barr 2009).

A useful Bereavement Assessment Tool for use with people with learning disabilities has been developed by Blackman (2008). This can be helpful to professionals in determining areas of support which may be required by the person with a learning disability who has been bereaved. The Bereavement Assessment Tool consists of three key questions which can be used. These are shown in Box 13.1.

Box 13.1   The Bereavement Assessment Tool

- Practical issues – Has the person's ability to communicate with others been affected by this loss?
- Social issues – What impact has the death had on the person's familial network?
- Emotional issues – Does the person recognise their emotions and can they express them?

(Blackman 2008, p. 165)

Read and Elliott (2007) suggest that the support required by someone with a learning disability who has been bereaved may involve educating the person about death, dying and bereavement, enabling them to actively participate in death rituals if that is what the person desires (such as attendance at the funeral or visiting the grave) and facilitating them to talk about what is happening. This may be the person's first time taking part in death rituals so an explanation of what this involves is important.

In supporting someone with a learning disability in a bereavement situation, information should be given in an accessible format and tailored to the person's understanding while being consistently open and honest. Bereavement counsellors may use a variety of approaches such as memory books, life story books, pictures, photographs, art work and family trees (Read 2007). In some settings, staff caring for people with learning disabilities over a long period of time may also experience grief following their death and strategies should be in place for self-care and staff support.

Case Study 13.1: Jane

Jane is a 56-year-old lady with a learning disability. She has recently been diagnosed with advanced stomach cancer and has been admitted from a residential home, where she has lived for almost 20 years, to the local palliative care unit for assessment and management of abdominal pain. Jane's sister and staff from the residential home visit regularly and are very familiar to her. The nursing staff in the palliative care unit are unsure how to assess and plan care for Jane as they have limited experience of working with people with learning disabilities at end of life. They are also unsure how to communicate with Jane or how much she understands about what is happening to her. Jane seems very uncomfortable, anxious and distressed following her admission to the palliative care unit.

- What should the nursing staff in the palliative care unit do to empower them to assess and plan care for Jane?
- What important information could they find out from Jane's sister and the staff from the residential home?
- What resources and/or websites could the palliative care team access to obtain information about palliative care for people with learning disabilities?
- As a nurse, have you ever been in this situation where you have been unsure how to assess and plan care for someone with a learning disability at end of life? How did you deal with this situation or how would you deal with it if faced with a situation like this in the future?
- In reading through this section of the chapter on palliative care and people with learning disabilities, what have you learned which you could transfer to your practice?

Key learning points

- People with learning disabilities have the same end of life care needs as the general population, but they have additional needs, thus services need to adjust the care and support offered and facilitate them to take part in their care.
- There is evidence that partnership working between services can be helpful in assessing, planning and delivering holistic care to people with learning disabilities at end of life.

- It is vital to work jointly with people familiar to and with the person with learning disability who have prior knowledge of their communication methods and can interpret what the person is communicating.
- Studies have shown that people with learning disabilities can have conversations about a taboo subject such as death and dying and can do so in an insightful and natural way.
- The capacity of a person with a learning disability to be a partner in decision-making, and to provide consent to examination, treatment and care, should be assumed unless proven otherwise.
- A person with learning disability can experience loss and grief and may require bereavement care and support.

The next discussion focuses on the homeless population and the challenges of providing palliative care for their end of life care needs.

Palliative care provision for homeless populations

People who are homeless (the homeless) are known for being 'allergic' to healthcare services. This apparent allergy can be explained by the fact that healthcare services and systems were historically developed with the needs of mainstream society at the centre (Podymow et al. 2006; DH 2010; Collier 2011; Nyatanga 2015; Webb 2015), and leave no established system of caring for people who are homeless who may also need palliative care. The homeless population are also marginalised from mainstream society and yet they probably need palliative care support more than most other groups (Collier 2011). This makes the homeless population elusive and challenging for provision of coherent palliative and end of life care.

The transient nature of those who are homeless makes it hard to ascertain exact numbers of homeless people (Atkinson 2000). Thus, it is difficult for nurses to know where, when and how to provide palliative care for them and there is a paucity of information about their palliative care needs or wishes (Collier 2011; Nyatanga 2012; 2015; Webb 2015). There is therefore an argument for viewing people who are homeless as marginalised and vulnerable.

Because of the complexities inherent in homelessness, it is not clear who would be best suited to provide palliative care for this population. In 2008, the Department of Health (DH) for England and Wales (UK) suggested that since homeless people frequent hostels, the staff within these establishments should provide essential palliative care. Hostel staff may not be best equipped in terms of resources, staffing levels and palliative care knowledge and skills to effectively support the homeless population (Webb 2015). The challenge is ensuring that hostel staff are competent to provide palliative care, and that there is access to specialist palliative care when required.

The barriers encountered by the homeless in accessing healthcare are widely recognised, and a number of different care models are used in different countries, for example:

- *Canada* uses emergency shelters, and temporary institution accommodation for the homeless (Gaetz et al. 2013). Canada also has 'violence against women' shelters specifically for abused women, the numbers of which can be high any given night.
- *Sweden* provides palliative care through the Swedish Support Homes (SSH) with staff being trained to offer person-centred care grounded in understanding health/illness literacy (perception) of the homeless as a determinant of life as a homeless person (Hakanson et al. 2016).
- *Germany* has a Constitution which requires the state to ensure every citizen can live in dignity (Meyers 2014). 'Life in dignity', as it is popularly known, is translated to mean everyone having food, clothes and a roof over their heads. For the homeless, the state agencies help them to find a new apartment, pay the rent and provide monthly spending money.

Understanding who is homeless

In the UK, the homeless are classified into different groups (Table 13.2).

This classification has problems of accuracy due to the transient nature of this population, such as the exclusion of single homeless people without children in the statutory group. In addition, there is little mention of abused women, when research by Goodman et al. (1991) and Gaetz et al. (2013) suggests that most women become homeless following physical and sexual abuse leading to psychological trauma. The low self-esteem often accompanied by stigmatisation by mainstream healthcare services (Hudson et al. 2016) may explain why these patients may not seek palliative care support for life-threatening conditions.

Table 13.2 Classification of homeless people

Classification group	Definition
Rough sleepers	Street counts or estimates by all local councils of people sleeping rough
Statutory homeless	Defined under the UK 1996 Housing Act to represent all those who apply to local council for homelessness assistance
Hostel and supported accommodation	Often single people without dependent children
Hidden homelessness	Do not appear on official figures and accurate numbers are not available
	Include those who become homeless, but find temporary solutions with family/friends

Palliative care need in homeless populations

People who are homeless can have a shortened life expectancy. The mean age of death can be as low as 40–42 years old (Podymow et al. 2006; Henwood et al. 2015), with deaths up to four times higher than the general population (Podymow et al. 2006; Henwood et al. 2015; Tobey et al. 2016). This requires well-planned palliative and end of life care to be provided to this population group at a much earlier time period than required for most adults. This means nurses finding a way of identifying the homeless who are dying, assessing their palliative care needs and supporting them in centres outside of mainstream healthcare.

Challenges of delivering palliative care

The homeless cannot choose to be cared for or die at home as their homes are predominantly the street family networks (Johnson 2015; Nyatanga 2015). These networks can be volatile, unpredictable and therefore unstable for effective palliative care delivery.

Team-based approaches are common in palliative care because of the complex and multiple needs patients frequently have. This is particularly important in homeless populations because of the likely co-morbidities particular to this group such as those associated with substance abuse and mental illness (Westermeyer and Lee 2013; Hakanson et al. 2016; Hakanson and Ohlen 2016).

While the homeless may prefer to remain in familiar hostel-type accommodation for their palliative and end of life care, healthcare professionals need to recognise that the same environment may also be a source of emotional trauma as it acts as a reminder of how they are marginalised and disadvantaged from mainstream healthcare and society (Podymow et al. 2006; Johnson 2015).

For most people, the first point of contact for health-related problems would normally be through the general practice. However, the homeless do not tend to access their general practitioner services, but are often rushed into hospital as emergencies (Daiski 2007; St Mungos 2009) where they may have longer periods as in-patients as they do not always have a fixed address for discharge (Podymow et al. 2006; Nyatanga 2015).

A source of meaningful hope for the homeless to receive palliative care is through charities and centres of care, like the Swedish Support Homes, Maggs Centres for the homeless in the UK, and Housing First in America. However, it is imperative that staff in these environments receive training on palliative and end of life care in order to benefit not only the homeless person, but themselves in terms of being able to self-care and regulate their emotional investment with such sensitive care. Chapter 19 in this volume has more information on burnout and stress in palliative care nursing.

Complexities of being homeless

The nature of many homeless people's lifestyles means that symptoms they present with can be related to alcohol, tobacco and drug abuse. Evidence suggests that alcohol abuse contributes to between 20 and 30 per cent of liver disease, oesophageal cancer, epileptic seizures, cardiovascular disease and cerebral vascular accidents (WHO 2004). Excessive alcohol consumption is also reported to severely impair mental functioning with significant impact of social ability to hold down effective family roles and relationships (WHO 2004). There is a positive correlation between excessive alcohol use and depression, and homeless people are nine times more likely to commit suicide than the general population (Fitzpatrick et al. 2015). It is likely that between a third and two-thirds of deaths among the homeless are attributed to drug and alcohol abuse (Page et al. 2012; Fitzpatrick et al. 2015).

Johnson (2015) claims that the relationships formed by the homeless tend to be mainly exploitative and characterised by dependence and counter-dependence. The lifestyle of many homeless people is closely related to a dependence on alcohol and drugs (Page et al. 2012; Rehm et al. 2014; Hutt et al. 2016), which can lead to impairment of mental functioning and with that, the loss of multiple abilities, including social etiquette and self-care (Hakanson et al. 2016; Hutt et al. 2016). Therefore, communicating with the homeless about healthcare is challenging, and accessing palliative care even more so (Hudson et al. 2016; Hutt et al. 2016). The role of nurses or a health facilitator becomes important in establishing continuity in relationships with the homeless, while being the link with healthcare services.

Learning exercise 13.1

Considering the transient nature of the homeless population, what steps should healthcare professionals and nurses take to help in the following areas?

- Integrating the homeless into mainstream healthcare service.
- Developing dedicated centres for the homeless.
- Helping to increase the life expectancy of the homeless population.
- Breaking down any barriers and stigmatisation to encourage access to palliative care services.
- Ensuring palliative care training is provided to hostel staff and others who care for the homeless population.

The way forward

Any successful plan to care for people who are homeless depends on how much is known about this population. However, from what is known now, the homeless can best be cared for by first understanding that homelessness is not a choice, but a social disaffiliation from the normality of society (Nyatanga 2015). Coupled with this is the need to recognise the negative impact of existing stigmatisation of the homeless population, and then a real desire to change this to promote inclusion in mainstream healthcare and society at large. The homeless may need to 'feel' this change in order to have the confidence to access health services. For palliative care nurses, there is a genuine need to recognise that our deeply held palliative care core values and their intentions may not always be acceptable to the homeless community. It is important that we understand the nature of values they may hold and how they interpret them in terms of life, health and death, thus suspending our judgement and allowing them to lead us in defining their own end of life desires. For example, since the homeless seem allergic to hospitals and even hospices, could their palliative care be delivered away from these institutions? The creation of health hubs linked to hostels and other centres that the homeless frequent may provide a welcome and less threatening solution for delivering palliative care to this group.

Increasing life expectancy

To help increase life expectancy among the homeless, nurses and other healthcare professionals need to understand and recognise fundamental barriers that stop the homeless accessing general healthcare and palliative care services. Pursuing good health may not be at the top of the homeless person's priorities, as the homeless tend to use health services when it becomes an emergency and is life-threatening (Johnson 2015). The homeless need help and support to break the cycle of psychological dependence on others. This can only be possible once the known barriers discussed above are broken down and they begin to feel confident/comfortable accessing health and palliative care services.

Accessing palliative care (breaking down barriers)

- Breaking down and eradicating stigmatisation of the homeless is one way of integrating them into mainstream society.
- Developing health hubs to serve the homeless community with health and palliative care-related needs, advice and rehabilitation.
- Having an experienced health facilitator as a first point of contact for the homeless in each hub and centre.
- The facilitator is key to developing a trusting relationship with this vulnerable population and in ensuring that there is a familiar face all the time. The facilitator can also escort homeless patients to hospital appointments and help break down hierarchies and authorities that the homeless resent (Johnson 2015).
- Finally, a clear functional link between the health hub and hostels and centres must be guaranteed.

Key learning points

- The transient nature of the homeless population makes it hard to establish exact numbers in this country and where, when and how to provide palliative care.

- The homeless can best be cared for by, first, understanding that homelessness is not a choice, but a social disaffiliation from normality of society for multiple reasons.
- The impact of existing stigmatisation of the homeless makes them less trusting of society and healthcare institutions (hospices and hospitals) that are meant to support and care for them.
- Homeless people may prefer to remain in familiar hostel-type accommodation for their palliative and end of life care, but the same environment may cause emotional trauma in reminding them they are marginalised and disadvantaged from mainstream healthcare and society.
- Staff in hostels may benefit from further training in the practice of palliative care to include communication skills, breaking bad news and self-care after witnessing dying and death.

Other disadvantaged groups

Similar challenges exist for other disadvantaged groups at the end of life which can be addressed in similar ways to those which have been previously highlighted. Some key points can be seen in Table 13.3.

Conclusion

This chapter discussed palliative and end of life care for disadvantaged groups and focused on two specific groups of people – people with learning disabilities and the homeless, while offering brief outlines on prisoners, those with mental illness and LGBT groups. These groups have become marginalised from mainstream society and healthcare and, therefore, disadvantaged in terms of accessing healthcare services such as palliative care. The communication difficulties and special needs that characterise people with learning disabilities and street life networks for the homeless culminate in a state of disaffiliation from mainstream society. Careful planning and input by nurses, and other healthcare professionals, can ameliorate this situation. This chapter has also highlighted similar key points in relation to other disadvantaged groups. Professionals should understand the additional needs, held values and priorities of disadvantaged groups in order to tailor care to their needs. It is clear from this chapter that the way health services are organised does not always attract or give confidence to disadvantaged groups to access them equitably. Therefore, a way of planning quality palliative and end of life care with disadvantaged groups in mind might be effective, integrated working between services and agencies across settings.

Table 13.3 Key points in end of life care for other disadvantaged groups

Prisoners	People with mental health needs	People who are lesbian, gay, bisexual or transgender (LGBT)
People with chronic disease can die in a number of settings including prisons The culture of prisons, limited space within a prison cell and lack of training for prison staff create challenges in enabling people in prisons to receive palliative care (Turner et al. 2011)	A population-based study in Canada found a lack of access to palliative care and pain management for people with mental health needs who tended to die in nursing homes (Chochinov et al. 2012)	An Australian study surveyed people who were LGBT (n = 305) and found a need for educational approaches to increase awareness around end of life care planning (Hughes and Cartwright 2014)
There is evidence from UK studies that key to enabling people in prisons to access quality palliative care are partnership working between nurses and prison staff and links with specialist palliative care teams (Turner et al. 2011; Papadopoulos and Lay 2016)	In Belgium, a study using a grounded theory approach, with people with mental health needs (n = 20), identified that talking about the end of life was seen as positive and not something that was feared (Sweers et al. 2013)	Nurses need to have an awareness of the isolating feeling which stigma can create and adapt the end of life care that they deliver to people who are LGBT in responding to their specific and holistic needs (Chidiac and Connelly 2016)
	There is evidence that people with mental health needs have similar end of life care needs as the general population (Sweers et al. 2013)	Findings from a systematic review, focusing on the bereavement experiences of people who are LGBT, highlighted the additional sources of stress which may occur creating a need for individualised support in grieving which may be disenfranchised (Bristowe et al. 2016)

References

Akker, M., Maaskant, M.A. and Meijden, R.J.M. (2006) Cardiac diseases in people with intellectual disability. *Journal of Intellectual Disability Research*, 50(7): 515–22.

Atkinson, J. (2000) Nursing homeless men: a study of proactive intervention. *Journal of Nursing Practice*, 16(2): 1–8.

Blackman, N. (2008) The development of an assessment tool for the bereavement needs of people with learning disabilities. *British Journal of Learning Disabilities*, 36: 165–70.

Bristowe, K., Marshall, S. and Harding, R. (2016) The bereavement experiences of lesbian, gay, bisexual and transgender people who have lost a partner: a systematic review, thematic synthesis and modelling of the literature. *Palliative Medicine*, 30(8): 730–44.

Chidiac, C. and Connelly, M. (2016) Considering the impact of stigma on lesbian, gay and bisexual people receiving palliative and end of life care. *International Journal of Palliative Nursing*, 22(7): 334–40.

Chochinov, H.M., Martens, P.J., Prior, H.J. and Kredentser, M.S. (2012) Comparative health care use patterns of people with schizophrenia near the end of life: a population-based study in Manitoba, Canada. *Schizophrenia Research*, 141: 241–6.

Collier, R. (2011) Bringing palliative care to the homeless. *CMAJ*, 183(6): E317–E318.

Cooke, L.B. (1997) Cancer and learning disability. *Journal of Intellectual Disability Research*, 41: 312–16.

Cross, H., Cameron, M., Marsh, S. and Tuffrey-Wijne, I. (2012) Practical approaches toward improving end-of-life care for people with intellectual disabilities: effectiveness and sustainability. *Journal of Palliative Care*, 15(3): 322–6.

Daiski, I. (2007) Perspectives of homeless people on their health and health needs priorities. *Journal of Advanced Nursing*, 53(5): 565–73.

Department of Health (2010) *End of Life Care: Achieving Quality in Hostels and for the Homeless People – A Route to Success*. London: Department of Health.

Doka, K.J. (2002) *Disenfranchised Grief: New Directions, Challenges and Strategies for Practice*. Springfield, IL: Research Press.

Dooley, K.J. (2006) History of management of congenital heart disease. In Rubin, I.L. and Crocker, A.C. (eds) *Cardiology in Medical Care for Children and Adults with Developmental Disabilities*. Baltimore, MD: Paul H. Brookes, pp. 373–9.

Douglas, N.A. (2010) Infectious diseases. In O'Hara, J., McCarthy, J. and Bouras, N. (eds) *Intellectual Disability and Ill Health*. Cambridge: Cambridge University Press, pp. 47–60.

Ferris-Taylor, R. (2007) Communication. In Gates, B. (ed.) *Learning Disabilities: Toward Inclusion* (5th edn). London: Churchill Livingstone, pp. 325–57.

Fitzpatrick, S., Pawson, H., Bramley, G. et al. (2015) The homelessness monitor: England 2015. *Crisis*, February 2015. London.

Gates, B. and Barr, O. (2009) *Learning and Intellectual Disability*. Oxford: Oxford University Press.

Gaetz, S., Donaldson, J., Richter, T. and Gulliver, T. (2013) The state of homelessness in Canada in 2013. Homeless Hub paper #4. Toronto: Canadian Homelessness Research Network Press.

Goodman, L., Saxe, L. and Harvey, M. (1991) Homelessness and psychological trauma: broadening perspectives. *The American Psychologist*, 46(11): 1219–25.

Gwyther, L., Brennan, F. and Harding, R. (2009) Advancing palliative care as a human right. *Journal of Pain and Symptom Management*, 38(5): 767–74.

Hakanson, C. and Ohlen, J. (2016) Illness narratives of people who are homeless. *International Journal of Qualitative Studies in Health and Well-being*, 11: 32924.

Hakanson, C., Sandberg, J., Ekstedt, M. et al. (2016) Providing palliative care in a Swedish support home for people who are homeless. *Qualitative Research*, 26(9): 1252–62.

Henwood, B.F., Byrne, T. and Scriber, B. (2015) Examining mortality among formerly homeless adults enrolled in Housing First: an observational study. *BMC Public Health*, 4(15): 1209.

Heslop, P., Blair, P., Fleming, P. et al. (2013) *Confidential Inquiry into Premature Deaths of People with Learning Disabilities*. Bristol: Norah Fry Research Centre, University of Bristol.

Holland, K. (2011) *Factsheet: Learning Disabilities*. British Institute of Learning Disabilities. Available at: www.bild.org.uk.

Hudson, B.F., Fleming, K., Shulman, C. and Candy, B. (2016) Challenges to access and provision of palliative care for people who are homeless: a systematic review of qualitative research. *BMC Palliative Care*, 3(15): 96.

Hughes, M. and Cartwright, C. (2014) LGBT people's knowledge of and preparedness to discuss end of life care planning options. *Health and Social Care in the Community*, 22(5): 545–52.

Hutt, E., Whitfield, E., Min, S.J. et al. (2016) Challenges of providing end-of-life care for homeless veterans. *American Journal of Hospital Palliative Care*, 33(4): 381–9.

Johnson, A. (2015) The word from the streets: an interpretive phenomenological analysis of the experiences of health-related services in the homeless. Unpublished Master's dissertation in Applied Psychology. University of Worcester, Worcester.

Lindsey, M. (2002) Comprehensive health care services for people with learning disabilities. *Advances in Psychiatric Treatment*, 8: 138–47.

Mash, E. and Wolfe, D. (2004) *Abnormal Child Psychology*. Belmont, CA: Thompson Wadsworth.

Meyers, F. (2014) How does Germany deal with the homeless and poor? Available at: https://www.quora.com/How-does-Germany-deal-with-the-homeless-and-the-poor (accessed 27 January 2017).

Michael, J. (2008) *Healthcare for All: Report of the Independent Inquiry into Access to Healthcare for People with Learning Disabilities*. London: NHS.

McCarron, M., Gill, M. and McCallion, P. (2005) Health co-morbidities in ageing persons with Down syndrome and Alzheimer's dementia. *Journal of Intellectual Disability Research*, 49: 560–6.

McConkey, R. (2006) Accessibility of healthcare information for people with a learning disability. A review and discussion paper. University of Ulster.

McLaughlin, D., Barr, O., McIlfatrick, S. and McConkey, R. (2014) Developing a best practice model for partnership practice between specialist palliative care and intellectual disability services: a mixed methods study. *Palliative Medicine*, 28(10): 1213–21.

McLaughlin, D., Barr, O., McIlfatrick, S. and McConkey, R. (2015) Service user perspectives on palliative care education for health and social care professionals supporting people with learning disabilities. *BMJ Supportive and Palliative Care*, 5(5): 531–7.

National Health Scotland (2004) *Health Needs Assessment Report: People with Learning Disabilities in Scotland*. Glasgow: NHS Scotland.

Nyatanga, B. (2012) Is there room at the inn? Palliative care for the homeless. *British Journal of Community Nursing*, 17(10): 473.

Nyatanga, B. (2015) Care for the homeless person. In Ingleton, C. and Larkin, P.J. (eds) *Palliative Care Nursing at a Glance*. Chichester: Wiley Blackwell.

ONS (2015) *Alcohol Related Deaths in the United Kingdom: Registered 2013, Statistical Bulletin*. London: HMSO.

Oswin, M. (1991) *Am I Allowed to Cry? A Story of Bereavement Amongst People Who Have Learning Difficulties*. London: WBC Print.

Page, S.A., Thurston, W.E. and Mahoney, C.E. (2012) Causes of death among an urban homeless population considered by the medical examiner. *Journal of Social Work and End of Life Palliative Care*, 8(3): 265–71.

Papadopoulos, I. and Lay, M. (2016) Current and emerging practice of end of life care in British prisons: findings from an on-line survey of prison nurses. *BMJ Supportive and Palliative Care*, 6(1): 101–4.

Patja, K., Eero, P. and Iivanainen, M. (2001) Cancer incidence among people with intellectual disability. *Journal of Intellectual Disability Research*, 45(4): 300–7.

Podymow, T., Turnbull, J. and Coyle, D. (2006) Shelter-based palliative care for the homeless terminally ill. *Palliative Medicine*, 20: 81–8.

Pomona (2008) *Health Indicators for People with Intellectual Disabilities: Using an Indicator Set*. Pomona 11 final report. Available at: http//www.pomonaproject.org/action1_2004_frep_14_en.pdf (accessed 8 September 2016).

Radbruch, L. and Payne, S. (2010) White Paper on standards and norms for hospice and palliative care in Europe: part 2. *European Journal of Palliative Care*, 17(1): 22–33.

Read, S. (2007) *Bereavement Counselling for People with Learning Disabilities*. London: Quay Books.

Read, S. and Elliott, D. (2007) Exploring a continuum of support for bereaved people with intellectual disabilities: a strategic approach. *Journal of Intellectual Disability*, 11(2): 167–81.

Regnard, C., Reynolds, J., Watson, B. et al. (2007) Understanding distress in people with severe communication difficulties: developing and assessing the Disability Distress Assessment Tool (DisDAT). *Journal of Intellectual Disability Research*, 51(4): 277–92.

Rehm, J. and Shields, K.D. (2014) Alcohol and mortality: global alcohol-attributable deaths from cancer, liver cirrhosis, and injury in 2010. *Alcohol Research: Current Reviews*, 35(2): 174–83.

Reiss, S. and Syzszko, J. (1983) Diagnostic overshadowing and professional experience with mentally retarded persons. *American Journal of Mental Deficiency*, 87: 396–402.

Ryan, K., McEvoy, J., Guerin, S. and Dodd, P. (2010) An exploration of the experience, confidence and attitudes of staff to the provision of palliative care to people with intellectual disabilities. *Palliative Medicine*, 24(6): 566–72.

Stein, G. (2008) Providing palliative care to people with intellectual disabilities: services, staff knowledge and challenges. *Journal of Palliative Medicine*, 11(9): 1241–8.

Stephens, C., Sackett, N., Pierce, R. et al. (2013) Transitional care challenges of rehospitalized veterans: listening to patients and providers. *Population Health Management*, 16(5): 326–31.

St Mungos (2009) *S.O.S. Sick of Suffering: St Mungos Report into the Health Problems of Homeless People*. Available at: www.mungosbroadway.org.uk (accessed 23 July 2016).

Sweers, K., Dierckx de Casterle, B., Detraux, J. and De Hert, M. (2013) End of life (care) perspectives and expectations of patients with schizophrenia. *Archives of Psychiatric Nursing*, 27: 246–52.

Thillai, M. (2010) Respiratory diseases. In O'Hara, J., McCarthy, J. and Bouras, N. (eds) *Intellectual Disability and Ill Health*. Cambridge: Cambridge University Press, pp. 78–87.

Tobey, M., Manasson, J., Decarlo, K. et al. (2016) Homeless individuals approaching the end of life: symptoms and attitudes. *Journal of Pain and Symptom Management*, 10: 364.

Todd, S. and Read, S. (2010) Thinking about death and what it means: the perspectives of people with intellectual disability. *International Journal of Child Health and Human Development*, 3(2): 207–14.

Tuffrey-Wijne, I., Bernal, J., Butler, G. et al. (2007) Using nominal group technique to investigate the views of people with intellectual disabilities on end of life care provision. *Journal of Advanced Nursing*, 58(1): 80–9.

Tuffrey-Wijne, I., Whelton, R., Curfs, L. and Hollins, S. (2008) Palliative care provision for people with intellectual disabilities: a questionnaire survey of specialist palliative care professionals. *Palliative Medicine*, 22: 281–90.

Tuffrey-Wijne, I. (2009) Am I a good girl? Dying people who have a learning disability. *End of Life Care*, 3(1): 35–9.

Tuffrey-Wijne, I. (2010) *Living with Learning Disabilities: Dying with Cancer*. London: Jessica Kingsley Publishers.

Tuffrey-Wijne, I. (2013) *How to Break Bad News to People with Intellectual Disabilities: A Guide for Carers and Professionals*. London: Jessica Kingsley Publishers.

Tuffrey-Wijne, I., McLaughlin, D., Curfs, L. et al. (2016) Defining consensus norms for palliative care of people with intellectual disabilities in Europe, using Delphi methods: a White Paper from the European Association of Palliative Care. *Palliative Medicine*, 30(95): 446–55.

Turner, M., Payne, S. and Barbarachild, Z. (2011) Care or custody? An evaluation of palliative care in prisons in North West England. *Palliative Medicine*, 25(4): 370–7.

Tyrer, F. and McGrother, C. (2009) Cause specific mortality and death certificate reporting in adults with moderate to profound intellectual disability. *Journal of Intellectual Disability Research*, 53(11): 898–904.

Webb, W. (2015) When dying at home is not an option: an exploration of the perception of hostel staff regarding the provision of hostel-based palliative care to homeless people. *BMJ Supportive and Palliative Care*, 5: A75–A76.

Westermeyer, J. and Lee, K. (2013) Residential placement for veterans with addiction: American Society of Addiction Medicine criteria vs veterans homeless program. *Journal of Nervous Mental Disability*, 201(7): 567–71.

World Health Organization (2004) *Global Status Report on Alcohol*. Geneva: World Health Organization.

World Health Organization (2011) *World Report on Disability*. Geneva: World Health Organization.

World Health Organization (2012) *Management of Substance Abuse: Alcohol*. Available at: http://www.who.int/substance_abuse/facts/alcohol/en/ (accessed 16 July 2016).

Advanced and expanded roles in palliative care nursing

Catriona Kennedy and Michael Connolly

Introduction

This chapter explores contemporary issues around advanced practice nursing roles and their contributions to palliative care. Our approach here is to consider advanced practice as a generic term which includes clinical nurse specialist and advanced nurse practitioner roles. These are extended roles and signify nurses who practise at a higher level than traditional nurses. The roles are shaped by the countries and context in which the nurse is practising. Our aim is to define the concepts and characteristics in advanced practice in order to provide insights into nursing contributions to palliative care.

In this chapter we identify the growing demands for palliative care due to demographic changes alongside the resulting implications for education, professional identity and the scope and development of advanced practice nursing roles. We draw on evidence which demonstrates a 'blurring of professional boundaries' and 'fluid role boundaries' in advanced practice roles and which place the person in need of care at the centre of the service model. We also highlight the difficulties in differentiating between specialist, expanded and advanced roles and suggest further work is required to name, value and assess the contributions of such nursing roles.

Making a difference to people who need palliative care and at the end of life, be they patients or those who support them, is an interdisciplinary endeavour. Nurses provide care as part of an interdisciplinary team so while this chapter has a focus on nursing roles, it does so in recognition of the nursing contribution to a team-based approach to palliative care. This is particularly important when considering the nature of advanced practice where advanced nursing roles may lie at the boundaries between nursing and medicine or other allied health professional roles.

Modernising nursing roles in palliative care

Health services providers internationally are concerned with ensuring that the nursing and midwifery resource is deployed to full advantage. This is driven by numerous factors, including the need to modernise health services to meet growing demands due to an increasing older population, as well as public expectations. Palliative care, as a relatively young specialty, has a particular need to develop flexible and responsive service models, given care provision should be based on needs rather than diagnosis and focused around the preferences of patients and their families.

There exists growing evidence on the important role of nurses in providing safe patient care. The Registered Nurse Forecasting (RN4CAST) study (2009–2011) scaled up evidence across European countries and demonstrated that good nursing workforce strategies are associated with improved patient outcomes (Sermeus et al. 2011). Good staff ratios and nurse qualifications were two key factors shown to improve patient care and safety and staff satisfaction. RN4CAST has generated a large evidence base of nurse workforce issues and has linked higher education attainment with improved patient outcomes (Sermeus et al. 2011). This is important evidence when planning the education needs of the nursing workforce to meet growing demands for palliative and end of life care.

Ensuring the nursing workforce can meet the growing demands for palliative care is challenging. Only a small proportion of palliative care is delivered in specialist settings such as hospices by specialists in palliative care. Most palliative care is delivered in a range of care settings by nurses with or without additional education in palliative care. The growth in numbers of clinical nurse specialists and advanced nurse practitioners, who work in disease-specific roles and have palliative care as part of their remit, complicates the process of identifying role boundaries and the preparation required for such roles. In addition, the development of palliative care specific specialist and advanced roles presents opportunities for both changes and challenges in professional nursing identity concerning the scope of roles in palliative care. In the next section we explore the links between levels of palliative care, education and advanced practice roles.

Levels of palliative care and education preparation for clinical nurse specialist and advanced nursing practice roles

Palliative care has been defined by both the World Health Organization (2002) and the European Association for Palliative Care (1998) as care which aims to improve the quality of life of an individual with a life-threatening illness through the management of physical, psychological, social and spiritual issues. That care is extended to the family of the individual concerned and can continue if required to the period after the death of the individual. Not only must the focus be on the physical, psychological, social and spiritual management of the individual and their family, but cognisance must also be taken of the level of service provided which, in turn, corresponds to the complexity of needs of patients and their families alongside levels of interaction with specialist

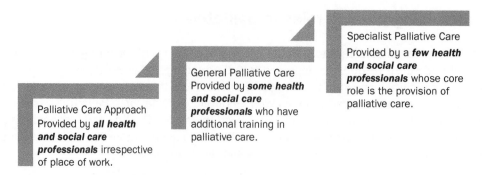

Figure 14.1 Levels of palliative care

palliative services (Radbruch and Payne 2009). The levels of service provision and interaction can be described as the palliative care approach, general palliative care and specialist palliative care, and can be used to identify and indicate the most appropriate level of education and resulting knowledge and skills required for practice, in order to meet patient and family needs (Figure 14.1).

A rapid appraisal of the literature identifies key components of effective models of palliative care which have relevance for the nursing contribution:

- *Case management* to meet the full range of an individual's palliative and other care needs and social well-being.
- *Shared care* which comprises a team around the patient and family from primary, community and specialist services. Shared care and case management are linked, often through nurse specialist roles, which provide an interface between primary, secondary and tertiary care services and also in the coordination of services.
- *Specialist outreach services* have been shown to improve health outcomes in primary care, although more comparisons of specialist palliative care outreach services are required.
- *Managed clinical networks* which may facilitate access for hard to reach or underserved groups. Integrated care which is based on the principles of advocacy and the provision of seamless, continuous care from referral through to bereavement.

(Adapted from Luckett et al. 2014)

It therefore follows that different levels of education and preparation for nurses providing palliative care, irrespective of care setting, will be required to meet the needs of the populations served, recognising the different roles they may undertake. It is notable that the numbers of clinical nurse specialist posts grew during the 1970s and 1980s as the numbers of academic programmes increased to address the growing need for specialisation. Despite this, there exists a lack of agreement about role preparation, role boundaries and the need for accreditation of such roles. For example, in the UK, the clinical nurse specialist or advanced nurse practitioner title is not regulated, unlike in the USA, Australia, Canada and Ireland where they are (Lowe et al. 2012).

The *palliative care approach* is the integration and use of palliative care principles in a range of general care settings such as acute hospitals and nursing/care homes. A range of healthcare and social care professionals, including general practitioners and nurses, provide care using this approach, which embodies excellent person-centred support for family carers. It is generally agreed that all healthcare professionals need to understand the principles of palliative care and their application to physical, psychological, social and spiritual care. Progress has been made in incorporating education about the palliative care approach in the curricula for medical, nursing and other healthcare and social care professionals (Ryan et al. 2014). Indeed, the Council of Europe recommends that all professionals working in healthcare should be confident in their understanding and use of the palliative care principles (Council of Europe 2003).

General palliative care is provided by professionals for patients with an advanced life-limiting condition, and incorporates the integration of the principles of palliative care with the use of advanced clinical skills and knowledge. Such professionals will have improved knowledge and skills in managing difficult symptoms and advance care planning. Many people who die in hospital or community settings require general palliative care provided by those healthcare and social care professionals working in clinical areas such as oncology, older person services or in the community. Healthcare and social care professionals, particularly nurses, working in these areas require good basic palliative care skills and knowledge, alongside some additional training and experience in palliative care (Council of Europe 2003; Department of Health and Children 2001; Radbruch and Payne 2009).

Specialist palliative care is provided by healthcare and social care professionals, whose core activity is the provision of palliative care. The specialist palliative care service is aimed at patients with complex care needs across a range of in-patient and community services. Consequently the provision of specialist palliative care requires staff who have undergone recognised specialist palliative care training, often to Master's level of study or beyond. Specialist palliative care services require a team approach, combining a multi-professional team with an interdisciplinary mode of work. The specialist palliative care team should have expertise in the clinical management of problems in multiple domains in order to meet the patient's complex needs (DOHC 2001; Clinical Standards Board for Scotland 2002; National Consensus Project for Quality Palliative Care 2004). Given the range and scope of competences required by nurses who work in specialist palliative care, advanced education up to and including a Master's degree or beyond should be the ideal.

In a number of jurisdictions, including the UK and Ireland, there is a clinical career pathway for nurses who choose to work and specialise in palliative care. Upon completion and initial registration as a nurse, the individual nurse will work towards attaining a level of experience in clinical care and, upon choosing to specialise in palliative care, can move to work in the area and commence further education in palliative care or may choose to obtain a higher education award in palliative care prior to moving into specialist practice.

What is clear is that those nurses who choose to specialise in palliative care are required to have a minimum of Level 7 (European Commission 2012) education award

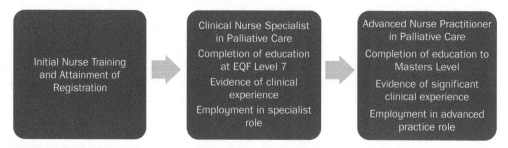

Figure 14.2 Levels of education and training for a clinical career

in order to qualify for specialist or advanced practice status as laid down by the Royal College of Nursing (2009) in the UK and the Nursing and Midwifery Board of Ireland respectively (Figure 14.2). A similar picture exists in the USA, Australia and, since 2010, New Zealand, where Master's degree level education or above is required by advanced nurse practitioners. However, in a number of countries across Europe (e.g. Germany, Poland, Romania), specialisation in palliative care nursing is in its infancy and although higher level education and continuing practice development programmes are available, there is no substantive requirement for a Master's degree level qualification to be obtained in order to practise in a specialist palliative care role (Sheer et al. 2008).

The broadening scope of palliative care and the challenges for advancing nursing roles

Nurses in specialist and advanced practice roles make a central and significant contribution to the delivery of palliative care. In particular, clinical nurse specialist posts are established across a number of disease-specific areas incorporating advanced skills in assessment, supportive care and technical skills, many of which may previously have required hospital attendance and/or admission. It is recognised that when a clinical nurse specialist has palliative care in their title or remit that a significant proportion of their time is likely to be devoted to palliative and end of life care. There is evidence from 12 developed countries that advanced nursing practitioners perform as well as doctors, given appropriate education and training for the tasks allocated to them. There is also evidence of high patient satisfaction, mainly due to the way advanced nurse specialists interact with patients and family members and a focus on education and counselling (Delamaire and Lafortune 2010).

As discussed earlier in this chapter, no universally agreed definitions exist of clinical nurse specialist or advanced nurse practitioner roles although it is recognised that such post-holders will have additional education (Figure 14.2). Currently different perspectives exist on whether clinical nurse specialist or advanced nurse practitioner roles differ or are similar. There are suggestions that the clinical nurse specialist role involves direct care provision informed by increased knowledge and skills and the advanced nurse practitioner role moves into areas of expanded practice such as diagnosis and treatment. However, the evidence is inconclusive and there exists a lack of clarity (Lowe et al. 2012).

As members of the multi-professional healthcare team, nurses spend most time caring for and being with the patient and their family, and so have an intimate picture of the individual and their needs, desires, concerns and fears. Given the major changes in the working patterns of junior doctors, in a number of jurisdictions, as a result of an EU directive, the role of the nurse is poised to further expand in order to meet service needs (Kennedy et al. 2015). Furthermore, the growing recognition of the palliative care needs of individuals with non-malignant diseases and the need for service providers to meet end of life care needs for those affected by non-malignant, life-limiting disease have implications for the development of the nursing workforce (Murray et al. 2006; Chahine et al. 2008; Bausewein et al. 2010; Pinnock et al. 2011; Higginson et al. 2012; McConigley et al. 2012; Higginson et al. 2014; Kimbell et al. 2015; Eriksson et al. 2016). This means there is potential to influence the further expansion of the palliative care advanced practice roles, irrespective of the care setting.

Professional identity and advanced clinical roles

An important aspect of moving to expanded advanced practice nursing roles is the need to ensure that nurses working in palliative care are not seen to extend their role to fulfil tasks and provide care that other professionals would have done in the past and are no longer willing to do so. This is particularly so in the nurse/doctor dyad where both professions may be concerned about role erosion or shifting the role boundaries from those considered traditional to that profession. Similarly there is some evidence that the presence of specialists may erode the opportunities for role expansion of other colleagues who are not in specialist roles. It is also recognised that advance practice roles provide opportunities for holistic care alongside some traditional medical roles around diagnosis and assessment (Lowe et al. 2012; Kennedy et al. 2015).

Effective team working makes best use of the skills and knowledge of its members. Over-zealous demarcation of role boundaries may hinder team working, however, effective team working also requires role clarity and understanding between members. Defining specialist and advanced roles in nursing is challenging due to the inherent differences that exist in such classifications. Nurses who work in hospice or palliative care units are not necessarily nurse specialists, although they may have undertaken some additional education in palliative care. Rather, they are working in a specialist area. This can be confusing for patients, their families and indeed other healthcare and social care professionals in that the same level of knowledge and expertise is used irrespective of place of care, but the titles of those providing the care differ.

The questions arise then as to what precisely defines an advanced practice role in specialist palliative care. Specialisation may be considered to occur as part of the advancement of a profession and in nursing is generally considered to be 'a good thing'.

Developing specialist and advanced roles contributes to both the advancement of the nursing profession and the delivery of patient-, family- and community-focused care through expanding and moving boundaries forward. Having said that, there is a lack of clarity around how practice might concentrate around a specialism and the knowledge and skills required to achieve this level of practice. Furthermore, we know little about the numbers of specialist and advanced practitioners required and the areas of practice suited to such roles. Linking levels of palliative care (Figure 14.1) to levels of education (Figure 14.2) provides a useful model for the development of specialist and advanced roles but there remains questions about balancing practice restriction with practice expansion, and defining the scope of advanced and specialist nursing practice (Gardner et al. 2007; Lowe et al. 2012; McConnell et al. 2013).

Irrespective of the setting, there are specific skills, attributes and competences associated with specialist practice. In some jurisdictions these are clearly articulated. In Ireland, the National Council for the Professional Development of Nursing and Midwifery (2007) articulated core concepts for the clinical nurse specialist role (Table 14.1). Similar concepts for clinical nurse specialist have also been identified by the Royal College of Nursing in the UK (2009).

The roles of nurses working at advanced practice level in Australia (ANMAC 2015), New Zealand (NZNO 2008), the United States (AANP 1993) and the UK (2012) are also described. Table 14.1 summarises clinical nurse specialist and advanced nurse practice key concepts and descriptors. It can be seen that there are areas of overlap and the key concepts underpinning both clinical nurse specialist and advanced practice roles are linked. The difference in these roles may lie in the levels of expectation and the reach and scope of the advanced nurse practice role as opposed to the clinical nurse specialist role, which lies mainly at the level of the patient and family.

These concepts when demonstrated by the clinical nurse specialist equate to the ability to practise with an increased level of competence and confidence. As such, what is observed is an individual who has clear leadership abilities and a capacity for collaboration, consultation and an ability to see 'the wider picture' when assessing and providing for the needs of the patient and their family. Advanced practice builds on the reach and scope of the clinical nurse specialist role to exert broader influence and development on clinical practice, education, research and leadership (Clinical Standards Board for Scotland 2002; Lowe et al. 2012; Ryan et al. 2014; Kennedy et al. 2015).

The combination of rising incidence of long-term conditions and ageing populations is increasing pressures in meeting the demand for palliative care, and creative use of the nursing workforce is vital. This rising need is in a context where economic and workforce resources are diminishing. The key contribution nurses make to the delivery of palliative care is recognised. Across Europe and internationally the clinical nurse specialist in palliative care is relatively well established although we do not know how many such roles exist. A natural and logical progression is therefore the investigation of the potential benefits and parameters of the advanced nurse practice role in palliative care, a role which is relatively unexplored (Reed 2010).

Table 14.1 Clinical nurse specialist/advanced nurse practitioner key concepts and descriptors

Concept	Clinical Nurse Specialist (CNS) descriptor	Concept	Advanced Nurse Practitioner (ANP) descriptor
Clinical focus	The work of the CNS must have a strong patient focus and must define itself as nursing and provide both direct and indirect care.	Autonomy in clinical practice	The autonomous ANP/AMP (advanced midwife practitioner) is accountable and responsible for advanced levels of decision-making which occur through management of specific patient/client caseload.
Patient advocate	The CNS role involves communication, negotiation and representation of patient values and preferences in care decisions.	Expert practice	Expert practitioners demonstrate practical and theoretical knowledge and critical thinking skills that are acknowledged by their peers as exemplary. They also demonstrate the ability to articulate and rationalise the concept of advanced practice. Education must be at Master's degree level (or higher) in a programme relevant to the area of specialist practice and which encompasses a major clinical component.
Education and training	The CNS holds a remit for education and training which consists of structured and impromptu educational opportunities to facilitate both staff development and patient education.	Professional and clinical leadership	ANPs/AMPs are pioneers and clinical leaders in that they may initiate and implement changes in healthcare service in response to patient/client need and service demand. They must have a vision of areas of nursing/midwifery practice that can be developed beyond the current scope of nursing/midwifery practice and a commitment to the development of these areas. They provide new and additional health services to many communities in collaboration with other healthcare professionals to meet a growing need that is identified both locally and nationally by healthcare management and governmental organisations.
			ANPs/AMPs participate in educating nursing/midwifery staff and other healthcare professionals through role-modelling, mentoring, sharing and facilitating the exchange of knowledge in the classroom, the clinical area and the wider community.

(Continued)

Table 14.1 (*Continued*)

Concept	Clinical Nurse Specialist (CNS) descriptor	Concept	Advanced Nurse Practitioner (ANP) descriptor
Audit and research	Audit of current nursing practice and evaluation of improvements in the quality of patient/client care are essential requirements of the CNS role. The CNS, as well as keeping up to date with relevant current research to ensure evidence-based practice and research utilisation, must also contribute to relevant nursing research.	Research	ANPs/AMPs are required to initiate and coordinate nursing/midwifery audit and research. They identify and integrate nursing/midwifery research in areas of the healthcare environment that can incorporate best evidence-based practice to meet patient/client and service need. They are required to carry out nursing/midwifery research which contributes to quality patient/client care and which advances nursing/midwifery and health policy development, implementation and evaluation. They demonstrate accountability by initiating and participating in audit of their practice. The application of evidence-based practice, audit and research will inform and evaluate practice and thus contribute to the professional body of nursing/midwifery knowledge both nationally and internationally.
Consultant	The CNS will provide both inter- and intra-disciplinary consultations, across sites and services. This consultative role contributes to improved patient management.		

Constructs of advanced practice and relevance to palliative care

The advanced nurse practice in palliative care is a relatively new phenomenon. Although advanced nurse practice roles have been developed across a range of healthcare settings which include primary care in the USA and Sweden, and acute hospital services in the UK, Australia and Ireland (Kennedy et al. 2015), the number of advanced nurse practitioners in palliative care has not reached the levels seen in other areas of specialty. There is also only limited evidence of research into the potential of the advanced nurse practitioner in palliative care (Reed 2010). That said, there appears to be agreement that advanced nurse practitioners in palliative care are distinguished by their highly developed clinical skills and knowledge, which are used to develop and deliver care. Key attributes of the advanced nurse practitioner in palliative care have also been identified as: critical thinking, autonomous decision-making, and an advanced ability to problem-solve, as well as impeccable assessment, diagnosis and treatment planning. It is also important to note that the advanced nurse practitioner role relates primarily to clinical care of patients and their families, but also encompasses research, education and leadership, making the reach and scope of the advanced nurse practitioner role different to that of the clinical nurse specialist (Wickham 2003; RCN 2008). The advanced nurse practitioner role is also likely to combine holistic care with advanced clinical skills around assessment and diagnosis (Lowe et al. 2012; Kennedy et al. 2015).

The term 'advanced nurse practitioner' has been used inconsistently across a number of roles and jurisdictions. There have been a number of attempts to define competencies, and standards for advanced practice (Lowe et al. 2012). As identified earlier, a degree of inconsistency persists despite the attempts to benchmark standards and competencies for advanced practice.

Optimal healthcare delivery which responds to patient and service needs is arguably dependent on empowering nurses and midwives to expand their scope of practice when patient and service needs make it prudent to do so (D'Amour et al. 2012). In palliative care there is an urgent need to develop new models of healthcare and service delivery to meet the needs of all patients with advanced illness and their families. Expanded levels of autonomy, skills and decision-making for nurses are central to this endeavour, although this has resulted in some confusion in the health service community internationally about the professional role and scope of the advanced nurse practitioner. Long-standing difficulties exist in relation to the scope of advanced nursing practice and such roles. In particular, the international literature identifies that balancing practice restrictions with practice expansion coupled with environmental and client-specific contextual factors, is problematic.

The most widely accepted definition of advanced practice is that proposed by the International Council of Nursing:

A Nurse Practitioner-advanced practice nurse is a registered nurse who has acquired the expert knowledge base, complex decision-making skills and clinical competencies for expanded practice, the characteristics of which are shaped by the context and/or country in which s/he is credentialed to practice. A master's degree is recommended for entry level.

(ICN 2013)

Despite some of the difficulties around defining advanced practice, there exists agreement that such practitioners require a number of attributes, including the ability to work autonomously, think critically and demonstrate expertise in complex decision-making. Positive role modelling in order to improve, change and deliver evidence-based practice is important for service delivery. Four spheres of advanced practice are identified: leadership, facilitating learning of others, research and advanced clinical practice. Expanded practice may include non-medical prescribing (NMP) and clinical skills in diagnosis which can be identified as an expansion of nursing practice. It is more complex to identify expanded practice in terms of clinical decision-making, leadership and the provision of holistic care.

This means that key issues for palliative care services, considering the introduction of advanced nurse practice roles, include the current lack of clarity regarding the contribution to holistic care provision and outcomes, where advanced nurse practitioners are positioned within multi-professional teams and the impact on team working (Reed 2010). The perspectives of patients and carers regarding this service model are also necessary. The increasing complexity and availability of options for palliative care and treatment and the needs of patients with non-cancer illness throughout the palliative phase of their illness mean the technical and diagnostic skills of the ANP have attracted attention. In addition, recent changes in UK legislation to allow NMP of controlled drugs (Home Office 2012) supports the successful operation of these roles in the palliative care setting. The UK is recognised as a leader in NMP and although there are developments across North America and Australasia, these jurisdictions do not have the same extended NMP rights as in the UK. A UK survey in 2015 to explore the current position of nurse prescribing in palliative care identified NMP working in palliative care, showing that the 2012 legislative changes have been embraced. However, the findings identified a need to improve the transition between becoming qualified and undertaking active NMP. The authors identified a lack of research in this area and recommended ensuring the provision of proper study leave for nurses and further research to include the patients' perspectives and economic implications (Ziegler et al. 2015).

Advanced nurse practitioners in palliative care

The numbers of advanced nurse practitioners providing specialist palliative care are relatively unknown. Furthermore, there exists a paucity of information about the nature of these roles and how these reflect the four spheres of advanced practice: leadership, facilitating learning of others, research and advanced clinical practice.

One example which illuminates attributes of the advanced practice role in palliative care is the evaluation of two advanced nursing practice roles in a specialist multi-professional palliative care service in Scotland (Kennedy et al. 2015). Two advanced nurse practitioners were supported to complete Master's level studies and worked between a specialist palliative care unit and the acute hospital where they had an advisory role. Three phases of qualitative data collection were conducted over a period of 10 months. Twenty-one participants spanning advanced nurse practitioners (n = 2), multi-professional staff (n = 14) and patients/carers (n = 5) took part. Individual and focus group interviews with key stakeholders, observation of the advanced nurse practitioners at work and analysis of their reflexive diaries were the data collection methods.

Overall, the findings of this evaluation demonstrate that if the advanced nurse practice role can flourish, it has the potential to shape 'new identities', re-construct the boundaries of nursing roles and emphasise the relationship-based elements of excellent nursing work (Box 14.1). In this study the advanced nurse practitioner roles offered *a unique contribution* to the service and these roles were characterised by *fluid role boundaries*. Throughout, the overarching notion of the *delivery of person-centred care* in the palliative care context was evident.

Box 14.1   Advanced practice in palliative care in action: a patient's perspective

[ANP named] answers all our questions, she doesn't avoid the difficult questions that we've wanted to ask, whether it's on treatment, whether it's on the progress, on the disease or the process or what the hospice can provide or what it can't provide. She's not averse to giving you a cuddle when she knows you're very down and you need it. She seems to have great insight into how you're feeling and she provides for you as an individual need. I've talked – we've talked – about all aspects about my demise, something I haven't done with anybody else . . . (a) because she's made herself available and (b) because we have confidence in her.

The findings showed that in this context the advanced nurse practice role incorporated aspects of nursing alongside the utilisation of skills not traditionally associated with nursing or specialist palliative nursing roles (Box 14.2). This included physical examination; independent non-medical prescribing; initiating, ordering and interpreting investigations, accepting and coordinating admissions/discharges. These skills were integrated with expertise in advanced communication and counselling, ethical and person-centred decision-making and care planning.

Box 14.2   Moving the boundaries of palliative nursing care

Research Observations: [ANP and Speciality Doctor reviewed the drug kardex together to note how much analgesia had been used over the last few days], cognitive status and changes, as well as wider disease and indications of sepsis, degree of response to antibiotics, fluids and bloods. During the face-to-face review, the Speciality Doctor followed up on points made by the ANP, gaining more information about how the patient felt. During this time, ANP at times prompted patient about information that patient had previously disclosed but that patient had not yet mentioned to the Speciality Doctor. The patient was reluctant for fluids but ANP and the Speciality Doctor gently negotiated this with the patient and the patient agreed. Following review, the ANP offered her perspective on current and appropriate analgesia which included adjuvant and second line opiates and diagnosis of toxicity, use of fluids, and the judgement that the patient was deteriorating despite antibiotic intervention – the issue of sepsis against a background of advancing disease and unpredictable but short prognosis. There appeared to be agreement from the Speciality Doctor and from this, the ANP amended the kardex and attended to fluids. ANP raised the issue of ensuring patient's family were aware of the situation as unpredictable but most likely deteriorating rapidly.

(Observation, In-Patient Unit, Ward Round, Phase Two)

The findings of this study suggest advanced nurse practice roles have the potential to blur the boundaries between caring and treating/curing although significant further work is required to identify which patient and family outcomes are best met by an advanced nursing role. This study identified and confirmed that the context in which advanced nurse practice roles are developed is important, as acceptance of the role by other members of the interdisciplinary team is linked to the co-construction of a different nursing identity.

Conclusion

There have been a number of attempts to identify distinct levels of palliative nursing care practice which correspond to the palliative and end of life care needs of patients and families across a range of healthcare settings. All nurses require education in palliative care and never more so than in an environment where palliative care should be available to all, regardless of diagnosis and care setting. There is a clear need to ensure that the nursing contribution to palliative and end of life care is supported and developed and that the expansion and advancement of professional nursing identities is supported. The expansion of palliative care nursing roles at each level of palliative care delivery; the palliative care approach; generalist palliative care and specialist palliative care is necessary.

At the specialist level, the nurse has the potential to enhance and improve the quality of care to patients and families while also acting as a resource for the inter-professional team, and other colleagues working in varying clinical settings. At the advanced level, palliative care nursing has a key role to play in the provision of person-centred, evidence-based care that uses the advanced skills and knowledge of the individual nurse and blurs the boundaries between treatment and care. The planning of advanced nurse practice roles should include prioritising the scope and focus of the post within the four recognised core domains. The introduction of advanced nurse practitioner roles needs to recognise the context in which the post will exist and the implications for key stakeholders as acceptance of the role is linked to the co-construction of a different nursing identity.

As palliative care nursing continues to evolve and expand, it is important that these advances be supported in both their design and development, in order to ensure that palliative care nursing remains person-centred and central to the provision of care to individuals with life-limiting conditions and their families. There exists a need to define, defend, evaluate and name the work of expanded and advanced nursing roles in palliative care if patient and family care outcomes are to be met.

Learning exercise 14.1

As a nurse providing palliative care, reflect on your current role and responsibilities taking time to consider how you currently articulate the key concepts and descriptors described in Table 14.1. Some questions to consider:

- What level of palliative care am I providing?
- Do I consider I am performing my current role at a specialist level?
- Do I consider I am performing my current role at an advanced level?
- What key activities do I undertake that I think represent holistic care in palliative care?
- What attributes do I have that I consider contribute to my professional identity as a palliative care nurse?

References

American Association of Nurse Practitioners (1993) Standards of Practice for Nurse Practitioners. Available at: https://www.aanp.org/images/documents/publications/standardsofpractice.pdf

ANMAC (Australian Nursing and Midwifery Accreditation Council) (2015) Nurse Practitioner Accreditation Standards. Available at: http://www.anmac.org.au/sites/default/files/documents/Nurse_Practitioner_Accreditation_Standard_2015.pdf

Bausewein, C., Daveson, B., Benalia, H. et al. (2010) PRISMA: a pan-European co-ordinating action to advance the science in end-of-life cancer care. *European Journal of Cancer*, 46(9): 1493–501.

Chahine, L.M., Malik, B. and Davis, M. (2008) Palliative care needs of patients with neurologic or neurosurgical conditions. *European Journal of Neurology*, 15: 1265–72.

Clinical Standards Board for Scotland (2002) *Clinical Standards for Specialist Palliative Care*. Edinburgh: NHS Scotland.

Council of Europe (2003) Recommendation Rec (2003) 24 of the Committee of Ministers to member states on the organisation of palliative care. Available at: www.coe.int/t/dg3/health/Source/Rec(2003)24_en.pdf

D'Amour, D., Dubois, C.A., Dery, J. et al. (2012) Measuring actual scope of nursing practice: a new tool for nurse leaders. *Journal of Nursing Administration*, 42(5): 248–55.

Delamaire, M. and Lafortune, G. (2010) Nurses in advanced roles: a description and evaluation of experiences in 12 countries. Contract No.: 54. OEDX Working Paper.

Department of Health and Children (2001) *Report of the National Advisory Committee on Palliative Care*. Dublin: Stationery Office. Available at: http://www.dohc.ie/publications/pdf/nacpc.pdf?direct=1

Department of Health, Western Australia (2008) *Palliative Care Model of Care*. Perth: WA Cancer and Palliative Care Network, Department of Health, Western Australia. Available at: http://www.healthnetworks.health.wa.gov.au/modelsofcare/docs/Palliative_Care_Model_of_Care.pdf (accessed 6 September 2016).

EAPC (European Association for Palliative Care) (1998) *Definition of Palliative Care*. Available at: www.eapcnet.org/about/definition.html (accessed 6 September 2016).

EAPC (European Association for Palliative Care) (2014) European Declaration on Palliative Care. Available at: http://palliativecare2020.eu/declaration/ (accessed 6 September 2016).

Eriksson, H., Milberg, A., Hjelm, K. and Friedrichsen, M. (2016) End of life care for patients dying of stroke: a comparative registry study of stroke and cancer. *PLoS One*, 11(2): e0147694.

European Commission (2012) Descriptors defining levels in the European Qualifications Framework. Available at: https://ec.europa.eu/ploteus/en/content/descriptors-page (accessed 27 June 2016).

Gardner, G., Chang, A. and Duffield, C. (2007) Making nursing work: breaking through the role confusion of advanced practice nursing. *Journal of Advanced Nursing*, 57(4): 382–91.

Higginson, I.J., Bausewein, C., Reilly, C.C. et al. (2014) An integrated palliative and respiratory care service for patients with advanced disease and refractory breathlessness: a randomised controlled trial. *The Lancet Respiratory Medicine*, 2(12): 979–87.

Higginson, I.J., Gao, W., Saleem, T.Z. et al. (2012) Symptoms and quality of life in late stage Parkinson syndromes: a longitudinal community study of predictive factors. *PLoS One*, 7(11): 46327.

Home Office (2012) Circular 009/2012: Nurse and pharmacist independent prescribing, 'mixing of medicines', possession authorities under patient group directions and personal exemption provisions for Schedule 4 Part II drugs. Available at: https://www.gov.uk/government/publications (accessed 6 September 2016).

International Council of Nurses (2013) *Scope of Nursing Position Statement*. Available at: http://www.icn.ch/publications/position-statements/ (accessed 6 September 2016).

Kennedy, C., Brooks Young, P., Nicol, J. et al. (2015) Fluid boundaries: exploring the contribution of the advanced nurse practitioner to multi-professional palliative care. *Journal of Clinical Nursing*, 24(21–2): 3296–305.

Kimbell, B., Boyd, K., Kendall, M. et al. (2015) Managing uncertainty in advanced liver disease: a qualitative, multiperspective, serial interview study. *BMJ Open*, 5: e009241. doi:10.1136/bmjopen-2015-009241.

Lowe, G., Plummer, V., O'Brien, A.P. and Boyd, L. (2012) Time to clarify – the value of advanced practice nursing roles in health care. *Journal of Advanced Nursing*, 68(3): 677–85.

Luckett, T., Phillips, J., Agar, M. et al. (2014) Elements of effective palliative care models: a rapid review. *BMC Health Services Research*, 14: 136.

McConigley, R., Aoun, S., Kristjanson, L. et al. (2012) Implementation and evaluation of an education program to guide palliative care for people with motor neurone disease. *Palliative Medicine*, 26(8): 994–1000.

McConnell, D., Slevin, O.D. and McIlfatrick, S.J. (2013) Emergency nurse practitioners' perceptions of their role and scope of practice: is it advanced practice? *International Emergency Nursing*, 21(2): 76–83.

Murray, S., Pinnock, H. and Sheikh, A. (2006) Palliative care for people with COPD: we need to meet the challenge. *Primary Care Respiratory Journal*, 15(6): 362–4.

National Consensus Project for Quality Palliative Care (2004) *Clinical Practice Guidelines for Quality Palliative Care*. Pittsburgh: National Consensus Project for Quality Palliative Care.

National Council for the Professional Development of Nursing and Midwifery (2007) *Framework for the Establishment of Clinical Nurse/Midwife Specialist Posts: Intermediate Pathway* (3rd edn). Dublin: National Council for the Professional Development of Nursing and Midwifery.

New Zealand Nursing Organisation (2008) Practice position statement: Advanced Nursing Practice. Available at: http://www.nzno.org.nz/Portals/0/publications/Advanced%20Nursing%20Practice,%202008.pdf

Pinnock, H., Kendall, M., Murray, S.A. et al. (2011) Living and dying with severe chronic obstructive pulmonary disease: multiperspective longitudinal qualitative study. *BMJ*, 342: d142.

Radbruch, L. and Payne, S. (2009) White Paper on standards and norms for hospice and palliative care in Europe: part 1. Recommendations from the European Association for Palliative Care. *European Journal of Palliative Care*, 16(6): 278–89.

Reed, S. (2010) A unitary-caring conceptual model for advanced nursing practice in palliative care. *Holistic Nursing Practice*, 24: 23–34.

Royal College of Nursing (2008) *Advanced Nurse Practitioners: An RCN Guide to the Advanced Nurse Practitioner Role, Competencies and Programme Accreditation*. London: RCN.

Royal College of Nursing (2009) *Specialist Nurses Make a Difference*. Policy Briefing 14/2009. London: RCN.

Royal College of Nursing (2012) Advanced nurse practitioners: an RCN guide to advanced nursing practice, advanced nurse practitioners and programme accreditation. Available at: https//www2.rcn.org.uk/__data/assets/pdf_file/0003/146478/003207.pdf

Ryan, K., Connolly, M., Charnley, K. et al. and Palliative Care Competence Framework Steering Group (2014) *Palliative Care Competence Framework*. Dublin: Health Service Executive.

Sermeus, W., Aiken, L., Van den Heede, K. et al. (2011) Nurse forecasting in Europe (RN4CAST): rationale, design and methodology. *BMC Nursing*, 10: 6.

Sheer, B., Kam, F. and Wong, Y. (2008) The development of advanced nursing practice globally. *Journal of Nursing Scholarship*, 40(3): 204–11.

Wickham, S. (2003) Development of nurse specialists/advanced practitioners in Ireland. *British Journal of Nursing*, 12(1): 28–33.

World Health Assembly (2014) Strengthening of palliative care as a component of comprehensive care throughout the life course. Available at: Apps.who.int (accessed 12 September 2016).

World Health Organization (2002) Definition of palliative care. Available at: http://www.who.int/cancer/palliative/definition/en/ (accessed 12 September 2016).

Ziegler, L., Bennett, M., Blenkinsopp, A. and Coppock, S. (2015) Non-medical prescribing in palliative care: a regional survey. *Palliative Medicine*, 29(2): 177–81.

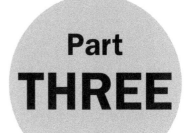

Part

THREE

CARING AROUND THE TIME OF DEATH

Introduction to Part Three

Catherine Walshe

While many current developments in palliative care nursing focus on expanding palliative care by providing it earlier, alongside palliative and curative treatments, and to a wider range of people with life-limiting illness, it still remains the case that many, if not most, of those we provide palliative care for will die during or soon after that episode of care (Clark et al. 2014). It is important that nurses providing palliative care appreciate how to enable people to prepare for their deaths, to care for people as they die, and to work with the grieving and bereaved. Such care can be challenging and stressful, and nurses need to appreciate how to care for themselves and their colleagues. In Part Three, we explore care at and around the time of death for those who are dying, their friends and family, and the nurses and other healthcare professionals providing care.

Understanding that someone is entering the last phase of their lives is challenging. It is hard for healthcare professionals to accurately predict impending death, but perhaps harder for friends and family to recognise that death may be close at hand (Griffiths et al. 2015; Amblas-Novellas et al. 2016). This challenge is compounded by the difficulties nurses and other healthcare professionals have in effectively communicating prognosis (Pontin and Jordan 2013; Broom et al. 2014). In Chapter 15, Maureen Coombs and Sarah Russell examine the impact and ramifications of these issues through exploring the theory and research around preparing for death, how this impacts on health policies (particularly focusing on advance care planning), and how to help people prepare for different types of death. They suggest patient-focused simple communication, exploring issues that matter to people such as their goals, fears and desires.

When death is imminent, most people wish comfort and peace, and to die in the manner they want in the place of their choice (Gomes et al. 2012; Virdun et al. 2016). In Chapter 16, Sarah Russell, Maureen Coombs and Jo Loney explore how to facilitate this, examining issues around place of death, how to enable individualised care, and important care areas such as achieving optimal symptom control and recognising that death is imminent. Nurses are key professionals in this phase of illness, frequently privileged to be alongside the person and their family before and at the point of death, and to care for the body after death. The skills and compassion that nurses show at this point can live long in the memories of friends and family and potentially influence future grief experiences.

Understanding how to assess grief and plan for a bereavement experience are the central issues addressed in Chapter 17, by Linda Machin. Grief is a fundamental human emotion, a normal expression of loss. However, for some, the grief response becomes overwhelming and can affect their capacity to function. In this chapter an evidence-based way of assessing responses and attitudes to grief and loss is presented; this can be used by nurses to both assess the grief of individuals and appraise the risk of poor outcomes. This enables nurses to use the most appropriate strategies to work with people who are grieving.

Interventions which may be helpful in the nurses' repertoire for people who are bereaved are presented by Lauren Breen and Samar Aoun in Chapter 18. They set the context of bereavement, examine different types of bereavement care interventions, and explore how these can be integrated into palliative care.

Providing care at or around the time of death (and earlier in the disease trajectory) can be difficult work. It is known that working in palliative care can be difficult, upsetting, but also inspiring. Nurses can be exposed to structural, professional and emotional stressors, through repeated exposure to death, distress, concern and suffering (Koh et al. 2015; Vargas et al. 2016). In Chapter 19, Lise Fillion and Mary Vachon explore stressors and risk factors, offer a framework for promoting well-being, and present evidence-based interventions to support nurses.

In a generally death-denying society it can be easy to ignore the needs of patients, family and friends, and nurses and other healthcare professionals around the time of death. These chapters re-focus attention on this important time in people's lives, and the importance of nursing care. There is still much to know about how to provide impeccable care at and around the time of death, and nurses need to be at the forefront of research in this field, and its implementation, to ensure the highest possible standards and outcomes from nursing the dying.

References

Amblas-Novellas, J., Murray, S.A., Espaulella, J. et al. (2016) Identifying patients with advanced chronic conditions for a progressive palliative care approach: a cross-sectional study of prognostic indicators related to end-of-life trajectories. *BMJ Open*, 6(9): e012340.

Broom, A., Kirby, E., Good, P. et al. (2014) The troubles of telling: managing communication about the end of life. *Qualitative Health Research*, 24(2): 151–62.

Clark, D., Armstrong, M., Allan, A. et al. (2014) Imminence of death among hospital inpatients: prevalent cohort study. *Palliative Medicine*, 28(6): 474–9.

Gomes, B., Higginson, I.J., Calanzani, N. et al. (2012) Preferences for place of death if faced with advanced cancer: a population survey in England, Flanders, Germany, Italy, the Netherlands, Portugal and Spain. *Annals of Oncology*, 23(8): 2006–15.

Griffiths, J., Ewing, G., Wilson, C. et al. (2015) Breaking bad news about transitions to dying: a qualitative exploration of the role of the District Nurse. *Palliative Medicine*, 29(2): 138–46.

Koh, M.Y.H., Chong, P.H., Neo, P.S.H. et al. (2015) Burnout, psychological morbidity and use of coping mechanisms among palliative care practitioners: a multi-centre cross-sectional study. *Palliative Medicine*, 29(7): 633–42.

Pontin, D. and Jordan, N. (2013) Issues in prognostication for hospital specialist palliative care doctors and nurses: a qualitative inquiry. *Palliative Medicine*, 27(2): 165–71.

Vargas, R.M., Mahtani-Chugani, V., Pallero, M.S. et al. (2016) The transformation process for palliative care professionals: the metamorphosis, a qualitative research study. *Palliative Medicine*, 30(2): 161–70.

Virdun, C., Luckett, T., Lorenz, K. et al. (2016) Dying in the hospital setting: a meta-synthesis identifying the elements of end-of-life care that patients and their families describe as being important. *Palliative Medicine*, 31(7): 587–601.

Preparing and planning for death

Maureen Coombs and Sarah Russell

Introduction

Take a moment to think about the following situations. A young man is informed that his wife would not survive following a large sub-arachnoid haemorrhage. An 80-year-old man with long-standing heart failure receiving maximal anti-failure therapy admitted in acute failure for the third time in 2 months. Young parents with an 8-year-old son diagnosed with advanced high-grade glioblastoma. Death is confronting all these people. As a nurse, what can you say to help them prepare for death and for their loss and bereavement?

This chapter explores preparing and planning for death in its many guises. It begins with an exploration of the empirical understanding of preparing for death, and its impact on patients and family members. There follows a discussion on current health policy strategies developed to help people live their life before death and make clear their wishes at end of life. The chapter explores the challenges of recognising the dying process and then closes with a practical focus on what to say to help others prepare for different types of death. In this way, it sets the scene for the next chapter that explores the last days and hours of life.

Why preparing and planning for death is important

Being prepared for death is about being ready for death and for the dying process that precedes it. Recognising that death is approaching, especially when it is the death of someone close to us, requires an internal shift in thinking. This change in cognition recognises that life will not go on forever. Such an adjustment is required by the patient who is dying, by their family, and by the healthcare and social care team involved. Recognising that death is impending can result from becoming aware of a weakening in a person's condition, perhaps appreciating that there is an increased need for care or interventions, or a realisation that medical therapies are no longer having the benefits intended.

When caring for patients at the end of life, we can be tempted to think that family members must be sensitive to the impending death. We may think that family members must have seen the physical deterioration in their family member. Perhaps we have heard families repeatedly say 'There is nothing more to be done', so they must understand that death is approaching. However, when preparing for death, there can be no assumptions. There are many challenges in this area of practice where the uncertainties inherent in the illness situation, the impact of inadequate communication by healthcare staff, and the lack of understanding of patients and family members (Hebert et al. 2006) all contribute to a lack of preparation for death.

Although practitioners make consistent claims about preparing patients and families for death, large numbers of people continue to be unprepared for death. In a study of patients 4 months from death, only 37 per cent of patients reported having end of life discussions with medical staff (Wright et al. 2008). While some patients may exercise choice in not wanting to discuss their illness and future, others will want the opportunity to understand and make choices about care. A commonly held view is that patients may be fearful of discussing dying and fearful of the unknown. However, research indicates that patients report feeling more at peace and have a better quality of life when involved in discussions about death and dying (Ray et al. 2006).

Family members are not always well prepared for death (Teno et al. 2004). This is concerning, given that the unexpected death of a family member is known to lead to increased risk in the bereaved of major depressive disorders, panic and anxiety, and post-traumatic stress disorders (Keyes et al. 2014). The consequences for family members following unexpected death are not limited to mental health: there is also risk of physical health problems. Symptoms reported range from general headache and dizziness, insomnia and loss of appetite (Sorensen and Pinquart 2005) to the more serious health issues of increased risk of cardiovascular events (Buckley et al. 2011). It is therefore important to consider how and when patients and families can prepare and plan for death.

Advance care planning and personalised plans of care

Traditionally, preparation and planning for death were activities undertaken in the last weeks or day of life. More recently, the concept of planning how best to live one's life up to the point of death has gained support in international health policy. 'Advance care planning' is an overarching term that describes conversations held about choices at end of life, decisions made about care (including the right to refuse treatments), and the appointment of proxy or surrogate decision-makers should decision-making capacity be lost (National End of Life Care Programme 2010). These can be documented to inform future treatments and care received.

There are benefits of advance care planning activity occurring early in the disease trajectory. A recent systematic review has identified that when decisions are made in line with patient values, patient goals are achieved more frequently, including preferred place of death and reduction in inappropriate hospital admissions (Brinkman-Stoppelenburg et al. 2014). Improvements are seen in the quality of end of life care received and in patient and family satisfaction, and the levels of stress, anxiety and depression in surviving relatives are reduced (Detering et al. 2010; Bischoff et al. 2013).

Internationally there are a number of different terms and definitions used in the area of advance care planning, each responding to the local legal frameworks. For example, in Scotland, anticipatory care planning for adults is positioned within the long-term conditions health policy (Scottish Government 2010) and in England and Wales, the Charity 'Together for Short Lives' (2016) advocates anticipatory planning for young people with unstable conditions and life-threatening complications. However, there are broad similarities, namely:

1 a written or verbal expression of wishes and preferences about care to be taken into account when discussing, planning and coordinating future care needs;
2 a formal, documented advance refusal of future treatments or interventions to be used if the person is unable to state their refusal of treatments or interventions;
3 a formally appointed surrogate decision-maker to act as the person's advocate;
4 a process or system to document and disseminate decisions.

Specific wishes and decisions such as Do Not Attempt Cardio Pulmonary Resuscitation (DNACPR), withdrawal and withholding of treatment, preferred place of care or death, treatment escalation plans as well as processes and legal jurisdictions for making decisions in the best interests of a person in the event of a loss of capacity, can also be contained within advance care planning. Advance care planning in children requires acknowledgement of other considerations, including the legal position concerning the age for decision-making authority, and the role of the parent in this (Lotz et al. 2015).

Advance care planning also requires systems and processes to be in place for documentation and dissemination of the decisions made; these must be regularly reviewed and refined. This is important as choices and preferences may change over time (Evans et al. 2014) with questions raised about whether advance decisions can consistently and accurately reflect individual preferences (Levi and Green 2010). While there are many benefits to making choices about future healthcare, advance care planning remains poorly adopted. This may result from contextual influencers, including the relationship between palliative care and patient ethnicity and culture (Russell 2015); patient's age (Institute of Medicine 2015); previous experience of illness (Fried et al. 2009); patient's health status or disability (Lovell and Yates 2014); and the patient's health literacy (Volandes et al. 2008).

Internationally, different approaches have been adopted to respect patient choice about treatment options closer to the end of life. In America, this has included use of 'Practitioner Orders for Life-Sustaining Treatments' (POLST), in Australia and New Zealand 'Goals of Care', with end-of-life care pathways being championed in the United Kingdom (Chan et al. 2016). One of the most profiled pathways, the Liverpool Care

Pathway, was phased out in the United Kingdom in 2014 (Neuberger et al. 2013), and replaced by a personalised plan of care. While the evidence for end of life pathways remains poor and further study is required, a recent Cochrane Review (Chan et al. 2016) concludes that the underlying principles of end of life pathways remain relevant, having favourable effects on care (Costantini et al. 2014; Verhofstede et al. 2016).

Perhaps most importantly, such pathways must be used in an informed way with focus on patient outcomes (Sleeman et al. 2015), rather than seen simply as a dehumanised care process or activity; this is clearly explored in the Leadership Alliance for the Care of Dying People's 'Five Priorities of Care' (2014).

Learning exercise 15.1

Think about your own workplace.

- How you would know if a patient had carried out advance care planning and discussed or documented their wishes and decisions about care?
- Where would you find details of this?
- How would you know if any documents still accurately reflected their wishes?
- How would you incorporate their advance care planning into a personalised plan of care?

How to prepare patients and family members for death

Even the most cursory of glances at healthcare research and the popular press reveals that a common concern for patients and families is how infrequently discussions are held about death and dying, and about what will, or will not happen, at end of life (Ellershaw and Ward 2003; Donnelly 2016). While some doctors and nurses may feel under-confident in this area and therefore unwilling to engage families in such discussions, patients and family members are clear on what will help prepare them for death.

Patients often want information about their disease and prognosis, on symptom management, the on-going care available, and what will happen to carer/family members after their death (Aldred et al. 2005). Perhaps more important to patients is not only to express their concerns, but also to have these listened to and heard by healthcare staff, and by staff familiar with their particular situation (Ventura et al. 2014). In one ethnographic study, bereaved caregivers and family members identified a range of medical, practical, psychological and spiritual questions that were important to prepare for death, but not always discussed with healthcare professionals (Hebert et al. 2008). Questions about what dying would look like, disclosure of medical errors, and how to arrange funerals were important areas for exploration. Factors that prevented these questions from being asked included feeling overwhelmed by circumstances, having a lack of trust in the clinical team, and concern that in asking questions, healthcare staff might consider them ignorant (Hebert et al. 2008). These findings provide a clear steer for doctors and nurses to do the following:

- recognise that clinical situations can be overwhelming for family members;
- reinforce the importance for families of establishing confidence in clinical teams;
- encourage families to verbalise their concerns.

The importance of skilled communication with families is clear – see more on communication in Chapter 7 in this volume. In a recent research review on preparing families for death, Loke et al. (2013) identified the importance of giving honest and accurate information to families about the prognosis of their family member. With many studies highlighting similar findings (Francke and Willems 2005; Stajuduhar et al. 2008; Hauksdottir et al. 2010), information not only helps family members prepare and make decisions at the end of someone's life (and death), it also improves communication between families and the dying person. Patients and families value information about death and the dying process (Hebert et al. 2008) and recognise that proactive, as opposed to reactive, communication is important when preparing for death (Francke and Willems 2005). Furthermore, there is evidence that greater clarity is needed in the words used to discuss and describe preparing for dying (Steinhauser et al. 2001).

While families clearly articulate the importance of information, this does not address how doctors and nurses can identify what information is important to meet individual needs, and help prepare patients and families for future events. Over the past decade, work undertaken in this area has explored the 'serious illness conversation'. This work recognises that patient, clinician and system factors affect the timing and content of these discussions (Bernacki et al. 2014). The patient's emotional state, patient expectations of doctors initiating health-related conversations, and preference about use of aggressive treatment at end of life are all factors affecting serious illness conversations. The level of physician training in communication skills at end of life, the established practice of only holding discussion about life expectancy near to death, and the hesitancy of clinicians to share uncertain prognostic information with patients and families are important physician-related issues. There are also organisational challenges in holding serious illness conversations. In hospital, the default position of driving towards sustaining life means that there is little acknowledgment of death and the care required by the dying and there is also a lack of clarity about who holds responsibility for holding such conversations 24/7 (Bernacki et al. 2014).

Against this complex backdrop, there are strategies to identify patients for whom it may be timely to hold the 'serious illness conversation'. Prognostic- and disease-related triggers help to identify which patients may benefit from discussions about what the future may hold. For example, healthcare staff using the 'Would you be surprised if this person died in the next year?' as a prognostic question when considering the risk of death for a patient with cancer. As disease-related triggers, examples would be noting the lack of further treatment options, functional decline or on-going oxygen requirement for patients with chronic obstructive disease (Janssen et al. 2012). Such approaches can be used to identify patients at high risk of death. Awareness of this group of patients may trigger serious illness conversations early, for example, in the outpatient clinic prior to any crisis or prior to transition to a phase of active dying.

In understanding that patients and families want honest communication, yet acknowledging that serious illness conversations can be anxiety-provoking for patients and healthcare staff, some guidance is available. One framework to structure conversations about preparing for death uses Gawande's (2014) five questions. These can easily be adapted for conversations held with patients and with families of seriously ill patients. The questions are:

1 What is your understanding of your current health or condition?
2 If your current condition worsens, what are your goals?
3 What are your fears?
4 Are there any trade-offs you are willing to make or not?
5 What would a good day be like?

Learning exercise 15.2

Reflect on the last time you talked with a patient about their death. What went well, and what areas could improve? Consider whether Gawande's framework could have been helpful.

In using such simple, direct and open questions, the agenda of any discussion held with patients or with families, shifts. The discussion becomes patient-/family-centred with the pace and direction of the conversation driven by the patient and family rather than healthcare staff (Back et al. 2009); this is important in order to respect patient autonomy and choice.

While this chapter is about preparatory care for patients of all ages, there is one population group for whom talking about death holds particular emotional burden. How to prepare children if they ask about their own death or about the death of others is always an area of concern. While there is little empirical work to guide practice in this area, many hospices and charities, for example, Marie Curie UK and the American Cancer Society, offer practice tips to support children at this distressing time. Box 15.1 lists some practical advice.

Box 15.1 How to prepare children for death

- Be honest and use clear, unambiguous language to explain what death and dying mean rather than 'going to sleep' or 'passing away'.
- Use a lead in sentence, for example, 'I have some sad news to tell you . . .'
- If the child knows that they/the person was unwell, build on this knowledge, 'You remember when we last saw Uncle Jack in hospital and he was very unwell?'
- After you have spoken about dying/death, pause and wait for questions to follow. This allows the child to indicate readiness for more information.
- Ask open-ended questions to allow the child to reply in their own way: 'How did you feel when Grandad died?' rather than 'Did you feel sad when Grandad died?'
- Ensure the child understands that the death is not because of something they did or did not do.
- For young children, explain death using appropriate terms, for example, 'Grandma's body was not working any more and it could not be fixed.'
- Be honest with children that death is a part of life and look for 'teachable moments', including the death of a pet or the illness of a character in a book or movie.

Aspects of death and dying that can be prepared for

Work on preparation for death and dying focuses on four areas of preparation: medical, psychological, spiritual and practical (Steinhauser et al. 2001; Loke et al. 2013). It is important to recognise that individuals can demonstrate a range of responses when preparing for death and dying, and that it is important to be culturally aware and sensitive at this time. The medical area of preparation describes how patients and families want information and support from healthcare professionals about the medical condition, prognosis, the signs and symptoms as death approaches, and at death itself. Such preparation encompasses talking about what dying may look like (as discussed later). These can be sensitive areas to discuss with patients and families. Clarifying the level of detail wanted by patients and families is important and achieved by saying: 'I can be very specific about what changes you will see at the end or you may be thinking about something else here. What information would be useful for you?'

Psychological preparation is about allowing time for discussion about the impending separation from others, grief about dying and loss, and of the emotions experienced. Attending to a review of the person's life, resolving interpersonal and family conflicts and saying good-bye are important aspects of psychological preparation. There will be individuals not ready to talk about, nor prepared for death, and this is explored in Case Study 15.1. Psychological preparation can be physically and emotionally tiring for patients and families. Nurses have an opportunity to assess how draining this situation is for patients and families and make suggestions about how to organise time for being together, and time for quiet and rest. Help patients and families understand that sitting in silence with someone as well as active involvement in care can all contribute to psychological preparation. While nurses may spend substantial time with patients and families, other experts in hospital and community settings can provide psychological bedside support and can be involved in care, including specialist palliative care and counselling professionals.

Attendance to spiritual matters is often an individual matter. For some, religious and spiritual matters are of little import, while for others, the opportunity for prayer and attendance to religious practices is crucial. It is important that there is time to reflect and re-examine life's purpose and finding meaning in the life, and the death, of the person. The inclusion of pastoral support staff can be significant. Use of questions such as 'Can you help me understand what I need to know about your beliefs and practices in order to take care of you?' can help nurses acknowledge and incorporate spiritual care into patient and family support.

Finally, there are practical aspects of preparation that refer to planning for events after death. For patients and families, this includes making funeral arrangements, organising of finances, making a will, and attending to issues of estate. It is important that clear information is available to help all parties prepare for this area. While some may view this as 'morbid', it is an important area that allows all to talk openly about the impending death, and serves to reassure the dying person that no burdens are left behind after their death. This in itself brings peace that all is in place before death occurs.

Diagnosing dying – and why it is important

At some stage in everyone's life, there is usually a moment where the imminent death is recognised. However, this is not always easy to identify. Diagnosing the last days or hours of life is challenging and can be referred to as 'actively dying' (Hui et al. 2014; Australian Commission on Safety and Quality in Health Care 2015). The signs of actively dying (Table 15.1), with more specific indications of death within 3 days, may include: decreased response to verbal and visual stimuli, inability to close eyelids, drooping of the nasolabial fold, and grunting of vocal cords (Hui et al. 2015). In paediatric palliative care, similar signs are reported, including circulatory and breathing changes, anorexia and neurological changes (Amery 2009; NICE 2016), together with disease trajectory changes and changes in attitude to disease and living (NICE 2016).

One of the challenges of diagnosing 'actively dying' is that there is no single validated tool to diagnose this period, with existing tools predominately based on cancer populations (Kennedy et al. 2014). Given such uncertainty, prognostic tools such as the Palliative Prognostic Score, the Palliative Prognostic Index and the Glasgow Prognostic Score can facilitate clinical decision-making by providing approximated timeframes (Hui 2015). Different disease populations demonstrate different physiological patterns

Table 15.1 Examples of signs of actively dying

United Kingdom	New Zealand	Australia
Agitation, Cheyne–Stokes breathing, deterioration in level of consciousness, mottled skin, noisy respiratory secretions and progressive weight loss. Increasing fatigue and loss of appetite. Changes in communication, deteriorating mobility or performance status, or social withdrawal. (NICE 2015)	Being bed-bound, semi-comatose, only able to take sips of fluids and no longer able to take oral medication. Increasing weakness and tiredness resulting in the person spending more and more of their time in bed, a period of withdrawal with the person spending less time awake and increasing time asleep, decreasing intake of food and medicine, and decreased interaction with others, a period of unconsciousness with no waking, cooling of peripheries as the blood circulation is diverted to central processes, irregularities of heart beat due to metabolic or vascular changes, stiffness caused by immobility and change in breathing patterns. (Ministry of Health New Zealand 2015)	Poor or incomplete response to medical treatment, continued deterioration despite medical treatment as well as decline in the patient's condition, or a clinical determination that they will not benefit from interventions. (Australian Commission on Safety and Quality in Health Care 2015)

in the actively dying stage and this further complicates the situation. Patients with cancer and amyotrophic lateral sclerosis may have increased dyspnoea (Plonk and Arnold 2005) and patients who have sustained a major stroke often show signs and symptoms of aspiration pneumonia (Mazzocato et al. 2010).

It is therefore important to recognise the uncertainty in diagnosing dying, and the need to work with and within this concept (Kennedy et al. 2014). However, this should not prevent clinicians from raising the possibility that the patient may be 'actively dying' to avoid potentially harmful and futile treatments as well as facilitating conversations about end of life care (Cardona-Morell and Hillman 2015) with patients, families and other clinical team members.

Learning exercise 15.3

Think about a recent patient you have cared for who was at the end of life.

- How did you recognise that they might be in the last days or hours of life?
- How did you make that judgement?
- Do you or your team/organisation have a process to assess, recognise and plan for the 'actively dying' period?

How to prepare people when death and dying are expected

With the incidence of chronic disease in developed countries rising, more people are dying expected deaths across care settings (Crawford et al. 2013). Most deaths from chronic disease often follow a pattern of frequent admission into hospital followed by adjustment to a new 'normal'. While this has historically been thought to help patients understand the dying trajectory, recent reports identify that patients with chronic illness, for example, heart failure and respiratory disease, may not perceive death as an anticipated consequence of their disease (Pinnock et al. 2011) with death not perceived as an imminent threat. However, other patients, for example, those with chronic renal failure, may have visual triggers of deterioration, for example, signs that the body is deteriorating, that lead to contemplation of the future (Axelsson et al. 2012).

Periods of family caregiving usually precede death from chronic disease (Figueiredoab et al. 2014). Some carers may feel overwhelmed and unable to make decisions about care choices as death approaches, or they may see death as a failure of their caring. Others may see death as a welcome release for their family member and feel relief, resulting in a sense of guilt at such thoughts and feelings. It is important that healthcare staff use supportive communication skills to identify what the patient and family are thinking and feeling at this time. This can then be used to inform how best to support patients and families.

Case Study 15.1: Preparing a patient for death

Kiki is a young Māori woman diagnosed with oligodendroglioma shortly after the birth of her fourth child. She has received intensive treatment over the past four years. She is admitted from home to an acute neurological ward as her pain and nausea are worsening. Kiki does not want to talk about dying and wants to be at home.

Assessment

It is difficult to know whether Kiki is aware that she is nearing the end of her life. Kiki may be experiencing lack of control over her life; concern as to whether she has been a good mother; perhaps, sadness and loss in not seeing her children grow up.

Plan

Care should focus on effective symptom control with explanation to enable Kiki to be comfortable and aid in understanding her symptoms and help in her medical preparation for events. Questions such as 'What is your understanding of what is happening to you?' will identify Kiki's awareness of events. Probing questions such as 'If you become sicker, how much are you willing to go through to possibly gain more time?' will direct care choices and help plan for future events.

Kiki's children and her family/whānau [Māori word for extended family] should be encouraged to visit, as directed by Kiki, to offer support, giving her a legitimacy to talk about her life and her family/whānau. This will assist with the emotional preparation.

Asking questions such as 'What are your biggest fears and worries about the future?' and 'If your health worsens, what are your most important goals?' can explore spiritual and existential issues for Kiki. Involving kaumātua [Māori word for respected elders or priest] may also help with spiritual preparation.

Asking questions such as 'How much does your family know about your priorities and wishes?' are helpful to address aspects of practical preparation and use of Whānau Care support services and social worker support are important.

How to prepare people when death is unexpected

The death of someone close may not be easy to cope with or to understand. However, a death that is sudden and unexpected is even more difficult to comprehend and raises strong emotions of shock, anger, denial and even guilt (Norton et al. 2011). Sudden death can occur in many care settings, at home, in the community, or in hospitals. The circumstances of unexpected death can range from a child who has taken an accidental fatal overdose, the adolescent who is a victim of a road traffic accident, or the adult who has an unexpected hospital cardiac arrest with unsuccessful cardio-pulmonary resuscitation. Sudden death can occur outside of hospital, with the person certified dead in the community. However, events precipitating unexpected death can occur in the community with the person surviving and admitted to hospital and receiving intensive medical management. Death then occurs some hours to days later when treatment is no longer effective or beneficial, and may involve withdrawal of life-sustaining therapies.

Unexpected deaths are more complex than expected ones with additional legal requirements associated with coroner and police investigation. There are also moral and ethical issues that arise from the need to respect patient autonomy and act in the patient's best interest. This can be difficult if the patient lacks capacity for decision-making and the wishes of the patient are unknown (Smith et al. 2009). As patients in this condition are often unconscious, an increased decision-making burden rests on the family members (Wendler and Rid 2011). Given the emotional distress families experience at this time, information about the patient is often staged and given over time (minutes/hours/days), with frequent updates and reinforcement of messages (Coombs et al. 2012). This helps family members assimilate and process information, enabling decision-making and preparing for what is ahead.

There are general evidence-based principles used to support bereaved families at this time (Roe 2011). Central to these are:

- ensure privacy for the family while considering family attendance at resuscitation;
- choose an appropriately skilled person who is knowledgeable about events to talk with the family;

- deliver information about the death compassionately, using clear language and using the person's name;
- allow families to express emotions and provide families with practical support for comfort needs;
- enable death customs and rituals to be conducted, including spending time with the deceased.

Nurses are in a unique position to support family understanding at this time, and yet caring for a person who has died unexpectedly is challenging. Nurses and other healthcare staff are often required to transition from delivering intense activity to resuscitate a person to a role of supporting and listening to a grieving family (Eberwein 2006). It is well recognised that working in such situations is challenging for nurses (Norton et al. 2011) and this is known to have an impact on burnout and retention. It is therefore important that support strategies such as debriefing and education about loss and bereavement are available for all staff working in this area.

Case Study 15.2: Preparing a carer for death

John is a 64-year-old man admitted to an acute medical ward following an extensive ischaemic stroke with profound irreversible brain damage. John is married to Carol and was preparing for retirement. They have no children. The medical team have spoken with Carol and confirmed that it is unlikely that John will ever gain consciousness and that death will probably occur in days.

Assessment

There has been no warning of this event for Carol. There may be many issues for Carol: no opportunity to say goodbye, no other close family nearby, a sense of loss, denial, anger, loneliness and grief.

Plan

While the priority in care is to ensure that John is comfortable, supporting Carol is important too. Regular updating of Carol using visual test results, for example, computerised tomography scan results will help her understand the severity of the situation and assist in medical preparation. Using techniques such as 'Ask-Tell-Ask' (Shannon et al. 2011) will help meet Carol's information needs and ensure understanding of information given. Development of rapid rapport and trust is needed to direct care choices and help plan for future events.

Talking with Carol about who can help her over the coming days/weeks is important to enable established support structures to help with Carol's emotional preparation. Personalising John's bed space with photos and music can help, as can sharing of memories. Asking Carol is she would like to participate in care, for example, face washing, combing of hair, hand massage may be helpful. Palliative care referral can be helpful.

Ascertaining what beliefs are important to John and Carol, and honouring these is part of spiritual preparation. Involvement with local pastoral support teams is important although this is an individual decision.

Understanding Carol's concerns about practical preparation for death will help guide the information given to her. Written information is helpful at this time as under stress, verbal information is forgotten. Social worker and family doctor support may be helpful as can follow-up bereavement services, if available.

Conclusion

Death and dying occur in many different ways and contexts. The experience of death is uniquely different for each person, the family, and for the healthcare staff involved. Death can sometimes come with advanced warning with time for preparation and adjustment. While, for some, death can be sudden. Whatever the circumstance, patients and their families should have an opportunity to prepare or plan for death, and nurses have an important contribution to this aspect of care.

Key learning points

- Death and dying are a unique and personal experience.
- Lack of preparedness for death can cause physical and psychological problems.
- Having discussions about death and dying in advance of the event is important and leads to patient-centred and family-centred care.
- Compassionate and honest communication skills and supply of clear information are key to assist patients and families prepare for death.

References

Aldred, H., Gott, M. and Gariballa, S. (2005) Advanced heart failure: impact on older patients and informal carers. *Journal of Advanced Nursing*, 49: 116–24.

Amery, J. (ed.) (2009) *Children's Palliative Care in Africa*. Oxford: Oxford University Press.

Australian Commission on Safety and Quality in Health Care (2015) *National Consensus Statement: Essential Elements for Safe High Quality End of Life Care*. Sydney: ACSQHC.

Axelsson, L., Randers, I., Hagelin, C.L. et al. (2012) Thoughts on death and dying when living with haemodialysis approaching end of life. *Journal of Clinical Nursing*, 21: 2149–59.

Back, A., Arnold, R. and Tulsky, J. (2009) *Mastering Communication with Seriously Ill Patients: Balancing Honesty with Empathy and Hope*. New York: Cambridge University Press.

Bernacki, R.E., Block, S.D., American College of Physicians High Value Care Task Force. (2014) Communication about serious illness care goals: a review and synthesis of best practices. *JAMA Internal Medicine*, 174: 1994–2003.

Bischoff, K.E., Sudore, R., Miao, Y. et al. (2013) Advance care planning and the quality of end-of-life care in older adults. *Journal of the American Geriatrics Society*, 61(2): 209–14.

Brinkman-Stoppelenburg, A., Rietjens, J.A. and van der Heide, A. (2014) The effects of advance care planning on end-of-life care: a systematic review. *Palliative Medicine*, 28: 1000–25. doi: 10.1177/0269216314526272.

Buckley, T., Mihailidou, A.S., Bartrop, R. et al. (2011) Haemodynamic changes during early bereavement: potential contribution to increased cardiovascular risk. *Heart, Lung and Circulation*, 20: 91–8.

Cardona-Morrell, M. and Hillman, K. (2015) Development of a tool for defining and identifying the dying patient in hospital: Criteria for Screening and Triaging to Appropriate aLternative care (CriSTAL). *BMJ Supportive and Palliative Care*, pp.bmjspcare-2014.

Chan, R.J., Webster, J. and Bowers, A. (2016) End-of-life care pathways for improving outcomes in caring for the dying. *Cochrane Database of Systematic Reviews*, 2: CD008006. doi: 10.1002/14651858.CD008006.pub2.

Coombs, M.A., Addington-Hall, J. and Long-Sutehall, T. (2012) Challenges in transition from intervention to end of life care in intensive care: a qualitative study. *International Journal of Nursing Studies*, 49: 519–27.

Costantini, M., Romoli, V., Di Leo, S. et al. (2014) Liverpool Care Pathway for patients with cancer in hospital: a cluster randomised trial. *The Lancet*, 383(9913): 226–37.

Crawford, G.B., Brooksbank, M.A., Brown, M. et al. (2013) Unmet needs of people with end-stage chronic obstructive pulmonary disease: recommendations for change in Australia. *Internal Medicine Journal*, 43: 183–90.

Detering, K.M., Hancock, A.D., Reade, M.C. and Silvester, W. (2010) The impact of advance care planning on end of life care in elderly patients: randomised controlled trial. *British Medical Journal*, 340: c1345.

Donnelly, H. (2016) 'Unforgivable' failings in end-of-life care revealed as 40,000 dying patients subject to secret 'do not resuscitate' orders every year. *The Telegraph*, 5 January. Available at: http://www.telegraph.co.uk/news/2016/05/01/unforgivable-failings-in-end-of-life-care-revealed-40000-dying-p/ (accessed 4 August 2016).

Eberwein, K.E. (2006) A mental health clinician's guide to death notification. *International Journal of Emergency Mental Health*, 8: 117–26.

Ellershaw, J. and Ward, C. (2003) Care of the dying patient: the last hours or days of life. *British Medical Journal*, 326: 30–4.

Evans, N., Pasman, H.R., Deeg, D. et al. (2014) How do general end-of-life treatment goals and values relate to specific treatment preferences? A population-based study. *Palliative Medicine*, 28(10): 1206–12.

Figueiredoab, D., Gabrielab, R., Jácomea, C. et al. (2014) Caring for relatives with chronic obstructive pulmonary disease: how does the disease severity impact on family carers? *Ageing and Mental Health*, 18: 385–93.

Francke, A.L. and Willems, D.L. (2005) Terminal patients' awareness of impending death: the impact upon requesting adequate care. *Cancer Nursing*, 28: 241–7.

Fried, T.R., Bullock, K., Iannone, L. and O'Leary, J.R. (2009) Understanding advance care planning as a process of health behavior change. *Journal of the American Geriatrics Society*, 57(9): 1547–55.

Gawande, A. (2014) *Being Mortal: Medicine and What Matters in the End.* New York: Metropolitan Books.

Hauksdottir, A., Valdimarsdottir, U., Furst, C.J. et al. (2010) Health care related predictors of husbands' preparedness for the death of a wife to cancer population-based follow-up. *Annals of Oncology*, 21: 354–61.

Hebert, R.S., Dang, Q. and Schulz, R. (2006) Preparedness for the death of a loved one and mental health in bereaved caregivers of patients with dementia: findings from the REACH study. *Journal of Palliative Medicine*, 9: 683–93.

Hebert, R.S., Schulz, R., Copeland, V. and Arnold, R.M. (2008) What questions do family caregivers want to discuss with health care providers in order to prepare for the death of a loved one? An ethnographic study of caregivers of patients at end of life. *Journal of Palliative Medicine*, 11: 476–83.

Hui, D., dos Santos, R., Chisholm, G. et al. (2015) Bedside clinical signs associated with impending death in patients with advanced cancer: preliminary findings of a prospective, longitudinal cohort study. *Cancer*, 121(6): 960–7.

Hui, D., Nooruddin, Z., Didwaniya, N. et al. (2014) Concepts and definitions for 'actively dying,' 'end of life,' 'terminally ill,' 'terminal care,' and 'transition of care': a systematic review. *Journal of Pain and Symptom Management*, 47(1): 77–89.

Institute of Medicine (2015) *Dying in America: Improving Quality and Honoring Individual Preferences Near the End of Life.* Washington, DC: National Academies Press.

Janssen, D.J., Spruit, M.A., Schols, J.M. et al. (2012) Predicting changes in preferences for life-sustaining treatment among patients with advanced chronic organ failure. *Chest*, 141: 1251–9.

Kennedy, C., Brooks-Young, P., Gray, C.B. et al. (2014) Diagnosing dying: an integrative literature review. *BMJ Supportive and Palliative Care*, 4(3): 263–70.

Keyes, K.M., Pratt, C., Galea, S. et al. (2014) The burden of loss: unexpected death of a loved one and psychiatric disorders across the life course in a national study. *American Journal of Psychiatry*, 171: 864–71. doi: 10.1176/appi.ajp.2014.130811320.

Leadership Alliance for the Care of Dying People (2014) One chance to get it right: how health and care organisations should care for people in the last days of their life. Available at: https://www.gov.uk/government/uploads/system/uploads/attachment_data/file/323188/One_chance_to_get_it_right.pdf

Levi, B.H. and Green, M.J. (2010) Too soon to give up: re-examining the value of advance directives. *American Journal of Bioethics*, 10(4): 3–22.

Loke, A.Y., Li, Q. and Sui Man, L. (2013) Preparing family members for the death of their loved one with cancer. a review of literature and direction for future research. *Journal of Hospice and Palliative Nursing*, 15(2): E1–E11.

Lotz, J.D., Jox, R.J., Borasio, G.D. and Führer, M. (2015) Pediatric advance care planning from the perspective of health care professionals: a qualitative interview study. *Palliative Medicine*, 29: 212–22. doi: 10.1177/0269216314552091.

Lovell, A. and Yates, P. (2014) Advance care planning in palliative care: a systematic literature review of the contextual factors influencing its uptake 2008–2012. *Palliative Medicine*, 28(8): 1026–35.

Mazzocato, C., Michel-Nemitz, J., Anwar, D. and Michel, P. (2010) The last days of dying stroke patients referred to a palliative care consult team in an acute hospital. *European Journal of Neurology*, 17(1): 73–7.

Ministry of Health New Zealand (2015) *Te Ara Whakapiri: Principles and Guidance for the Last Days of Life*. Wellington, NZ: Ministry of Health.

National End of Life Care Programme (2010) *Capacity, Care Planning and Advance Care Planning in Life Limiting Illness. A Guide for Health and Social Care Staff*. National End of Life Programme. London: Public Health England.

Neuberger, J., Aaronovitch, D. and Bonserv, T. (2013) More care, less pathway: a review of the Liverpool Care Pathway. Available at: https://www.gov.uk/.../file/212450/Liverpool_Care_Pathway.pdf

NICE (National Institute for Health and Care Excellence) (2015) *Care of Dying Adults in the Last Days of Life*. NICE Guideline no. 31. London: NICE. Available at https://www.nice.org.uk/guidance/ng31/resources/care-of-dying-adults-in-the-last-days-of-life-1837387324357

NICE (National Institute for Health and Care Excellence) (2016) *End of Life Care for Infants, Children and Young People: Planning and Management*. NICE Guideline no. 61. London: NICE. Available at https://www.nice.org.uk/guidance/ng61

Norton, C.K., Hobson, G. and Kulm, E. (2011) Palliative and end-of-life care in the emergency department: guidelines for nurses. *Journal of Emergency Nursing*, 37: 240–5.

Pinnock, H., Kendall, M., Murray, S.A. et al. (2011) Living and dying with severe chronic obstructive pulmonary disease: multi-perspective longitudinal qualitative study. *British Medical Journal*, 342: d142.

Plonk, Jr, W.M. and Arnold, R.M. (2005) Terminal care: the last weeks of life. *Journal of Palliative Medicine*, 8(5): 1042–54.

Ray, A., Block, S.D., Friedlander, R.J. et al. (2006) Peaceful awareness in patients with advanced cancer. *Journal of Palliative Medicine*, 9: 1359–68.

Roe, E. (2011) Practical strategies for death notification in the emergency department. *Journal of Emergency Nursing*, 38: 130–4.

Russell, S. (2015) Why diversity matters in advance care planning. *International Journal of Palliative Nursing*, 21(5): 234–5.

Shannon, S.E., Long-Sutehall, T. and Coombs, M. (2011) Conversations in end-of-life care: communication tools for critical care practitioners. *Nursing in Critical Care*, 16: 124–30.

Sleeman, K.E., Koffman, J., Bristowe, K. et al. (2015) 'It doesn't do the care for you': a qualitative study of health care professionals' perceptions of the benefits and harms of integrated care pathways for end of life care. *BMJ Open*, 5: e008242.

Smith, A.K., Fisher, J., Schonberg, M.A. et al. (2009) Am I doing the right thing? Provider perspectives on improving palliative care in the emergency department. *Annals of Emergency Medicine*, 54: 86–93.

Sorensen, S. and Pinquart, M. (2005) Racial and ethnic differences in the relationship of caregiving stressors, resources, and sociodemographic variables to caregiver depression and perceived physical health. *Aging and Mental Health*, 9: 482–95.

Stajuduhar, K.I., Martin, W.L., Barwich, D. and Fyles, G. (2008) Factors influencing family caregivers' ability to cope with providing end-of-life cancer care at home. *Cancer Nursing*, 31: 77–85.

Steinhauser, K.E., Christakis, N.A., Clipp, E.C. et al. (2001) Preparing for the end of life: preferences of patients, families, physicians, and other care providers. *Journal of Pain and Symptom Management*, 22: 727–37.

Teno, J.M., Clarridge, B.R., Casey, V. et al. (2004) Family perspectives on end-of-life care at the last place of care. *Journal of the American Medical Association*, 291: 88–93.

Ventura, A.D., Burney, S., Brooker, J. et al. (2014) Home-based palliative care: a systematic literature review of the self-reported unmet needs of patients and carers. *Palliative Medicine*, 28: 391–402.

Verhofstede, R., Smets, T., Cohen, J. et al. (2016) Implementing the care programme for the last days of life in an acute geriatric hospital ward: a phase 2 mixed method study. *BMC Palliative Care*, 15: 27.

Volandes, A.E., Paasche-Orlow, M., Gillick, M.R. et al. (2008) Health literacy not race predicts end-of-life care preferences. *Journal of Palliative Medicine*, 11(5): 754–62.

Wendler, D. and Rid, A. (2011) Systematic review: the effect on surrogates of making treatment decisions for others. *Annals of Internal Medicine*, 154: 336–46.

Wright, A.A., Zhang, B., Ray, A. et al. (2008) Associations between end-of-life discussions, patient mental health, medical care near death, and caregiver bereavement adjustment. *Journal of the American Medical Association*, 8(300): 1665–73. doi: 10.1001/jama.300.14.1665.

The last days and hours of life

Sarah Russell, Maureen Coombs and Jo Loney

Introduction

What help and support do patients and their families need or want in the last days or hours of life? Chapter 15 discussed how to prepare and plan for death. Here, we will explore nursing care in the more immediate period before death for an adult, young person, child and their family.

A peaceful and dignified end of life is the goal of care in the last days and hours of life (Ministry of Health 2015). This is achived through attending to the emotional, physical, spiritual and social needs of each person, including conversations with them, those that matter to them and care providers. Inquiries about previous advance care planning and current wishes can then ensure that care reflects the person's on-going personal choices and preferences. In such discussions, it is helpful to consider the age-specific development needs of children and young adults (Bennett 2012; Amery 2016) and explore and act upon personal, cultural, religious or spiritual preferences (QEOLCC 2010; National Strategy for Palliative Care Implementation Task Force 2015).

Preferred place of care or death

Achieving the preferred place of death is often cited as a goal of palliative care (De Roo et al. 2014). Studies report that dying at home is the preferred place for most adults (Gomes et al. 2012) and children (Amery 2016). This is more likely with end of life home-care programmes, rapid response teams (Gomes et al. 2013) and general practitioner involvement (Neergaard et al. 2009). However, not everyone will die at home (Gomes et al. 2012), with children and young people more likely to die in hospital or a hospice (Gao et al. 2016). Therefore, conversations and planning tailored to the individual are essential. The evidence tells us that understanding the factors regarding individual preferences about care or place of death (wherever that may be) is important (Burge et al. 2015; Gomes et al. 2015; Costa et al. 2016) . For example, home may not be the preferred place of death for everyone (Collier et al. 2015; Hoare et al. 2015; Pollock 2015) and future care preferences and choices may not always be stable (Auriemma et al. 2014), influenced by changes in health status, social circumstances, functional ability (Lobo 2011) or dependent on available support (Thomas et al. 2004).

Dying at home is not just about a physical care setting. A preferred place of death may have personal, social and symbolic meaning. Studies tell us that people may worry about being a burden or are concerned about seeing families distressed and exposed to intimate aspects of care (Gott et al. 2004; Shepperd et al. 2011). The emotional and practical burden of care is often under-recognised and under-researched (Collier 2013). Dying at home (and elsewhere) needs careful consideration of the complex social and emotional factors experienced by the dying person and their family (Morris et al. 2015; Milligan et al. 2016). Exploring previous wishes about preferred care or place of death within the context of the reality of the last days of life is part of discussing, planning and providing care.

Other considerations include reviewing care, services, equipment as well as coordination and communication with medical, health, social care services, community/hospital/hospice teams and 'out of hours' services (Lacey 2015). There are often local protocols as to how information is shared and distributed, for example, shared electronic records (Petrova et al. 2016). Discussion with families that death is approaching is helpful (The Australian and New Zealand Paediatric Palliative Care Reference Group 2015; Lacey 2015) and ensuring that families have details about who can be contacted for advice or support during the day, overnight and at weekends.

Conversations with the patient, family and clinical teams about the management of any future causes of concern can help a shared understanding of goals for care (Perkins et al. 2016). These include reasons for deterioration, such as infections, dehydration, opioid toxicity, steroid withdrawal, hypercalcaemia, hypo- or hyperglycaemia as well as discussions and documentation about Do Not Attempt Cardio Pulmonary Resuscitation (DNACPR) and withholding or withdrawing of treatment.

Learning exercise 16.1

What policies, procedures or guidelines do you have in your work setting to plan and provide care?

Individualised care

Individualised care is underpinned by the principles of choice, autonomy, shared decision-making, dignity and respect. In the past, clinical pathways (e.g. the Liverpool

Care Pathway) have been used widely around the world to manage end of life care (Chan et al. 2016). Recent reviews conclude that although strong evidence supporting end of life care pathways is lacking, the principles underpinning such pathways remain relevant (Chan et al. 2016). Furthermore, end of life planning should be carried out in consultation with patients and significant others.

These person-centred principles are seen in many paediatric and adult guidelines, for example, those of the Australian and New Zealand Paediatric Palliative Care Reference Group (2015), NICE (2016), Quality End-of-Life Care Coalition of Canada (2010), Singapore's National Strategy for Palliative Care Implementation Task Force (2015) and in recent UK policy (Box 16.1).

Box 16.1 Five priorities for care for adults in the last days and hours of life

1 The possibility that a person may die within the coming days and hours is recognised and communicated clearly, decisions about care are made in accordance with the person's needs and wishes, and these are reviewed and revised regularly.
2 Sensitive communication takes place between staff and the person who is dying and those important to them.
3 The dying person, and those identified as important to them, are involved in decisions about treatment and care.
4 The people important to the dying person are listened to and their needs are respected.
5 Care is tailored to the individual and delivered with compassion – with an individual care plan in place. This priority includes the fact that a person must be supported to eat and drink as long as they wish to do so, and their comfort and dignity prioritised.

(The Leadership Alliance for the Care of Dying 2014)

Recognising that death is imminent

Recognising the final days of life is extremely difficult given the uncertainties concerned with prognostication (Taylor et al. 2017). However, guidance advises that death is likely when the person is bed-bound, semi-comatose, only taking sips of fluid or unable to take tablets or food (Hospice Friendly Hospitals 2008). While each person's final moments are individual in nature, there are common features reported in a number of international guides for adults, young people and children included in Box 16.2.

Box 16.2 Common signs of dying

- Reduced functional and physical ability
- Increase in fatigue and weakness
- Withdrawal from day-to-day activities and interaction
- Decreasing levels of consciousness
- Reduced appetite
- Loss of ability to swallow

- Increase or changes in physical signs and symptoms
- Blue colour or mottling in peripheries
- Bowel and bladder changes and reduced or darker urine
- Cardio-vascular changes such as thready pulse
- Shallow and long pauses in between breathing (Cheyne Stokes)
- Noisy, rattling breathing ('death rattle')

Based on Amery (2016); Downing et al. (2015); Hockley (2015); Kehl and Kowalkowski (2013); NICE (2015; 2016); Plonk and Arnold (2005); The Australian and New Zealand Paediatric Palliative Care Reference Group (2015); Watson et al. (2016).

Pharmacological management of physical symptoms

All healthcare and social care providers have a part to play in the holistic assessment and management of symptoms. Collaboration and discussions with hospice and specialist palliative care teams are also helpful if further advice or support is required. Common symptoms reported include: anorexia, drowsiness, fatigue, dyspnoea, excessive respiratory secretions, agitation, nausea and vomiting, dysphagia, fluid and urinary incontinence, as well as delirium and pain (Hui et al. 2015; Steindal et al. 2015). Regular assessment of the cause of symptoms and benefits of pharmacological or other interventions will be necessary, and discontinuation of medicines that are not providing symptomatic benefit (QEOLCC 2010; The Australian and New Zealand Paediatric Palliative Care Reference Group 2015; NICE 2015; 2016; Watson et al. 2016).

There are a number of drugs used in symptom control. It is important to use the most appropriate route of administration. The preferred route is oral (QEOLCC 2010; Watson et al. 2016), but if a person is unable to swallow, then an alternative route such as subcutaneous is recommended. Intramuscular injections are usually avoided because of pain (QEOLCC 2010; Watson et al. 2016). If using buccal medication, a moist mouth is required to enable absorption. Some countries have the availability of transdermal patches to deliver opioid analgesia (e.g. Fentanyl), but these should not be introduced at this stage unless they have already been used before (due to strength of opioid and challenges in titration and delivery rate). Some people and cultures accept administration by the rectal route while others may not, and the nurse must review if this is the most appropriate route.

Non-pharmacological interventions can be of benefit, albeit the evidence base, for example, for hypnotherapy, aromatherapy and relaxation, is unproven (Coelho et al. 2016).

There are anecdotal reports of the benefits of patient positioning, use of fans and adopting familiar routines. There is also emerging evidence of the use of music therapy, for example, for improving quality of life and relief of pain (McConnell, Scott and Porter 2016).

Anticipatory prescribing and use of continuous subcutaneous infusions

One of the ways to provide symptom control is the use of anticipatory/just in case prescribing as well as continuous subcutaneous infusions (e.g. via a syringe pump). These can be used to administer medications for symptom control when a person is no longer able to swallow (e.g. due to weakness, fatigue, semi-consciousness, nausea or vomiting).

The objective of 'anticipatory' or 'just in case' prescribing is to have made a patient assessment and planned and prescribed for future symptoms usually via the intramuscular or subcutaneous route but sometimes intravenously or the buccal/nasal/oral route.

The objective of 'continuous subcutaneous infusions' is to administer medications continuously to control symptoms. This is usually via a portable, battery-operated device used to deliver a continuous subcutaneous infusion of medication over 24 hours, i.e. syringe pump or driver device. Mixing of several medications (for example, analgesia and sedative agents) is not uncommon. While off-label prescriptions or the prescription of a registered medicine for a use that is not included in the product information (Gazarian et al. 2006) are unlicensed, it is quite common practice in syringe drivers and palliative care (Toscani 2013).

When assessing and prescribing 'anticipatory' or 'just in case' prescribing as well as 'continuous subcutaneous infusions', it is prudent for the nurse to also assess for 'break through' or 'as required' medications. These are medications prescribed for additional symptom control. For example, if a patient is receiving the opioid Diamorphine for pain control via a 24-hour continuous subcutaneous infusion (e.g. a syringe pump), then a 'break through' or 'as required' dose of subcutaneous dimorphine may be prescribed for use if pain is not controlled.

When using such medication approaches, there are a number of considerations that nurses need to consider (Box 16.3).

Box 16.3   Considerations for anticipatory, subcutaneous infusions, as required prescribing

1   Assess current symptoms and effectiveness of medications.
2   Assess ability to take oral medications.
3   Consider future symptoms.
4   Discuss with patient and/or family purpose of anticipatory, subcutaneous, as required prescribing.

5 Discuss and agree with prescriber, prescriptions for drug, mode of administration, dose, range and frequency.

6 Ensure prescription and dispensing of medications and equipment required (e.g. needles, syringes).

7 Ensure up-to-date documentation and care plan for re-assessment and monitoring of symptoms.

8 Discuss and explore any questions or concerns with the patient and/or family about the care and plan.

Table 16.1 Generic examples of drugs and indications

Drug (class of drug)	Indications
Diamorphine (Opioid analgesic)	Pain, dyspnoea, cough, diarrhoea
Morphine (Opioid analgesic)	
Oxycodone (Opioid analgesic)	
Fentanyl Alfentanil (Opioid analgesic)	Pain in patients with renal failure
NSAID e.g. Diclofenac (Non-opioid analgesic)	Pain (particularly associated with tissue inflammation or bone pain/movement-related pain)
Parecoxib (COX-2 inhibitor)	Pain (especially in presence of inflammation)
Cyclizine (Antihistaminic, antimuscarinic, antiemetic)	Nausea and vomiting associated with motion sickness, anticipatory nausea, pharyngeal stimulation, mechanical bowel obstruction, raised intracranial pressure
Levomepromazine (Antiemetic phenothiazine antipsychotic)	Nausea and vomiting, insomnia, terminal agitation (useful as antiemetic and sedation, can be very sedating)
Metoclopramide (Prokinetic antiemetic)	Nausea and vomiting caused by gastric irritation, delayed gastric emptying, stimulation of the CTZ, obstructive bowel symptoms without colic
Dexamethasone (Corticosteroid)	Antiemetic, pain relief, raised intracranial pressure, spinal cord compression, intestinal obstruction, liver capsule pain
Glycopyrronium bromide (Quaternary ammonium antimuscarinic)	Noisy, rattling breathing ('death rattle'), colic in inoperable bowel obstruction (does not cross the blood–brain barrier so does not cause drowsiness)

(Continued)

Table 16.1 (Continued)

Drug (class of drug)	Indications
Hyoscine butylbromide (Antimuscarinic, antispasmodic, antisecretory)	Intestinal obstruction, crampy abdominal pain, noisy, rattling breathing ('death rattle')
Hyoscine hydrobromide (Antimuscarinic)	Death rattle, colic, reduces salivation, some antiemetic action
Midazolam Benzodiazepine (Anxiolytic)	Sedation for terminal agitation, multifocal myoclonus, epilepsy, intractable hiccup, muscle spasm
Octreotide (Somatostatin analogue)	Intestinal obstruction associated with vomiting, intractable diarrhoea, symptoms associated with hormone secreting tumours, bowel fistulae.
SEEK SPECIALIST ADVICE	Injection can be painful
Phenobarbital (Barbiturate)	Seizures, refractory terminal restlessness

Sources: Amery (2016); Bennett (2012); Lacey (2015); NICE (2015; 2016); Watson et al. (2016).

When prescribing and delivering medications in this way, it is advisable to follow guidance and assess indications, note contraindications and possible side effects. Table 16.1 is a generic guide for indications and mediations. A useful international resource is http://www.palliativedrugs.com/

Clinically assisted hydration and nutrition

The intake of fluids and food normally reduces in the last days of life (Good et al. 2014a; 2014b; Fritzson et al. 2015). This can lead to inquiries about the use of subcutaneous or intravenous infusions, i.e. clinically assisted hydration (CAH), or nasogastric and parental feeding, i.e. artificial nutrition (CAN). The aim of CAH and CAN is to relieve symptoms of thirst, dehydration, hunger and myoclonus, rather than to prolong life.

The evidence for use or non-use of CAH is uncertain (NICE 2015). While symptoms can be relieved, unpleasant side effects may occur including oedema, effusions, ascites and cannula site inflammation (NICE 2015). This is a difficult area of decision-making. For example, concerns over people dying of thirst was one of the issues raised in the UK review of the Liverpool Care Pathway for the Dying Patient (Neuberger 2013; Chan et al. 2016). Furthermore, current research is predominately adult-focused, with a paucity of pediatric evidence to guide decision-making (Rapoport et al. 2013).

There is also a lack of high quality evidence for the use of CAN, with clinicians needing to make decisions based on perceived individual benefits and harms (Good et al. 2014a; 2014b). CAH and CAN are medical interventions, and as such require an indication for use, a therapeutic goal, and the consent of a competent patient (Druml et al. 2016). Views on individual benefits and harms of such treatment may also be influenced by culture and context. There may be concerns about a family member 'giving up or starving to death' and worries about making the right decision. These concerns need to be approached sensitively with case-by-case individual assessment of benefit (or potential harm).

Learning exercise 16.2

Thinking about the evidence regarding artificial hydration and nutrition, what do you need to consider about your policies, procedures and practice?

Management of cardiac devices

Management of cardiac devices requires attention from when devices are implemented to when they may need to be deactivated; in particular, use of implanted cardioverter defibrillators (ICDs) and pacemakers.

ICDs are devices that monitor cardiac activity and deliver programmed pacing and/or electrical cardioversion for life-threatening tachyarrhythmias. While ICDs can extend and improve the quality of life for patients, continued activation of ICDs in patients at end of life results in the delivery of electric shocks as the patient's cardiac rhythm deteriorates. Twenty per cent of patients in the last week of life experience ICD shocks (Goldstein et al. 2004). This not only causes pain and distress for patient and family (Russo 2011), it may be inconsistent with goals of care at end of life (Thanavaro 2013).

Conversations with patients and their families should include the management of the ICD and whether deactivation is necessary. Deactivation of the defibrillator function of an ICD is painless and does not affect the pacing function of the device. Deactivation of the defibrillator will not cause sudden death, but will not prevent death should the patient experience a life-threatening tachycardia. Reprogramming of the ICD by a cardiologist or specialist technician will disable the defibrillation function and this is the preferred and most guaranteed method of deactivation (Goldstein et al. 2010). Temporary deactivation of the ICD, for example, as death is approaching, occurs by placement of a deactivation magnet (doughnut magnet) on the chest surface (Braunschweig et al. 2010). Placing a magnet over the ICD device temporarily suspends tachycardia detection and the shock therapy. In these instances, adhesive tape is used to secure the magnet on the chest to ensure patient and staff safety.

Details of the ICD deactivation are documented as per local clinical guidelines and consideration may need to be given for those in rural areas with long distances to travel. Any clinical setting where patients with ICDs are cared for should have access to deactivation magnets. Staff should have training to understand deactivation procedures and care. If patients with deactivated ICDs are transferred to other clinical settings, clear written and verbal information about the ICD status should be handed over to staff.

It is important that permanent deactivation of the device occurs post mortem by re-programming of the device so that mortuary and funeral staff are not exposed to the risk of an electric shock.

There are different issues for patients with cardiac pacemakers in situ. Discontinuing pacemaker therapy can occur at end of life. There may be questions about what happens when the pacemaker is discontinued. However, if the person is dependent on the pacemaker for cardiac rhythm and cardiac output, then stopping the pacemaker may make the person feel unnecessarily unwell at this time. Discontinuation of pacemakers at end of life is not required as the pacemaker device only provides an electrical impulse to stimulate the myocardium to contract. Once cell death occurs, for example, as hypoxia and anoxia occur during the natural process of dying and death, the cardiac muscle dies and does not respond to the electrical impulse of the pacemaker.

It is important that any implanted electrical heart rhythm device is explanted from the body prior to cremation. Cremating a body with such electrical devices in situ can cause lithium battery explosion when exposed to extreme heat and pressure (Medicines and Healthcare Products Regulatory Agency 2008). As ICDs and pacemakers are removed post mortem in funeral homes or by morticians, it is important that there is clear documentation about these in situ devices in the last offices documentation.

Organ and tissue donation

A recently recognised important area in end of life is tissue and organ donation. With global demand for organs continuing to exceed supply (International Registry in Organ Donation and Transplantation 2014), increasing the number of organs and tissues available for donation is important. However, the focus of maximising the function of the potential organs and tissues for donation can be perceived to be at odds with the goals of care for the dying person (Coombs and Woods 2017).

In brief, organs donated after death include heart, lungs, liver, pancreas and kidneys. Donated tissues include corneas, heart valves, skin and bone. Procedurally donation is a complex area requiring specialist knowledge and skill. Many countries have national policies and governing bodies to ensure ethical practice in this area. In the UK, there is the NHS Blood and Transplant Service, and in the United States of America, the Government Information on Organ Donation and Transplantation. There are also many cultural and ethical barriers to donation. In one systematic review (Irving et al. 2012), distrust of the medical system, misunderstandings about religious stances, and ignorance about the donation process all influenced decisions to donate. These are areas for consideration given the increasing recognition of organ donation as an important component of end of life care (Serri and Marsolais 2017).

There is limited evidence to guide organ donation at end of life in children and young people. The need for the views of children and young people, as well as their parents and healthcare professionals, to inform this area has been recognised (NICE 2016). Existing recommendations include use of sensitive communication and information in discussions about organ donation and respecting the choices and preferences of all those involved in organ donation decisions (Bennett 2012; Amery 2016; NICE 2016). As discussions in this area need to be clearly understood, support and expertise from donation coordinators and nurse specialists in this area are beneficial to patients, families and healthcare staff (Mullins, Simes and Yuen 2012).

Deceased organ donation can occur in patients following brain stem death and circulatory death. Most organ donors are patients who die from brain stem death, also known as brain death, usually following a catastrophic brain injury. These donors are mainly cared for in intensive care and ventilated to supply oxygen to the tissues and organs. Once death in this circumstance is confirmed by the undertaking of a strict and repeated set of tests, discussions are held with family members about the donation wishes of the patient. If organ donation proceeds, the physiological state of the patient is optimised to maintain organ function and organ removal occurs in the operating theatre (McKeown, Bonser and Kellum 2012). Once all suitable organs are removed, ventilatory and cardiovascular support discontinues.

Donation can also occur after cardiac death. This type of death is commonly recognised as absent palpable pulses, absent heart sounds, absent breath sounds, and the absence of respiratory effort or chest wall motion (Shemie et al. 2014). Patients who die in settings outside of intensive care can donate kidneys and, in certain situations, other organs, but these must be removed within minutes of the heart stopping to prevent hypoxic damage. Both types of donors can donate their corneas and other tissue, if specific conditions are met. Most healthcare organisations have well-established processes to ensure timely information and expertise are available to support these practices.

Identifying potential tissue and organ donors is a detailed process, requiring attendance to ethical, physiological, and communication processes and attention to the individual national legislative framework for donation. Healthcare professionals must be compassionate in their approach to patients and families, and make decisions about when is best to discuss potential tissue and organ donation matters, and indeed who may be best equipped to discuss and support patients and families.

Care and comfort measures

As death approaches, meticulous nursing care is necessary as the person may be more dependent on others for care and comfort. Measuring and recording patient data not directly related to comfort (such as weighing, pulse and blood pressure) may no longer be appropriate (Lacey 2015; National Strategy for Palliative Care Implementation Task Force 2015).

Mobility and skin care

Joints can become stiff and uncomfortable with the person being unable to move independently. Lying immobile over time applies pressure on the skin, increasing the risk of ischaemia leading to the development of pressure sores. There are a number of recommendations (Box 16.4).

Box 16.4   Mobility and skin care recommendations

1   Keep skin clean and dry and assess regularly.
2   Consider a polyurethane foam dressing for bony prominences (e.g. heels, sacrum) to prevent pressure ulcers in areas frequently subjected to friction and shear.
3   Consider a skin moisturiser to hydrate and massage dry skin in order to reduce risk of skin damage (but do not rub vigorously).
4   Redistribute weight by turning and repositioning – but consider the patient's personal preferences.
5   Assess for pressure-relieving mattress, being mindful that some find the alternating pressure changes of selective electric mattresses nauseating and distressing.
6   Assess the need for pain control before turning.
7   Use opportunities such as personal hygiene care to gently and passively move joints.
8   Use opportunities to teach/encourage family to participate in care.

Based on European Pressure Ulcer Advisory Panel (EPUAP) and
National Pressure Ulcer Advisory Panel (2009); Langemo and
Black (2010); Lacey (2015).

Mouth care

Frequent mouth and lip care including cleaning teeth or dentures is important for comfort and dignity (NICE 2015). The person should be supported to drink if they wish and are able to; but checks should be made for any difficulties, for example, swallowing problems or risk of aspiration (NICE 2015). Oral fluids (especially those with the consistency of jelly or ice cream) are often well tolerated (Hockley 2015) and assessments should be made for dry or cracked lips and signs of oral candida. The mouth should be kept moist and clean with a water-based gel. Oral candida can be treated with an anti-fungal treatment and sips of fluid or ice slithers may aid patient comfort. Family members should be given opportunity to undertake mouth care, enabling them to be part of care.

Terminal secretions or 'death rattle'

Noisy breathing or the 'death rattle' occurs in 23–92 per cent of people who are dying (Wee and Hillier 2008). This may arise from (Type 1) pooling of saliva and secretions in the upper airways along with reduced swallowing reflexes, dysphagia, and inability to expectorate and/or (Type 2) pooling of bronchial secretions (Lacey 2015). Type 1 is associated in some studies with being a predictor of imminent death and somewhat responsive to antimuscarinic agents (Lacey 2015). However, while the death rattle is common, it is doubtful if patients suffer with it (Lokker et al. 2014). A focus on supporting potential family distress in the witnessing of death rattle (Lacey 2015), as well as mouth care, positioning and dignity is recommended. The routine use of antimuscarinic drugs is not supported (Wee and Hillier 2008; Lokker et al. 2014).

Delirium, agitation and restlessness

Delirium is a syndrome characterised by a disturbance of often fluctuating consciousness, cognition and perception (Candy et al. 2012). It can be present in up to 88 per cent of patients at the end of life (Lacey 2015). Terminal restlessness is an agitated delirium that occurs in some people during the last days of life (Doyle and Woodruff 2008). While antipsychotic drugs may be widely used (Agar et al. 2017), sedation should not automatically be the first line response, especially for symptoms of delirium that are known to be associated with distress in mild to moderately severe delirium (Agar et al. 2017). Individualised management of delirium is key (Agar et al. 2017), as is paying attention to underlying causes (Candy et al. 2012), such as pain, urinary or faecal retention, general discomfort or psychological, emotional or spiritual distress. A role for nurses is to discuss with the patient or their family about possible causes and strategies, including the potential use of sedating medications. Non-pharmacological interventions include nursing the patient in a stable environment with continuity of care, positioning, familiar routines, appropriate lighting for time of day and reduction of noise (Candy et al. 2012).

Bowel and bladder function

Loss of bowel and bladder function, including urinary retention and faecal impaction, are likely in the last days of life (Lacey 2015; Watson et al. 2016). This can be distressing for both patient and family. Incontinence pads and a urinary catheter can minimise the frequent need for toileting and cleaning. It can be helpful to prepare families that following death there may be complete relaxation of the sphincter muscles, causing incontinence.

Constipation is characterized by infrequent bowel evacuations with hard, small faeces or difficulty or pain on defecation. Medications such as opioids may increase the likelihood of constipation and attention to constipation eases pain and distress. Larkin et al. (2008) recommend considering diet, fibre, fluid intake, immobility and toileting as well as using stimulant and softener laxatives to ease defecation (rather than increase regularity). Other considerations include using suppositories or enemas to stimulate evacuation or soften faeces to ease passage from rectum or stoma.

Diarrhoea is the passage of more than three unformed stools a day. This can be embarrassing, undignified and increases skin fragility. Nursing care includes identifying the cause, maintaining skin integrity by keeping skin clean, dry and applying barrier creams as well as considering medications that might minimise flow.

For both constipation and diarrhoea, odour can be controlled by keeping the skin and care areas clean and using fragrances attractive to the person (e.g. through toiletries or aromatherapy). If the patient has some mobility, the toilet or commode should be easily accessible. Any specific cultural or personal toileting rituals should also be followed.

Emotional and spiritual care

Dying is as much a social experience as it is a biomedical event. The nurse can encourage and empower the family to continue to take part in the care of and relationship with the dying person. Anecdotal evidence suggests that hearing is the last sense to be lost (Worcester 1935), so advising continued (appropriate) conversations or quietly holding a hand (Hockley 2015) is useful in providing a link between the dying person and their family.

Emotional support includes assessment, specialised psychological interventions as well as listening and communication skills. In the last days of life, such support is as important for the person who is dying as it is for their families and friends. For example, the dying person may be concerned about the emotional needs of their families or worry about how they will manage after they have died (Russell 2016). There may be anxiety about dying alone, in pain, experiencing breathlessness, or fear about how and when death will occur. Hockley (2015) suggests that one of the roles of the nurse is to be present and engaged in the process of dying, for example, knowing how to drop the professional role 'mask' and relate to others simply and richly as a human being (Roy 1988). By comforting interactions, verbally affirming statements and touch, nurses can provide ongoing emotional support (Skilbeck and Payne 2003).

Religious beliefs and spirituality can be central to how many people cope with terminal illness (Alcorn et al. 2010). Spirituality is different from religion and includes

the dynamic dimension of human life that relates to the way persons (individual or community) experience, express and/or seek meaning, purpose and transcendence, and the way they connect to the moment, self, to others, to nature, to the significant and/or sacred.

(Nolan et al. 2011, p. 88)

As an adult or child is dying, they may experience spiritual distress or a feeling of emptiness (Bennett 2012; Selman et al. 2014). Studies report the value of effective communication skills in order to respond to a child's spiritual questioning and help parent and child understand the spiritual meaning of their illness (Ferrell et al. 2016a; 2016b). For both adults and children there may be questions about the meaning of life and death; loss of purpose; being afraid to fall asleep at night; anger at their belief systems or feelings of being abandoned. Part of the role of a nurse is to be non-judgemental, compassionate, kind and empathic as well as enabling discussions with others, for example, a spiritual leader or professional.

Learning exercise 16.3

Florence is 11 years old and dying. She and her family do not participate in any type of religious practice. Florence is asking questions about what happens to 'her' when she dies and how will she know that she is still 'part of her family'.

What advice or support would you offer to her and her family?

Care at the moment of death

Death, as it is traditionally understood (that is, not brain death), occurs when there is an absence of a carotid pulse or heart sounds, absence of breath or respiratory sounds, and fixed, dilated pupils that are unreactive to light. The moment of death is treated with respect for the deceased and their family. Families vary in the degree of professional support necessary at this time (Lacey 2015) and there will be many different international and cultural policies and traditions for when a person has died.

Care after death

Sometimes known as 'last offices or last rites', care after death is the physical preparation of a person's body, the psychological care of their family and friends and the undertaking of formal/legal processes associated with death (Hospice UK and National Nurse Consultant Group 2015). The physical preparation of the body is often done by nurses and carers. While care of the body is used to mark the transition from living being to the dead person, it is important that all the principles associated with respectful, person-centred care are maintained. There are several international documents providing guidance for adults, children and young people (see Bennett 2012; Hospice UK and National Nurse Consultant Group 2015; Ministry of Health 2015; The Australian and New Zealand Paediatric Palliative Care Reference Group 2015; Amery 2016; NICE 2016). Box 16.5 illustrates the common principles found in guidance.

Box 16.5   Common principles for care after death

1   Compassionate dignified care

- Preparing the body and ensuring the person looks dignified in the way that they would want to be seen and remembered (e.g. dressing in own clothes or shroud or similar).
- Respecting cultural, religious, spiritual and personal preferences and practices.

2   Family support

- Opportunity to view the deceased person and say goodbye.
- Opportunity for family members to participate in care after death.
- Bereavement support and supporting the expression of grief (in whatever personal or cultural form in which that might occur).

3   Clinical considerations

- If the death has occurred in a care setting, identify the deceased person with a named label or as indicated in local procedures.
- Wounds and stomas: Cover with clean absorbent dressings and stomas with a clean bag.

- If the death is being reported to the coroner (or similar) due to circumstances surrounding the death, medical devices such as syringe pumps, catheters and cannulae are usually left in place.
- Organ and tissue donation.
- Cardiac devices and disposal of medications.
- Informing other services and teams involved in care.

4   Legal and formal considerations

- Informing medical and/or nursing services within a few hours of death so that verification of death can take place.
- Legal requirements if the death is suspicious or may need to be investigated.
- Information about registering the death and funeral directors.
- Transferring the body to the funeral directors (or similar).
- Financial and funeral issues.

Reflective practice

Nursing care in the last days and hours of life is not solely concerned with symptomology and clinical tasks. It also means attuning ourselves (as nurses) to the psycho-spiritual and existential dynamics of day-to-day care (Hockley 2015). It is good practice to recognise this and the impact of the death on ourselves and others through reflection, clinical supervision and peer support (Lacey 2015).

Learning exercise 16.4

- What are the policies and procedures for care after death in your setting?
- Reflecting upon your own experience, what do you need to do to be more knowledgeable or competent when caring for a person after death?

Conclusion

Nurses are instrumental in enabling and providing care during the last hours of a person's life, and at the moment of death. Nursing care in the last days and hours of life requires knowledge and skills (e.g. assessment and management of symptoms), practical and technical awareness (e.g. administering personal care or medications), compassion (e.g. spiritual and emotional support) and an appreciation of the holistic needs of patients and families. As nurses, we also have an obligation to contribute to the evidence base of end of life care in the last days and hours of life through research and service evaluation, and have a responsibility to be the advocate for patients and families, and to support others through education and mentorship as well as contribute to the design of service models, strategy and policy. Nursing combines the art and science of care; connecting evidence and compassion in one of the most intimate, personal times of a person's life, the time of a person's dying. In this chapter we have explored care considerations at this time so that nursing practice is compassionate, evidence-based, valued and sustainable.

Grief, mourning and bereavement are covered elsewhere in this book. However, it is pertinent to be mindful that the last days of life are part of the bereavement experience.

Key learning points

Individualised care in the last days of life includes:

- reviewing previous advance care planning wishes or decisions;
- physical symptom control as well as practical comfort measures and coordination with other services;
- considering organ donation, cardiac devices and artificial nutrition or hydration;
- spiritual and emotional assessment and care;
- care after death should be treated with the same respect as care during life;
- care extends to family/friends of the dying person.

References

Agar, M.R., Lawlor, P.G., Quinn, S. et al. (2017) Efficacy of oral risperidone, haloperidol, or placebo for symptoms of delirium among patients in palliative care: a randomized clinical trial. *JAMA Internal Medicine*, 177(1): 34–42.

Alcorn, S.R., Balboui, M.J., Pigerson, H.G. et al. (2010) 'If God wanted me yesterday, I wouldn't be here today': religious and spiritual themes in patients' experiences of advanced cancer. *Journal of Palliative Medicine*, 13(5): 581–8.

Amery, J. (2016) *Really Practical Handbook of Children's Palliative Care for Doctors and Nurses Anywhere in the World*. Raleigh, NC: Lulu Publishing Services.

Auriemma, C.L., Ngugen, C.A., Bronehim, R. et al. (2014) Stability of end-of-life preferences: a systematic review of the evidence. *JAMA Internal Medicine*, 174(7): 1085–92.

Bell, C.L., Somogyi-Zalud, E. and Masaki, K.H. (2010) Factors associated with congruence between preferred and actual place of death. *Journal of Pain and Symptom Management*, 39(3): 591–604.

Bennett, H. (2012) *Guide to End-of-life Care*. London: Together for Short Lives.

Braunschweig, F., Boriani, G., Bauer, A. et al. (2010) Management of patients receiving implantable cardiac defibrillator shocks: recommendations for acute and long-term patient management. *Europace: European Pacing, Arrhythmias, and Cardiac Electrophysiology: Journal of the Working Groups on Cardiac Pacing, Arrhythmias, and Cardiac Cellular Electrophysiology of the European Society of Cardiology,* 12(12): 1673–90.

Burge, F., Lawson, B., Johnston, G. et al. (2015) Preferred and actual location of death: what factors enable a preferred home death? *Journal of Palliative Medicine,* 18(12): 1054–9.

Candy, B., Jackson, K.C., Jones, L. et al. (2012) Drug therapy for delirium in terminally ill adult patients. *Cochrane Database of Systematic Reviews,* 11: CD004770.

Chan, R.J., Webster, J. and Bowers, A. (20160 End-of-life care pathways for improving outcomes in caring for the dying. *Cochrane Database of Systematic Reviews,* 2: CD008006.

Coelho, A., Parola, V., Cardoso, D. et al. (2017) Use of non-pharmacological interventions for comforting patients in palliative care: a scoping review. *JBI Database of Systematic Reviews and Implementation Reports,* 15(7): 1867–904.

Collier, A. (2013) *Deleuzians of Patient Safety: A Video Reflexive Ethnography of End of Life Care.* Adelaide, SA, Australia: Flinders University.

Collier, A., Phillips, J.L. and Iedema, R. (2015) The meaning of home at the end of life: a video-reflexive ethnography study. *Palliative Medicine,* 29(8): 695–702.

Coombs, M.A. and Woods, M. (2017) Organ donation practices and end-of-life care: unusual bedfellows or comfortable companions? In Shaw, R.M. (ed.) *Bioethics Beyond Altruism: Donating and Transforming Human Biological Material.* Sydney: Palgrave Macmillan Australia, pp. 239–63.

Costa, V., Earle, C.C., Esplen, M.J. et al. (2016) The determinants of home and nursing home death: a systematic review and meta-analysis. *BMC Palliative Care,* 15: 8.

De Roo, M.L., Miccinesi, G., Onwuteaka-Philipsen, B. et al. (2014) Actual and preferred place of death of home-dwelling patients in four European countries: making sense of quality indicators. *PLoS One,* 9(4): e93762.

Downing, J., Jassal, S.S., Matthews, L. et al. (2015) Pain. *Pediatric Pain Management in Palliative Care,* 5(1): 23–35.

Doyle, D. and Woodruff, R. (2008) *The IAHCP Manual of Palliative Care.* Houston, TX: IAHPC Press.

Druml, C., Ballmer, P.E., Druml, W. et al. (2016) ESPEN guideline on ethical aspects of artificial nutrition and hydration. *Clinical Nutrition (Edinburgh, Scotland),* 35(3): 545–56.

European Pressure Ulcer Advisory Panel (EPUAP) and National Pressure Ulcer Advisory Panel (2009) *Prevention and Treatment of Pressure Ulcers: Quick Reference Guide.* Available at: www.epuap.org

Ferrell, B., Wittenberg, E., Battista, V. et al. (2016a) Exploring the spiritual needs of families with seriously ill children. *International Journal of Palliative Nursing,* 22(8): 388–94.

Ferrell, B., Wittenberg, E., Battista, V. et al. (2016b) Nurses' experiences of spiritual communication with seriously ill children. *Journal of Palliative Medicine,* 19(11): 1166–70.

Fritzson, A., Tavelin, B. and Axelsson, B. (2015) Association between parenteral fluids and symptoms in hospital end-of-life care: an observational study of 280 patients. *BMJ Supportive and Palliative Care*, 5(2): 160–8.

Gao, W., Verne, J., Peacock, J. et al. (2016) Place of death in children and young people with cancer and implications for end of life care: a population-based study in England, 1993–2014. *BMC Cancer*, 16(1): 727.

Gazarian, M., Kelly, M., McPhee, J.R. et al. (2006) Off-label use of medicines: consensus recommendations for evaluating appropriateness. *Medical Journal of Australia*, 185(10): 544–8.

Goldstein, N.E., Lampert, R., Bradley, E. et al. (2004) Management of implantable cardioverter defibrillators in end-of-life care. *Annals of Internal Medicine*, 141(11): 835–8.

Gomes, B., Higginson, I.J., Calanzani, N. et al. (2012) Preferences for place of death if faced with advanced cancer: a population survey in England, Flanders, Germany, Italy, the Netherlands, Portugal and Spain. *Annals of Oncology*, 23(8): 2006–15.

Gomes, B., Calanzani, N., Curiale, V. et al. (2013) Effectiveness and cost-effectiveness of home palliative care services for adults with advanced illness and their caregivers. *Cochrane Database of Systematic Reviews*, 6: CD007760.

Gomes, B., Calanzani, N., Koffman, J. et al. (2015) Is dying in hospital better than home in incurable cancer and what factors influence this? A population-based study. *BMC Medicine*, 13: 235.

Good, P. Richard, R., Syrmis, W. et al. (2014a) Medically assisted hydration for adult palliative care patients. *Cochrane Database of Systematic Reviews*, 4: CD006273.

Good, P. Richard, R., Syrmis, W. et al. (2014b) Medically assisted nutrition for adult palliative care patients. *Cochrane Database of Systematic Reviews*, 4: CD006274.

Gott, M., Seymour, J.E., Bellamy, G. et al. (2004) Older people's views about home as a place of care at the end of life. *Palliative Medicine*, 18(5): 460–7.

Higginson, I.J. and Sen-Gupta, G.J. (2000) Place of care in advanced cancer: a qualitative systematic literature review of patient preferences. *Journal of Palliative Medicine*, 3(3): 287–300.

Hoare, S., Slote Morris, A., Kelly, M.P. et al. (2015) Do patients want to die at home? A systematic review of the UK literature, focused on missing preferences for place of death. *PloS One*, 10(11): e0142723.

Hockley, J. (2015) Intimations of dying: a visible and invisible process. *Journal of Palliative Care*, 31(3): 166–71.

Hospice Friendly Hospitals (2008) *When a Patient is Dying*. Limerick, Ireland.

Hospice UK and National Nurse Consultant Group (2015) *Care After Death: Guidance for Staff Responsible for Care After Death*. Available at: https://www.hospiceuk.org/media-centre/press-releases/details/2015/

Hui, D., Dos Santos, R., Chisholm, G. et al. (2015) Bedside clinical signs associated with impending death in patients with advanced cancer: preliminary findings of a prospective, longitudinal cohort study. *Cancer*, 121(6): 960–7.

Hui, D., Hess, K., Dos Santos, R. et al. (2015) A diagnostic model for impending death in cancer patients: preliminary report. *Cancer*, 121(21): 3914–21.

International Registry in Organ Donation and Transplantation (2014) Final numbers 2013. International Registry in Organ Donation and Transplantation.

Irving, M.J., Tong, A., Jan, S. et al. (2012) Factors that influence the decision to be an organ donor: a systematic review of the qualitative literature. *Nephrology Dialysis Transplantion*, 27: 2526–33. doi: 10.1093/ndt/gfr683.

Kehl, K. and Kowalkowski, J.A. (2013) A systematic review of the prevalence of signs of impending death and symptoms in the last 2 weeks of life. *American Journal of Hospice and Palliative Care*, 30(6): 601–16.

Kohut, N., Sam, M., O'Rourke, K. et al. (1997) Stability of treatment preferences: although most preferences do not change, most people change some of their preferences. *Journal of Clinical Ethics*, 8(2): 124–35.

Lacey, J. (2015) Management of the actively dying patient. In Cherny, N. et al. (eds) *Oxford Textbook of Palliative Medicine*. Oxford: Oxford University Press.

Langemo, D.K. and Black, J. (2010) Pressure ulcers in individuals receiving palliative care: a National Pressure Ulcer Advisory Panel White Paper. *Advances in Skin and Wound Care*, 23(2): 59–72.

Larkin, P.J., Sykes, N.P., Centeno, C. et al. (2008) The management of constipation in palliative care: clinical practice recommendations. *Palliative Medicine*, 22(7): 796–807.

Lobo, B. (2011) Advance Decisions to Refuse Treatment (ADRT). In Thomas, K. and Lobo, B. (eds) *Advance Care Planning in End of Life Care*. Oxford: Oxford University Press, pp. 101–12.

Lokker, M.E. , van Zuylen, L., van der Rijt, C., van der Heide, A. (2014) Prevalence, impact, and treatment of death rattle: a systematic review. *Journal of Pain and Symptom Management*, 47(1): 105–22.

McConnell, T., Scott, D. and Porter, S. (2016) Music therapy for end-of-life care: an updated systematic review. *Palliative Medicine*, 30(9): 877–83.

McKeown, D.W., Bonser, R.S. and Kellum, J.A. (2012) Management of the heart beating brain-dead organ donor. *British Journal of Anaesthesia*, 108: i96–i107.

Medicines & Healthcare Products Regulatory Agency (2008) Medical Device Alert (MDA/2008/068). Available at: http://www.mhra.gov.uk/home/groups/dts-bs/documents/medicaldevicealert/con025836.pdf

Milligan, C., Turner, M., Blake, S. et al. (2016) Unpacking the impact of older adults' home death on family care-givers' experiences of home. *Health and Place*, 38(March): 103–11.

Ministry of Health (2015) *Te-Ara-Whakapiri-Principles: Guidance Last Days of Life*. Wellington, New Zealand: Ministry of Health.

Morris, S.M., King, C., Turner, M. et al. (2015) Family carers providing support to a person dying in the home setting: a narrative literature review. *Palliative Medicine*, 29(6): 487–95.

Mullins, G.C., Simes, D. and Yuen, K.J. (2012) Approaching families for organ donation-intensivists' perspectives. *Anaesthesia and Intensive Care*, 40: 1035–9.

National Strategy for Palliative Care Implementation Task Force (2015) *National Guidelines for Palliative Care*. Singapore.

Neergaard, M., Vedsted, P., Olesen, F. et al. (2009) Associations between home death and GP involvement in palliative cancer care. *British Journal of General Practice*, 59(566): 671–7.

Neuberger, J. (2013) *More Care: Less Pathway: A Review of the Liverpool Care Pathway*. Available at: https://www.gov.uk/.../file/212450/Liverpool_Care_Pathway.pdf

NICE (National Institute for Health and Care Excellence) (2015) *Care of the Dying Adult.* NICE guideline (NG31). London: NICE.

NICE (National Institute for Health and Care Excellence) (2016) *End of Life Care for Infants, Children and Young People with Life-Limiting Conditions: Planning and Management.* NICE guideline (NG61). London: NICE.

Nolan, S., Saltmarsh, P. and Leget, C. (2011) Spiritual care in palliative care: working towards an EAPC Task Force. *European Journal of Palliative Care,* 18(2): 86–9.

Northern England Clinical Networks (2016) *Palliative and End of Life Care Guidelines Symptom Control For Cancer and Non-Cancer Patients* (4th edn). Available at: http://www.necn.nhs.uk/wp-content/uploads/2016/09/NECNXPALLIATIVEXCAREX2016.pdf. Accessed 9 March 2018.

Perkins, G.D., Griffiths, F., Slowther, A. et al. (2016) Do-not-attempt-cardiopulmonary-resuscitation decisions: an evidence synthesis. *Health Services and Delivery Research,* 4(11).

Petrova, M. , Riley, J., Abel, J., Barclay, S., (2016) Crash course in EPaCCS (Electronic Palliative Care Coordination Systems): 8 years of successes and failures in patient data sharing to learn from. *BMJ Supportive and Palliative Care.* doi: 10.1136/bmjspcare-2015-001059.

Plonk, W. and Arnold, R. (2005) Terminal care: the last weeks of life. *Journal of Palliative Medicine,* 8(2): 1042–55.

Pollock, K. (2015) Is home always the best and preferred place of death? *BMJ,* 351: h4855.

QEOLCC (2010) *Blue Print for Action 2010 to 2020.* Toronto, Canada: QEOLCC.

Rapoport, A., Shaheed, J., Newman, C. et al. (2013) Parental perceptions of forgoing artificial nutrition and hydration during end-of-life care. *Pediatrics,* 131(5): 861–9.

Roy, D. (1988) Ethics and aging: trends and problems in the clinical setting. In Thornton, J.E. and Winkler, E.R. (eds) *Ethics and Aging: The Right to Live, the Right to Die.* Vancouver: UBC Press.

Russell, S. (2016) *Advance Care Planning and Living with Dying: The Views of Hospice Patients.* Doctoral thesis, University of Hertfordshire.

Russo, J.E. (2011) Original research: deactivation of ICDs at the end of life: a systematic review of clinical practices and provider and patient attitudes. *American Journal of Nursing,* 111: 26–35.

Selman, L., Young, T.E., Vermandere, M. et al. (2014) Research priorities in spiritual care: an international survey of palliative care researchers and clinicians. *Journal of Pain and Symptom Management,* 48(4): 518–31.

Serri, K. and Marsolais, P. (2017) End-of-life issues in cardiac critical care: the option of organ donation. *Canadian Journal of Cardiology,* 33(1): 128–34.

Shemie, S.D., Hornby, L., Baker, A. et al. and The International Guidelines for Determination of Death phase 1 participants, in collaboration with the World Health Organization (2014) International guideline development for the determination of death. *Intensive Care Medicine,* 40: 788–97.

Shepperd, S., Wee, B. and Straus, S.E. (2011) Hospital at home: home-based end of life care. *Cochrane Database of Systematic Reviews,* 7: CD009231.

Skilbeck, J. and Payne, S. (2003) Emotional support and the role of Clinical Nurse Specialists in palliative care. *Journal of Advanced Nursing*, 43(5): 521–30.

Steindal, S.A., Bredal, I., Ranhoff, A.H. et al. (2015) The last three days of life: a comparison of pain management in the young old and the oldest old hospitalised patients using the Resident Assessment Instrument for Palliative Care. *International Journal of Older People Nursing*, 10(4): 263–72.

Taylor, P., Dowding, D. and Johnson, M. (2017) Clinical decision making in the recognition of dying: a qualitative interview study. *BMC Palliative Care*, 16(1): 11.

Thanavaro, J.L. (2013) ICD deactivation: review of literature and clinical recommendations. *Clinical Nursing Research*, 22: 36–50.

The Australian and New Zealand Paediatric Palliative Care Reference Group (2015) *Paediatric Palliative Care*. Canberra.

The Leadership Alliance for the Care of Dying (2014) *One Chance to Get it Right: Improving People's Experience of Care in the Last Few Days and Hours of Life*. London.

Thomas, C., Morris, S.M. and Clark, D. (2004) Place of death: preferences among cancer patients and their carers. *Social Science and Medicine*, 58(12): 2431–44.

Toscani, F. (2013) Prescribing in palliative care: a quest for appropriateness. *Palliative Medicine*, 27(4): 293–4.

Wee, B. and Hillier, R. (2008) Interventions for noisy breathing in patients near to death. *Cochrane Database of Systematic Reviews*, 1: CD005177.

Worcester, A. (1935) *The Care of the Aged, the Dying and the Dead*. Springfield, IL: Charles C. Thomas.

Understanding and assessing grief and bereavement

Linda Machin

Introduction

Life is punctuated with many losses but none are more affecting than those associated with death, dying and bereavement. As people face their own end of life journey or that of someone close, heightened emotions and thoughts, together with social change and reflection on life's meaning, are poignant reactions at the forefront of experience. These reactions to loss produce complex and hugely varied individual manifestations of grief. This is a challenge for practitioners in palliative and bereavement care who face not only the varied expressions of grief in patients and families but confrontation with their own personal existential questions. Understanding the impact and expression of grief, as part of a universally shared human experience, will influence the quality and effectiveness of the communications between patients, their carers, bereaved people and professional practitioners.

While national, local and organisational policies and procedures determine the framework for care provision, being able to assess both resilience and risk is an important prelude to offering appropriate and effective care throughout the pre- and post-bereavement journey of loss. This chapter explores a theoretical model, which emerged from research and practice and which provides a structure for understanding the spectrum of reactions and responses to loss. Developed alongside it is a tool used to identify and assess the characteristics of grief expressed by individuals experiencing loss. The model, the Range of Response to Loss (RRL) model, together with the conceptually linked Adult Attitude to Grief (AAG) scale, provide a framework for appraising resilience and vulnerability in grieving people. Together these have been found to be conceptually accessible and helpful for practitioners. The practice implications and application of this approach to assessment will be explored.

Background

In a UK Department of Health-funded project, national providers and practitioners have been addressing the challenge of ensuring continuity of care between end of life and bereavement services through the 'Gold Standard Bereavement Care project' (Bereavement Care Service Standards 2013). It has identified the pathway and multiple services engaged in care provision at points along the patient and carer journey. Implementing joined-up care demands collaboration across statutory health services and community voluntary services to ensure the changing needs of patients, their families and carers are met sensitively and effectively. 'End-of-life and bereavement care delivery remains etched on the memories of bereaved relatives. The importance of delivering this final care appropriately cannot be overemphasised ... [it] can influence grieving and the longer-term health of bereaved people' (Chaplin 2009, p. 2). What is clear is that the complex range of services need to be bridged by a common understanding of the needs of patients, their families and carers during the end of life phase and into bereavement. Practitioners within those services need to be able to offer care with expertise and sensitivity, working collaboratively and consistently. What do we need to know and how can we implement that knowledge to provide an integrated journey of care from end of life to bereavement?

Loss at the end of life and in bereavement

As a prelude to considering grief and its manifestations, it is important to set out the nature of end of life and bereavement losses for the dying, for those most closely related and for those who provide clinical care.

The losses and changes for the dying person (Parkes 1998; Aujoulat et al. 2007) may include:

- loss of personal and social reference points with the disturbance in the continuity of the 'taken-for-granted' aspects of life such as home, health, relationships, etc.;
- sympathy/empathy in responding to the losses being felt by family and friends;
- impending death involving the loss of everything in the present and in the future.

Loss and change for carers pre-bereavement (Braine and Wray 2016) may include:

- personal loss and change with the impending death of a significant relative/friend;
- dealing with other people's losses; feeling for the dying relative as s/he faces end of life changes and death; and responding to the impact on other family members;
- changes in the caring role by working alongside or giving up the caring role to professionals;
- confronting one's own death.

Loss and change for practitioners as end of life care providers (Papadatou 2009) may include:

- sympathy/empathy for the dying person and their carers, family and friends;
- being the bearer/sharer of 'bad news' and facing the challenge to one's skill when feeling the pain and helplessness of the situation;
- travelling the journey of loss with the dying person and being the witness of their pain and end of life transitions;
- the losses witnessed can be a mirror of losses already experienced and a reminder of what might be lost in the future.

Loss and change for family/friends post-bereavement (Lewis 1961; Didion 2005) may include:

- loss of a significant relative/friend;
- responding to other people's loss reactions;
- loss of relationship role, for example, partner, child, parent and the social significance of these roles;
- changes in lifestyle, i.e. financial and social.

Confronting loss and change for the practitioner providing bereavement care (Machin [2009] 2014) may include:

- dealing with a sense of one's own powerlessness in the face of another's grief;
- identification with the losses being witnessed as a mirror of losses already experienced and/or as a reminder of what might be lost in the future.

These losses can be challenging and will be variably grieved. Grief, especially where circumstantial or personal factors lead to increased risk of a poor outcome, is something to be fully understood by practitioners if they are to offer good end of life and bereavement care.

Understanding grief

Grief is a normal reaction to a significant life loss and is experienced in a number of ways. For example, at an emotional level, sadness, anger, guilt, etc. may be expressed through crying; physically, there is likely to be tiredness, irritability, and perhaps disturbed eating and sleeping patterns; cognitively, concentration may be difficult with singular attention to thoughts about the deceased; the search for answers to loss and its meaning may touch on the spiritual dimension of experience. However, for an estimated 10–15 per cent of people, grief can more profoundly affect the capacity to function well over a more extended period with increased risk of depression, generalised anxiety, substance abuse and increased use of medications, sudden cardiac events, suicidal thinking, abnormalities in immune functioning with associated risks of cardiovascular disease and cancer (Shear 2015).

The study of grief was dominated in the twentieth century by the psychodynamic school of thought and particularly by the work of John Bowlby (1980) and his influential theory of attachment; an influence which continues within contemporary research (Cassidy, Jones and Shaver 2013). His theory focused on relationships and their quality as indicators of personality development. Along with his colleagues (Ainsworth et al. 1978), an attachment classification was established which provided a model for understanding the nature and variability of reactions to separation and loss, or the threat of it. This has provided a foundation for research and practice developments in the field of loss and bereavement (Parkes [1972] 1996; 2006; Parkes and Weiss 1983; Raphael 1984; Mikulincer and Florian 1998; Cassidy and Shaver 1999; Fraley and Shaver 1999). Associated with this theoretical perspective was a bias towards a predominantly emotion-focused view of grief which has influenced the nature of support and intervention thought to be needed by grieving people.

A challenge to this classic theory of 'grief work' came with the development of the Dual Process Model (DPM) (Stroebe 1992). This model provided a more comprehensive account of the nature of grief (Stroebe and Schut 1999; 2010) by giving equal attention to on-going life demands (restoration orientation) as to the emotional distress caused by loss (loss orientation). The capacity to move between these two orientations (oscillation) demonstrates adjustments to loss taking place across the cognitive/behavioural/social domain as well as the emotional domain. This shift in emphasis has been widely used in contemporary bereavement and palliative care practice (Archer 1999; Payne et al. 1999; Thompson 2002; Quinn 2005; Dallos 2006; Hindmarch 2009).

Additionally, a growing body of research suggests that an apparent absence of grief is not necessarily indicative of pathology, as previously maintained, and that resilience in the face of loss is more common than believed (Bonanno 2004).

The impact of grief

Over half a million people die in Britain each year and each of these deaths is usually felt by a number of people. While death, dying and bereavement will confront people with some of the most stressful challenges that humans experience (Folkman 2001), new understanding about the human capacity for resilience suggests that characteristics of personal resourcefulness, a positive life perspective and effective social support are key factors in the capacity to emerge from traumatic or disturbing life events (Frankl 1959; Seligman and Csikszentmihalyi 2000; Greene 2002; Machin [2009] 2014). However, this still leaves an estimated 10–15 per cent of the general bereaved population potentially susceptible to complicated grief (Prigerson and Jacobs 2001); some of these complications are likely to have their origin in a 'bad' end of life/death experience (Chaplin 2009). Mitigating the negative outcomes of loss and bereavement is, therefore, a significant issue for professionals in healthcare and social care. Identifying those people whose vulnerability makes them most in need of help is crucial in the development of appropriate care provision.

Risk and complications

Circumstances that have been shown to increase the risk of complications in bereavement include: sudden unexpected deaths, including suicide and murder; parental bereavement; concurrent crises, such as divorce, unemployment, financial problems, health problems; and perceived lack of social support (Sanders 1993; Shear et al. 2011). Personal life experience and personality are also factors which contribute to whether a person is able to cope effectively with loss. The circumstances and the nature of a stress, such as bereavement, test the strength and limitations of a person and affect their capacity to cope with the consequences of loss (Folkman 2001; Lazarus and Folkman 1984; Stroebe et al. 2006).

Complicated grief, which is also called prolonged grief disorder, is characterised by difficulty in functioning in work and in social relationships, a sense of meaninglessness, prolonged yearning for the deceased, disruption in personal beliefs, and a potential for the misuse of drugs and alcohol, and antisocial behaviour (Parkes and Weiss 1983; Stroebe and Stroebe 1987) and a higher suicide risk (Shear 2015). Foremost in the field of research of complicated grief has been Prigerson and colleagues who produced an Inventory of Complicated Grief (Prigerson et al. 1995) and a measure of Prolonged Grief Disorder (PGD) (Prigerson et al. 2009). It is worth noting that, while measures of depression (Kroenke and Spitzer 2002) and anxiety (Spitzer et al. 2006) are frequently used to provide symptomatic evidence of complicated grief, these psychometric tests are not designed to identify the spectrum of grief responses which might make a person vulnerable.

The Adult Attitude to Grief (AAG) scale will be described below as a measure which provides a grief-specific measure of vulnerability and resilience. The AAG emerged from research and practice (Machin 2001; [2009] 2014), has been statistically validated (Sim et al. 2014) and been well received by practitioners. Measures, including the AAG, which have been used in practice and recorded in a survey by the European Association of Palliative Care (Guldin et al. 2015) include the Bereavement Risk Index, the Inventory of Complicated Grief, the Family Risk Index and the Prolonged Grief scale.

The Range of Response to Loss model of grief

The Adult Attitude to Grief scale is based on the theoretical concepts identified in the Range of Response to Loss (RRL) model (Machin 2001; [2009] 2014). These concepts emerged from listening to grieving people in both research and practice.

A framework for defining key grief components

The characteristics of grief conceptualised within the RRL model were initially made up of three elements:

1   an overwhelmed reaction to loss;
2   a controlled reaction to loss;
3   a balanced/resilient coping response

(Machin 2001; [2009] 2014).

To this was added the concept of vulnerability as a fourth and opposite coping response to resilience. This framework, while reflecting the language used by clients, parallels the concepts of both attachment theory (Ainsworth et al. 1978) (anxious/ambivalent attachment and the overwhelmed response to loss, avoidant attachment and the controlled response, and secure attachment and the balance/ resilient response) and the Dual Process Model (Stroebe and Schut 1999) (loss orientation parallels the state of being overwhelmed, restoration orientation reflects the state of control and the capacity to oscillate between the two reflects the balanced/resilient state). The state of resilience is a dynamic one in which there is a successful management of the competing forces of overwhelming feelings created by the powerlessness of loss, and the pull to (re)establish control in thinking and behaving.

It became clear that the model was describing two distinct dimensions in response to loss. The first of these consists of the core loss impact (stressor), producing variable overwhelmed and controlled reactions. The second of these is the coping dimension in which the capacity to respond to grief with equilibrium (resilience) is contrasted with a limited capacity or incapacity to manage grief: a state of vulnerability (Figure 17.1).

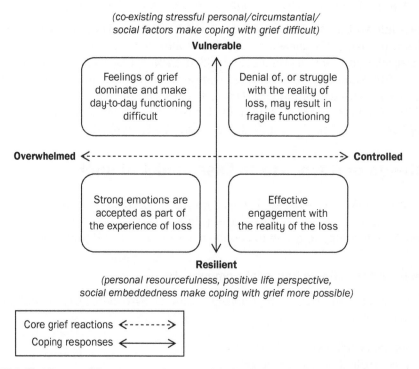

Figure 17.1 The Range of Response to Loss model: the interacting dimensions of core grief reactions and coping responses

Learning exercise 17.1

Engage in a process of self-reflection by asking yourself the following questions:

- What are my natural ways of reacting to loss, i.e. do I tend to express or suppress my feelings?
- In what ways have I coped with life's losses?
- What helps me to cope well?
- How might my style of reacting to loss and coping with grief affect my support of grieving people?

The Adult Attitude to Grief scale: providing a profile of individual grief

The Adult Attitude to Grief (AAG) scale was devised to test the validity of three of the categories originally making up the RRL model. In the scale, three items reflect qualities associated with being overwhelmed – stressful, irreversible and uncontrollable (Mikulincer and Florian 1998); three items represent control – restricted acknowledgement of distress, an exaggerated need for self-reliance and an avoidance of grief through overly engaging in day-to-day life (Mikulincer and Florian 1998); and three items reflect resilience – courage, resourcefulness and optimism (Seligman 1998; Greene 2002) (Table 17.1).

Responses to the nine-item scale are on a five-point Likert scale from 'strongly agree' to 'strongly disagree'. The 2001 research provided support for the concepts in the RRL model and also demonstrated the complex blend of all of the grief components in the model – overwhelmed, controlled and balanced/resilient – in the responses of bereaved study participants (Machin 2001). This suggested that the scale might usefully be used to profile grief reactions and responses in people seeking help in their bereavement. Subsequent studies (Machin and Spall 2004; Machin 2007) have supported the practical usefulness of the AAG scale as a measure able to provide a picture of individual grief and its changes over time. The findings from those studies confirmed the

Table 17.1 The Range of Response to Loss model concepts reflected in the Adult Attitude to Grief Scale

Overwhelmed	Controlled	Balanced/resilient
2. Disturbingly intrusive	4. Valuing stoicism	1. Courage in facing the loss
5. Unremittingly painful	6. Denial of, or covering	3. Sense of personal
7. Robbing life of meaning	distress	resourcefulness
	8. Focus on day-to-day living	9. Hopefulness

Themes are numbered as the items appear in the AAG scale.

Table 17.2 Adult Attitude to Grief scale
Practitioner Record Sheet
Client number.................. Date .... Session number............

Adult Attitude to Grief scale	Strongly agree	Agree	Neither agree nor disagree	Disagree	Strongly disagree	Additional responses/ comments
R 1. I feel able to face the pain which comes with loss.	0	1	2	3	4	
O 2. For me, it is difficult to switch off thoughts about the person I have lost.	4	3	2	1	0	
R 3. I feel very aware of my inner strength when faced with grief.	0	1	2	3	4	
C 4. I believe that I must be brave in the face of loss.	4	3	2	1	0	
O 5. I feel that I will always carry the pain of grief with me.	4	3	2	1	0	
C 6. For me, it is important to keep my grief under control.	4	3	2	1	0	
O 7. Life has less meaning for me after this loss.	4	3	2	1	0	
C 8. I think it's best just to get on with life and not dwell on this loss.*	4	3	2	1	0	
R 9. It may not always feel like it but I do believe that I will come through this experience of grief.	0	1	2	3	4	

R = Resilient items 1, 3, 9; **C** = Controlled items 4, 6, 8; **O** = Overwhelmed items 2, 5, 7.

Vulnerability Indicator score = total score for the 9 items.

N.B. resilient scores reversed to indicate vulnerability.

© Linda Machin 2010 (* modified 2013)

value to practitioners of using the AAG scale as a prompt in exploring clients' experiences of loss in greater depth and in highlighting the areas which were most troubling to them. Increasing practitioner interest and enthusiasm for the model and the measure have been seen in their adoption in palliative and bereavement care contexts (Relf et al. 2010), and in the recognition given to their contribution to contemporary theories of assessment (Agnew et al. 2009).

Identifying vulnerability in grief

The AAG scale explores the degree to which a person is reacting to grief: emotionally, through the overwhelmed scores; cognitively/behaviourally, through the controlled scores; and the ability to balance these elements, through the resilient scores. An inability to balance the feeling and the functioning, i.e. a lack of or limited resilience, is indicative of a measure of vulnerability. Identifying vulnerability as a separate component is done quantitatively by adding the scores for the overwhelmed items on a scale of 4–0 (from strongly agree to strongly disagree) and reversing the score for the resilient items, i.e. 0–4. This provides an overall scale of 0–36 where a score of above 24 is indicative of severe vulnerability, 21–23 high vulnerability, and less than 20 low vulnerability (Sim, Machin and Bartlam 2014; Machin, Bartlam and Bartlam 2015) (Table 17.2 and Box 17.1).

Box 17.1 AAG practice protocol

(a) Providing information for service users

1 *Explain* how the AAG is used in the service/by the practitioner.
2 *Explain the purpose of the scale,* i.e. to help the service user understand something about the nature of their grief and for the practitioner to have a clear picture of how grief is being experienced and expressed.
3 *Gain consent* to use the scale.
4 *Give a copy of the scale to the service user;* explain the five choices associated with each item on the scale (from strong agreement to strong disagreement) and decide who will read out each statement.
5 *Assure* the service user that there are no right or wrong answers.
6 When the scale is used, in addition to identifying levels of agreement/ disagreement with the 9 items in the scale, *encourage* the service user to say more about each of the 9 statements to increase an understanding of their individual experience and perspective on grief.

(b) The Vulnerability Indicator score

The Vulnerability Indicator score is to help the practitioner have an overview of the service user's level of vulnerability and together with other formal/informal assessment information is a guide to appropriate support. It is important NOT to use a score/numbers sheet with service users as this can convey a sense of being tested and may prevent honest responses.

(c) On completion of the AAG
When the AAG has been completed, discuss the responses to the scale with the service user:

1 Ask how the service user felt using the scale.
2 Ask whether there were particular themes in the scale which stood out as being *significant* **or** *troubling* to them.
3 Give feedback on any *evident bias*, i.e. an overview of the tendency towards being overwhelmed, controlled or resilient.
4 Give more detailed feedback, reflecting on where there seems to be *tension/contradictions* between the overwhelmed, controlled and resilient responses, suggesting possible vulnerability, for example, where the desire to be in control and get on with life is undermined by strong emotions.

Training and practice are desirable for interpreting the scale.

(d) Use the evidence from the AAG responses and Vulnerability Indicator scores

1 Determine *what kind of support* service is most appropriate for the client.
2 Enable the practitioner and the service user to jointly *set goals* for support/ intervention.
3 As part of the help process, *review* the service user's changing grief reactions and responses.
4 As a tool in supervision and multidisciplinary meetings to determine appropriate and effective therapeutic/support strategies.
5 Evaluate the outcome of the support provided for the service user.

Research developments

Originally the AAG was designed and validated for use in bereavement. More recently two pre-bereavement versions of the AAG have been developed for use: (1) with patients and (2) with their carers. Face validity for these versions of the scale has come from practice experience but fuller validation of the psychometric properties is currently being undertaken. As part of this research, testing is also focusing on the capacity of the AAG to enhance end of life conversations as practitioners seek to facilitate effective decision-making and appropriate support for patients and their carers.

At the time of writing, the University of Iceland is also undertaking research to evaluate nurses' experience of the effectiveness of 'therapeutic conversations' across the end of life and bereavement journey as a way to improve outcomes for family caregivers (Petursdottir et al. 2016). The AAG has been used in the bereavement phases of this research and while the quantitative data is still to be analysed, the researchers report that the scale was of great value in improving bereavement assessment and building on the pre-bereavement discussions with the family. It was a helpful source of information about how family members were coping and in assessing the need for further services (personal correspondence, July 2016).

It is important that recognition is given to cultural differences in pursuit of common care goals. It is essential to focus on understanding cultural variations in practices and perspectives associated with loss and grief together with appropriate translation of assessment tools such as the AAG (Sumathipala and Murray 2000).

Assessment

The intuition of experienced practitioners has always been central to assessment but the demand for systematic and evidence-based assessment is growing as commissioners require demonstrable support to show care interventions match need. The RRL model and the AAG scale, described in this chapter, provide a structure and a tool for assessment. The assessment process is made up of four steps:

1   Exploring the wider context of grief.
2   The Range of Response to Loss model as a theoretical 'compass'.
3   The Adult Attitude to Grief scale in practice.
4   Implications for practice.

Step 1 Exploring the wider context of grief

The focus of assessment is the individual, whether patient, carer, or bereaved person, but the wider influences on their grief need to be understood. In a multicultural society, the place of ethnicity, culture, religion/beliefs needs to be recognised. Understanding this more fully may only be possible by asking the person whose care needs are being addressed about their life perspectives. This is likely to have a significant bearing on how they make sense of their experience of loss. More specific to their own experience will be the nature of family, its relationships and networks, together with their educational and employment history. All of these factors may contribute to current social circumstances, which may either add to the vulnerability of the individual because of the demands or complexity of their situation or provide a stable supportive base from which to cope with grief (Rosenblatt 2001; Sheehy 2013) (Figure 17.2).

Step 2 The Range of Response to Loss model as a theoretical 'compass'

The RRL model provides a theoretical perspective for thinking about the expressions and experiences of grief being described by the grieving person, in pre- and post-bereavement states (Relf et al. 2010; Brocklehurst et al. 2014). Figure 17.1 identified the characteristics resulting from the intersection of core grief reactions and coping responses. This helps identify the relative nature of feelings and functioning, and the degree of vulnerability and resilience. These are guides for thinking and may be the prelude to more systematic assessment using the AAG.

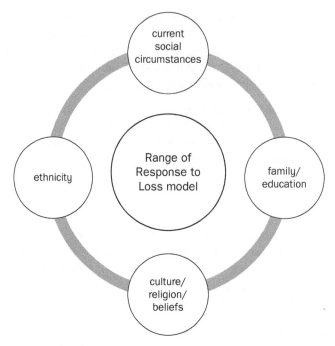

Figure 17.2 The wider context of grief which influences the Range of Response to Loss

Learning exercise 16.2

Think of someone you are currently providing nursing care for and consider:

- How much do you know about the wider context of their life situation?
- How much do you know about the current circumstances which might be adding complexity to their grief?
- Is their reaction to loss inclined to be overwhelmed or controlled?
- Do you see evidence of their resilient coping, i.e. an ability to manage both feelings and day-to-day functioning, or do you observe elements of vulnerability in coping with loss?
- What factors may be contributing to their vulnerability?

Step 3 The Adult Attitude to Grief scale in practice

Box 17.1 is a protocol for implementing the AAG. The AAG can be used as a standard form of assessment within a service or used selectively, i.e. where it is seen to be appropriate.

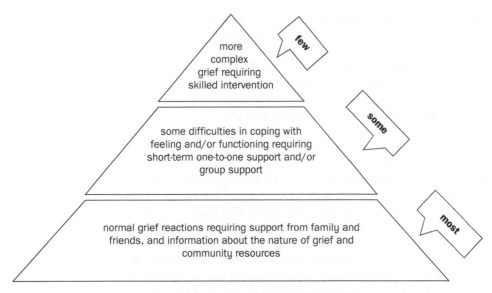

Figure 17.3 The three-tier level of grief need and matched intervention

Step 4 Implications for practice

The final section of the AAG protocol, section (d), sees the AAG as providing a triage system for directing people to the care appropriate to their need and then appraising their pathway through the helping process. Increasingly, practice is being based on three components of need/intervention (NICE 2004) (see Figure 17.3). No longer does a one-size-fits-all approach or recourse to counselling for everyone either meet service user needs or help limited resources. Most grieving people require only limited help and sign-posting to practical services together with support from family and friends. Some people may require more support on a one-to-one basis or in a grief-specific group of the kind offered by many voluntary services. Only 10–15 per cent of people require more intensive intervention such as counselling. Distinguishing these different levels of need is essential to providing appropriate and effective levels of care. It challenges service providers of end of life and bereavement care to give greater attention to the practice procedures necessary to achieve this. Nurses are front-line practitioners who need to be able to assess levels of need, provide assurance to most people of the normality of their grief, and, where necessary, refer to more specialist help.

The knowledge and skill we bring to caring

It is foundational to work in end of life and bereavement care that nurses have knowledge of grief theory based on up-to-date evidence. In addition there are three practice approaches, which all have their own well-developed psychotherapy theory, but which can be applied more broadly by all practitioners (nurses, doctors, social workers, etc.), offering meaningful support to patients and families:

- a person-centred approach as a way of being – accepting, empathic and genuine;
- a narrative approach, focusing on the story of grief and loss;
- a systems approach which recognises and understands the complexity of relationships, roles and responsibilities.

Relating to people in a way which values them and keeps their concerns central is embodied in a person-centred approach (Rogers 1980). It holds to the principle of keeping the person to the foreground, ahead of any of the other 'agendas' brought by the practitioner in meeting with a patient/client or their relative. Sustaining that focus is further facilitated by giving full attention to the 'story' of loss, which is described from a narrative perspective as consisting of three elements (Angus and Hardke 1994):

- the facts – what happened/is happening, when and how;
- the impact of what happened/is happening on the teller;
- the meaning(s) attached to the experience of loss.

This provides a structure for listening which can help increase an understanding of what is heard and provide prompts to helping the story of loss unfold. To maximise support for an individual, a nurse needs also to explore the social context in which the loss is occurring by facilitating the telling of a wider story which includes relationships, roles and responsibilities; a systems approach (Shapiro 2001). Within the social frame of the family, it is especially important to identify different communication styles and grief perspectives, as this significantly influences how grief is experienced and expressed. Support needs to take into account the varied and potentially conflicting aspects of family communications (Table 17.3).

All three of the helping approaches we have discussed above can be adopted to provide a structure for creating and sustaining good interpersonal relationships in nursing practice. They will enhance the skill base and capacity for sensitivity upon which all end of life and bereavement care conversations depend. These conversations, confronting painful and distressing life and death concerns, reflect three potentially varying perspectives: that of the nurse, the patient (or the deceased person represented by their bereaved relative) and the family/friends network. Papadatou (2009) has explored the personal and professional impact on nurses, of working with dying patients and their family. Figure 17.4 looks at this dynamic and the factors which need to be understood and skilfully accommodated by the nurse.

Increasing attention is being given to setting up those end of life situations where stressful or bad news is to be given. A six-step protocol has been devised to give full recognition to the sensitivity of these communications (Baile et al. 2000):

1   Set the physical scene with reference to comfort and privacy and with appropriate family support for the patient.
2   'Ask' the patient how they understand their situation, treatment, etc.

3 Invite the patient to indicate what and how much they would like to know.
4 Provide information – prepare the patient if the news is not good and explain in
   terms that can be understood.
5 Respond to the patient's emotional reaction to the 'news' they have been given.
6 If the patient is ready and able, begin to form a treatment plan and/or continuity
   of care.

Table 17.3 Family systems and grief

Examples of different communication styles in grieving families	
Open communication style	*Role-specific communication style*
All family members are able to express feelings and thoughts openly with each other	Traditional family roles are reflected in communicating reactions and responses to grief, e.g. dad is the strong angry person, mum is the quiet tearful person, etc.
Grief is understood and recognised	Conflicting perspectives about the nature of grief and how to cope with it
Communication focused on adult grief:	*Communication focused on children's grief:*
Children are excluded from expressions of grief in the family context • Rationalised as 'they don't understand' • There is too much adult grief to allow space for attention to the children	Little recognition of adult grief • Children may vicariously carry the grief of adults • In a context where control is the adult way of coping, children who express grief more expressively (and normally) may be misunderstood and thought to have a 'problem'

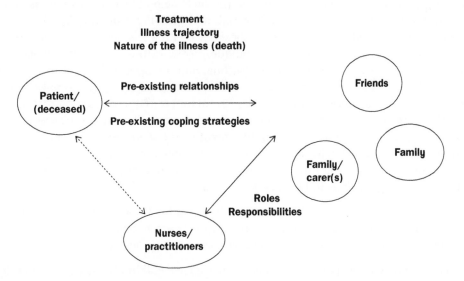

Figure 17.4 The triadic relationship dynamics in end of life and (bereavement) care

This kind of structured approach can help counter end of life uncertainty and can contribute to a climate in which assessment and shared decision-making can occur effectively. Conversely, uncertainty will influence patient experience and potentially lead to adverse outcomes (Etkind et al. 2016).

Learning exercise 17.3

Think about a situation where you were a bereaved relative:

- In the last days of your relative's life, did you feel that important concerns were heard?
- If not, what didn't happen that you would have liked to have happened?
- What do you remember as an example of good practice?

Examples of the AAG in practice

Currently research and practice use of the RRL model and AAG scale are adding to earlier support for this approach (Machin and Spall 2004; Machin 2007; Machin [2009] 2014) and there is evidence of its wider use in healthcare and social care settings (see website: www.keele.ac.uk/mappinggrief).

While the predominant use of the AAG is among practitioners whose role is the provision of psychosocial care, increasing recognition is being given to its wider assessment potential in screening for mental health risk and grieving vulnerability, for example, in generalist care. One GP who has used the AAG with a few selected patients pre- and post-bereavement found it provided a unique profile of their grief experience and its change over time. 'I think it is both educational and therapeutic in itself for the patient and provides an excellent structure for telling their grief story' (personal correspondence, November 2015). She saw this as a useful tool for GPs with an interest in mental health and allied professionals in contact with patients suffering any loss or change in circumstance, for example, loss of employment or the diagnosis of a long-term condition such as diabetes, which may cause a grief reaction. If it is repeated over time, it may demonstrate to the patient how their coping skills may alter and how they themselves may develop coping skills to become more resilient.

The pre-bereavement grief trajectory will reflect the fluctuations in physical health, changes or withdrawal of treatment, and shifting care needs. Assessment of altering grief perspectives, using the AAG, may form part of the journey of care.

This pre-bereavement approach has been used in a children's hospice (Naomi House, Winchester, UK) to look at how parental responses to a child's illness and its changes/

deterioration might inform likely bereavement needs (see case example in Machin [2009] 2014, pp. 89–91). The senior family support worker/counsellor reported that:

> Our experience almost universally was that parents found the way the AAG was constructed meant they had free rein to tell their story and they could venture into areas (especially end-of-life) that they may have avoided previously. The careful wording in the AAG, and the fact these are shared overtly with the parent, meant the 'telling of the story' created more of an equal relationship, rather than 'I am the helper, you are in need'. In our experience, this allowed a freer exchange both in terms of factual detail and in terms of emotional responses.
>
> (personal correspondence, July 2016)

The pre-bereavement version for patients and carers (now called the Attitude to Health Change) is used systematically at the Heart of Kent Hospice, Aylesford, UK. Social workers, counsellors and volunteers all use the scale for formal assessment and therapeutic purposes and are comfortable with this approach which works well in facilitating conversations with patients and family members. The feedback from these practitioners attests to the face validity of these scales, reporting that it provides a structure for appraising the impact of change/deterioration in health, it helps normalise end of life and pre-bereavement experience by articulating reactions and coping responses, and encourages exploration of grief issues which can sometimes be difficult to reach.

A Canadian bereavement hospice programme (Victoria Hospice, Vancouver) using the AAG with bereaved clients found that the Vulnerability Indicator scores equate with their clinical impression of client need and is consistent with the Inventory of Complicated Grief scores (Prigerson 1995) where both measures were used pre- and post-intervention.

Conclusion

The National End of Life Strategy (DH 2008) sets out the pathway in which open and honest communication, assessment, treatment with dignity and the emotional, practical and spiritual support of carers as well as patients, are crucial. However, in a survey of end of life communications, Parry, Land and Seymour (2014, p. 1) concluded from a review of journal articles and published book chapters, that 'practices vary in how strongly they encourage patients to engage in talk about matters such as illness progression and dying'. Without the strategies and skills to engage with these key issues, being able to gauge risk and vulnerability will remain problematic. Unresolved and unsatisfactory end of life communications will be inherited in bereavement as experiences to be grieved in sadness and anger over and above the loss of the relative or friend.

Translating theories and strategies into practice is a challenge and one requiring constant review and revision. This is especially true in end of life and bereavement care where new concepts and initiatives demand the acquisition of new knowledge and newly articulated skills. This chapter has described the RRL model and the associated AAG scale which can be used by nurses to assess individual grief and appraise the level of vulnerability and hence risk of poor outcomes. It has linked the theoretical concepts of the model and the use of the scale with strategies for enhancing the conversations and engagement with people who are grieving and has the potential to be added to the nurses' repertoire of skills and tools.

Acknowledgements

I would like to thank the staff of the following organisations for feedback on their experiences of using the concepts of the Range of Response to Loss model and the Adult Attitude to Grief scale:

- Naomi House Hospice, Winchester
- Heart of Kent Hospice, Aylesford
- Victoria Hospice, Vancouver, Canada
- University of Iceland School of Health Sciences
- Dr Anthea Robinson, Luton GP

References

Agnew, A., Manktelow, R., Taylor, B.J. and Jones, L. (2009) Bereavement needs assessment in specialist palliative care: a review of the literature. *Palliative Medicine*, 24: 46–59.

Ainsworth, M.D.S., Blehar, M.C., Waters, E. and Wall, S. (1978) *Patterns of Attachment: A Psychological Study of the Strange Situation*. Hillsdale, NJ: Erlbaum.

Angus, L. and Hardke, K. (1994) Narrative processes in psychotherapy. *Canadian Psychology*, 35: 190–203.

Archer, J. (1999) *The Nature of Grief*. London: Routledge.

Aujoulat, I., Luminet, O. and Decache, A. (2007) The perspective of patients on their experience of powerlessness. *Qualitative Health Research*, 17(6): 772–85.

Baile, W.F., Buckman, R., Lenzi, R. et al. (2000) SPIKES: a six-step protocol for delivering bad news: application to the patient with cancer. *The Oncologist*, 5: 302–11.

Bereavement Care Service Standards (2013) Bereavement Services Association and Cruse Bereavement Care.

Bonanno, G.A. (2004) Loss, trauma and human resilience. *American Psychologist*, 59(1): 20–8.

Bowlby, J. (1980) *Attachment and Loss: Vol. 3. Loss: Sadness and Depression*. Harmondsworth: Penguin.

Braine, M.E. and Wray, J. (2016) *Supporting Families and Carers: A Nursing Perspective*. Boca Raton, FL: CRC Press.

Brocklehurst, T., Hearnshaw, C. and Machin, L. (2014) Bereavement needs assessment – piloting a process. *Progress in Palliative Care*, 22(3): 143–9.

Cassidy, J., Jones, J.D. and Shaver, P.R. (2013) Contributions of Attachment Theory and Research: a framework for future research, translation and policy. *Developmental Psychopathology*, 402: 1415–34.

Cassidy, J. and Shaver, P.R. (eds) (1999) *Handbook of Attachment: Theory, Research and Clinical Application.* New York: Guilford Press.

Chaplin, D. (2009) Developing an end-of-life care pathway to improve nurses' bereavement care. *Nursing Times,* 105(1): 20–1.

Dallos, R. (2006) *Attachment Narrative Therapy.* Maidenhead: Open University Press.

Department of Health (2008) *End of Life Care Strategy.* London: Department of Health.

Didion, J. (2005) *The Year of Magical Thinking.* London: Fourth Estate.

Etkind, S.N., Bristowe, K., Bailey, K. et al. (2016) How does uncertainty shape patient experience in advanced illness? A secondary analysis of qualitative data. *Palliative Medicine.* doi:10.1177/0269216316647610.pmj.sagepub.com.

Folkman, S. (2001) Revised coping theory and the process of bereavement. In Stroebe, M.S., Hansson, R.O., Stroebe, W. and Schut, H. (eds) *Handbook of Bereavement Research.* Washington, DC: American Psychological Association, pp. 563–84.

Fraley, R.C. and Shaver, P.R. (1999) Loss and bereavement: attachment theory and recent controversies concerning grief work and the nature of detachment. In Cassidy, J. and Shaver, P.R. (eds) *Handbook of Attachment: Theory, Research, and Clinical Applications.* New York: Guilford Press, pp. 735–59.

Frankl, V. (1959) *Man's Search for Meaning.* Boston: Beacon Press.

Greene, R. (2002) Holocaust survivors: a study in resilience. *Journal of Gerontological Social Work,* 37: 3–18.

Guldin, M-B., Murphy, I., Keegan, O. et al. (2015) Bereavement care provision in Europe: a survey by the EAPC Bereavement Care Taskforce. *European Journal of Palliative Care,* 22(4): 185–9.

Hindmarch, C. (2009) *On the Death of a Child.* Oxford: Radcliffe Publishing.

Kroenke, K. and Spitzer, R.L. (2002) The PHQ-9: a new depression and diagnostic severity measure. *Psychiatric Annals,* 32: 509–21.

Lazarus, R.S. and Folkman, S. (1984) *Stress, Appraisal and Coping.* New York: Springer.

Lewis, C.S. (1961) *A Grief Observed.* London: Faber & Faber.

Machin, L. (2001) Exploring a framework for understanding the range of response to loss: a study of clients receiving bereavement counselling. Unpublished PhD thesis, Keele University, UK.

Machin, L. (2007) *The Adult Attitude to Grief Scale as a Tool of Practice for Counsellors Working with Bereaved People.* A study report sponsored by Age Concern, Tameside and Keele University.

Machin, L. ([2009] 2014) *Working with Loss and Grief* (2nd edn). London: Sage.

Machin, L., Bartlam, R. and Bartlam, B (2015) Identifying levels of vulnerability in grief using the Adult Attitude to Grief scale: from theory to practice. *Bereavement Care,* 34(2): 59–68.

Machin, L. and Spall, R. (2004) Mapping grief: a study in practice using a quantitative and qualitative approach to exploring and addressing the range of response to loss. *Counselling and Psychotherapy Research,* 4(1): 9–17.

Mikulincer, M. and Florian, V. (1998) The relationship between adult attachment styles and emotional and cognitive reactions to stressful events. In Simpson, J.A. and Rholes, W.S. (eds) *Attachment Theory and Close Relationships.* New York: Guilford Press, pp. 143–65.

NICE (National Institute for Clinical Excellence) (2004) *Improving Supportive and Palliative Care for Adults with Cancer: Three Component Models of Bereavement Support*. London: NICE.

Papadatou, D. (2009) *In the Face of Death*. New York: Springer.

Parkes, C.M. (1996) *Bereavement: Studies of Grief in Adult Life*. London: Routledge.

Parkes, C.M. and Weiss, R.S. (1983) *Recovery from Bereavement*. New York: Basic Books.

Parkes, C.M. (1998) The dying patient. *BMJ*, 316 (7140): 1313–15.

Parry, R., Land, V. and Seymour, J. (2014) How to communicate with patients about future illness progression and end of life: a systematic review. *BMJ Supportive and Palliative Care*. Available at: http://spcare.bmj.com/content/early/2014/10.24/bmjspcare-2014-000649

Payne, S., Horn, S. and Relf, M. (1999) *Loss and Bereavement*. Buckingham: Open University Press.

Petursdottir, A.B., Svavarsdottir, E.K., Sigurdardóttir, V. et al. (2016) Family nursing in specialized palliative home care: the benefits of a therapeutic conversation intervention. Poster presentation at the European Association of Palliative Care Congress, Dublin.

Prigerson, H.G., Horowitz. M.J., Jacobs, S.C. et al. (2009) Prolonged grief disorder: psychometric validation of criteria proposed for DSM-V and ICD-11. Available at: http://dx.doi.org/10.1371/journal.pmed.1000121

Prigerson, H.G. and Jacobs, S.C. (2001) Traumatic grief as a distinct disorder: a rationale, consensus criteria, and a preliminary empirical test. In Stroebe, M.S., Hansson, R.O., Stroebe, W. and Schut, H. (eds) *Handbook of Bereavement Research*. Washington, DC: American Psychological Association, pp. 613–45.

Prigerson, H.G., Maciejewski, P.K., Reynolds, C.F. III. et al. (1995) Inventory of Complicated Grief: a scale to measure maladaptive symptoms of loss. *Psychiatry Research*, 59: 65–79.

Quinn, A. (2005) The context of loss, change and bereavement in palliative care. In Firth, P., Luff, G. and Oliviere, D. (eds) *Loss, Change and Bereavement in Palliative Care*. Maidenhead: Open University Press.

Raphael, B. (1984) *The Anatomy of Bereavement*. London: Unwin Hyman.

Relf, M., Machin, L. and Archer, N. (2010) *Guidance for Bereavement Needs Assessment in Palliative Care* (2nd edn). London: Help the Hospices.

Rogers, C.R. (1980) *A Way of Being*. Boston: Houghton Mifflin.

Rosenblatt, P.C. (2001) A social constructionist perspective on cultural differences in grief. In Stroebe, M.S., Hansson, R.O., Stroebe, W. and Schut, H. (eds) *Handbook of Bereavement Research*. Washington, DC: American Psychological Association, pp. 285–300.

Sanders, C.M. (1993) Risk factors in bereavement outcome. In Stroebe, M.S., Stroebe, W. and Hansson, R.O. (eds) *Handbook of Bereavement*. Cambridge: Cambridge University Press, pp. 255–67.

Seligman, M.E.P. (1998) Building human strength: psychology's forgotten mission, *American Psychological Association Monitor*, 29(1).

Seligman, M.E.P. and Csikszentmihalyi, M. (2000) Positive psychology: an introduction. *American Psychologist*, 55: 5–14.

Shapiro, E.R. (2001) Grief in interpersonal perspectives: theories and their implications. In Stroebe, M.S., Hansson, R.O., Stroebe, W. and Schut, H. (eds) *Handbook of Bereavement Research*. Washington, DC: American Psychological Association, pp. 301–27.

Shear, M.K. (2015) Complicated grief. *New England Journal of Medicine*. 372: 153–60.

Shear, M.K., Boelen, P.A. and Neimeyer, R.A. (2011) Treating complicated grief: converging approaches. In Neimeyer, R.A., Harris, D.L., Winokuer, H.R. and Thornton, G.F. (eds) *Grief and Bereavement in Contemporary Society*. New York: Routledge, pp. 139–62.

Sheehy, L. (2013) Understanding factors that influence the grieving process. *End of Life Journal*, 3(1): 1–9.

Sim, J., Machin, L. and Bartlam, B. (2014) Identifying vulnerability in grief: psychometric properties of the Adult Attitude to Grief Scale. *Quality of Life Research*, 23(4): 1211–15.

Spitzer, R.L., Kroenka, K., Williams, J.B. and Löwe, B. (2006) A brief measure for assessing generalised anxiety disorder: the GAD-7. *Archives of Internal Medicine*, 166: 1092–7.

Stroebe, M. (1992–93) Coping with bereavement: a review of the grief work hypothesis. *Omega*, 26(1): 19–42.

Stroebe, M.S., Folkman, S., Hansson, R.O. and Schut, H. (2006) The prediction of bereavement outcome: development of an integrative risk factor framework. *Social Science and Medicine*, 63: 2440–51.

Stroebe, M. and Schut, H. (1999) The dual process model of coping with bereavement: rationale and description. *Death Studies*, 23: 197–224.

Stroebe, M.S. and Schut, H. (2010) The dual process model of coping with bereavement: a decade on. *Omega*, 61(4): 273–89.

Stroebe, W. and Stroebe, M.S. (1987) *Bereavement and Health*. Cambridge: Cambridge University Press.

Sumathipala, A. and Murray, J. (2000) New approach to translating instruments for cross-cultural research: a combined qualitative and quantitative approach for translation and consensus generation. *International Journal of Methods in Psychiatric Research*, 9(2): 87–95.

Thompson, S. (2002) Older people. In Thompson, N. (ed.) *Loss and Grief*. Basingstoke: Palgrave, pp. 162–73.

Bereavement care

Lauren J. Breen and Samar M. Aoun

Introduction

Bereavement care is an important component of palliative care policy (National Institute for Clinical Excellence 2004; Palliative Care Australia 2005; World Health Organization 2007; National Hospice and Palliative Care Organization 2008) but can be challenging to implement in practice. Palliative care services may grapple with issues, including having limited resources to devote to bereavement care, not knowing whom to offer support – and for how long – with the bereavement care resources they do have, and a desire for clear evidence to underpin their bereavement care services (Breen et al. 2014).

It has long been recognised that nurses have a central role in providing bereavement care (Cooley 1992). This chapter explores practical bereavement care interventions across a range of settings, with a particular focus on how nurses might provide appropriate and responsive care around the time of death. The chapter has three sections:

- The first section sets the context of bereavement by providing an overview of key concepts, the actors that are likely to mollify or exacerbate the grief response, grief trajectories, and complications in grief. (Note that specific issues of bereavement risk assessment are provided in Chapter 17.)
- The next section examines the different types of bereavement care interventions and summarises the evidence for their effectiveness.
- In the third section, various bereavement care strategies are described to demonstrate how bereavement care can be provided in partnership with the palliative care sector.

The context of bereavement

Key concepts

Following the seminal work of Parkes (1970), the terms bereavement, grief, and mourning are defined in the following manner:

- bereavement is the situation of having lost a significant person through death;
- grief is the response to being bereaved and is multidimensional in that it includes emotional, physical, behavioural, and social domains;
- mourning is the manner in which grief is expressed.

However, there is no consensus in the literature in defining these terms. For example, mourning is often defined as the psychological or intra-psychic process of grief (Rando 1993). Moreover, grief is often defined as the emotional reaction to loss (Raphael 1984) while bereavement is a broader term encompassing the entire experience of anticipating the death, the death itself, and the subsequent adjustment to living without the deceased (Stroebe et al. 2008). Further, the terms grief and bereavement are often used synonymously (Center for the Advancement of Health 2004), as are grief and mourning, particularly by those with a psychoanalytic background (Stroebe et al. 2001).

Factors affecting grief responses

There are numerous factors that can promote adaptive grief responses or exacerbate distress (Center for the Advancement of Health 2004; Breen and O'Connor 2007; Lobb et al. 2010; Blackburn and Dwyer 2017). These include:

- the relationship to the deceased, with closer or difficult relationships between the deceased and the bereaved yielding a potentially more distressing grief response;
- the circumstances of the death, such as whether or not the death was anticipated by the bereaved; was it violent/traumatic, or preventable?;
- the characteristics of the bereaved individual, including age, gender, coping strategies, previous losses, and concurrent stressors;
- the availability of interpersonal support received by the bereaved, and whether or not the support is perceived as helpful by the bereaved;
- sociocultural factors that include the presence and perceived relevance of mourning rituals, customs, and traditions and whether or not the loss is 'disenfranchised' (Doka 2002).

The combination and complex interplay of these factors underpin each grief experience and are what makes it unique. An important point to consider is that a bereaved individual might have several 'risk' factors and yet adapt to and accommodate the loss with seeming ease, while another bereaved person might not have many 'risk' factors yet may experience distressing and debilitating grief (Lobb et al. 2010).

Grief trajectories

The grief response was at one time considered to be the same for all grievers or, at least, all adult grievers within a Western context. Several theories posited grief as a generic pattern comprising stages or phases that culminated in recovery. However, grievers grieve in many different ways, informed by those factors described in the previous section, and these ways have been described as grief trajectories.

A prospective study of spousal bereavement identified the most common trajectories of adjustment to loss (Bonanno et al. 2002). Perhaps surprisingly, given the salience of complicated grief reactions, the most common pattern was described as resilient. Most of the bereaved spouses' grief experiences could be described as one of five trajectories:

- Common grief or recovery (11 per cent) – This group exhibited low pre-loss depression and a grief response at 6 months that was resolved by 18 months post-bereavement.
- Chronic grief (16 per cent) – Like the common grief trajectory, this group exhibited low pre-loss depression. However, the grief response was elevated at both 6 and 18 months post-bereavement.
- Resilient (46 per cent) – This group showed low levels of distress that was stable from pre-loss and to both 6 and 18 months post-bereavement.
- Depressed-improved (10 per cent) – This group included individuals who improved in functioning after the death of their spouse, due to relief following a period of considerable carer burden or the end of an oppressive spousal relationship.
- Chronic depression (8 per cent) – This group exhibited high levels of depression that was stable from pre-loss to both 6 and 18 months post-bereavement.

Similar trajectories have been described in other studies of bereaved spouses (e.g. Galatzer-Levy and Bonanno 2012; Tang et al. 2013). Grief experiences and their relation to factors underpinning grief responses and trajectories are explored in Learning exercise 18.1.

Learning exercise 18.1

At this point it is useful to reflect on the role of nurses in working with bereaved people in palliative care. Consider the following vignettes.

- Cora is 12 years old. Her mum, who is very close to death, has instructed the palliative care staff not to let Cora know what is going on. The staff knows that Cora's aunt will soon be arriving at the hospital and that she will become Cora's legal guardian. Cora's aunt lives on the other side of the country and Cora will have to move immediately with her aunt after her mother's death. The situation means that every aspect of Cora's life is about to change but she just doesn't know it yet.

- Frank is a 65-year-old man whose wife died 2 weeks ago. Frank is very satisfied with his wife's healthcare and particularly the palliative care she received in the last few months of her life. He is stoic, doesn't dwell much on the emotional side of things, but is expressing enjoyment in developing his skills in cooking and housekeeping. His adult daughter and her family live nearby and Frank sees them about twice a week, and always for Sunday roast.

Using Table 18.1, identify the factors in each vignette that might promote adaptive grief responses or exacerbate distress.

Table 18.1 Factors affecting grief

	Factors that might promote an adaptive response	Factors that might exacerbate distress
Cora		
Frank		

- How might your thoughts on Cora's grief differ if, instead of being 12, she was 22? Or, instead of her mother dying, it was her aunt?
- How might your thoughts on Frank's grief differ if, instead of having a daughter who lives nearby, he had no family nearby? Or, instead of his wife dying peacefully, she died following an unexpected, major haemorrhage?
- Are there any issues in either scenario that might be difficult for the palliative care nursing staff to deal with?
- Bonanno and colleagues (2002) described five trajectories of grief. Which trajectory do you think best describes Frank's experience so far? Which do you think will best describe Cora's experience?
- Think of the bereaved family members you have seen while working in palliative care. Have you seen all five trajectories? Are you surprised by any of the trajectories and/or their proportion of the sample?

Complications in grief

A small subset of bereaved people experience prolonged and unremitting distress known as Prolonged Grief Disorder (PGD; Prigerson et al. 2009) or Complicated Grief (Shear et al. 2011). PGD is is distinguishable from mood and anxiety disorders and is characterised by persistent yearning for the deceased, social and occupational impairment,

Table 18.2 Criteria for Prolonged Grief Disorder

A. Event Criterion	The individual has experienced bereavement (i.e. the loss, via death, of a person).
B. Separation Distress	At least daily, the individual must experience longing or yearning for the deceased and/or intense feelings of emotional pain, sorrow, or pangs of grief related to the lost relationship.
C. Duration Criterion	The above symptoms of separation distress must be elevated at least 6 months after the bereavement.
D. Cognitive, Emotional, and Behavioural Symptoms	The individual must experience at least 5 of the following symptoms at least 'once a day' or 'quite a bit': 1. attempts to avoid reminders that the person is gone 2. feeling stunned, shocked, or dazed by the loss 3. feeling confused about his/her role in life or feeling that a part of the self has died 4. trouble accepting the loss 5. difficulty trusting others since the loss 6. feeling bitter over the loss 7. feeling that moving on (e.g. making new friends, pursuing new interests) would be difficult 8. feeling emotionally numb since the loss 9. feeling that life is unfulfilling, empty, or meaningless since the loss.
E. Impairment Criterion	A significant reduction in social, occupational, or other important areas of functioning (e.g. domestic responsibilities).

Note: Adapted from http://endoflife.weill.cornell.edu/research/assessments_and_tools

Each of the requirements for Criteria A–E must be met for a diagnosis of PGD.

and various behavioural and cognitive symptoms (Table 18.2). These symptoms are associated with a considerably elevated risk of suicidality and, as such, grief assessment is best complemented with an assessment of suicidal ideation (Breen, Hall and Bryant 2017). PGD is proposed for inclusion in the forthcoming International Statistical Classification of Diseases and Related Health Problems (ICD; Maercker et al. 2013) and the American Psychiatric Association (2013) included Persistent Complex Bereavement Disorder in the latest *Diagnostic and Statistical Manual of Mental Disorders* (DSM-5) as a condition requiring further study.

Two recent population-based studies reported an almost identical prevalence of PGD – 6.7 per cent in Germany (Kersting et al. 2011) and 6.4 per cent in Australia (Aoun et al. 2015a). Similarly, a population-based survey of Danish bereaved family carers demonstrated that 7.6 per cent met diagnostic criteria for PGD (Nielsen et al. 2017). Within general samples (i.e. not bereaved samples), the prevalence of PGD was reported to be 1.8 per cent in China (He et al. 2015), 2.4 per cent in Japan (Fujisawa et al. 2010), and 2.8 per cent in The Netherlands (Saavedra Pérez et al. 2014).

Some subsets of bereaved people show higher incidences of disordered grief. For instance, the incidence appeared elevated following large-scale disasters such as the 2004 Southeast Asian tsunami (12 per cent; Kristensen et al. 2015) and the 2010 Japanese earthquake and tsunami (9.8 per cent; Tsutsui et al. 2014). Bereaved parents might be at particular risk – in a sample of perinatally-bereaved mothers in Australia, 12.4 per cent met diagnostic criteria for PGD (McSpedden et al. 2017) and it was 30 per cent of a sample of parents, predominantly mothers in the United States, bereaved via a range of causes of death (Keesee, Currier and Neimeyer 2008).

Despite concern over the potential for misdiagnosis, over-diagnosis, and the medicalisation of grief (Thieleman and Cacciatore 2013), an international survey of the general public demonstrated that 75 per cent of respondents believed that certain expressions of grief could be considered a mental disorder (Breen et al. 2015). Importantly, a survey of bereaved people showed that they believed that a diagnosis would likely decrease experiences of stigma and self-blame (Johnson et al. 2009).

Types of bereavement care

Evidence for bereavement care interventions

The aim of bereavement care is to restore functioning and promote well-being for bereaved people. However, the efficacy of bereavement care interventions has been the subject of much debate. Much of this is a result of earlier studies of interventions that were provided indiscriminately, rather than targeting bereaved people who would likely benefit from intervention. As a result, many studies demonstrated little to no effect and the data suggested that in some cases, the bereaved individuals might have been better off without intervention (Hansson and Stroebe 2003; Jordan and Neimeyer 2003).

As a consequence of improved sampling and study design, studies of bereavement care interventions with targeted bereaved samples (i.e. those individuals displaying higher levels of distress and those who self-referred to the intervention), have shown positive results. For instance, a meta-analysis of 61 controlled studies revealed that interventions offered to bereaved people with higher levels of distress yielded results similar to those found for psychotherapies for other difficulties (Currier, Neimeyer and Berman 2008). A meta-analysis of 14 interventions targeting complicated forms of grief showed that the interventions reduced symptomatology in the short and long term (Wittouck et al. 2011). However, the variability in results across studies is likely due to the differences in samples and recruitment methods, follow-up time points, and outcome measures (Waller et al. 2016).

In recognising that various bereavement care interventions demonstrate different levels of efficacy, Neimeyer (2008) differentiated between grief support (informal compassion and information from people who do not have professional bereavement training), grief counselling (provided by trained professionals to counteract future mental health concerns), and grief therapy (provided by a trained professional to people with mental health concerns), and it is important to explore these components of bereavement care more fully.

Grief support

Grief support includes a range of strategies that might benefit all bereaved people. For support in the context of bereavement to be effective, the need for it must be recognised, the support must be provided, and the support must be perceived as helpful by the receiving individual (Rando 1993). Grief support may be divided into two main types – structural and functional. Structural support refers to the number, pattern, and interconnectedness of interpersonal relationships, while functional support encompasses the extent to which these relationships serve particular functions such as reassurance and practical assistance (Gottlieb and Bergen 2010). Despite social support being one of the few factors affecting the grief response that is amenable to intervention following bereavement, the body of literature examining factors determining the offer of supportive behaviours following bereavement is hampered by methodological and sampling limitations (Logan, Thornton and Breen, 2017).

Grief counselling

Grief counselling can range from an opportunity to tell the story to a 'listening ear' (Connor and Monroe 2011) through to the provision of a therapeutic context within which bereaved people have sustained interaction with a practitioner who understands and addresses grief and promotes healthy adaptation (Neimeyer 2010). Grief counsellors – many of whom have nursing backgrounds (Breen 2011) – normalise grief reactions, help the bereaved remain emotionally connected to the deceased, foster integration of the loss into the life story of the bereaved, and promote hope, meaning, and posttraumatic growth (Gamino and Ritter 2009; Neimeyer and Sands 2011). Grief counselling recipients benefit from the opportunity to express their thoughts and feelings (Simonsen and Cooper 2015), which is particularly important when expression is not possible with family and friends (Breen and O'Connor 2011).

One study used a questionnaire to survey bereaved clients after they had completed bereavement counselling (Gallagher, Tracey and Millar 2005). Participants reported that they had experienced reductions in the intensity of their loss and improvements in their coping and confidence and valued the counsellors' listening skills, trustworthiness, honesty, and competence. Another study investigated the mechanisms of grief counselling in addressing loss and facilitating positive outcomes for clients (Klasen et al. 2017). The participants asserted that grief counselling reduced their thoughts of self-harm, dampened the intensity of their grief, helped to restore positive functioning in their day-to-day lives, and facilitated a future orientation. The findings demonstrated the importance of the client and counsellor working together to foster a therapeutic relationship in which interventions were tailored to individual client needs.

Grief therapy

Grief therapy encompasses a range of psychotherapies that are designed specifically with the aim of reducing the symptomatology of grief complications and promoting restorative functioning. Targeted interventions designed to address PGD include elements of exposure to traumatic memories, repetitive recall of stories, restructuring maladaptive thoughts, and behavioural activation, and have demonstrated efficacy (Shear et al. 2005; Boelen et al. 2007; Papa et al. 2013; Bryant et al. 2014; Shear et al. 2016). While most of the trials have been on individual therapy, there is also evidence for treatment in group modalities (Piper et al. 2007; Supiano and Luptak 2014), internet-based delivery (Wagner and Maercker 2007; Kersting et al. 2013; Eisma et al. 2015) and indicated prevention for those at risk of developing PGD (Litz et al. 2014).

There is still a need to refine these interventions further, given that not all participants achieve clinically relevant reductions in symptoms (Doering and Eisma 2016). Additionally, little is known about the therapeutic components or mechanism(s) within the interventions that are most beneficial or for whom they will most benefit (Breen, Hall et al., in press). Metacognitive grief therapy is a new intervention adapted from metacognitive therapy and may prove useful in targeting the mechanisms of rumination and worry that underpin PGD (Wenn et al. 2015).

Bereavement care strategies for nurses in palliative care

In many countries, the most comprehensive strategy for bereavement care is advocated within palliative care, which emphasises the care of patients with terminal illnesses and their family carers before and after the patient's death. Policies and guidelines on standards of care propose that supports should be offered according to need (Palliative Care Australia 2005; World Health Organization 2007; National Hospice and Palliative Care Organization 2008; Hall, Hudson and Boughey 2012). Thus, to optimise benefit, bereavement care interventions must be tailored to the needs of the bereaved. Given that palliative care nurses tend to establish relationships with patients and their family carers, they are well positioned to assist with the assessment of need (Cooley 1992). However, despite such policies and guidelines, studies demonstrate that palliative care services in general adopt an undifferentiated approach to supporting bereaved families (Abbott, O'Connor and Payne 2008; Agnew et al. 2010; Foliart, Clausen and Siljestrom 2001). Furthermore, where some assessments are made, the usefulness of these assessments varies widely and often depends upon the subjective opinion of service providers or the use of non-validated screening tools (Mather et al. 2008; Sealey et al. 2015a).

Public Health Model of Bereavement Care

A public health approach to bereavement support in palliative care was advanced to offer an evidence-based and cost-effective approach to the provision of bereavement care (Aoun et al. 2012). The Public Health Model of Bereavement Care (Figure 18.1) comprises a three-tiered approach to bereavement risk and need for support wherein the low risk group would need support principally from family and friends, the moderate risk group would need additional support from the wider community, and the high risk group would need support from mental health services. A population-based survey of bereaved clients of four funeral providers in Australia revealed that the proportions in the three groups were a close fit with the model. The predicted and actual proportions of low risk were 60 per cent vs 58.4 per cent respectively; the moderate risk proportions were 30 per cent vs 35.2 per cent, and the high risk proportions were 10 per cent vs 6.4 per cent respectively (Aoun et al. 2015a). Both percentages are shown in Figure 18.1.

The majority of the bereaved respondents accessed support from family and friends, followed by funeral directors and GPs (see Figure 18.2). Access to mental health professionals (counsellors, social workers, psychologists and psychiatrists) was more frequently reported by the high risk group. The moderate risk group was particularly visible in the support accessed from community groups and palliative care services. On the whole, the bereaved respondents in the low risk group reported being satisfied that they received enough support and did not need more. A third of those in the moderate risk group and nearly two-thirds of those in the high risk group perceived that they did not receive enough support (Aoun et al. 2015a). Typically, the low risk group had the support they needed already in place from their social networks. The moderate group needed some additional support from the wider community, including support from various professionals, while the high risk group needed support from mental health professionals.

The implementation of this model into practice requires partnerships between palliative care services and primary care practitioners, and also strong links with community groups and services (Aoun et al. 2012; Aoun et al. 2015a). Rather than attempting to deliver a comprehensive suite of services that encompasses all forms of bereavement care, palliative care providers are best placed to concentrate their resources on developing community capacity for bereavement care (Rumbold and Aoun 2014). Drawing and building upon existing community resources such as mutual help support groups, volunteers, and community workers would ensure that initiatives are cost-effective and sustainable (Rumbold and Aoun 2014, 2015).

The following sections return to Worden's three types of bereavement care and discuss how each might be offered in relation to palliative care settings.

Grief support and palliative care

Descriptions of bereavement care strategies offered by palliative care services demonstrate that many of these strategies would best be described as grief supports. These include newsletters and pamphlets containing grief information as well as memorial services (Breen, Aoun et al. 2014). The delivery of these strategies is best offered if underpinned by the principles of information and compassion as outlined in the Public Health Model of Bereavement Care. However, while family carers indicate a need for more information about bereavement, there is little evidence to guide what this information might contain. One study documented bereaved family carers' experiential knowledge of grief and highlighted the importance of preparations for bereavement, harnessing social networks, and developing strategies for dealing with grief (Breen, Aoun et al., in press). The authors argued that this wisdom could be used to develop information brochures and other strategies that would be helpful to future carers, as well as in upskilling palliative care bereavement volunteers and the wider community so that bereaved people are better supported.

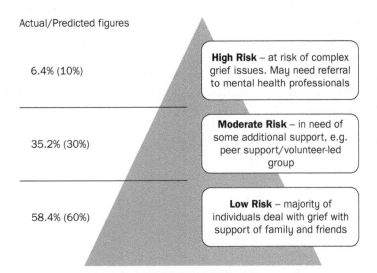

Actual/Predicted figures

6.4% (10%)

High Risk – at risk of complex grief issues. May need referral to mental health professionals

35.2% (30%)

Moderate Risk – in need of some additional support, e.g. peer support/volunteer-led group

58.4% (60%)

Low Risk – majority of individuals deal with grief with support of family and friends

Figure 18.1 The Public Health Model of Bereavement Care
Source: Aoun et al. (2015a).

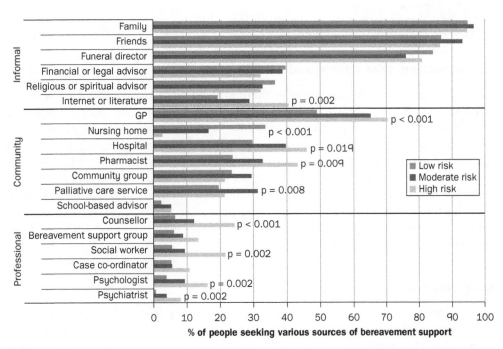

Figure 18.2 Sources of bereavement care accessed grouped according to types of support
Source: Aoun et al. (2015a).

Nurses may use their communication skills to convey compassion to bereaved carers as well as provide them with information about the death, grief responses, and relevant resources in the community (Walsh 2008). However, it is important to recognise that, in order to provide grief support, nurses require the appropriate training to understand grief responses, risk factors, and referral pathways (Matzo et al. 2003; Johnson 2015). Education on these issues is best complemented by nurses being aware of their own reactions, potential for compassionate fatigue, and self-care needs (Breen, O'Connor et al. 2014; Walsh 2008; Wenzel et al. 2011). Questions enabling you to reflect on implementing bereavement care strategies are in Learning exercise 18.2.

Learning exercise 18.2

- What types of bereavement care do you currently provide?
- What are the limitations of these approaches?
- What are the strengths that you would wish to retain?
- What would you like to add or do differently?
- What helps you provide bereavement care?
- Are there any barriers?

Grief counselling, grief therapy and palliative care

Providing grief counselling and/or grief therapy to all bereaved people irrespective of need is neither effective nor affordable (Aoun et al. 2012; Breen, Aoun et al. 2014). Palliative care services are well positioned to be involved in the development of strategies that would assist the identification and treatment of the more vulnerable carers. This is likely to be in the form of assessment of those with elevated distress/PGD symptomatology. Rather than providing specialist grief therapy, palliative care services could lead the development of pathways to enable the active referral of these vulnerable carers, both while caring and also following bereavement, so that they can receive relevant interventions, especially given the evidence that people with PGD tend not to seek out bereavement care (Lichtenthal et al. 2011).

Family caring and bereavement

As the majority of deaths worldwide are currently caused by life-limiting illnesses in older age, attention also needs to turn to family carers during the end of life phase (Stroebe and Boerner 2015). Currently, there is limited evidence to guide the pre-death assessment of post-bereavement distress or interventions that could benefit informal carers in terms of reducing their grief distress following the death of their care recipient (Breen 2012; Breen, Aoun and O'Connor 2015). Existing measurement tools tend to exhibit good psychometric priorities but may not be feasible for use in palliative care (Sealey et al. 2015a). However, there is evidence to suggest that reducing the burden of caregiving can prevent post-death psychiatric morbidity (Schulz et al. 2006; Boerner and Schulz 2009; Hudson et al. 2009; Guldin et al. 2012). The Carer Support Needs Assessment Tool (CSNAT) trials in Australia and the UK showed that this nurse-led intervention resulted in a significant reduction in carer strain pre-bereavement, lower levels of early grief, and better psychological and physical health post-bereavement in comparison to the control group (Aoun et al. 2015b; Grande et al. 2015). (Note that further information about carer needs and their assessment, including the CSNAT, is provided in Chapter 12 in this volume.)

In light of this emerging evidence, the 'window of opportunity' to assess grief responses and bereavement care needs prior to the care recipient's death can be optimised within palliative care. This assessment is critically important, given that carers' prolonged grief symptomatology is associated with their post-bereavement prolonged grief symptomatology (Nielsen et al. 2017). Therefore, there is a need to look at the continuum of the pre- and post-bereavement phases (Stroebe and Boerner 2015), engage carers in early and direct assessment of their support needs pre-bereavement (Aoun et al. 2015b; Grande et al. 2015), and develop strategies to assist carers in feeling more prepared for the death and their bereavement (Schulz et al. 2006).

Conclusion

This chapter began with an overview of the context of bereavement and established that grief responses are underpinned by numerous factors that promote adaptive grief responses or exacerbate distress. Next, the different types of bereavement care interventions and the evidence for their effectiveness were examined. Finally, various bereavement care strategies were explored to demonstrate the various ways that partnerships between the palliative care sector and community services can assist nurses to provide bereavement care. Effective bereavement care requires evidence-based assessments and interventions. Within the context of palliative care, bridging the gaps between the policy and practice of bereavement care requires working together to provide evidence-based assessment along the pre- and post-bereavement continuum, as well as the referral pathways to support the use of bereavement care interventions. Box 18.1 summarises the key learning points from this chapter.

Box 18.1 Key learning points

- There is no one way to grieve; instead, grief responses are underpinned by numerous factors that may promote adaptive grief responses or exacerbate distress.
- Grief is commonly characterised by resilience.
- Bereavement care comprises grief support, grief counselling, and grief therapy.

- The offer of bereavement care aims to restore functioning and promote well-being for bereaved people.
- Studies of bereavement care interventions offered indiscriminately show little benefit while interventions offered to individuals displaying higher levels of distress are beneficial.
- In many countries, palliative care services provide the most comprehensive strategy for bereavement care.
- Bereavement care is an important component of palliative care policy.
- Implementing evidence-based and cost-effective bereavement care can be challenging.
- It is important to align the care offered with the needs of the bereaved, so that the salient needs of bereaved people are respected and addressed.
- There is value in engaging family carers in early and direct assessment of their support needs pre-bereavement in order to gain post-bereavement benefits.
- Palliative care services need to develop strategies in partnerships with other providers in the community to assist family carers in feeling more prepared for the death.

References

Abbott, J., O'Connor, M. and Payne, S. (2008) An Australian survey of palliative care and hospice bereavement services. *Australian Journal of Cancer Nursing*, 9(2): 12–17.

Agnew, A., Manktelow, R., Taylor, B. and Jones, L. (2010) Bereavement needs assessment in specialist palliative care: a review of the literature. *Palliative Medicine*, 24(1): 46–59.

American Psychiatric Association (2013) *Diagnostic and Statistical Manual of Mental Disorders* (5th edn). Washington, DC: American Psychiatric Association.

Aoun, S.M., Breen, L.J., Howting, D.A. et al. (2015a) Who needs bereavement support? A population based survey of bereavement risk and support need. *PLoS ONE*, 10(3). doi: 10.1371/journal.pone.0121101.

Aoun, S.M., Breen, L.J., O'Connor, M. et al. (2012) A public health approach to bereavement support services in palliative care. *Australian and New Zealand Journal of Public Health*, 36(1): 14–16.

Aoun, S.M., Grande, G., Howting, D. et al. (2015b) The impact of the Carer Support Needs Assessment Tool (CSNAT) in community palliative care using a stepped wedge cluster trial. *PLoS ONE*, 10(4). doi: 10.1371/journal.pone.0123012.

Blackburn, P. and Dwyer, K. (2017) A bereavement common assessment framework in palliative care: informing practice, transforming care. *American Journal of Hospice and Palliative Care*, 34(7): 677–84.

Boelen, P.A., de Keijser, J., van den Hout, M.A. and van den Bout, J. (2007) Treatment of complicated grief: a comparison between cognitive-behavioral therapy and supportive counseling. *Journal of Consulting and Clinical Psychology*, 75(2): 277–84.

Boerner, K. and Schulz, R. (2009) Caregiving, bereavement and complicated grief. *Bereavement Care*, 28(3): 10–13.

Bonanno, G.A., Wortman, C.B., Lehman, D.R. et al. (2002) Resilience to loss and chronic grief: a prospective study from pre-loss to 18 months post-loss. *Journal of Personality and Social Psychology*, 83(5): 1150–64.

Breen, L.J. (2011) Professionals' experiences of grief counseling: implications for bridging the gap between research and practice, *Omega: Journal of Death and Dying*, 62: 285–303.

Breen, L.J. (2012) The effect of caring on post-bereavement outcome: research gaps and practice priorities. *Progress in Palliative Care*, 20(1): 27–30.

Breen, L.J., Aoun, S.M. and O'Connor, M. (2015) The effect of caregiving on bereavement outcome: study protocol for a longitudinal, prospective study. *BMC Palliative Care*, 16(6). doi: 10.1186/s12904-015-0009-z.

Breen, L.J., Aoun, S.M., O'Connor, M. and Rumbold, B. (2014) Bridging the gaps in palliative care bereavement support: an international perspective. *Death Studies*, 38(1): 54–61.

Breen, L.J., Aoun, S.M., Rumbold, B. et al. (2017) Building community capacity in bereavement support: lessons learnt from bereaved former caregivers. *American Journal of Hospice and Palliative Medicine*, 34: 275–81.

Breen, L.J., Hall, C.W. and Bryant, R. (2017) A clinician's quick guide of evidence-based approaches: prolonged grief disorder. *Clinical Psychologist*, 21: 153–4.

Breen, L.J. and O'Connor, M. (2007) The fundamental paradox in the grief literature: acritical reflection. *Omega: Journal of Death and Dying*, 55(3): 199–218.

Breen, L.J. and O'Connor, M. (2011) Family and social networks after bereavement: experiences of support, change and isolation. *Journal of Family Therapy*, 33(1): 98–120.

Breen, L.J., O'Connor, M., Hewitt, L.Y. and Lobb, E.A. (2014) The 'specter' of cancer: exploring secondary trauma for health professionals providing cancer support and counseling. *Psychological Services*, 11: 60–7.

Breen, L.J., Penman, E.L., Prigerson, H.G. and Hewitt, L.Y. (2015) Can grief be a mental disorder? An exploration of public opinion. *Journal of Nervous and Mental Disease*, 203(8): 569–73.

Bryant, R.A., Kenny, L., Joscelyne, A. et al. (2014) Treating prolonged grief disorder: a randomized clinical trial. *JAMA Psychiatry*, 71(12): 1332–9.

Center for the Advancement of Health (2004) Report on bereavement and grief research. *Death Studies*, 28(6): 491–575.

Cooley, M.E. (1992) Bereavement care: a role for nurses. *Cancer Nursing*, 15(2): 125–9.

Connor, S.R. and Monroe, B. (2011) Bereavement services provided under the hospice model of care. In Neimeyer, R.A., Harris, D.L., Winokuer, H.R., Thornton, G.F. (eds) *Grief and Bereavement in Contemporary Society: Bridging Research and Practice*. New York: Routledge, pp. 325–37.

Currier, J.M., Neimeyer, R.A. and Berman, J.S. (2008) The effectiveness of psychothera-peutic interventions for bereaved persons: a comprehensive quantitative review. *Psychological Bulletin*, 134(5): 648–61.

Doering, B.K. and Eisma, M.C. (2016) Treatment for complicated grief: state of the science and ways forward. *Current Opinion in Psychiatry*, 29(5): 286–91.

Doka, K.J. (ed.) (2002) *Disenfranchised Grief: New Directions. Challenges. and Strategies for Practice*. Champaign, IL: Research Press.

Eisma, M.C., Boelen, P.A., van den Bout, J. et al. (2015) Internet-based exposure and behavioral activation for complicated grief and rumination: a randomized controlled trial. *Behavior Therapy*, 46(5): 729–48.

Foliart, D.E., Clausen, M. and Siljestrom, C. (2001) Bereavement practices among California hospices: results of a statewide survey. *Death Studies*, 25(5): 461–7.

Fujisawa, D., Miyashita, M., Nakajima, S. et al. (2010) Prevalence and determinants of complicated grief in general population. *Journal of Affective Disorders*, 127: 352–8.

Galatzer-Levy, I.R. and Bonanno, G.A. (2012) Beyond normality in the study of bereavement: heterogeneity in depression outcomes following loss in older adults. *Social Science and Medicine*, 74: 1987–94.

Gallagher, M., Tracey, A. and Millar, R. (2005) Ex-clients' evaluation of bereavement counselling in a voluntary sector agency. *Psychology and Psychotherapy: Theory. Research and Practice*, 78(1): 59–76.

Gamino, L.A. and Ritter, R.H. Jr. (2009) *Ethical Practice in Grief Counseling*. New York: Springer.

Gottlieb, B.H. and Bergen, A.E. (2010) Social support concepts and measures. *Journal of Psychosomatic Research*, 69(5): 511–20.

Grande, G.E., Austin, L., Ewing, G. et al. (2015) Assessing the impact of a Carer Support Needs Assessment Tool (CSNAT) intervention in palliative home care: a stepped wedge cluster trial. *BMJ Supportive and Palliative Care*. doi: 10.1136/bmjspcare-2014-000829.

Guldin, M.B., Vedsted, P., Zachariae, R. et al. (2012) Complicated grief and need for professional support in family caregivers of cancer patients in palliative care: a longitudinal cohort study. *Supportive Care in Cancer*, 20(8): 1679–85.

Hall, C., Hudson, P. and Boughey, A. (2012) *Bereavement Support Standards for Specialist Palliative Care Services*. Melbourne: State Government of Victoria. Available at: http://centreforpallcare.org/assets/uploads/Bereavement%20support%20standards(1).pdf

Hansson, R.O. and Stroebe, M.S. (2003) Grief, older adulthood. In Bloom, M. and Gullotta, T.P. (eds) *Encyclopedia of Primary Prevention and Health Promotion*. New York: Kluwer Academic, pp. 515–21.

He, L., Tang, S., Yu, W. et al. (2015) The prevalence, comorbidity and risks of prolonged grief disorder among bereaved Chinese adults. *Psychological Medicine*, 45: 1389–99.

Hudson, P., Thomas, T., Quinn, K. et al. (2009) Teaching family carers about home-based palliative care: final results from a group education program. *Journal of Pain and Symptom Management*, 38(2): 299–308.

Johnson, J. (2015) Role of district and community nurses in bereavement care: a qualitative study. *British Journal of Community Nursing*, 20(10): 494–501.

Johnson, J.G., First, M.B., Block, S. et al.(2009) Stigmatization and receptivity to mental health services among recently bereaved adults. *Death Studies*, 33: 691–711.

Jordan, J.R. and Neimeyer, R.A. (2003) Does grief counseling work? *Death Studies*, 27(9): 765–86.

Keesee, N.J., Currier, J.M. and Neimeyer, R.A. (2008) Predictors of grief following the death of one's child: the contribution of finding meaning. *Journal of Clinical Psychology*, 64(10): 1145–63.

Kersting, A., Brahler, E., Glaesmer, H. and Wagner, B. (2011) Prevalence of complicated grief in a representative population-based sample. *Journal of Affective Disorders*, 131: 339–43.

Kersting, A., Dölemeyer, R., Steinig, J. et al. (2013) Brief Internet-based intervention reduces posttraumatic stress and prolonged grief in parents after the loss of a child during pregnancy: a randomized controlled trial. *Psychotherapy and Psychosomatics*, 82: 372–81.

Klasen, M., Bhar, S., Ugalde, A. and Hall, C.W. (2017) Clients' perspectives on outcomes and mechanisms of bereavement counselling: a qualitative study. *Australian Psychologist*, 52: 363–71.

Kristensen, P., Weisaeth, L., Hussain, A. and Heir, T. (2015) Prevalence of psychiatric disorders and functional impairment after loss of a family member: a longitudinal study after the 2004 Tsunami. *Depression and Anxiety*, 32(1): 49–56.

Lichtenthal, W.G., Nilsson, M., Kissane, D.W. et al. (2011) Underutilization of mental health services among bereaved caregivers with prolonged grief disorder. *Psychiatric Services*, 62(10): 1225–9.

Litz, B.T., Schorr, Y., Delaney, E. et al. (2014) A randomized controlled trial of an internet-based therapist-assisted indicated preventive intervention for prolonged grief disorder. *Behaviour Research and Therapy*, 61: 23–34.

Lobb, E.A., Kristjanson, L.J., Aoun, S.M. et al. (2010) Predictors of complicated grief: a systematic review of empirical studies. *Death Studies*, 34: 673–98.

Logan, E.L., Thornton, J.A. and Breen, L.J. (2017) What determines supportive behaviours following bereavement? A systematic review and call to action. *Death Studies*. doi: 10.1080/074811872017.1329760

Maercker, A., Brewin, C.R., Bryant, R.A. et al. (2013) Proposals for mental disorders specifically associated with stress in the International Classification of Diseases-11. *The Lancet*, 381(9878): 1683–5.

Mather, M.A., Good, P.D., Cavenagh, J.D. and Ravenscroft, P.J. (2008) Survey of bereavement support provided by Australian palliative care services. *Medical Journal of Australia*, 188(4): 228–30.

Matzo, M.L., Sharman, D.W., Lo, K. et al. (2003) Strategies for teaching loss, grief, and bereavement. *Nurse Educator*, 28(2): 71–6.

McSpedden, M., Mullan, B., Sharpe, L. et al. (2017) The presence and predictors of complicated grief symptoms in perinatally-bereaved mothers from a bereavement support organization. *Death Studies*, 41: 122–27.

National Hospice and Palliative Care Organization (2008) *Guidelines for Bereavement Care in Hospice* (2nd edn). Alexandria, VA: National Hospice and Palliative Care Organization.

National Institute for Health and Clinical Excellence (2004) *Guidance on Cancer Services: Improving Supportive and Palliative Care for Adults with Cancer. The Manual*. London: NICE.

Neimeyer, R.A. (2008) *Grief and bereavement counseling.* Available at: http://web.mac. com/neimeyer/Home/Scholarship.html

Neimeyer, R.A. (2010) Grief counselling and therapy. *Bereavement Care,* 29(2): 13–16.

Neimeyer, R.A. and Sands, D.C. (2011) Meaning reconstruction in bereavement: from principles to practice. In Neimeyer, R.A., Harris, D.L., Winokuer, H.R. and Thornton, G.F. (eds) *Grief and Bereavement in Contemporary Society: Bridging Research and Practice.* New York: Routledge, pp. 9–22.

Nielsen, M.K., Neergaard, M.A., Jensen, A.B. et al. (2017) Predictors of complicated grief and depression in bereaved caregivers: a nationwide prospective cohort study. *Journal of Pain and Symptom Management,* 53: 540–50.

Palliative Care Australia (2005) *Standards for Providing Quality Palliative Care for All Australians* (4th edn). Canberra: Palliative Care Australia.

Papa, A., Sewell, M.T., Garrison-Diehn, C. and Rummel, C. (2013) A randomized open trial assessing the feasibility of behavioral activation for pathological grief responding. *Behavior Therapy,* 44: 639–50.

Parkes, C.M. (1970) 'Seeking' and 'finding' a lost object: evidence from recent studies of the reaction to bereavement. *Social Science and Medicine,* 4: 187–201.

Piper, W.E., Ogrodniczuk, J.S., Joyce, A.S. et al. (2007) Group composition and group therapy for complicated grief. *Journal of Consulting and Clinical Psychology.* 75: 116–25.

Prigerson, H.G., Horowitz, M.J., Jacobs, S.C. et al. (2009) Prolonged grief disorder: psychometric validation of criteria proposed for DSM-IV and ICD-11. *Public Library of Science Medicine,* 6(8): 1–12.

Rando, T.A. (1993) *Treatment of Complicated Mourning.* Champaign, IL: Research Press.

Raphael, B. (1984) *The Anatomy of Bereavement: A Handbook for the Caring Professions.* London: Hutchinson.

Rumbold, B. and Aoun, S. (2014) Bereavement and palliative care: a public health perspective. *Progress in Palliative Care,* 22(3): 131–5.

Rumbold, B. and Aoun, S. (2015) An assets-based approach to bereavement care. *Bereavement Care,* 34(3): 99–102.

Saavedra Pérez, H.C., Ikram, M.A., Direk, N. et al. (2014) Cognition, structural brain changes and complicated grief: a population-based study. *Psychiatry Research,* 217: 67–71.

Schulz, R., Boerner, K., Shear, K. et al. (2006) Predictors of complicated grief among dementia caregivers: a prospective study of bereavement. *American Journal of Geriatric Psychiatry,* 14(8): 650–8.

Schut, H. (2010) Grief counselling efficacy. *Bereavement Care,* 29(1): 8–9.

Sealey, M., Breen, L.J., O'Connor, M. and Aoun, S.M. (2015a) A scoping review of bereavement risk assessment measures: implications for palliative care. *Palliative Medicine,* 29(7): 577–89.

Sealey, M., O'Connor, M., Aoun, S.M. and Breen, L.J. (2015b) Exploring barriers to assessment of bereavement risk in palliative care: perspectives of key stakeholders. *BMC Palliative Care,* 14(49). doi: 10.1186/s12904-015-0046-7.

Shear, K., Frank, E., Houck, P. and Reynolds, C.F. (2005) Treatment of complicated grief: a randomized controlled trial. *JAMA,* 293(21): 2601–8.

Shear, M.K., Reynolds, C.F., Simon, N.M. et al. (2016) Optimizing treatment of complicated grief: a randomized clinical trial. *JAMA Psychiatry*, 73: 685–94.

Shear, M.K., Simon, N., Wall, M. et al. (2011) Complicated grief and related bereavement issues for DSM-5. *Depression and Anxiety*, 28: 103–17.

Simonsen, G. and Cooper, M. (2015) Helpful aspects of bereavement counselling: an interpretative phenomenological analysis. *Counselling and Psychotherapy Research*, 15: 119–27.

Stroebe, M. and Boerner, K. (2015) Caregiving and bereavement research: bridges over the gap. *Palliative Medicine*, 29(7): 574–6.

Stroebe, M., Hansson, R., Schut, H. and Stroebe, W. (2008) *Handbook of Bereavement Research and Practice: Advances in Theory and Intervention*. Washington, DC: American Psychological Association.

Stroebe, M.S., Hansson, R.O., Stroebe, W. and Schut, H. (2001) Introduction: concepts and issues in contemporary research on bereavement. In Stroebe, M.S., Hansson, R.O., Stroebe, W. and Schut, H. (eds) *Handbook of Bereavement Research: Consequences, Coping, and Care*. Washington, DC: American Psychological Association, pp. 3–22.

Supiano, K.P. and Luptak, M. (2014) Complicated grief in older adults: a randomized controlled trial of complicated grief group therapy. *The Gerontologist*, 54: 840–56.

Tang, S.T., Huang, G.H., Wei, Y.C. et al. (2013) Trajectories of caregiver depressive symptoms while providing end of life care. *Psychooncology*, 22(12): 2702–10.

Thieleman, K. and Cacciatore, J. (2013) The DSM-5 and the bereavement exclusion: a call for critical evaluation. *Social Work*, 58: 277–80.

Tsutsui, T., Hasegawa, Y., Hiraga, M. et al. (2014) Distinctiveness of prolonged grief disorder symptoms among survivors of the Great East Japan Earthquake and Tsunami. *Psychiatry Research*, 217: 67–71.

Wagner, B. and Maercker, A. (2007) A 1.5-year follow-up of an Internet based intervention for complicated grief. *Journal of Traumatic Stress*, 20: 625–9.

Waller, A., Turon, H., Mansfield, E. et al. (2016) Assisting the bereaved: a systematic review of the evidence for grief counselling. *Palliative Medicine*, 30(2): 132–48.

Walsh, H.C. (2008) Caring for bereaved people 2: nursing management. *Nursing Times*, 104(1): 32–3.

Wenn, J., O'Connor, M., Breen, L.J. et al. (2015) Efficacy of metacognitive therapy for prolonged grief disorder: protocol for a randomised controlled trial. *BMJ Open*, 5(12). doi: 10.1136/bmjopen-2014-007221.

Wenzel, J., Shaha, M., Klimmek, R. and Krumm, S. (2011) Working through grief and loss: oncology nurses' perspectives on professional bereavement. *Oncology Nursing Forum*, 38(4): E272–E282.

Wittouck, C., Van Autreve, S., De Jaegere, E. et al. (2011) The prevention and treatment of complicated grief: a meta-analysis. *Clinical Psychology Review*, 31: 69–78.

Worden, J.W. (2009) *Grief Counseling and Grief Therapy: A Handbook for the Mental Health Practitioner* (4th edn). New York: Springer.

World Health Organization (2007) *Palliative Care*. (Cancer control: Knowledge into action: WHO guide for effective programmes; module 5). Geneva: WHO.

Chapter
19

The costs and rewards of caring in palliative care

Lise Fillion and Mary L.S. Vachon

Introduction

Working in palliative care can be challenging, distressing, but also very reward-ing. Palliative care involves several types of stressors: organisational, professional, and emotional. By the very nature of their work, palliative care clinicians encounter emotional demands and ethical challenges. They have to deal with repeated deaths, the distress of patients and family, ethical concerns, and their own personal suffering and stress, in a work environment which may be less supportive and more demanding than other settings. This chapter offers a reflection on and some suggestions relating to these clinicians' particular challenges. First, an understanding of workplace stress, the stress-ors specific to palliative care, and the psychosocial risks factors at work that may lead to burnout or job engagement is provided. It offers a framework for preventing burnout and promoting well-being and engagement at work. Second, examples of burnout inter-ventions published in the literature to support palliative care nurses are presented.

Palliative care and work-related stress

Palliative care research repeatedly suggests that clinicians are exposed to different stressors and could be at risk of experiencing work-related stress and burnout.

Work-related stress

The first step in preventing negative consequences such as burnout is recognition of work-related stress. The European Agency for Safety and Health at Work states: 'There is increasing consensus around defining work-related stress or occupational stress in terms of the "interactions" between employees and their work environment' (Cox et al. 2000). Accordingly, stress reactions can be said to be experienced by nurses when the demands from the work environment (stressors at work) exceed the employee's ability to cope with them.

Negative and positive outcomes of work-related stress

Work-related stress contributes to negative outcomes at both the individual and organisational levels. Clinicians can show stress symptoms, such as elevated levels of depression, anxiety, compassion fatigue, burnout, job dissatisfaction, poorer physical health and self-care, substance use and, in some instances, elevated rates of suicide (Shanafelt and Dyrbye 2012; Vachon and Fillion 2015). The distress or the emotional stress reaction experienced by nurses has the potential to impact adversely on patient care, with reported associations with poorer quality of care, higher rates of clinical errors, diminished empathy in care, and adverse impact on professionalism (Vachon and Harris 2016). For the organisation, stress is associated with a negative impact on quality of care and job performance, greater absenteeism, and decisions to leave healthcare or consider early retirement (Verhaeghe et al. 2004; Dyrbye et al. 2010).

The same exposure to workplace stressors, when one's abilities are well matched to demands, may, however, be associated with a positive experience of job engagement. Whether the stress consequence is a harm or benefit depends in part on the individual's cognitive appraisal of the stressors and the coping skills with stressors at work (Lazarus and Folkman 1984). Coping skills refer to the ability to manage demands that are perceived as stressful. When coping is ineffective, stress reactions are high. Conversely, use of effective coping is associated with less distress and burnout (Koh et al. 2015) and better spiritual quality of life and vigour (Desbiens and Fillion 2007).

Burnout, engagement, person-environment fit model and resilience

Maslach et al. (2001) define burnout as a psychological syndrome in response to chronic stressors on the job, and report three key dimensions:

1 Emotional exhaustion refers to feelings of being overextended and depleted of one's emotional and physical resources.
2 Feelings of cynicism and detachment from the job refers to a negative, callous, or excessively detached response to various aspects of the job.
3 A sense of ineffectiveness refers to feelings of incompetence and a lack of achievement and productivity at work.

In contrast, job engagement can be conceptualised as the opposite of burnout (Leiter and Maslach 2004; Maslach 2011). Job engagement is a persistent, positive-affective-motivational state of fulfilment characterised by vigour, dedication, and absorption. Job engagement entails energy and involvement. It encompasses the individual's relationship with work.

Leiter and Maslach (2004) propose a person-environment fit model to prevent or reverse burnout and reinforce job engagement. This suggests that burnout and job engagement are interrelated concepts. While burnout feels like emotional exhaustion, job engagement feels like energy; burnout manifests as cynicism, job engagement as involvement; and, burnout feels like inefficacy, engagement feels like efficacy. Leiter and Maslach suggest that the two concepts could be explained by the same six work conditions: (1) workload (amount of work); (2) control (participation in decisions); (3) reward (recognition); (4) community (supportive work interaction); (5) fairness (equal consideration, transparency); and (6) values (meaningfulness).

Their model also describes individual characteristics, such as age, life experience, personality and preferences. Individual characteristics also involve coping skills and resilience to stressful events (Back et al. 2016). Coping and resilience are terms that describe how people respond to the work-related stressors. Unlike coping which may be adaptive or maladaptive, resilience refers to the ability to cope effectively. Resilience is defined as the capacity to respond to stressors in a healthy way or to bounce back (Epstein and Krasner 2013) and to the ability to return to a zone of stability in the midst of challenging circumstances (Zwack and Schweitzer 2013). Resilience skills promote constructive and healthy engagement with (rather than withdrawal from) the challenges at work and can be trained (see Box 19.1).

Box 19.1   Resilience skills that can be learned to prevent burnout

- Working from strengths (being aware of personal and external resources).
- Tracking activation (paying attention to body sensations and monitoring them).
- Healthy boundaries (recognising and maintaining boundaries that establish appropriate limits).
- Regulating emotions (e.g. using breathing techniques and deliberately slowing down).
- Recognising distortions (e.g. working on reducing 'should' thoughts).
- Having reasonable expectations (practising being gentle with yourself, and self-empathy).
- Finding meaning (knowing your values; making mindful choices and actions).
- Committing to long term (having meaningful objectives; socialising and participating).

Adapted from Back et al. (2016).

Psychosocial risk factors and mismatch framework

Increasing resilience skills alone will not necessarily result in burnout prevention. The person-environment fit model recognises the importance of directly addressing work conditions or organisational factors in order to respond proactively to common stressors. The French Ministry offer a definition of work-related stress as the sustained presence of psychosocial risk factors at work (Collège d'expertise sur le suivi des risques psycho-sociaux au travail, 2011). These factors are close to the six work conditions described by Maslach, and can be grouped around six axes: (1) emotional demands; (2) social climate (poor social support); (3) conflicts of values (moral conflicts); (4) lack of autonomy; (5) workload or intensity of work (high workload); (6) and lack of safety/justice issues.

Inspired by the six areas of psychosocial risk factors, and by the person-environment fit approach suggested by Maslach et al., we define burnout as the result of a chronic mismatch between the characteristics of the work environment and the individual. Conversely, engagement at work could be associated with better goodness of fit between individual and organisational characteristics.

Psychosocial risk factors could provide a useful framework to classify the characteristics of individuals as well as the characteristics of the work environment that could be targeted to prevent burnout and promote job engagement. For instance, and for all workers, burnout may arise from chronic mismatches between individuals and their work settings in some or all of these six axes summarised in the first two columns of Table 19.1.

The framework is useful to explore individual strategies to improve resilience skills as well as organisational strategies targeting work conditions that can prevent burnout and promote engagement. For each axis, a listing of organisational and individual strategies, aimed at preventing burnout and promoting well-being and satisfaction, are provided as examples of what can be done to decrease risk factors or by individuals to increase resilience skills.

Emotional demands or capacity to find meaning in suffering

The first axis concerns emotional demands. They are related to the need to self-regulate, and control one's emotions at work. Having to regulate, control, repress or hide emotions is demanding. Palliative care is associated with high emotional demands. Our palliative care research in acute care settings demonstrates the link between having to cope with high patient and family distress, and showing higher distress and lower job satisfaction (Fillion et al. 2007). Conversely, 'being with the dying' has been described by caregivers as one of the most rewarding part of their work. Clinicians often report less emotional burden and better work satisfaction than care providers from other care settings (Huggard 2008; Fillion et al. 2011). Clinicians report that these issues are manageable as long as there are sufficient and appropriate organisational support practices, such as acknowledgement of the deaths, the use of rituals, and the availability of debriefing sessions.

Some situations are particularly difficult and may sometimes be considered as being a traumatic exposure, also known as secondary or vicarious traumatisation or compassion fatigue (Figley 2002). Figley describes compassion fatigue as 'the natural consequent behaviours and emotions resulting from knowing about a traumatizing event experienced or suffered by the persons'. Some authors suggest that compassion fatigue may occur when caregivers unconsciously absorb the distress, anxiety, fears, and trauma of the patient (Bush 2009). Others, including neuroscientists, prefer

Table 19.1 Six axes of psychosocial risk factors, and examples of organisational and individual strategies to increase palliative care clinicians' support and resilience skills

Psychosocial risk factors at work	Organisational/individual mismatch	Organisational strategies (support)	Individual strategies (resilience skills)
Emotional demands (frequent needs to self-regulate, control, and shape one's emotions at work)	Feeling overwhelmed by: • Patient and family distress/suffering • Repeated griefs • Death of young patients • Identification with patients	– Support groups (group format/ bereavement/debriefing) – Psychoeducation (distress/stress management, dying process, compassion fatigue, grief, skills in communication, psychosocial care, spiritual care) – Counselling/spiritual care for staff, patients, and families (knowledge) – Bulletin board for sympathy/funeral cards, and thank-you notes	– Self-regulation of emotion (awareness, relaxation, meditation, breathing, cognitive restructuration, healthy boundaries) – Emotional expression (music therapy, art therapy) – Stress management and self-care (coping skills, stressor management, healthy lifestyle, energy conservation) – External counselling/coaching/ complementary medicine
Social climate (lack of support from colleagues and organisation, communication problem and loss of community belonging)	Feeling disconnected: • From the rest of the team • Feeling like an outsider • Feelings of isolation and loneliness	– Encouraging staff to voice feelings – Enhanced teamwork and interdisciplinary competences (knowledge) – Increasing interactions in daily routines, groups activities, staff meetings, or activities outside work – Reduce interdisciplinary conflict and reinforce interdisciplinary network	– Training courses in interpersonal or communication skills (attentive presence; listening skills) – Cultivating compassion towards staff, patient and self – Professional relationship – Facilitating exchange with other nurses – Participation in activities outside work
Conflicts of values/loss of meaning (incoherence between values and actions)	Feeling caught in conflicting values, constrained to do something unethical and not in accord with values	– Access to counselling, ethical guidance – Ongoing opportunities for professional learning, supervision and support – Expressive therapies like art, music to clarify values and cultivate moral sensitivity/encouraging reflection – Creating space (group format) to discuss cases (cultural/ethical/moral)	– Taking a pause and self-reflecting – Meaning centred therapy – Mindfulness – Yoga classes, healing touch – Humour – Enhance introspection related to death anxiety

Table 19.1 (Continued)

Psychosocial risk factors at work	Organisational/individual mismatch	Organisational strategies (support)	Individual strategies (resilience skills)
		– Group sessions to clarify shared values and cultivate moral sensitivity – Mobilising staff around meaningful causes; celebration of successes – Regular feedback to staff – Ethical decision-making support	– Empathic confrontation – Resilient responding (grounding + resourcing) – Empowerment – Coping and assertiveness skills
Lack of autonomy (lack of control, flexibility, capacity to make mindful choices, recognition, professional development)	Feeling hopeless or powerless, not recognised, not heard	– Recognition and appreciation of staff – Participation in decisions that affect work – Quality of leadership from upper management – Flexibility in scheduling or assignment to work setting – Appropriate recruitment – Accurate job descriptions	– Making meaningful choices and actions according to values – Feelings of choice and control – Clarifying and expressing personal needs and assertiveness for them – Looking for other jobs offering more benefits
Workload or intensity of work (psychological demand/effort)	Feeling physically and emotionally drained at the end of the day Doing it all alone Skipping lunches and breaks	– Adequate staffing, reduced work hours or patient contact – Advanced technology and training to help reduce workload – Teamwork to share care – Reallocation of selected tasks or conflicting responsibilities – Employment requiring to take block of 2 weeks' consecutive leave/year	– Meaningful choices (time management) – Developing realistic expectations for one's own performance – Request for support (assertiveness) and delegation – Increase personal days/vacation time
Lack of safety/justice (economic uncertainty, unfairness)	Feeling personal safety compromised or outside the favoured group	– Annual retreat for staff and management – Management education – Health and safety policies that are not only focusing on physical safety	– Problem-solving with colleagues and managers – Reach for support, e.g. union or other collective or professional support

not to name this problem as compassion fatigue and would rather suggest it should be described as a difficulty in being aware of and being able to self-regulate their empathic reactions (Klimecki and Singer 2012). For Halifax (2013), compassion does not lead to fatigue, rather, it can contribute to resilience and includes self-regulation of emotion. Without self-regulation capacity, emotional demands, stress reactions and compassion fatigue (or problem with empathy reactions) may lead to burnout (Klimecki et al. 2013; Vachon, Huggard and Huggard 2015). In contrast, when clinicians have developed a capacity to recognise, accept, face, and cope with their own emotion and suffering, they may experience compassion satisfaction (Huggard, Stamm and Pearlman 2013).

Not surprisingly, most interventions to prevent burnout in palliative care settings target ways to improve capacity to cope with emotional demands and mainly focus on individual coping strategies and resilience skills. Interventions may include single or multimodal components such as self-regulation techniques or expression of emotions, or a variety of strategies to improve emotional and meaning-based coping strategies.

Social climate or the importance of human connections

Social climate corresponds, on one hand, to the relationships between workers and, on the other, to the relationship between the worker and the employing organisation. It involves good communication, and a sense that the social environment is supportive, collaborative and positive. Social climate must also be considered in connection with the concepts of integration into the community (in the sociological sense), and recognition from others. Social support from people with whom one shares praise, comfort, happiness, and humour affirms membership in a group with a shared sense of values (Vachon 2011, Maslach, Schaufeli, Leiter, 2001).

A mismatch may arise when people lose their sense of personal connection with others in the workplace. Team communication problems have long been identified as an issue in palliative care, as in other specialties. Payne (2001) found that conflict with staff contributed to both the emotional exhaustion and depersonalisation subscales of the Maslach Burnout Inventory. In palliative care interventions to prevent burnout, social climate is mostly addressed in targeting communication skills or in offering group format activities (see Table 19.1). Table 19.1 suggests a variety of other interventions that could be implemented.

Values and coherence, or being aware of what really matters and meaning

The third axis refers to values and meaning at work. Meaning at work may be defined according to three dimensions:

1 *Significance* refers to 'the value of work in the subject's view and his definition or representation of it'.
2 *Orientation* corresponds to 'what the subject is seeking in work and the purposes that guide his actions'.
3 *Coherence* is 'the effect between the subject and the work he performs, between his expectations, his values and the actions he performs daily in the work environment' (Morin 2008).

Being with dying people and their families is often rich in significance for nurses. When nurses reflect on their motivations for choosing palliative care, they may recall their profound intention of helping people along their journey. Meaning can have positive outcomes for workers and organisations, in terms of increased resilience and other forms of well-being. Meaningful work is related to higher organisational commitment. Moreover, providing a sense of meaning from work is a desirable characteristic when recruiting job applicants and more effective teamwork (Wrzesniewski et al. 1997; Duffy et al. 2011).

A mismatch may arise particularly when clinicians feel caught in conflicting values. Such situations may be associated with a discord between workers' beliefs and the aim of the work, or a pressure to act in opposition to their conscience. People might feel constrained by their job's setting to do something unethical and not in accord with their own values. There may also be a mismatch between their personal career goals and the values of the organisation. For instance, when there is a discrepancy between a cost-efficacy culture and a high-quality service, or when the values are in conflict. A variety of organisational pressures can lead to staff not being able to do the job properly, a decrease in quality patient care, and an increase in moral distress or ethical suffering.

Moral distress can be defined as:

> the pain or anguish affecting the mind, body or relationships in response to a situation in which the person is aware of a moral problem, acknowledges moral responsibility, and makes a moral judgment about the correct action; yet, as a result of real or perceived constraints, participates in perceived moral wrongdoing.
>
> (Nathaniel 2002)

Moral distress in the workplace occurs when there is an experience of conflict between one's beliefs and one's actions, and possibly also outcomes.

Being aware of what constitutes our core values and motivation at work is useful to help us to develop a capacity to act accordingly. An article providing strategies to reduce burnout among oncologists reported that optimisation of career fit (balance between personal and professional values) led to increased job satisfaction (Shanafelt et al. 2006). Psycho-educational and meaning-based approaches often include a component on value clarification and ethical issues (see Table 19.2).

Autonomy and control, or capacity to make mindful choices

Autonomy at work involves the worker as an active participant in the production of wealth and in the driving of one's professional life. It refers to the capacity to make mindful choices, have flexibility in work situations, participate in decision-making, and have opportunities to use and develop skills and competencies. The notion of autonomy includes the idea of professional development and achievement, and the ability to take some pleasure in one's achievements.

A mismatch occurs when there is no recognition, there is low control or lack of autonomy, insufficient resources or other disruptions that preclude the individual from properly doing the work, or a lack of personal reward at work. The issue of control

Table 19.2 Summary of burnout interventions

Study	Interventions	Individual strategies	Organisational strategies	Interventions
SUPPORT GROUPS				
Feld (2006)	Support group	Emotional expression	Professionally led support groups	Inspired by Balint model. Sharing experiences – develop confidence in their work and themselves; Establishing relationships – Confidentiality – support each other, bond as a group, valuing the group; Time allocation – time set aside to discuss stressful issues.
Keene (2010)	Support group	Emotional expression	Bereavement debriefing groups	Bereavement debriefing sessions offered after all patient deaths but are not mandatory. Session facilitated by bereavement coordinator following a structured format: welcoming, information, case review, grief responses, emotional aspect, strategies for coping, lessons learned, and conclusion. For each segment of the session, open questions were posed as a way to invite emotional expression.
Rushton (2006)	Support group and others	Emotional expression Conflict resolution Knowledge	Bereavement debriefings groups Interdisciplinary PC rounds Interdisciplinary conflict solving	Four interdisciplinary activities facilitated by the paediatric palliative care team: Interdisciplinary networking and education to support palliative and end of life care; Palliative Care Rounds (spiritual care for patients, encourage staff to voice feelings); Patient Care Conferences (reduce interdisciplinary conflict); and Bereavement Debriefing Sessions. One of the key questions asked in each session was: What was the most difficult aspect of the case? Most common theme in response was that the death ended a long-term relationship with the patient.
Sands (2008)	Narrative and emotional expression	Emotional expression	Group format Team building	Narrative intervention and written emotional expression conducted with an inter-disciplinary group of healthcare professionals in paediatric oncology.

Table 19.2 (Continued)

Study	Interventions	Individual strategies	Organisational strategies	Interventions
LeBlanc (2007)	Support group + problem-solving	Support Problem-solving	Participatory approach Balancing demands/ resources	One Introductory session and 3-hour session each month for 6 months. Programme topics included building social support, balancing job-related investments and outcomes, solving problems through team actions. Programme counsellors met with participants prior to the intervention to gather information on organisational structure, policies, management's perception of the sources of stress.
STRESS MANAGEMENT				
Kravrit (2010)	Stress management plan	Goal setting Coping skills	Group format	Assisting nurses who work in high-stress areas to develop personalised stress management plans that rely on the use of adaptive coping strategies to reduce stress and cultivate a resilience focusing on setting creative and achievable goals and maintaining positive mood.
Edmonds (2012)	Stress management	Relaxation/ meditation Self-care Yoga	Group format	'Care for the Professional Caregiver' programme. Discussions in the morning about: grief, short- and long-term consequences of burnout and self-care strategies. Experiential in the afternoon: relaxation, guided imagery, body movement and mindful breathing.
Hilliard (2006)	Stress management/ music therapy	Relaxation Coping skills Cultivating compassion	Group format Team building	Group 1: Ecological instrumental music therapy approach with open, structure-free format, with encouragement for toning and chanting. Group 2: A didactic music therapy approach with a structured format wherein interventions were planned and facilitated by the music therapist *a priori*. Such interventions included guided meditation with live music, lyric analyses, and music and movement. Each group began with breathing exercises paired with live music.
Potash (2015)	Stress management/art therapy	Self-regulation of emotions	Group format Encourage staff to voice feelings	6-week art therapy-based supervision group specifically addressed three broad areas: self-care and stress management, case sharing and clinical skills, and grief and bereavement.

(Continued)

Table 19.2 (Continued)

Study	Interventions	Individual strategies	Organisational strategies	Interventions
EDUCATION				
Rogers (2008)	Education	Knowledge in PC	Group format	Training sessions to increase comfort level with dying children. Modified version of the ELNEC and IPPC programmes. Pain/symptom management, ethical/legal issues, communication/ culture, spirituality/anxiety issues at end of life, prevention and compassion.
Melo and Oliver (2011)	Education + practical exercises	Introspection/ death anxiety Communication skills	Group format	1st module: group therapy for personal introspection on death anxiety. 2nd module: theoretical infomation and practical exercises to improve communication skills and understand dying patients' spiritual and psychological needs
Whitehead (2010)	Education	Knowledge in PC	Group format Ongoing education opportunities	ELNEC training programme.
Wessel (2005)	Education + narrative exercises	Knowledge in PC	Group format	Ethics issues resolving, communication techniques, issues of spirituality, grief, and bereavement. Narrative exercises.
MEANING-BASED COPING				
Fillion (2009)	Meaning-centred therapy (MCI) (didactics + experiential + coping)	Meaningful choices/actions Sharing experiences Coping	Group format Encourage staff to voice feelings and share experiences	Logotherapy based on Frankl. Four weekly sessions of half-day or two full days. The topics include: (a) characteristics of meaning at work; (b) sources of meaning and clarification of values; (c) creative values explored in terms of personal historical perspective (intention to be a nurse) and a sense of accomplishment at work (benefits of working in PC); (d) suffering, attitudinal change and presence; (e) affective experiences and humour. Participants are encouraged to find meaning in their work in cultivating presence and making meaningful choices and actions based on personal and organisational values.

Table 19.2 (*Continued*)

Study	Interventions	Individual strategies	Organisational strategies	Interventions
McPherson (2008)	Storytelling	Meaning-making coping Benefits finding	Group format	Peer-supported storytelling for grieving paediatric oncology nurses.
Wasner (2005)	Spiritual care (didactics+ experiential)	Cultivate compassion	Workshops on spiritual care	'Wisdom and Compassion in Care for the Dying' including: active and compassionate listening, recognition of and dealing with emotional and spiritual suffering, contemplation and meditation.
Meredith (2010)	Spiritual care (experiential)	Meaning-making	Workshops on spiritual care	Poems, music, quotes, movie clips, interviews, reflection journal and photo montages about spirituality.
Rushton (2009)	BWD programme (experiential exercises + meditation)	Quality of attention Compassion Self-care Mindfulness	One-week retreat often suggested by organisation	Being with dying (BWD) – Integrative approaches to dying and death; ethical, spiritual, psychological, and social aspects of care of the dying; application of contemplative practices to the care of the dying, their families, and professional caregivers; community-building around dying people and relationship-centred care; cross-cultural issues related to dying; exploration of pain, suffering, and peri-death phenomena; care of the caregiver; integration of psychosocial and spiritual content into conventional medical settings.
MINDFULNESS				
Cohen-Katz (2005)	MBSR programme	Meditation Communication skills, didactics, Coping skills	Group format	An 8-week programme; 2.5 hours/week; + 6 hours daily retreat; mindfulness-based stress reduction (MBSR) meditation, formal didactic instructions, communication skill, stress reactivity, self-compassion and experiential exercises (developed by J. Kabat-Zinn).
Gerhart (2016)	ACCEPTS Mindfulness and others	Mindfulness Self-regulation of emotion Communication	Group format	Formal meditation practices, communication role plays, and value clarification exercises. Group format, improve communication, engage with peers, didactics about death and values.

(Continued)

Table 19.2 (Continued)

Study	Interventions	Individual strategies	Organisational strategies	Interventions
Hevezi (2015)	Meditation	Self-regulation – Meditation – Cultivating compassion		Specific meditations (with an audio-CD) designed to establish a sense of calm, relaxation, and self-compassion, 5 days/week for 4 weeks. An educational PowerPoint with terms description and an author-made audio CD are given to participants. Content of the CD: 4-minute mindful breathing technique for immediate stress reduction, 8-minute breathing meditation for relaxation and 4 minutes designed to cultivate self-compassion.
McKenzie (2006)	Brief MBSR	– Mindfulness + coping skills	Group format-session offered six times/week	Shortened version of MBSR programme. Four 30-minute group sessions including didactics and experiential exercises. Audio-guided meditations on CD, instructed to practise at least 10 mins/day, 5 days/week. Manual that summarized key points.
Moody (2013)	Mindfulness (adapted from MBSR)	– Meditation – Communication skills – Self-care – Compassion	Group format	Mindfulness-based course (MBC): Didactic material topics included cultivating awareness of body sensations, thoughts, and emotions during pleasant and unpleasant events, identifying perceptual biases and filters, exploring individual reactivity to stress, reflecting on meaningful experiences and practice, training in skilful listening and communication and exploring self-care. A total of 15 hours (6 hours intro; six weekly 1-hour sessions and one 3-hour final session), co-leaded by MBSR clinicians.

is related to lack of efficacy or reduced personal accomplishment. Mismatches often indicate that individuals have insufficient control over the resources necessary to do their work, or insufficient authority to pursue the work in what they believe is the best manner. How can autonomy and rewards of accomplishment be activated?

One of our previous qualitative studies described how the perception of being able to make a difference for a person and a family at the end of life was a personal reward for nurses providing palliative care (Fillion and Saint Laurent 2003). Meaning-based coping interventions that develop decision-making processes and the capacity to make meaningful choices and actions according to values can increase feelings of choice and control. Similarly, support groups that clarify and facilitate the expression of personal needs, and educational interventions that improve communication and assertiveness skills, constitute other examples of strategies to improve autonomy and a sense of accomplishment (see Table 19.2). This may even include looking for other jobs which are offering more benefits, particularly when the work conditions also conflict with one's own values.

Workload or the intensity of work

Work intensity is expressed in terms of psychosocial risk factors through concepts such as those of 'psychological demands' or 'effort'. Perceptions of a heavy workload may arise when the sense of responsibility becomes overwhelming, obscuring the sense of self and losing the boundaries necessary for healthy professional and personal relationships (Weissman 2011). In contrast, experiencing 'flow' or a state of absorption in which one's abilities match the demands, describes the fluid process of creative effort and is characterised by an intense concentration, a feeling of there being the perfect level of challenge (neither being bored nor overwhelmed), and a sense of time flying (Csikszentmihalyi 1998).

The mismatch is often observed when workload and lack of resources interfere with the quality of work. Excessive workload exhausts the individual to the extent that recovery becomes difficult. Direct patient care activities have an impact on stress through a heavy workload of complex care, a shortage of staff, and a feeling of lack of competence (van Staa et al. 2000). In the palliative care literature on interventions on burnout, we noticed few interventions to deal with workload.

Safety and justice

The last axis refers to safety and justice. This includes economic uncertainty, unexpected change in tasks or working conditions. Economic insecurity can come from the risk of losing one's job, the associated income reduction, or loss of benefits observed in a more 'normal' career pathway. Working conditions can also generate other safety and justice issues. The concept of justice can be seen as being related to the issues of 'values', 'fairness', and 'community' in burnout. As the individual does not feel integrated into the community, perceptions of unfairness or injustice and uncertainty about the future may emerge.

A mismatch occurs when economic and personal safety may be compromised or when the individual feels outside the favoured group. For example, nurses working in a hospice in South Africa were uncomfortable going into some settings, particularly at night. As a group, they explored with the administration the option of refusing to go into some areas.

Brainstorming together, the nurses suggested working with the police when the nurses were going into a potentially dangerous situation. The nurses asked the police to accompany them if they were uncomfortable visiting certain areas but felt they should visit for the sake of the patient (Vachon 2001). As for the previous axis, it appears that there is a paucity of interventions to deal with safety/justice issues in palliative care domains.

Interventions to decrease occupational risk factors in healthcare settings

This section briefly describes a variety of interventions to prevent burnout grouped into five categories: (1) support groups; (2) stress management; (3) education; (4) meaning-based coping; and (5) mindfulness. Most of the interventions are designed at the individual level, although the interventions often use a group format. A brief description of strategies and content is provided in Table 19.2.

Support groups

Many hospices and palliative care units offer staff support groups. Support groups allow clinicians to share work-related affective experiences and discuss the clinical management of patients. Support groups could also be offered to discuss bereavement issues and timely critical incidents. For instance, Keene et al. (2010) proposed a structured format for conducting bereavement debriefing sessions. Bereavement debriefing sessions were offered most frequently after unexpected deaths or deaths of long term patients.

Combining staff support groups with a participatory action research approach, Le Blanc et al. (2007) conducted a quasi-experimental study among staff of oncology wards on the effects of a team-based burnout intervention programme. Staff in the experimental wards experienced less emotional exhaustion and less depersonalisation, compared with the control wards. Changes in burnout levels were significantly related to changes in the perception of the job characteristics over time.

Stress management

To deal with emotional demands and increase coping and resilience skills, stress management programmes, sometimes called self-care or resilience interventions, are often suggested. A meta-analysis of 48 occupational stress-reducing interventions (van der Klink et al. 2001) described that cognitive-behavioural therapy (CBT) appears to be the most effective strategy in improving perceived quality of work life, enhancing psychological resources and responses and reducing complaints. Similarly, a recent Cochrane systematic review (Ruotsalainen et al. 2015) concluded that CBT as well as mental and physical relaxation all reduce stress in healthcare workers. Also in the domain of oncology, Mimura and Griffiths (2003) conducted a systematic review of the literature addressing nursing stress management. The results indicate that the self-care programme components that appear to be effective include relaxation training, social support, cognitive techniques, exercise, and music.

Education

Educational interventions aim at enhancing job competences, often focused on communication skills training. A meta-analysis on communication training in oncology settings showed a moderate effect on communication skills (Barth and Lannen 2001). Although useful to improve communication skills, reviews of the impact of this training on burnout have reached varied conclusions, with a recent review finding inadequate evidence to support a positive impact of this training on clinicians' burnout (Moore et al. 2013).

Similarly, an educational intervention responding to the moral distress of neonatal nurses and provided by hospital ethics committee members and hospice specialists was evaluated by Rogers et al. (2008). Only an improvement on ethical/legal issues and symptom management knowledge was observed from pre- to post-test. Whitehead et al. (2010) evaluated the impact of the End-of-life Nursing Education Consortium (ELNEC) at the Institutional Level on death anxiety, concerns about dying and knowledge of the dying process. Participants improved their knowledge of the dying process at post-test and 12-months follow-up. However, no differences were noted on death anxiety and concerns about dying, suggesting that education alone on palliative care competencies is not enough to decrease emotional demands.

When education is combined with reflective practices, a positive impact could be observed on clinicians' well-being. For instance, the impact of a 6-day course for clinicians that provided training in communication and in introspection on death anxiety was evaluated with a pre- and post-intervention design by Melo and Olivier (2011). Results show a reduction in burnout and death anxiety, and an increase in personal well-being and professional fulfilment. Similarly, combining palliative care education and writing a reflective end of life narrative seems to improve outcomes related to death and dying (Wessel and Rutledge 2005). Both studies suggest the combination of education (didactics) with experiential exercises as a way to improve emotional outcomes.

Meaning-based coping

The workplace positive elements (i.e. rewards and benefits) could stimulate clinicians to find meaning in their work and, consequently, enhance their well-being and job satisfaction (Fillion et al. 2007). A meaning-centred intervention (MCI), combining didactic and process-oriented strategies, was tested to address emotional demands and existential issues (Fillion et al. 2009). Palliative care nurses in the experimental group reported more perceived benefits of working in palliative care after the intervention and at follow-up. A subsequent qualitative study demonstrated that MCI expanded nurses' spiritual and existential awareness by increasing their awareness of life's finiteness, opening them up to new meanings and purposes of suffering, having them become more aware of sources of meaning and purpose in life, and by having them access a state of mindfulness (Vachon et al. 2011).

Focusing on spiritual care as a broad concept, as opposed to as a religious interpretation, two studies combined education and spiritual workshops. Wasner et al. (2005) evaluated the effects of spiritual care training for clinicians on spiritual quality of life, self-transcendence and level of religiosity. Spirituality increased significantly after the training and was still present after 6 months. Self-transcendence increased significantly after the training but not after 6 months. Level of religiosity did not change significantly over time. In the second study (Meridith et al., 2010), the Spirituality in Palliative Care Training Package enabled increases in spirituality, spiritual care, and confidence in providing spiritual care.

Likewise, targeting palliative care staff, an in-depth intervention called Being with Dying (BWD) is based on the development of mindfulness and receptive attention through contemplative practice. Four main themes emerged: the power of presence, cultivating balanced compassion, recognising grief, and the importance of self-care. The interviewees considered BWD's contemplative and reflective practices to be meaningful, useful, and valuable and reported that BWD provided skills, attitudes, behaviours, and tools to change how they worked with the dying and bereaved (Rushton et al. 2009).

Mindfulness

Other studies conducted with healthcare providers are giving some support to the usefulness of mindfulness in the context of palliative care. Rooted in Buddhism, mindfulness-based stress reduction (MBSR) is a structured therapy package combining mindfulness-based meditation with yoga. It consists of an 8-week course in which participants meet once a week for a 2.5-hour session and one 8-hour day (Praissman, 2008; Irving, Dobkin, and Park, 2009). It has been found to have an effect on exhaustion and depersonalisation when part of a multifaceted strategy including organisational components, such as forming a nursing advisory council, enhancing a model of shared governance, and increasing opportunities for education and professional development (Cohen-Katz et al. 2005).

Shorter (less than 10 minutes) structured meditations may increase compassion satisfaction, decrease burnout and secondary trauma (Hevezi 2016), and a brief MBSR format may improve burnout symptoms, relaxation and life satisfaction (McKenzie et al. 2006). In both cases, the authors conclude that mindfulness training is a promising method for helping those in the nursing profession to manage stress and prevent burnout, even when provided in a brief format. However, one pilot study using a brief format of mindfulness-based intervention failed to show any effects of the training on burnout, perceived stress, or depression (Moody et al. 2013). The authors explained the lack of benefits by the severity of the stress in their sample. Some of the participants even found that the intervention added stress to their day by requiring them to carry out another task. The authors of the study conclude by emphasising the need to revise the intervention in integrating a multimodal component, notably death and dying issues, and caregiver feelings of failure. In addition to individual resilience, organisational factors should also be addressed.

A literature review on burnout interventions conducted by Awa et al. (2010) revealed that 68 per cent were person-directed interventions, 8 per cent were organisation-directed and 24 per cent were a combination of both intervention types. Eighty per cent of all programmes led to a reduction in burnout. Person-directed interventions reduced burnout in the short term (6 months or less), while a combination of both person- and organisation-directed interventions had longer-lasting positive effects (12 months and over). In all cases, positive intervention effects diminished in the course of time. Institutions should recognise the need for and make burnout intervention available (see Box 19.3).

Box 19.3   Implications for nursing practice

- Help prevent or correct palliative care nursing burnout by knowing the importance of psychosocial risk factors and what can be done at the individual and organisational level.
- At the individual level, nurses from their initial training should become aware of the stress process and their own stress vulnerabilities. Ideally, they have to learn to transform stress reactions into resilience in learning how to respond more adequately. This involves personal development and emotional coping. They can be invited to seek out emotional support and healthy programmes where they can develop a repertoire of coping strategies, resilience skills and self-care activities. Learning mindfulness meditation techniques in their initial education can be helpful.
- At the organisation level, organisations are encouraged to implement support interventions, such as support groups, retreats, or other activities creating space to share experiences and emotions. In addition to emotional demands, the social climate and other risk factors have to be considered. Team building, interdisciplinary support and help to manage conflicts are important as well as emotional support. Furthermore, having a definition of clear values and ethical consultation services is essential.

Conclusion

Most interventions developed for nurses target specific components to increase individual resilience to stress. The integration of organisational components still appears limited. Being aware of the lack of tested interventions integrating organisational and individual factors, we have been conscious of presenting a variety of key ingredients that can be combined. The choice of components is important and may depend on the needs of the targeted units.

Learning exercise 19.1

You are a nurse in charge of a busy palliative care in-patient unit. Things have been difficult recently, as well as the recent deaths of some patients which the staff found clinically challenging, your organisation is also about to implement some changes which the nursing staff are finding difficult, including a new rostering and shift system and new nursing paperwork. Your staff are starting to be concerned about how they will cope. Think about:

- What are the issues here which may contribute to stress or burnout?
- Where does responsibility lie for addressing issues (tip: they may not all be your responsibility).
- Are there any interventions you would suggest to reduce workplace stress, and why do you think they may be effective?

References

Awa, W.L., Plaumann, M. and Walter, U. (2010) Burnout prevention: a review of intervention programs. *Patient Education and Counseling*, 78(2): 184–90. doi: 10.1016/j.pec.2009.04.008

Aycock, N. and Boyle, D. (2009) Interventions to manage compassion fatigue in oncology nursing. *Clinical Journal of Oncology Nursing*, 13(2): 183–91. doi: 10.1188/09.CJON.183–191

Back, A.L., Steinhauser, K.E., Kamil, A.H. and Jackson, V.A. (2016) Building resilience for palliative care clinicians: an approach to burnout prevention based on individual skills and workplace factors. *Journal of Pain and Symptom Management*, 52(2): 284–91. doi: 10.1016/j.jpainsymman.2016.02.002.

Barth, J. and Lannen, P. (2001) Efficacy of communication skills training courses in oncology: a systematic review and meta-analysis. *Annals of Oncology*, 22(5): 1030–40. doi: 10.1093/annonc/mdq441.

Bush, N.J. (2009) Compassion fatigue: are you at risk? *Oncology Nursing Forum*, 36: 24–8. doi:10.1188/09.ONF.24–28.

Cohen-Katz, J., Wiley, S., Capuano, T. et al. (2005) The effects of mindfulness-based stress reduction on nurse stress and burnout: a qualitative and quantitative study, Part III. *Holistic Nursing Practice*, 19(2): 78–86.

Collège d'expertise sur le suivi des risques psychosociaux au travail (2011) *Mesurer les facteurs psychosociaux de risque au travail pour les maîtriser*. Available at: www.college-risquespsychosociaux-travail.fr. Published April 2011 (accessed November 2015).

Cox, T., Griffiths, A. and Rial-Gonzalez, E. (2000) *Research on Work-Related Stress*. Luxembourg: European Agency for Safety and Health at Work; Office for Official Publications for the European Communities.

Csikszentmihalyi, M. (1998) *Finding Flow: The Psychology of Engagement with Every-day Life*. New York: Basic Books.

Day, A. and Hurrell, J.J. (2014) Building a foundation for psychologically healthy workplaces and well-being. In Day, A., Kelloway, E.K. and Hurrell, JJ. (eds) *Workplace Well-being: How to Build Psychologically Healthy Workplaces*. Chichester: John Wiley and Sons, Ltd.

Desbiens, J.F. and Fillion, L. (2007) Coping strategies, emotional outcomes and spiritual quality of life among palliative care nurses. *International Journal of Palliative Nursing*, 13(6): 291–300.

Duffy, R.D., Dik, B.J. and Steger, M.F. (2011) Calling and work-related outcomes: career commitment as a mediator. *Journal of Vocational Behavior*, 78(2): 210–18. doi: 10.1016/j.jvb.2010.09.013.

Dyrbye, L.N., Massie, S., Eacker, A. et al. (2010) Relationship between burnout and professional conduct and attitudes among US medical students. *JAMA*, 304(11): 1171–80.

Edmonds, C., Lockwood, G.M., Bezjak, A. and Nyhof-Young, J. (2012) Alleviating emotional exhaustion in oncology nurses: an evaluation of Wellspring's 'Care for the Professional Caregiver Program'. *Journal of Cancer Education*, 27(1): 27–36. doi: 10.1007/s13187-011-0278-z.

Epstein, R.M. and Krasner, M.S. (2013) Physician resilience: what it means, why it it matters, and how to promote it. *Academic Medicine*, 88: 301–3. doi: 10.1097/ACM.0b013e318280cff0.

Feld, J. and Heyse-Moore, L. (2006) An evaluation of a support group for junior doctors working in palliative medicine. *American Journal of Hospice and Palliative Medicine*, 23(4): 287–96. doi: 10.1177/1049909106290717.

Figley, C.R. (ed.) (2002) *Treating Compassion Fatigue*. New York: Brunner-Routledge.

Fillion, L., Desbiens, J.F., Truchon, M. et al. (2011) Le stress au travail chez les infirmières en soins palliatifs de fin de vie selon le milieu de pratique. *Psycho-Oncologie*, 5(2): 127–36.

Fillion, L., Dupuis, R., Tremblay, I. et al. (2006) Enhancing meaning in palliative care practice: a meaning-centered intervention to promote job satisfaction. *Palliative Support Care*, 4: 333–44.

Fillion, L., Duval, S., Dumont, S. et al. (2009) Impact of a meaning-centered intervention on job satisfaction and on quality of life among palliative care nurses. *Psycho-Oncology*, 18: 1300–10.

Fillion, L. and Saint-Laurent, L. (2003) Les conditions favorables liées à la pratique infirmière en soins palliatifs: les points de vue des infirmières. *Les Cahiers de Soins Palliatifs*, 4(2): 5–42.

Fillion, L., Tremblay, I., Truchon, M. et al. (2007) Job satisfaction and emotional distress among nurses providing palliative care: empirical evidence for an integrative occupational stress-model. *International Journal of Stress Management*, 14(1): 1–25. doi: 10.1037/1072-5245.14.1.1.

Fillion, L., Truchon, M., L'Heureux, M. et al. (2014) *Impact of Work Environment on Nurses' Job Satisfaction and Well-Being: Improving End-of-Life Care and Services*. Final report. Montreal: IRSST. Available at: http://www.irsst.qc.ca/publications-et-outils/publication/i/100782/n/work-environment-on-nurses-job-r-846 (accessed November 2015).

Gerhart, J., O'Mahony, S., Abrams, I. et al. (2016) A pilot test of a mindfulness-based communication training to enhance resilience in palliative care professionals. *Journal of Contextual Behavioral Science*, 5(2): 89–96. doi: 10.1016/j.jcbs.2016.04.003.

Halifax, J. (2013) Understanding and cultivating compassion in clinical settings: the A.B.I.D.E. compassion model. In Singer, T. and Bolz, M. (eds) *Compassion: Bridging Practice and Science*. ebook. Munich: Max Planck Society, pp. 208–26,

Henry, B.J. (2014) Nursing burnout interventions: what is being done? *Clinical Journal of Oncology Nursing*, 18(2): 211–14.

Hevezi, J.A. (2016) Evaluation of a meditation intervention to reduce the effects of stressors associated with compassion fatigue among nurses. *Journal of Holistic Nursing*, 34(4): 343–50. doi: 10.1177/0898010115615981.

Hilliard, R.E. (2006) The effect of music therapy sessions on compassion fatigue and team building of professional hospice caregivers. *The Arts in Psychotherapy*, 33(5): 395–401. doi: 10.1016/j.aip.2006.06.002.

Hospice Friendly Hospitals Program (2013) *End-of-Life Care and Supporting Staff: A Literature Review*. Available at: http://hospicefoundation.ie/wp-content/uploads/2013/04/End-of-Life-Care-Supporting-Staff-a-literature-review.pdf (accessed August 2016).

Huggard, J. (2008) A national survey of the support needs of interprofessional hospice staff in Aotearoa/New Zealand. Unpublished Master's thesis, University of Auckland, Auckland, New Zealand.

Huggard, J. and Nichols, J. (2011) Emotional safety in the workplace: one hospice's response for effective support. *International Journal of Palliative Nursing*, 17(12): 611–17. doi: 10.12968/iipn.2011.17.12.611.

Huggard, P.K., Stamm, B.H. and Pearlman, L.A. (2013) Physician stress: compassion satisfaction, compassion fatigue and vicarious traumatization. In Figley, C.R., Huggard, P.K. and Rees C. (eds) *First Do No Self-Harm*. New York: Oxford University Press, pp. 127–45.

Irving, J.A., Dobkin, P.L and Park, J. (2009) Cultivating mindfulness in health care professionals: a review of empirical studies of mindfulness-based stress reduction (MBSR). *Complementary Therapies in Clinical Practice*, 15(2): 61–6. doi: 10.1016/j.ctcp.2009.01.002.

Keene, E.A., Hutton, N., Hall, B. and Rushton, C. (2010) Bereavement debriefing sessions: an intervention to support health care professionals in managing their grief after the death of a patient. *Pediatric Nursing*, 36(4): 185–9.

Kerney, M.K., Weininger, R.B., Vachon, M.L.S. et al. (2009) Self-care of physicians caring for patients at the end of life. *JAMA*, 301(11): 1155–64. doi: 10.1001/jama.2009.352.

Klimecki, O. and Singer, T. (2012) Empathic distress fatigue rather than compassion fatigue? Integrating findings from empathy research in psychology and social neuroscience. In Oakley, B., Knafo, A., Madhavan, G. and Wilson, D.S. (eds) *Pathological Altruism*. New York: Oxford University Press, pp. 368–83.

Klimecki, O., Ricard, M. and Singer, T. (2013) Empathy versus compassion: lessons from the 1st and 3rd person methods. In Singer, T. and Bolz, M. (eds) *Compassion: Bridging Practice and Science*. eBook: Munich: Max Planck Society, pp. 272–87.

Koh, M.Y., Chong, P.H., Neo, P.S.H. et al. (2015) Burnout, psychological morbidity and use of coping mechanisms among palliative care practitioners: a multi-centre cross-sectional study. *Palliative Medicine*, 29: 633–42.

Kravit, K., McAllister-Black, R., Grant, M. and Kirk, C. (2010) Self-care strategies for nurses: a psycho-educational intervention for stress reduction and the prevention of burnout. *Applied Nursing Research*, 23(3): 130–8. doi: 10.1016/j.apnr.2008.08.002.

Lazarus, R.S. and Folkman, S. (eds) (1984) *Stress, Appraisal and Coping*. New York: Springer Publishing Company.

Le Blanc, P.M., Hox, J.J., Schaufeli, W.B. et al. (2007) Take care! The evaluation of a team-based burnout intervention program for oncology care providers. *Journal of Applied Psychology*, 92(1): 213–27. doi: 10.1037/0021-9010.92.1.213.

Leiter, M. and Maslach, C. (2004) Areas of worklife: a structural approach to organizational predictors of job burnout. In Perrewe, P. and Ganster, D. (eds) *Research in Occupational Stress and Well Being*, vol. 3, *Emotional and Physiological Processes and Positive Intervention Strategies*. Oxford: JAI Press/Elsevier, pp. 91–134.

Macpherson, C.F. (2008) Peer-supported storytelling for grieving pediatric oncology nurses. *Journal of Pediatric Oncology Nursing*, 25(3): 148–63. doi: 10.1177/1043454208317236.

Maslach, C. (2011) Engagement research: some thoughts from a burnout perspective. *European Journal of Work and Organizational Psychology*, 20(1): 47–52.

Maslach, C., Schaufeli, W.B. and Leiter, M.P. (2001) Job burnout. *Annual Review of Psychology*, 52: 397–422.

McKenzie, C.S., Poulin, P. and Seidman-Carlson, R. (2006) A brief mindfulness-based stress reduction intervention for nurses and nurse aides. *Applied Nursing Research*, 19: 105–9.

Melo, C.G. and Olivier, D. (2011) Can addressing death anxiety reduce health care workers' burnout and improve patient care? *Journal of Palliative Care*, 27(4): 287–95.

Meredith, P., Murray, J., Wilson, T. et al. (2010) Can spirituality be taught to health care professionals? *Journal of Religion and Health*, 51(3): 879–89. doi: 10.1007/s10943-010-9399-7.

Mimura, C. and Griffiths, P. (2003) The effectiveness of current approaches to work place stress management in the nursing profession: an evidence based literature review. *Occupational and Environmental Medicine*, 60(1): 10–15.

Moody, K., Kramer, D., Santizo, R. et al. (2013) Helping the helpers: mindfulness training for burnout in pediatric oncology: a pilot program. *Journal of Pediatric Oncology Nursing*, 30(5): 275–84. doi: 10.1177/104345421350449.

Moore, P.M., Rivera Mercado, S., Grez Artigues, M. and Lawrie, T.A. (2013) Communication skills training for healthcare professionals working with people who have cancer. *Cochrane Database of Systematic Reviews*, 3: CD003751. doi: 10.1002/14651858.CD003751.pub3.

Morin, E. (2008) *The Meaning of Work, Mental Health and Organizational Commitment*. Montréal: IRSST. Available at: http://www.irsst.qc.ca/publications-et-outils/publication/i/100415/n/sens-du-travail-sante-mentale-et-engagement-organisationnel-r-585 (accessed November 2015).

Nathaniel, A. (2002) Moral distress among nurses. *American Nurses Association Ethics and Human Rights Issues Updates*, 1(3a).

Payne, N. (2001) Occupational stressors and coping as determinants of burnout in female hospice nurses. *Journal of Advanced Nursing*, 33(3): 396–405. doi: 10.1046/j.1365-2648.2001.01677.x.

Potash, J.S., Chan, F., Ho, A.H.Y. et al. (2015) A model for art therapy-based supervision for end-of-life care workers in Hong Kong. *Death Studies*, 39(1): 44–51. doi: 10.1080/07481187.2013.859187.

Praissman, S. (2008) Mindfulness-based stress reduction: a literature review and clinician's guide. *Journal of the American Academy of Nurse Practitioners*, 20(4): 212–16. doi: 10.1111/j.1745-7599.2008.00306.x.

Rogers, S., Badgi. A. and Gomez, C. (2008) Educational interventions in end-of-life care: part 1: an educational intervention responding to the moral distress of NICU nurses provided by an ethics consultation team. *Advances in Neonatal Care*, 8(1): 56–65. doi: 10.1097/01.ANC.0000311017.02005.20.

Ruotsalainen, J., Verbeek, J., Marine, A. and Serra, C. (2015) Preventing occupational stress in healthcare workers. *Cochrane Database of Systematic Reviews*, 4: CD002892. doi: 10.1002/14651858.CD002892.pub5.

Rushton, C.H., Reder, E., Hall, B. et al. (2006) Interdisciplinary interventions to improve pediatric palliative care and reduce health care professional suffering. *Journal of Palliative Medicine*, 9(4): 922–33. doi: 10.1089/jpm.2006.9.922.

Rushton, C.H., Sellers, D.E., Heller, K.S. et al. (2009) Impact of a contemplative end-of-life training program: being with dying. *Palliative and Supportive Care*, 7(4): 405–14. doi: 10.1017/s1478951509990411.

Sands, S.A., Stanley, P. and Charon, R. (2008) Pediatric narrative oncology: interprofessional training to promote empathy, build teams, and prevent burnout. *Journal of Supportive Oncology*, 6(7): 307–12.

Shanafelt, T. and Dyrbye, L. (2012) Oncologist burnout: causes, consequences and responses. *Journal of Clinical Oncology*, 30(11): 1235–41.

Shanafelt, T., Chung, H., White, H. and Lyckholm, L.J. (2006) Shaping your career to maximize personal satisfaction in the practice of oncology. *Journal of Clinical Oncology*, 24(24): 4020–6. doi: 10.1200/JCO.2006.05.8248.

Vachon, M.L.S. (1999) Reflections on the history of occupational stress in hospice/palliative care. *The Hospice Journal*, 14(3–4): 229–46.

Vachon, M.L.S. (2001) The nurse's role: the world of palliative care nursing. In Ferrell, N. and Coyle, N. (eds) *The Oxford Textbook of Palliative Nursing*. New York: Oxford University Press, pp. 647–62.

Vachon, M.L.S. (2011) Four decades of selected research in hospice/palliative care: have the stressors changed? In Renzenbrink, I. (ed.) *Caregiver Stress and Staff Support in Illness, Dying, and Bereavement*. Oxford: Oxford University Press, pp. 1–24.

Vachon, M.L.S. and Fillion, L. (2015) Staff stress and burnout in palliative care. In Bruera, E., Higginson, I.J., von Gunten, C.F. and Morita, T. (eds) *Textbook of Palliative Medicine* (2nd edn). London: Hodder Arnold, pp. 1033–46.

Vachon, M., Fillion, L., Achille, M. et al. (2011) An awakening experience: an interpretive phenomenological analysis of the effects of a meaning-centered intervention shared amongst palliative care nurses. *Qualitative Research in Psychology*, 8, 66–80.

Vachon, M.L.S. and Harris, D. (2016) The liberating capacity of compassion. In Harris, D. and Bordere, T. (eds) *Handbook of Social Justice in Loss and Grief.* New York: Routledge, pp. 265–81.

Vachon, M.L.S., Huggard, P.K. and Huggard, J. (2015) Reflections on occupational stress in palliative care nursing: is it changing? In Ferrell, B., Coyle, N. and Paice, J. (eds) *Oxford Textbook of Palliative Nursing* (4th edn). New York: Oxford University Press, pp. 969–86. doi: 10.1093/med/9780199332342.003.0064.

van der Klink, J.J.L., Blonk, R.W.B., Schene, A.H. and van Dijk, F.J.H. (2001) The benefits of intervention for work-related stress. *American Journal of Public Health*, 91(2): 270–6.

van Staa, A.L., Visser, A. and van der Zouwe, N. (2000) Caring for caregivers: experiences and evaluation of interventions for a palliative care team. *Patient Education and Counseling*, 41(1): 93–105.

Verhaeghe, R., Mak, R., Van Maele, G. et al. (2004) Job stress among middle-aged health care workers and its relation to sickness absence. *Stress and Health*, 19(5): 265–74.

Wasner, M., Longaker C., Feqq, M.J. and Borasio, G.D. (2005) Effects of spiritual care training for palliative care professionals. *Palliative Medicine*, 19(2): 99–104.

Weissman, D. (2011) Martyrs in palliative care. *Journal of Palliative Medicine*, 14(12): 1278–9. doi: 10.1089/jpm.2011.0293.

Wessel, E.M. and Rutledge, D.N. (2005) Home care and hospice nurses' attitude toward death and caring for the dying. *Journal of Hospice and Palliative Nursing*, 7(4): 212–17.

Whitehead, P.B., Anderson, E.S., Redican, K.J. and Stratton, R. (2010) Studying the effects of the End-of-Life Nursing Education Consortium at the institutional level. *Journal of Hospice and Palliative Care Nursing*, 12(3): 184–93.

Wrzesniewski, A., McCauley, C., Rozin, P. and Schwartz, B. (1997) Jobs, careers, and callings: people's relations to their work. *Journal of Research in Personality*, 31(1): 21–33.

Zwack, J. and Schweitzer, J. (2013) If every fifth physician is affected by burnout, what about the other four? Resilience strategies of experienced physicians. *Academic Medicine*, 88: 382–9. doi: 10.1097/ACM.0b013e318281696b.

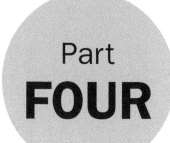

Part
FOUR

CHALLENGING ISSUES IN PALLIATIVE CARE NURSING

Introduction to Part Four

Nancy Preston

Palliative care has developed considerably over the last 20 years. But as care evolves further, staff will face new challenges. In Part Four, we look at some of the areas where change is happening or where it needs to happen and will consider the response palliative care nurses may make to it.

The decisions we make in regards to how we want to live our lives right up until the very end are important, and, in palliative care, advance care planning has been crucial to helping people gain a voice to express the type of care they wish to have. In Chapter 20, Philomena Swarbrick and Gary Rycroft discuss the issues around advance care planning, including what it means to the individual and to nurses caring for people who may want to share their views with both family and other carers including nurses. The legal ramifications of these kinds of situations are explained, including what happens when we lose competence. Advance care planning is recommended as an integral part of the UK's End of Life Care Strategy (Department of Health 2008), and while there is a growing evidence base to support its use, we need to look to research to see what the benefits to patients, their carers and the health service are in practice, and importantly how and who we should approach (Rietjens et al. 2016).

In some countries, legislation permits different forms of assisted dying, including euthanasia and physician-assisted suicide. In Chapter 21, Deborah Lewis, Sheri Mila Gerson and Claudia Gamondi explain the different systems from a range of countries which support the use of some form of assisted dying, and look at the place of palliative care particularly in systems where palliative care works alongside assisted dying practices. Palliative care has an uneasy relationship with any form of assisted dying, particularly in the UK, and this is also reflected in position statements from palliative care organisations such as the European Association of Palliative Care (Radbruch et al. 2016) and the International Association of Hospice and Palliative Care (De Lima et al. 2017). While not legal in the UK, we know that British people do use clinics such as Dignitas in Switzerland. Nurses need to know how to respond in these situations; whether it is by having a conversation on this topic themselves with the patient and their family or recognising the need to refer to others. As palliative care includes the bereaved, we need to consider our response to them too, which can be difficult particularly if the family feel the need to keep such actions a secret, and this may lead to feelings of isolation.

How we learn about and manage changes in palliative care is discussed by Laura Green and Sue Spencer in Chapter 22, which, together with John Costello's Chapter 23 on education, helps nurses establish how they might develop individually but also how nursing as an institution or within an institute might respond. With the growing reality that not everyone will receive specialist palliative care, the greater the need there is to educate generalists, as these are the nurses who will care for most people in their last year of life. Laura Green and Sue Spencer's chapter includes examples of how social media, for example, can be used to share knowledge and help to bring about change.

As a relatively new speciality, research into the clinical application of palliative care is still developing. Morag Farquhar and Jane Phillips write about these developments in Chapter 24. They draw on guidance such as the MORECare statement which suggests ways to design and conduct research (Higginson et al. 2013). Nurses have always been leaders in developing palliative care and examples of nurse-led clinically based research are given, including breathlessness clinics.

The final 'challenge' chapter looks at the development of palliative care worldwide but particularly from an African standpoint. Written by Richard Harding and Julia Downing, Chapter 25 is enhanced by co-authorship with Mackuline Atieno working in Africa. Challenges to palliative care delivery are highlighted, not least the large numbers of patients who present with advanced disease in Africa. New advances are being developed, for instance, in mobile health. This involves the use of mobile phones to share information with patients and between healthcare workers, similar to telemedicine in the UK.

These different chapters start to give an idea of the future for palliative care. Indeed, there is now research looking at different models of care which can be drawn on to develop palliative care, with den Herder-van der Eerden et al. (2017), for example, demonstrating that for patients to receive good continuity in their care, having a small number of trusted nurses working with a multi-disciplinary team is key. These researchers identified examples of best practice which showed good integration of palliative care services with other services. Crucial to this has been how information is shared and good information technology systems are crucial to this, to deliver a more streamlined approach. Palliative care in the UK is trying to change its model of care delivery which developed from cancer care. In countries starting to develop palliative care now, they can learn from our mistakes and hopefully will not get entrenched into palliative care only being for cancer patients.

How these ideas are incorporated into clinical practice is a further challenge. Following the media outcry after the difficulties faced using the Liverpool Care Pathway, palliative care has had to respond in a measured way and embrace the challenges of implementation research to ensure the advances that have been made can be consolidated. Palliative care nurses need some understanding of research to achieve this. A report by the Hospice Commission (Payne et al. 2013) gives examples of the ways hospices and other palliative care organisations might do this as we move forward into the new century.

References

De Lima, L., Woodruff, R., Pettus, K. et al. (2017) International Association for Hospice and Palliative Care Position Statement: Euthanasia and Physician-Assisted Suicide. *Journal of Palliative Medicine*, 20(1): 8–14.

den Herder-van der Eerden, M., Hasselaar, J., Payne, S. et al. (2017) How continuity of care is experienced within the context of integrated palliative care: a qualitative study with patients and family caregivers in five European countries. *Palliative Medicine*, 31(10): 946–55.

Department of Health (2008) *End of Life Care Strategy: Promoting High Quality for All at the End of Life*. London: Department of Health.

Higginson, I.J., Evans, C.J., Grande, G. et al. (2013) Evaluating complex interventions in end of life care: the MORECare statement on good practice generated by a synthesis of transparent expert consultations and systematic reviews. *BMC Medicine*, 11: 111.

Payne, S., Preston, N., Turner, M. et al. (2013) *Research in Palliative Care: Can Hospices Afford Not to Be Involved? A Report for the Commission into the Future of Hospice Care*. London: Hospice UK.

Radbruch, L., Leget, C., Bahr, P. et al (2016) Euthanasia and physician-assisted suicide: a White Paper from the European Association for Palliative Care. *Palliative Medicine*, 30(2): 104–16.

Rietjens, J.A., Korfage, I.J., Dunleavy, L. et al. (2016) Advance care planning – a multi-centre cluster randomised clinical trial: the research protocol of the ACTION study. *BMC Cancer*, 16(1): 264.

Decision-making and capacity: principles relating to ethical issues in palliative care nursing

Philomena Swarbrick and Gary Rycroft

Introduction

Before the advancement of modern medical techniques in life-saving treatments that could be used both for palliation of symptoms and for the extension of life beyond what was previously viewed as natural, decisions concerning how to die were less complex. In this chapter, we will consider how advance care planning (ACP) has developed in the West as a response to the burgeoning interventions and treatment options (Emanuel 2000). This chapter will focus on ACP in England and Wales, exploring its components and explaining how the ethics of clinical decision-making at end of life are intertwined with the laws of these countries.

ACP has been legally supported in varying degrees in other countries across the West. The European Convention on Human Rights has enshrined the right to self-determination. But whereas in England and Wales Advanced Directives are legal, if written and witnessed correctly, in Scotland they have no statutory underpinning, but are legally binding under common law. (For more information on this and other countries, see IHF Perspectives 2016.)

The most quintessential ethical concerns for terminally ill patients would probably be thought of as those surrounding questions of euthanasia, physician-assisted suicide or suicide itself. These issues will be discussed in Chapter 21 of this volume, but it is notable here that the 'Living Will' movement (Kutner 1969), which sought to advise people on how to create expressed wishes around the mode of dying, and which can be regarded as the forerunner of what we now call ACP, began because its proponents wished to avoid the over-medicalisation of death and, furthermore, to support the notion of euthanasia as an autonomous right of the person. This, of course, is far from the emphasis of modern ACP in the UK.

Autonomy and its status as an ethical principle

The now commonly accepted four principles of medical bioethics are: autonomy, beneficence, non-maleficence and justice (Beauchamp and Childress 2013). Beneficence (doing good), non-maleficence (not doing harm) and justice (equal access to care for all) cannot always be used as stand-alone, overriding principles and as separate from one another, but must be weighed constantly against each other, and each can also be sidelined by other impinging factors. For instance, beneficence and non-maleficence are often placed in a balance where, for example, the harm caused by strong treatment, such as chemotherapy, is weighed against the hoped-for overall beneficence of the treatment in the long term. The principle of justice is regularly transgressed because financial considerations limit access to many beneficent procedures and treatments and, furthermore, often limit these in a patchwork manner even in those countries which claim to uphold the principle of justice (in its bioethical sense).

In contrast to these three principles, the principle of autonomy of the person has come to be upheld even more strongly today, particularly in the West where bioethical principles have been developed and argued (Corrigan 2003). In the more recent editions of their classical text, Beauchamp and Childress (2013) are at pains to point out that their original account of autonomy has been criticised as being seen to give to autonomy an overriding importance within the framework of the four principles. The philosopher Dworkin maintains that although it is important to respect a person's autonomy, there are other qualities to take account of: 'their welfare, or their liberty, or their rationality'(1988, p. 32). There appears therefore to be a move towards the perception of personal autonomy being just one of a number of qualities that a person could consider employing during decision-making. Nedelsky first described the feminist construct of 'relational autonomy' in 1989 (Mackenzie and Stoljar 2000). It criticises definitions of autonomy which appear structural and hierarchical and which rely on the idea of the rational intellect alone being able to reflect and deliberate on internal desires and spontaneous feelings and instead requires that all aspects of a person's psyche be given credence and become integrated within the concept of autonomy. Beauchamp and Childress (2013) have tempered their position of absolute personal autonomy saying that: 'Individuals autonomously accept moral notions that derive from cultural traditions.'

Acknowledgement should be given to the fact that our moral norms are decided largely by the setting in which we grow up and in which we are educated; our moral codes are likely to differ between countries, cultures, religions and families, but may also differ *within* these domains, depending on our interpretations and understandings as individuals. For a more detailed debate on the challenge to the autonomy argument, see Herring (2012, pp. 514–17).

Informed consent

The development of the importance of modern-day autonomy accelerated after the atrocious infringements against persons held captive by the Nazis in the Second World War, who were subjected to experimentation in the name of research. Out of the Nuremberg trials emerged a clearer understanding of the 'rights' of individuals not to suffer subjugation for medical or other research aims. The code of practice enshrined in the Declaration of Helsinki (World Medical Association 1964) made the gaining of consent from individuals an absolute necessity (for all those countries that signed the code). The idea of 'informed consent' was mooted first at this time and became widespread in the 1970s. At first, it applied only to research participants but gradually the modern Western world has found the need to apply informed consent more formally to many aspects of social interaction; the worlds of finance, law, education, and so on, are continuing to formalise the practice of informed consent and the domain of health has taken the lead. O'Neill (2002b; 2003) sees the spread of litigation and compensation as accelerating this need.

It could be argued that nurses and other healthcare professionals (HCPs) might have a vested interest in promoting the autonomy of patients and to have exaggerated the potential of 'fully informed consent' in order to relieve them of some of the burden of decision-making. Corrigan (2003) refers to an 'empty ethics' model, where an attempt to indulge a person's autonomy is too often an insistence on individuals being asked to make decisions out of context, thus nullifying the ethical principle. O'Neill (2003) argues that the older trust-based model of the doctor–patient relationship has been replaced by the formalised requirement for achieving informed consent. She argues that the very nature of giving information in quantities sufficient to reduce the possibility of litigation creates a barrier to the relationship and poses undue strain on the vulnerable individual who is now more likely to feel that it is their decision alone which will influence the path of their future well-being. There would appear, therefore, to be a need for nurses and other HCPs to understand the balance between both informed consent and trust, and between autonomy and trust, and to appreciate that these concepts are intertwined. The patient requiring palliative care may wish assistance in making decisions about their care, otherwise the information being given to them could be considered overwhelming and technical. However, the pitfall of a 'paternalistic' attitude, where nurses and other HCPs 'prescribe' treatment for their patients, should always be tempered with the modern requirement for shared decision-making, for the 'nothing about me without me' principle that is now accepted in UK healthcare settings. Finding the balance that gives a patient control over their own life, even and especially towards its ending, while maintaining respect and trust between all parties, is a complex task that can be supported by communication skills training.

The Mental Capacity Act (MCA)

The 1995 Mental Incapacity Bill sat on a shelf for 10 years in Westminster before it became the Mental Capacity Act (MCA) 2005; it then did not come into force until 2007. It has been criticised as being a law which reflects the thinking of the mid-1990s on incapacity and that has retained the vestiges of paternalism in the concept of 'best interests' (Lush 2015). The counter-argument is that it was and remains revolutionary in providing both protection and rights for individuals who are or who become mentally incapacitated. It is certainly relevant for patients requiring palliative care who become increasingly unwell and therefore unable to make decisions about their own end of life healthcare.

The MCA allows patients to put in place a Lasting Power of Attorney (LPA) that names persons, called Attorneys, who are able to make decisions about health and welfare in the event of the patient becoming mentally incapacitated. Ideally, the named Attorneys would make decisions in accordance with a document made by the patient prior to loss of capacity, setting out their wishes with regard to future care. The LPA can be seen as the legal instrument that gives the Attorneys the authority to make decisions; while the patient's ACP serves to ensure the decisions made are in accordance with their wishes.

There are two types of written documents relevant to advance care planning. First, an Advance Decision to Refuse Treatment (ADRT), which is a legally binding statement of circumstance, where the patient would want medical treatment to be refused. A patient cannot refuse to have basic nursing care. An ADRT can be verbal as long as it does not relate to potentially life-saving treatment. If a person wishes to refuse the latter, then the ADRT must be written and witnessed with signatures and must state clearly what type of treatment is being refused and under what circumstances. The statement must also make it clear that the person understands that the lack of the treatment could lead to loss of their life. When a nurse or other HCP is making a decision based on an ADRT, they must be satisfied that all these conditions are met, otherwise they may choose to ignore it, but must be prepared to defend their decision to do so. Second, an Advance Statement (AS) is a more general document that may include details of the patient's medical history, the patient's philosophy with regard to ACP, spiritual beliefs (if any) and more prosaic (but nevertheless highly important) matters such as food and drink preferences.

The MCA 2005 is applicable to persons aged 18 years or over who have capacity and wish to plan for their future. Prior to the MCA 2005, there was a legal tradition of an Attorney being appointed to make decisions about property and finances, but it was revolutionary for an Attorney to have jurisdiction to make decisions about health and welfare. The MCA 2005 provides that those who have no Attorneys should have access to an Independent Mental Capacity Advocate (IMCA) appointed for them by the NHS or local authority body taking care of them, who should be consulted about important medical treatments.

Case Study 20.1: When the patient says 'NO'

In *Re T 'Adult: Refusal of Medical Treatment'* [1992] 4 ALL ER645, CA, Lord Donaldson made it clear that an adult patient 'has an absolute right to choose whether to consent to having medical treatment, to refuse it or to choose one rather than another of treatments being offered'. He went on to say that the absolute right to autonomy 'exists notwithstanding the reasons for making the choice are rational or irrational, unknown or even non-existent'. T was a young woman involved in a serious road traffic accident when her pregnancy was nearly full-term; she consented to a caesarean section the following day. Before the operation took place, she was visited by her mother, a devout Jehovah's Witness. T herself was not baptised as a Jehovah's Witness but after her mother's visit she told doctors that she would not agree to any blood transfusion before or during surgery. Her child was born stillborn and T herself lapsed into a coma. T's boyfriend and father sought a Court Order authorising a life-saving blood transfusion. Lord Donaldson granted that Order on the basis that T's refusal of treatment was not an autonomous decision. Her decision was flawed because of: (1) the effect of her injuries and medication she was taking; (2) she lacked sufficient information to make a decision; and (3) she was put under undue pressure by her mother. In essence, therefore, capacity is central to autonomy; it is the capacity of an individual to make a valid choice which matters.

The MCA 2005 also reformed the Court of Protection (COP). Under the MCA 2005, the jurisdiction of the COP was extended to health and welfare decisions and the Court may now appoint a 'Deputy' for incapacitated adults to make decisions about health and welfare for the patient. However, the experience of solicitors applying to the COP for an Order to appoint such a Deputy, is that the Court is reluctant to grant permission in many circumstances because of the significant power that the Deputy would wield. The Court takes the view that significant decisions about health and welfare should be made by the Court on a case-by-case basis; appointing a Deputy would, in many circumstances, aim to limit the scope and duration of the appointment as much as reasonably practical in the circumstances (www.gov.uk/power-of-attorney/make-lasting-power). In other words, the granting of a Deputyship Order is a last resort when the Court cannot make a one-off Order. In the case of palliative care, an application to the COP for Health and Welfare Deputies to be appointed would almost certainly be impractical, given the length of time it takes for an application to be heard at the COP and an Order made.

The MCA 2005 guarantees, from a legal viewpoint, that the words of individuals writing or speaking for themselves in the past will be acted upon as if they were speaking with capacity at that moment. With health and welfare decisions, the patient will always be asked to make decisions for themselves wherever possible. However, allowing individuals to appoint an Attorney to speak for them in the future inevitably goes further in extending personal autonomy into situations that could not have been predicted or that individuals do not wish to contemplate when fully capacitated. Accordingly, so that a person making a decision on behalf of an incapacitated patient may truly make a 'best interests' decision on behalf of that patient, the clinical team involved in the care of the patient should be encouraging discussions about ACP in accordance with the MCA 2005 at the earliest opportunity.

Box 20.1   The MCA 2005

Principles of decision-making using the MCA 2005

The five statutory principles of the MCA 2005 are the benchmark of the Act and underpin all actions carried out and decisions taken in relation to the Act:

1   A presumption of capacity. Every adult has the right to make his or her own decisions and be assumed to have capacity to do so unless it is proved otherwise.
2   An individual being supported to make their own decisions must be given all practical help before anyone treats them as not being able to make their own decisions.
3   People have the right to make decisions that others might regard as unwise or eccentric. No one can treat someone as lacking capacity for this reason.
4   Anything done for or on behalf of the person who lacks mental capacity must be done in their 'best interests'.
5   Someone making a decision or acting on behalf of a person who lacks capacity must consider whether it is possible to decide or act in a way that would interfere less with the person's rights and freedom of actions; in other words, take the least restrictive option.

The test for capacity

The clinical team caring for a patient should 'think capacity' at all times. The test to assess capacity is a two-stage functional test:

- Stage 1 Is there an impairment of or disturbance in the function of a person's mind or brain?
- Stage 2 If so, is the impairment of disturbance sufficient that the person lacks the capacity to make a particular decision?

The MCA 2005 states that a person is unable to make their decision if they cannot do one or more of the following four things:

- Understand information given to them.
- Retain the information long enough to be able to make the decision.
- Use the information available to make the decision.
- Communicate their decision. This could be by talking, using sign language or even simple muscle movement, such as blinking an eye or squeezing a hand.

If a patient can manage all of these for a specific decision, then they have the capacity for that particular care decision. You cannot override a decision for this patient even if you believe it to be an 'unwise' decision.

Learning exercise 20.1

You are looking after an 85-year-old woman on a general medical ward. She is deemed medically fit to be moved to longer-term care. She has no family living at home but she needs support for daily living. What questions will you ask her to ascertain whether or not she has mental capacity to make a decision?

Case Study 20.2: 'Best interests', the Tony Bland case (*Airedale NHS Trust v Bland*, 1993)

Tony Bland was injured in the Hillsborough Disaster in 1989 when he was 17 years old. Afterwards he was in a persistent vegetative state. He could breathe by himself but required a feeding tube and numerous antibiotics as well as full nursing care, to ensure that he remained in relatively good health. By 1992 his parents decided that Tony would not want this to continue and asked the doctors to remove the feeding tube to put an end to his life. The case was heard in Court where it was decided that the medical team had a duty to treat Tony in a way that was in his 'best interests'. The judge concluded that it was not in his best interests to have his life prolonged in this way because there was no prospect of any improvement in his condition.

Best interests

The notion of 'best interests' is central to medical decision-making in the case of the incompetent patient. The conflicting viewpoints of: (1) the objective account of best interests and (2) the subjective account of best interests is clearly outlined by Dawson (2002). The objective view is obtained when the clinical teams look at the patient's case from a medical viewpoint, weighing pros and cons of treatment to achieve an assumed 'best' course of action. This decision is based on the medical need of the patient and in its pure form does not consider the wishes of the patient or the views of close relatives and carers, regarding what might be best for the patient. The subjective view is what has come to be used in the USA, where 'substituted' decisions have been regularly sought from carers who have been nominated as the proxy for the patient there. In the subjective account, all interested parties who know the patient would have a say in suggesting how the patient might want the clinical teams to respond. The nominated proxy would have the final decision and any advance statement would be fully taken into account.

In the UK, the British Medical Association (BMA) produced guidance for doctors concerning how to understand 'best interests' (BMA 1995). In practice, medical teams consider the 'objective' view, but then the more 'subjective' view is ascertained by interviewing the people who know the patient well. More information for the wider objective view, in terms of the patient's social, psychological and spiritual well-being can also be collected from close carers by clinical teams. All the information so gathered is then pooled and some-times discussed in 'family conferences' with the intention of achieving consensus. Until the MCA (2005), there was no ethical or legal obligation to take the opinions of carers into consideration when treatment options were made. The MCA (2005) builds on these crite-ria by recording a series of specific actions to be followed before a 'best interests' decision can be made and enshrines good practice (see RCP 2009, Figure 2).

The MCA (2005) has made this process of 'best interests' of the patient clearer by for-malising the use of the 'advance statement'. Any competent person may produce informa-tion for others to take into account in the future, if they were to lose their mental capacity. This information can be given verbally or can be written, and, if written, does not need to be witnessed and is not a legally binding document (RCP 2009; NHS End of Life Care Programme 2011). Family and friends of the patient, and any nurses and other HCPs, who have cared for the patient, should give evidence concerning what they have heard that the patient would have wanted and how they would wish to be treated. Anything that the patient wrote, audiotaped or videotaped should be considered as having relevance to the decision to be made. Of course, if the patient is currently competent, then their present wishes override anything previously said or documented.

The future for the MCA 2005

In 2006, the United Nations General Assembly adopted the Convention on the Rights of Persons with Disabilities and its optional protocol. The purpose of the Convention is 'to promote, protect and ensure the full and equal treatment of all human rights and fundamental freedoms by all persons with disabilities and to promote respect for their inherent dignity' (Article 1) (www.un.org/development/desa/disabilities). The Conven-tion represents a 'paradigm shift' (Lush 2015) in attitudes and approaches towards per-sons with a disability, in terms of ceasing to regard people with disabilities as 'objects' of charity, medical treatment and social protection and views them instead as 'sub-jects' with rights who are capable of asserting those rights and making decisions for their lives based on their free and informed consent. The Supreme Court of the United Kingdom referred to the Convention for the first time in its landmark judgment of *P v Cheshire West and Chester Council* [2014] (Box 20.2).

Box 20.2   The judgment of *P v Cheshire West and Chester Council*

The judgment was a landmark in terms of extending the scope of the Deprivation of Liberty Safeguards (DoLS) set out in the MCA in that it widened the previously understood circumstances where DoLS would apply. The case introduced the 'acid test' which stated that there is a deprivation of liberty where a person is 'under continuous supervision and control' and 'is not free to leave' and 'the person lacks capacity to consent to these arrangements'.

The increase in circumstances where the deprivation of liberty safeguards apply was one factor in the Law Commission being asked to review the law in this area leading to the publication of a report 'Mental Capacity and Deprivation of Liberty' published on 13 March 2017. The report recommended that DoLS be replaced with a new scheme called 'The Liberty Protection Safeguards' and included a draft Bill to be considered by the UK Government.

In 2014, the Ministry of Justice commissioned the Essex Autonomy Project to prepare a report on whether the MCA 2005 was compliant with the United Nations Convention on the Rights of Persons with Disabilities (https://autonomy.essex.ac.uk). The main findings were that the MCA 2005 was not fully compliant but was in fact discriminatory in its restriction of mental capacity to those who suffer from 'an impairment of or a disturbance in the functioning of mind or the brain'. The report also criticised 'best interest' decision-making as failing to satisfy the requirement for safeguards respecting rights, will and preference of disabled persons in matters pertaining to the exercise of legal capacity. It recommended an amendment to allow the 'best interests' decision-maker to make the decision that accords best with the known wishes of the patient. This may impact on the process for all those with mental incapacity.

Advance care planning: history and evolution

As discussed earlier, the term 'advance care planning' (ACP) refers to a person's stated wishes concerning any type of care, clinical or otherwise, that they will be given either towards the end of their life or at times of critical, life-threatening illness. ACP presumes the possibility of loss of mental capacity leading to that person being unable to give instructions to nurses or other HCPs at important times of serious, even terminal illness.

In the USA

Early American documents were witnessed and signed as a standard will and testimony would be. What followed in the USA was a discourse around the concept of ACP, which also had other drivers behind its development including large medico-legal cases that were proving costly, in both financial and emotional terms. One of these landmark US cases is summarised in Case Study 20.3.

Case Study 20.3: Nancy Cruzan

Nancy Cruzan was left in a persistent vegetative state after a road traffic accident in 1983. Her case appeared before the Missouri court in 1990. This court refused to allow removal of a life support measure (feeding tube) because they required written evidence, in the form of an advance directive, of the patient's wishes for herself. They disallowed verbal evidence of her wishes from parents and friends (*Cruzan v. Director, Missouri Department of Health* 1990). This challenging case led to the US Supreme Court declaring that competent adults had a right to make advance decisions about their own medical treatment (Colby 2006), placing the autonomy of the competent person as the primary ethical consideration in medical decision-making in the US. The Patient Self-Determination Act 1991 has since required US nurses and other HCPs to ask patients on admission to healthcare institutions about any advance directives, but there is no requirement to help patients to create these (Greco et al. 1991).

In the USA, living wills or 'instructional advance directives' now allow for a named person to be the decision-maker for healthcare on behalf of another person if incapacitated. Durable powers of attorney have been used in the USA since 1983. The 'medical directive' evolved into a variety of questionnaire formats that became highly complex, scenario-based worksheets (Emanuel and Emanuel 1989; Emanuel 2000). Their narrow focus and the difficulty in applying concepts to actual practical situations meant that uptake was disappointing (Cantor 1998). Document usage was 9.8 per cent (Hanson and Rodgman 1996) and the large SUPPORT study (1995) attempted, but failed, to improve clinical outcomes by educating doctors and nurses in their use and by supplying them with information about their patients' prognoses. This landmark research signalled a sea change for the American perception of ACP (Street and Gottmann 2006).

Doukas and McCullough (1991) mooted the concept of the 'values history', and since then the direction of ACP in the USA has been developing down the route of being a 'process' rather than simply a 'product' that can be written and referred to. The 'process' model requires physicians to initiate end of life discussions with patients and families together, when appropriate, which may proceed on to the drafting of a written 'product' in the form of a directive or statement of will (Hammes and Rooney 1998; Teno 1998; Crane et al. 2005). This iterative and inclusive method was shown to be able to achieve a 95 per cent completion rate for advance directives (Hammes and Rooney 1998). Subsequent research has confirmed that participants prefer ACP that is individualised, voluntary, social, and which does not have to create a written outcome. This evolving history in the USA illustrates some of the reasons for significant cultural differences remaining between the two countries, in terms of ACP. While ACP in the UK focuses on patients with life-shortening illness, this is not the case in the USA (Stein and Cohen Fineberg 2013), and documentation there has followed a largely different route.

In the UK

The guidelines (RCP 2009) are clear that the process of engaging with ACP is voluntary and that HCPs should approach patients and families who appear to be ready to undergo such discussions and not be reliant on form-filling. ACP should not be a single temporal experience but needs to be an iterative process that is returned to and updated (Schwartz et al. 2003; Seymour et al. 2004; Lambert et al. 2005; RCP 2009). Patients should be allowed to have whoever else they wish to be present with them and they should give consent for any documentation to be made or passed to others. It is also advised that facilitators of ACP understand the patient's illness and have all necessary information to hand that might assist the patient to make decisions ahead of time. Nurses and other HCPs should be trained in good communication skills so that the process is effective and supportive, and should have sufficient time to conduct it, in an environment conducive to developing rapport.

Box 20.3   The ACP

Components of advance care planning (ACP)

- Preferred Priorities of Care statement: http://endoflifecareambitions.org.uk/wp-content/uploads/2016/09/preferred_priorities_of_care_pdf.pdf
- Advance Decisions to Refuse Treatment: www.compassionindying.org.uk
- Lasting Power of Attorney: www.gov.uk/power-of-attorney
- Do Not Attempt Cardio-Pulmonary Resuscitation: www.respectprocess.org.uk/_pdfs./ReSPECT-Specimen-Form.pdf
- Emergency Healthcare Plan: www.nescn.nhs.uk/wp-content/uploads/2014/06/EHCP-NHS-Fillable-form-v14-April-2013.pdf

Henry and Seymour (2007); Compassion in Dying (2015);
Resuscitation Council (2016): www.resus.org.uk; Deciding Right (2017):
www.nescn.nhs.uk ReSPECT (2017): respectprocess.org.uk.

Table 20.1 outlines the status of the components of the ACP.

Table 20.1 Status of components of ACP

Component	Legally binding	Guidance	Valid ACP?
1. Preferred Priorities for Care Statement (PPC)	No	Yes	Yes
OR			
2. Advance Statement (AS) of philosophy, spiritual belief, food preferences and anything else desired by the patient	No	Yes	Yes
3. Advance Decision to Refuse Treatment (ADRT)	Yes	Yes	Yes
4. Making a Lasting Power of Attorney (LPA) for Health and Welfare	Yes	Sometimes*	Yes
5. DNACPR form	No	Yes	Yes
6. Emergency Healthcare Plan (EHCP)	No	Yes	Yes
7. Talking to loved ones/carers/clinical team	No	Yes	Yes

*The LPA form allows the Donor of the LPA to set out details of 'preferences' and 'instructions'. Care needs to be taken, as the Office of the Public Guardian (OPG) will strike out preferences and instructions that they consider to be incompatible with the MCA 2005. An alternative would be to include such preferences and instructions in a 'Letter of Wishes' to accompany the LPA, rather than make them part of the LPA instrument.

Learning exercise 20.2

Look at specimen documentation for each of the components in Table 20.1 and familiarise yourself with what each entails.

'Advance care planning is now defined as a process of discussion between a patient and professional carer, which sometimes includes family and friends' (Murray et al. 2006, p. 868). The Gold Standards Framework (GSF) had already begun to be introduced widely into general practice (Thomas 2003). This was a schema that was devised to assist primary care teams to care for patients receiving palliative care. One of the principles it upheld included early ideas on the need to create not just a care plan for each patient but also to consider ACP for the future (Thomas and Lobo 2011). Alongside this new intervention, a separate team of clinical practitioners was developing the notion of a hand-held record that patients receiving palliative care could keep with them and write down details concerning their wishes for end of life care. This document was eventually named the 'Preferred Priorities for Care' (PPC) document and has been available for use in the UK in a variety of healthcare settings (Storey and Betteley 2011). Comprehensive guidance for UK healthcare practitioners is available (NHS 2007; RCP 2009).

The MCA (2005) further focused the understanding of how ACP could be used, identifying two potential major benefits. First, to allow people to discuss openly with others how they wished various aspects of their care to develop, creating the opportunity to prevent fewer unacceptable events from occurring, even in circumstances where the patient retained capacity. Second, to allow the creation of a record of a person's wishes in case they became incapacitated, so that others would be able to honour the patient's autonomous desires. It is now clear that ACP can increase compliance with a patient's end of life care wishes and improve their satisfaction with care (Brinkman-Stoppelenburg et al. 2014).

Requesting care interventions

Patients cannot insist that any specific medical treatment should be given to them, but can only accept or refuse the care that is offered (BMA 1995; 2007a); the final decision for active treatment rests with the medical team. This is because doctors are expected to have greater knowledge and understanding of the limitations of medical interventions; it is their duty to help patients gain this understanding to the best of their abilities

(GMC 2008). If a patient still insists on treatment which the doctors regard as 'futile', that is, treatment that cannot have any likelihood of benefit for the patient and is therefore not in their best interests, then it is within the rights of the doctor to refuse this treatment. The doctor must be sure that their decision is in accordance with other medical peer opinion and make a thorough examination of the balance of risk and benefits (*Bolitho v City and Hackney HA* 1998).

Medical decisions are now often made within multi-disciplinary teams, where doctors and nurses, as well as other HCPs, can voice opinions. This is especially the case for complex interventions and medical treatments, such as those regarding cancer diagnoses. Patients' advance statements of care cannot insist on the continuation of specific treatments for a time when the patient has become incapacitated. This restriction on advance statements was tested in court (*R (Burke) v GMC* 2004) when a patient requested that 'artificial nutrition and hydration' should be allowed to continue once his ability to communicate was lost; he believed that it would always be in his best interests for this to occur and he wanted his opinion to be noted (Biggs 2007). This was initially upheld, however, the Appeal Court ruled that an advance statement requesting treatment could only be taken into consideration, that it could not be allowed to be determinative and it was therefore over-ruled (Samanta and Samanta 2006).

Withholding or withdrawing treatment

When the patient is incompetent and is already receiving medical life-sustaining support, such as ventilation or clinically assisted nutrition and hydration, removing that support can be a difficult decision for medical teams even with the agreement of family members. The Courts (of England, Wales and Northern Ireland) must be applied to in the cases of patients who are in a 'persistent vegetative state' (PVS) or for patients whose condition closely resembles PVS (GMC 2010), or when consensus cannot be achieved (see Case Study 20.2). In arriving at a decision concerning withholding or withdrawing treatment for an incompetent patient, the medical team has the responsibility to weigh the benefits and disadvantages of the treatment under consideration and can only give it if it is thought to have overall beneficence. They should consider the patient's 'best interests' and should garner opinions from all parties involved in the care of the patient. If consensus cannot be achieved, then further help may be sought from expert second opinion, from medical ethical review bodies or ultimately from the Courts. Professional UK guidelines (BMA 2007; GMC 2010) note that limited resources may mean that health teams cannot always provide those treatments that are both requested by the patient and which appear beneficial.

Learning exercise 20.3

You are looking after a 75-year-old man on your acute hospital ward. He has a diagnosis of end-stage cancer of the prostate. He is frail, at risk of falls, needs a lot of care for his weeping, oedematous legs and help with taking his medication. He wants to go home to his cramped caravan to be looked after by his elderly wife, and he is deemed to have mental capacity for this decision. His wife, however, feels that she can no longer take care of him safely. The caravan is in both of their names.

What are the rights of both the patient and his wife? How will you proceed with decisions about his future place of care? Who else might need to be involved in these conversations?

Barriers to ACP

The spoken word versus the written word

Some patients appear to doubt that their spoken words during ACP would be heeded by HCPs, while others maintain that speaking to family members would be of benefit to carers when discussing options on their behalf in the future (Swarbrick 2013). The notion that ACP has to be written prevents some patients from exploring this process (Rosenfield et al. 2000; Clayton et al. 2005; Lambert et al. 2005; Barnes et al. 2007). The perceived finality and potential irreversibility of written statements concern some people and the process of discussion was also worrying to some who discussed their ideation of 'magical thinking' (Swarbrick 2013); this can be defined as a conviction that thinking is equivalent to doing, or happening, and therefore that the foretelling of their death might cause it to happen.

The uncertain future

Several patients decline to contemplate what might happen to them in the future, preferring to live in the present and to concentrate on the concrete practices of daily living, which seemed easier to focus upon than an array of possible future occurrences (Carrese et al. 2002; Horne et al. 2012). For some, this is a method of allowing hope to be maintained, for others, it is a question of their faith, allowing God or fate to take care of events.

One of the inherent principles of ACP is that a person is able to 'adequately imagine themselves in that state and predict accurately what their preferences will be should they actually experience it' (Ditto and Hawkins 2005, p. S64). But for some patients, the details of future events are difficult to focus on. So this prerequisite appears to pose a problem even for patients who are close to dying (Fried and Bradley 2003; Davison 2006). This threatens the authenticity of any narrowly focused advance statements and suggests that values statements and a more general approach to future decision-making might be more productive and reliable (Ditto et al. 2006).

The uncertain trajectory of illness may be even more marked in non-cancer terminal diseases (Gott et al. 2009). Patients' views often change as they perceive their health status to be deteriorating (Fried and Bradley 2003; Voogt et al. 2005) and there is evidence that undergoing procedures or interventions changes people's perceptions and decisions about having them again in the future (Ditto and Hawkins 2005).

Who should talk about ACP?

Patients in many studies in different countries appear uncertain as to who they would most like to conduct ACP with them, some wanting experts in their condition (Pearlman et al. 1995), others only wanting clinicians that they already knew well (Parker et al. 2007), others stipulating the need for facilitators trained in communication skills (Hammes 1996; Schwartz et al. 2002; Rodriguez and Young 2005; Horne et al. 2006; Barnes et al. 2007; Barnes et al. 2011). Generally, patients appear to trust their doctors to make good decisions about their care, however, many patients would not choose their doctors to conduct ACP (Samsi and Manthorpe 2011) either because of time constraints or lack of continuity problems. Some participants struggle to believe in the value of performing ACP because of a lack of trust in nurses, other HCPs and the healthcare service in general (Swarbrick 2013).

When should ACP be broached?

Research into the question of when ACP should be done has revealed different answers. Some conclude that, rather than contemplating too much of the process at a first meeting, the concept of ACP might be broached early on, initially seeking to ascertain exactly who the patient would feel most comfortable with for end of life discussions and creating a plan for a more ideal situation in the future (Barnes et al. 2007; Horne et al. 2012; Samsi and Manthorpe 2011).

Maintaining control

Patients are seen to struggle with the dilemma of having personal control over events and decisions, while also taking into account the effects of their decisions upon those closest to them (Singer et al. 1998; Volker and Wu 2011) and the desire of many to lessen the burden on their family and friends (Steinhauser et al. 2001; Vig and Pearlman 2003; Seymour et al. 2004; Winter and Parks 2011). Some feel uncomfortable sharing decision-making with family or friends (Samsi and Manthorpe 2011), while others cannot identify anyone to do this with. Across Europe the desire for involvement of family and friends in decision-making is prevalent and under-researched (Daveson et al. 2013).

Conclusion

Any kind of written ACP should be a living document that is open to being updated at any time. A patient considering how to be cared for at a time when they have not been diagnosed with a particular illness would likely produce a different outcome regarding

ACP once a diagnosis has taken place. As life moves forward, priorities change and goalposts move; a patient who has given up on living may suddenly want to keep going if there is a new event on the horizon, such as the expected birth of a new family member or other celebration. The custodian of a written ACP document should be the patient so that the patient may update the document as and when desired and so that a nurse or other HCP being given the document, or coming across it on the patient, is satisfied that it is an original and up-to-date version. From a legal standpoint, the 'counsel of perfection' would be achieved when a patient has made a LPA for Health and Welfare decisions and prepared both an ADRT and an Advance Statement. But it must be remembered that ACP is always voluntary, whether verbal or written, while also acknowledging that anything is better than nothing; conversations are not legally binding but can be highly informative. ACP that enables respect for the wishes of the patient so far and however they may be ascertained is the ideal that a clinical team should be aiming for.

References

Barnes, K., Barlow, C.A., Harrington, J. et al.. (2011) Advance care planning discussions in advanced cancer: analysis of dialogues between patients and care planning mediators. *Palliative and Supportive Care*, 9: 73–9.

Barnes, K., Jones, L., Tookman, A. and King, M. (2007) Acceptability of an advance care planning interview schedule: a focus group study. *Palliative Medicine*, 21: 23–8.

Beauchamp, T.L. and Childress, J.F. (2013) *Principles of Biomedical Ethics* (7th edn). Oxford: Oxford University Press.

Biggs, H. (2007) 'Taking account of the views of the patient', but only if the clinician (and the court) agrees – R (Burke) v General Medical Council. *Child and Family Law Quarterly*, 19(2): 225–38.

Brinkman-Stoppelenburg, A., Rietjens, J.A.C. and van der Heide, A. (2014) The effects of advance care planning on end-of-life care: a systematic review. *Palliative Medicine*, 28(8): 1000–25.

British Medical Association (1995) *Advance Statements about Medical Treatment*. London: BMJ Books.

British Medical Association (2007) *Advance Decisions and Proxy Decision-Making in Medical Treatment and Research: Guidance from the BMA's Medical Ethics Department*. London: BMA. Available at: www.bma.org.uk

Cantor, N.L. (1998) Making advance directives meaningful. *Psychology, Public Policy and Law*, 4(3): 629–52.

Carrese, J.A., Mullaney, J.L., Faden, R.R. and Finucane, T.E. (2002) Planning for death but not serious future illness: qualitative study of housebound elderly patients. *BMJ*, 325: 125–9.

Clayton, J.M., Butow, P.N., Arnold, R.M. and Tattersall, M.H.N. (2005) Discussing end-of-life issues with terminally ill cancer patients and their carers: a qualitative study. *Supportive Care in Cancer*, 13: 589–99.

Colby, W.H. (2006) From Quinlan to Cruzan to Schiavo: what have we learned? *Loyola University Chicago Law Journal*, 37: 279–96.

Compassion in Dying: Supporting your Choices (2015) Making and implementing advance decisions: a toolkit for healthcare professionals. Available at: www.compassionindying.org.uk

Corrigan, O. (2003) Empty ethics: the problem with informed consent. *Sociology of Health and Illness*, 25(3): 768–92.

Crane, M., Wittink, M. and Doukas, D. (2005) Respecting end-of-life treatment preferences. *American Family Physician*, 72(1270): 1263–8.

Curtis, J.R. (2008) Palliative and end-of-life care for patients with severe COPD. *European Respiratory Journal*, 32(3): 796–803.

Daveson, B.A., Bausewein, C., Murtagh, F.E. et al. (2013) To be involved or not to be involved: a survey of public preferences for self-involvement in decision-making involving mental capacity (competency) within Europe. *Palliative Medicine*, 27(5): 418–27.

Davison, S.N. (2006) Facilitating advance care planning for patients with end-stage renal disease: the patient perspective. *Clinical Journal of the American Society of Nephrology*, 1: 1023–8.

Dawson, A. (2002) Section 1. Best Interests. Non-treatment decisions: the need to define best interests. In *Vital Judgements: Ethical Decision Making at the End of Life*. London: National Council for Hospice and Specialist Palliative Care Services.

Deciding Right (2017) Northern England Strategic Clinical Networks. Available at: www.nescn.nhs.uk (accessed 7 January 2017).

Ditto, P.H. and Hawkins, N.A. (2005) Advance directives and cancer decision making near the end of life. *Health Psychology*, 24(4 suppl. 1): S63–70.

Ditto, P.H., Hawkins, N.A. and Pizarro, D.A. (2006) Imagining the end of life: psychology of advance medical decision making. *Motivation and Emotion*, 29(4): 475–96.

Doukas, D. and McCullough, L.B. (1991) The values history: the evaluation of the patient's values and advance directives. *Journal of Family Practice*, 32(2): 145–53.

Dworkin, G. (1988) *The Theory and Practice of Autonomy*. Cambridge: Cambridge University Press.

Emanuel, L.L. (2000) How living wills can help doctors and patients talk about dying: they can open the door to a positive, caring approach to death. *BMJ*, 320(7250): 1618–19.

Emanuel, L.L. and Emanuel, E.J. (1989) The medical directive: a new comprehensive advance care document. *JAMA*, 261: 3288–93.

Fried, T.R. and Bradley, E.H. (2003) What matters to seriously ill older persons making end-of-life treatment decisions? A qualitative study. *Journal of Palliative Medicine*, 6(2): 237–44.

General Medical Council (2008) *Consent Guidance: Patients and Doctors Making Decisions Together*. London: GMC. Available at: www.gmc-uk.org.uk

General Medical Council (2010) *Treatment and Care Towards the End of Life: Good Practice in Decision Making*. London: GMC.

Gott, M., Gardiner, C., Payne, S. et al. (2009) Barriers to advance care planning in chronic obstructive pulmonary disease. *Palliative Medicine*, 23: 642–8.

Greco, P.J., Schulman, K.A., Lavizzo-Mourey, R. and Hansen-Flaschen, J. (1991) The Patient Self-Determination Act and the future of advance directives. *Annals of Internal Medicine*, 115: 639–43.

Hammes, B. (ed.) (1996) *Respecting Your Choices: Training Manual*. La Crosse, WI: Lutheran Hospital.

Hammes, B.J. and Rooney, B.L.L. (1998) Death and end-of-life planning in one Midwestern community. *Archives of Internal Medicine*, 158: 383–90.

Hanson, L.C. and Rodgman, E. (1996) The use of living wills at the end of life: A national study. *Arch Int Med*, 156(9): 1018–22.

Henry, C. and Seymour, J.E. (2007) *Advance Care Planning: A Guide for Health and Social Care Professionals*. NHS End of Life Care Programme.

Herring, J. (2012) *Medical Law and Ethics* (4th edn). Oxford: Oxford University Press.

Horne, G., Seymour, J. and Shepherd, K. (2006) Advance care planning for patients with inoperable lung cancer. *International Journal of Palliative Nursing*, 12(4): 172–8.

Horne, G., Seymour, J. and Payne, S. (2012) Maintaining integrity in the face of death: a grounded theory to explain the perspectives of people affected by lung cancer about the expression of wishes for end of life care. *International Journal of Nursing Studies*, 49: 718–26.

IHF Perspectives (2016) *A Perspective on Advance Planning for End-of-life*. No. 4. Dublin: IHF Perspectives.

Kutner, L. (1969) Due process of euthanasia: the living will, a proposal. *Indiana Law Journal*, 44(539): 550–4.

Lambert, H.C., McColl, M.A., Gilbert, J. et al. (2005) Factors affecting long-term-care residents' decision-making processes as they formulate advance directives. *The Gerontologist*, 45(5): 626–33.

Lush, D. (2015) 'A gilded cage is a cage no less.' The Mental Capacity Act interfaced with the UN Convention on Human Rights of Disabled People and the EU Convention on Human Rights. Available at: https://www.5sah.co.uk/news-and-events/articles/2015-11-27/a-gilded-cage-is-a-cage-no-less-the-mental-capacity-act-interfaced-with-the-un-convention-on-human-rights-of-disabled-people-and-the-eu-convention-on-human-rights (accessed 15 March 2017).

Mackenzie, C. and Stoljar, N. (2000) Autonomy refigured. In *Relational Autonomy: Feminist Perspectives on Autonomy, Agency, and the Social Self*. New York: Oxford University Press.

Mental Capacity Act (2005) London: HMSO. http://www.legislation.gov.uk/ukpga/2005/9/pdfs/ukpga_20050009_en.pdf (accessed 22.3.2018).

Murray, S.A., Sheikh, A. and Thomas, K. (2006) Advance care planning in primary care. *BMJ*, 333: 868–9.

National Research Ethics Service (2006) *Guidance for Applicants to the NRES*. National Patient Safety Agency, NHS. Available at: www.nres.npsa.nhs.uk

NHS End of Life Care Programme (2007) *Advance Care Planning: A Guide for Health and Social Care Staff*. London: NHS. Available at: www.endoflifecare.nhs.uk

NHS End of Life Care Programme (2011) *Capacity, Care Planning and Advance Care Planning in Life Limiting Illness: A Guide for Health and Social Care Staff*. Leicester: NHS.

O'Neill, O. (2002) *A Question of Trust: The BBC Reith Lectures 2002*. Cambridge: Cambridge University Press.

O'Neill, O. (2003) Some limits of informed consent. *Journal of Medical Ethics*, 29: 4–7.

Parker, S.M., Clayton, J.M., Hancock, K. et al. (2007) A systematic review of prognostic/end-of-life communication with adults in the advanced stages of a life-limiting illness: patient/caregiver preferences for the content, style and timing of information. Review article. *Journal of Pain and Symptom Management*, 34(1): 81–93.

Pearlman, R.A., Cole, W.G., Patrick, D.L. et al. (1995) Advance care planning eliciting patient preferences for life-sustaining treatment. *Patient Education and Counselling*, 26: 353–61.

Resuscitation Council (UK) (2016) *Decision Relating to Cardiopulmonary Resuscitation* (3rd edn; 1st review). Guidance from the BMA, the Resuscitation Council (UK) and the RCN.

Resuscitation Council (UK) (2017) ReSPECT: Recommended Summary Care Plan for Emergency Care and Treatment. Available at: www.resus.org.uk

Rodriguez, K.L. and Young, A.J. (2005) Perspectives of elderly veterans regarding communication with medical providers about end-of-life care. *Journal of Palliative Medicine*, 8(3): 534–44.

Rosenfield, K.E., Wenger, N.S. and Kagawa-Singer, M. (2000) End-of-life decision making: a qualitative study of elderly individuals. *Journal of General Internal Medicine*, 15: 620–5.

RCP (Royal College of Physicians) (2009) *Concise Guidance to Good Practice, Number 12: Advance Care Planning. National Guidelines*. London: RCP.

Samanta, A. and Samanta, J. (2006) Advance directives, best interests and clinical judgement: shifting sands at the end of life. *Clinical Medicine*, 6(3): 274–8.

Samsi, K. and Manthorpe, J. (2011) 'I live for today': a qualitative study investigating older people's attitudes to advance planning. *Health and Social Care in the Community*, 19(1): 52–9.

Schwartz, C., Lennes, I., Hammes, B. et al. (2003) Honing an advance care planning intervention using qualitative analysis: The Living Well interview. *Journal of Palliative Medicine*, 6(4): 593–603.

Schwartz, C.E., Wheeler, H., Brownell, M.D. et al. and UMass End-Of-Life Working Group. (2002) Early intervention in planning end-of-life care with ambulatory geriatric patients: results of a pilot trial. *Archives of Internal Medicine*, 162(14): 1611–18.

Seymour, J., Gott, M., Bellamy, G. et al. (2004) Planning for the end of life: the views of older people about advance care statements. *Social Science and Medicine*, 59(1): 57–68.

Singer, P.A., Martin, K.M., Lavery, J.V. et al. (1998) Reconceptualizing advance care planning from the patient's perspective. *Archives of Internal Medicine*, 158(8): 879–84.

Stein, G.L. and Cohen Fineberg, I. (2013) Advance care planning in the USA and UK: a comparative analysis of policy, implementation and the social work role. *British Journal of Social Work*, 43(2): 1–16.

Steinhauser, K.E., Christakis, N.A., Clipp, E.C. et al. (2001) Preparing for the end of life: preferences of patients, families, physicians and other care providers. *Journal of Pain and Symptom Management*, 22(3): 727–37.

Storey, L. and Betteley, A. (2011) Preferred priorities for care: an advance care planning process. In Thomas, K. and Lobo, B. (eds) *Advance Care Planning in End of Life Care*. Oxford: Oxford University Press.

Street, A. and Gottmann, G. (2006) *State of the Science Review of Advance Care Planning Models*. Bundoora: La Trobe University.

SUPPORT Principal Investigators (1995) A controlled trial to improve care for seriously ill hospitalized patients: the study to understand prognoses and preferences for outcomes and risks of treatments (SUPPORT). *JAMA*, 274: 1591–8.

Swarbrick, P.M. (2013) Advance Care Planning with patients requiring palliative care: an exploration of perceptions and tension engendered by end of life conversations. Unpublished PhD.

Teno, J.M. (1998) Looking beyond the 'form' to complex interventions needed to improve end-of-life care. *Journal of the American Geriatrics Society*, 46: 1170–1.

Thomas, K. (2003) *Caring for the Dying at Home: Companions on the Journey*. Oxford: Radcliffe Medical Press Ltd.

Thomas, K. and Lobo, B. (eds) (2011) *Advance Care Planning in End of Life Care*. Oxford: Oxford University Press.

Vig, E.K. and Pearlman, R.A. (2003) Quality of life while dying: A qualitative study of terminally ill older men. *Journal of the American Geriatrics Society*, 51(11): 1595–1601.

Volker, D.L. and Wu, H-L. (2011) Cancer patients' preferences for control at the end of life. *Qualitative Health Research*, 21(12): 1618–31.

Voogt, E., van der Heide, A., Rietjens, J.A.C. et al. (2005) Attitudes of patients with incurable cancer toward medical treatment in the last phase of life. *Journal of Clinical Oncology*, 23(9): 2012–19.

Winter, L. and Parks, S.M. (2011) The reluctance to burden others as a value in end-of-life decision making: a source of inaccuracy in substituted judgment. *Journal of Health Psychology*, 17(2): 179–88.

World Medical Association (1964) *Declaration of Helsinki; Ethical Principles for Medical Research Involving Human Subjects*. Helsinki, Finland: World Medical Association.

Cases cited

Airedale NHS Trust v Bland (1993) AC 789 (HL).

Bolitho v City and Hackney HA [1998] AC 232.

Cruzan v. Director, Missouri Department of Health. [1990] 110 S. Ct. 2841.

P v Cheshire West and Chester Council [2014] UKSC 19 [2014] MHLO 16.

R (Burke) v General Medical Council (defendant) and Disability Rights Commission (interested party) and the Official Solicitor (intervener) [2004] EWHC1879.

Assisted dying: a global overview

Deborah Lewis, Sheri Mila Gerson
and Claudia Gamondi

Introduction

Assisted dying (AD) legislation is increasing globally, but how AD is interpreted and implemented varies in each jurisdiction. There has been some disquiet about how palliative care fits within these frameworks. This chapter presents a global overview of assisted dying practice and research in jurisdictions where there is legislation permitting its practice. It will highlight terminological variations globally, and briefly identify the features of legislation where it exists. As a variety of terms are used globally to avoid confusion in some sections, the generic term 'assisted dying' is used which the Commission for Assisted Dying (CAD 2012) in the United Kingdom defined as 'a generic term that refers to both assisted suicide and voluntary euthanasia when a person receives assistance from a third party to end their life'.

While all forms of assisted dying are unlawful in the UK, the findings of research in the Low Countries of the Netherlands, Belgium and Luxembourg, Switzerland, and North and South America where AD is practised will be presented. This is followed by a consideration of the impact of an assisted death for families and the dilemmas it causes for palliative care. We conclude by providing guidance for nurses and other professionals when asked to respond to hasten death requests in clinical practice.

Learning exercise 21.1

You may have heard of the term assisted dying:

- What practices are permitted?
- Can you name them?
- Where are they permitted?

Terminology

The word euthanasia, rooted in the ancient languages of Latin and Greek, means literally 'a good death' (Vink 2016). The delivery of lethal medication, however, with the intention of causing death is a controversial and sensitive topic (Gardner 2012) with ethical, legal and practical challenges. A practice recorded since antiquity (Manning 1998), in the early twentieth century it became the focus of political debates in Britain and the United States (Emanuel 1994). Historically, the word 'euthanasia' has often been prefixed by terms such as 'voluntary' and 'involuntary' (Manning 1998). In legislative terms (Emanuel et al. 2016), however, voluntary euthanasia relates to the explicit request by a mentally competent patient for a lethal injection to be administered by a physician or nurse practitioner. The Government of Canada is currently the only country that allows a nurse practitioner to prescribe or administer lethal medications to a patient who requests it. Table 21.1 provides definitions of the most commonly used terms in modern practice.

In the United States, the word 'suicide' is now generally avoided (Death with Dignity National Center 2016), with terms such as 'death with dignity' or 'aid in dying' (Death with Dignity National Center 2016) being used. There is some evidence that terminology matters, at least with the public, with higher levels of public support for physicians 'ending a life' rather than assisting a 'suicide' (Emanuel et al. 2016). Also arising are umbrella terms, encompassing both 'euthanasia' and 'physician-assisted dying' such as 'medical assistance in dying' in Canada (PoC 2016). Opinions differ, however, as to whether assisted dying should be considered a part of medical practice with arguments for (Tucker 2015) and against (Boudreau and Somerville 2013).

Table 21.1 Defining key legislative terms

Term	Country	Definition
Euthanasia	Belgium Canada (Province of Quebec) Luxembourg The Netherlands	A physician or nurse practitioner directly administers a substance that causes the death of the mentally competent person who has requested it
Physician-assisted suicide (PAS)	Canada Luxembourg The Netherlands Switzerland	A physician or nurse practitioner prescribes a substance that the requesting individual can self-administer to cause their own death
Assisted suicide (AS) Assisted dying (AD) Death with dignity (DWD) Physician-assisted dying (PAD)	United States	Term includes both self-administered and medically administered medications to cause death
Medical aid in dying Medical assistance in dying (MaID)	Canada	

Table 21.2 Locations where assisted dying is legal or a medical provider is not prosecuted for prescribing lethal medications

Assisted dying in a global context

Country	Term used in legislation	Self-administered	Lethal injection by professional	Advanced disease only	Minimum age limit	Year implemented
Europe						
Belgium	The Belgian Act on Euthanasia of 28 May 2002	No	Yes	No	none	2002
Luxembourg	Euthanasia and Assisted Suicide Law of 16 March 2009	Yes	Yes	No	18	2009
The Netherlands	Termination of Life on Request and Assisted Suicide Act	Yes	Yes	No	12	2002
Switzerland	Assistance au Suicide/Sterbehilfe/suicidio aswsistito	Yes	No	No	none	1942
North America						
Canada						
All provinces	Medical Assistance in Dying	Each province/territory to decide	No	No	18	2016
Quebec	Medical Aid to Die	No	Yes	No	18	2015
United States						
California	End of Life Option Act	Yes	No	Yes	18	2016
Colorado	End of Life Option Act	Yes	No	Yes	18	2016
DC	Death with Dignity Act	Yes	No	Yes	18	2017
Montana	Rights of the Terminally Ill Act	Yes	No	Yes	No data	2009
Oregon	Death with Dignity Act	Yes	No	Yes	18	1997
Vermont	Patient Choice and Control at End of Life	Yes	No	Yes	18	2013
Washington	Death with Dignity Act	Yes	No	Yes	18	2009
South America						
Columbia	Statutory Bill on Ending Life in a Decent and Human Way and Assistance to Suicide	No	Yes	Yes	18	2015

Global overview of assisted dying

Assisted dying has become lawful in a number of jurisdictions globally as summarised in Table 21.2. The term 'jurisdictions' is used because where AD legislation exists, it may apply to a country, but also to a state such as Oregon in the United States, or a province such as Quebec in Canada. There are also variations in the practices. In the Netherlands, the term 'physician-assisted suicide' applies to the self-administration of lethal medication by the patient with a physician present (TLRAS 2002). In the US, however, physicians do not need to be present when a patient self-administers the drugs. Common to all jurisdictions, however, is the right of all healthcare professionals to object to participation on moral or ethical grounds. This is called 'conscientious objection' in the UK (Goligher et al. 2016), an 'objection in principle' in the Netherlands (KNMG 2011) or 'freedom of conscience' in Luxembourg (MS 2009).

Europe

The Netherlands, Belgium and Luxembourg

In the Low Countries, AD legislation exists in the Netherlands (TLRAS 2002), Belgium (Kidd 2002) and Luxembourg (MS 2009). Permitted AD practices include 'euthanasia' which, by definition, applies to a voluntary request by a patient (KNMG 2012,) and physician-assisted dying. Common to all legislation in the Low Countries is the need to demonstrate enduring unbearable physical or mental suffering (Kidd 2002; TLRAS 2002; MS 2009) with no prospect of improvement (Emanuel et al. 2016) rather than a terminal illness. Table 21.3 illustrates the practices permitted, the due care criteria and the notifiable authorities.

The granting of an AD request, however, is not guaranteed and over half of all Dutch requests will not result in such a death (Pasman 2012). Refusal is more common if it relates to being 'tired of life', depression, or a fear of being a burden (Brinkman-Stoppelenburg et al. 2014). Despite a refusal, the desire for AD may remain, however, and such patients still require psychological support (Pasman et al. 2013). Research with Dutch staff (Lewis n.d.) suggests that patients with incurable chronic illness play an active role in timing their death, talking it through and revising their timelines with nursing staff. More research is needed, but this phenomenon may be limited to jurisdictions such as the Low Countries where a fixed likely prognosis is not an essential criterion.

Age restriction

Global variations exist in the age of a patient for whom an assisted death is permitted, but having reached the age of majority is the most common (Emanuel et al. 2016). Dutch patients, however, can request an assisted death from the age of 12, but parental consent is required (TLRAS 2002). Between ages 17 and 18, Dutch legislation specifies parental inclusion in the decision-making process (TLRAS 2002). However, such assisted deaths are extremely rare with Griffiths et al. (2008) reporting three children aged between 1 and 16 each year with a first report in 2005.

Controversially, since 2014, there has been no age barrier in Belgium to AD for minors with mental capacity and an adequate level of discernment (Friedel 2014). 'Discernment' means the ability to judge the issue involved and its implications, which is considered more important than chronological age (Dan et al. 2014). This extension to the existing law, however, excludes psychiatric disorders and requires a multi-disciplinary paediatric team assessment, including a clinical psychologist (Dan et al. 2014) and parental consent.

Reporting and scrutiny of cases

Scrutiny of cases occurs in all the Low Countries (Table 21.3). The reporting of deaths to a multidisciplinary 'Regional Euthanasia Review Committee' in the Netherlands (Kimsma and van Leeuwen 2012) or a Commission in Belgium and Luxembourg (Kidd 2002; MS 2009) is mandatory if a case is to be considered lawful. Such review committees and commissions collate statistics and report on the incidence, suggesting adjustments to practice and existing laws (TLRAS 2002; MS 2009). Individual case scrutiny includes the controversial End-Of-Life Clinic (Levenseinde Clinic 2016), founded in 2012 by the Dutch Right to Die Society to assist patients whose initial request has been rejected by their regular physician (Snijdewind et al. 2015).

The role of nurses

There are differences between the Low Countries in the role of nurses within the terms of legislation. Dutch nurses have no official role, with a lack of representation in law or in Review Committee Reports (Griffiths et al. 2008). Professional guidance is provided, however, in joint medical and nursing guidelines (AVVV, NU'91 and KNMG 2006). In Belgium and Luxembourg (Kidd 2002; MS 2009), the laws, however, explicitly require physicians to consult with nurses or the care team of the patient requesting AD. Moreover, Belgian research (Dierckx de Casterlé et al. 2010; Bilsen et al. 2014) reports that nurses are often consulted, particularly in settings with an ethos of multidisciplinary working. Outside of such settings, however, consultation may only involve the most senior nurse (Dierckx de Casterlé et al. 2010).

Studies relating to the role of nurses in AD, however, are limited. In one of the few Dutch papers (van Bruchem-van de Scheur et al. 2008), in 37 per cent of cases, the hospital nurse was the first person to hear the patient's AD request. Nurses were also involved in the decision-making in over half of all cases, but the prevalence varied between care settings and was more common in nursing homes and hospitals than homecare. Controversially, nurses also administered lethal medication, although this was a relatively rare occurrence being 2.4 per cent of 205 cases (van Bruchem-van de Scheur et al. 2008). A 2016 paper (Francke et al. 2016), however, suggests this illegal activity still occurs at a similar rate. Also of concern was that 7 per cent of Dutch nurses surveyed (n = 587) were unclear about the legal boundaries of their role which forbids any action, such as turning on a drip, that initiates the flow of lethal drugs into the patient.

Table 21.3 Permitted practices, due care criteria and notification of assisted dying cases

The Netherlands (TLRSA 2002; KNMG 2011)	Belgium (Kidd 2002)	Luxembourg (MS 2009)
Permitted practices: Euthanasia (by physician only) and physician-assisted suicide (self-administered)	*Permitted practices:* Euthanasia (by physician only)	*Permitted practices:* Euthanasia and physician-assisted suicide (self-administered)
The physician must: Ensure the request is voluntary and well considered	*The physician must:* Ensure the patient has attained the age of majority or is an emancipated minor (no age restrictions since 2014)	*The physician must:* Ensure the patient has attained the age of 18
Hold the conviction that the patient's suffering is lasting and unbearable	The request is voluntary, well considered, repeated and not the result of external pressure	Make sure request is voluntary, written if possible, well considered and non-coerced
Have informed the patient about their condition and prospects	The patient has a medically futile condition, with physical and mental suffering that cannot be alleviated, caused by a serious, incurable condition	The patient is capable and conscious at time of request
Must hold the conviction with the patient there is no other reasonable solution		Ensure the patient has a medically futile, incurable condition with constant unbearable suffering
Have consulted with at least one independent physician who has seen the patient and has given a written opinion on the case	Agree with the patient's decision	Consult with another physician and, if the patient does not object, the regular care team
	Consult with another independent physician and the nursing team in regular contact with the patient	
Notification: Assisted deaths are 'unnatural'. Referred to local prosecutor for investigation. Cases are reviewed by a Regional Euthanasia Review Committee (RERC)	*Notification:* Assisted deaths are 'natural' Physicians report cases to the Federal Control and Evaluation Commission	*Notification:* Case report sent for review by the Federal Control and Evaluation Committee Euthanasia

Useful guidelines for nurses on record-keeping, however, do exist (AVVV 2006, in Dutch) and may be relevant to nurses in jurisdictions implementing similar legislation to the Low Countries such as Canada (PoC 2016). Box 21.1 includes the information suggested for inclusion in nursing records (Griffiths et al. 2008), which is largely derived from the terms of the Dutch legislation.

> ## Box 21.1 Suggested items for nursing records in the Netherlands
>
> - The nature of the request and its consistency.
> - Views of family and friends and any influence on the nature of the patient's request.
> - Physical symptoms.
> - The emotional outlook of the patient.
> - The patient's social and spiritual aspects.

Switzerland

In Switzerland, where the terminology 'assisted suicide' is used, such deaths represent less than 1 per cent of total Swiss deaths per annum, with a small consistent increase over the last few years (Gamondi et al. 2014). Most patients accessing AD are members of a right to die organisation (Bosshard et al. 2003). There is, however, no specific legislation and such deaths occur with minimal physician participation (Gamondi et al. 2016) apart from an assessment of medical capacity and of the existence of incurable illness and prescription drugs. Active euthanasia is against the law, but if certain conditions are met, such deaths are not subject to prosecution. Under Articles 115 and 114 of the Swiss Penal Code, the act must be unselfish with practical assistance usually provided by volunteers who may be other health practitioners or laypersons. The wish to die must be deliberate, stable and linked to unbearable suffering, a hopeless prognosis or unreasonable disability (Fischer et al. 2009). Right to die associations, however, are also lobbying for 'tired of living' as a criterion (Exit Deutsche Schweiz 2014).

Self-administration of the medication (Dyer et al. 2015) is required, usually taking place in the patient's own home, as few healthcare facilities allow it on site (Dyer et al. 2015). Historically such deaths were not allowed on hospital premises, but in a few hospitals this has changed, although most maintain existing bans (Bosshard 2008), preferring not to be associated with this practice. Two French Swiss cantons (Vaud and Neuchâtel), however, have enacted laws allowing AD in public hospitals and nursing homes (Borasio 2015).

Foreign nationals

Four of the six Swiss right to die organisations (Dyer et al. 2015) allow non-residents of Switzerland to access assisted suicide through their associations (Gauthier et al. 2014). Although often associated with patients travelling to Switzerland from the UK, annual statistics from Dignitas (Dignitas 2016) suggest approximately half of their clients are German. The tourism phenomenon is also starting to be of concern in Belgium where the assisted dying legislation does not specifically exclude non-residents (BioEdge 2016).

Reporting of cases

Swiss law considers suicide an unnatural violent death and all AD cases are reported to the police for investigation (Lewis and Black 2013). This reporting practice for assisted deaths appears to be total (Lewis and Black 2013) with police investigation usually leading to a 'judgment of dismissal' after enquiries have been made.

North and South America

The United States

First legally permitted in the State of Oregon in 1997 (Ganzini et al. 2002), similar legislation exists in the States of Washington (Washington State Death with Dignity Act 2008), Vermont (Vermont General Assembly 2013), California (California Department of Public Health 2016), Colorado (Colorado Government 2016), and the District of Columbia (Death with Dignity Act of 2015). In Montana, formal AD legislation is lacking, and there are no guidelines or regulation of the procedures, but a precedent in case law (*Baxter v. State of Montana* 2009) may lessen the likelihood of prosecution for physicians for cases coming before the courts (Jackson and Bowman 2011). Where legal, the patient's illness is listed as the cause of death on the death certificate and not a suicide death from the lethal medication. Table 21.4 contains the general required criteria for assisted dying in the United States.

Table 21.4 General criteria in the US States of California, Colorado, Montana, Oregon, Vermont and Washington and District of Columbia

The individual requesting assisted dying must:	The physician must:
Be 18 years of age or older	Determine the patient to have a terminal illness with a 6-month prognosis
Be a resident of the state where they are requesting a legal lethal dose of medications	Determine the patient to be mentally capable, and to be acting voluntarily
Provide two verbal requests to their attending physician a minimum of 15 days apart	Request a mental health assessment if mental disorder indicated
Provide a written request to their attending physician	Refer to a consulting physician who must confirm the 6-month prognosis and mental competence
Be able to self-administer the lethal medications	Offer alternatives including comfort, hospice and palliative care
Physicians and pharmacists must file documentation with the state health authorities (Montana is an exception)	
The death certificate completed by the attending physician lists the disease as cause of death for individuals who die with 'aid in dying' medications	

Reported deaths

Official reports from Oregon and Washington indicate that patients seek to control timing over their death due to a fear of loss of autonomy, a loss of ability to engage in enjoyable activities, and loss of dignity (Oregon Public Health Division 2016; Washington State Department of Health 2016). Such patients are disproportionately white, have some college education, and live in the western parts of both Oregon and Washington. Individuals who live in more rural communities may have limited access due to the availability of physicians and pharmacies participating in the process. In addition, not all health insurance pays for the physician visits or the prescribed aid in dying medications that have costs reporting to be up to $5000 (Dembosky 2016).

Other countries

In Canada, following the Province of Quebec in 2014 (ANQ 2013), the Canadian Supreme Court voted for AD in June 2016 (PoC 2016). A country with limited home care services, almost 70 per cent of Canadian patients will die in hospital (Taylor and Martin 2014) and only 16–30 per cent will be able to access palliative care services depending on where they live (Canadian Hospice Palliative Care Association 2014). The Medical Assistance in Dying Bill C-14 (MAiD) (PoC 2016) more closely resembles the Low Countries, including voluntary euthanasia and physician-assisted dying. Regulatory guidelines drawn up by provinces, territories and institutions will determine how and where such deaths can take place, at the time of this writing (Canadian Hospice Palliative Care Association 2016).

In Columbia, South America, the Constitutional Court declared it unconstitutional to prosecute a physician who carries out the wish to die of the terminally ill (Michlowski 2009). Palliative care quality in Columbia has been questioned (Moyano 2008), but guidelines for staff were published in 2015 (Commission for Assisted Dying 2017, in Spanish). Intravenous injection by a physician at the voluntary request of a terminally ill patient with unresolved suffering is permitted after assessment by a physician, lawyer, and psychiatrist or a clinical psychologist (Dyer et al. 2015). In contrast to all other jurisdictions in Columbia, prior approval by an independent committee is required prior to the death taking place (Emanuel et al 2016).

Assisted dying and families

An assisted death can have an impact on family survivors. Families are acknowledged as important partners in the decision-making process, often being deeply involved in the decision-making as well as giving practical support (Dees et al. 2013; Gamondi et al. 2013). There is also evidence their support, or not, may have a bearing on the patient's final decision (Ganzini et al. 2009).

Research by Dees et al. (2013) suggests that decision-making is a complex task, demanding for families, patients and healthcare professionals alike. On top of the usual tasks of caregivers (Starks et al. 2007), families need to agree to respect the patient's view, support the patient's request, and may work to find a collaborating physician. They ponder their assistance in dying, including whether or not it is ethical (Starks et al. 2007), and value open dialogue with physicians during the decision-making process (Dees et al. 2013; Gamondi et al. 2013).

Grieving and bereavement

Evidence from the Netherlands (Swarte et al. 2003) and the US (Ganzini et al. 2009) indicates that families of AD patients are better prepared for the death than those experiencing the natural death of a loved one. Families were no more likely to experience an adverse mental health outcome than for a natural death (Swarte et al. 2003; Ganzini et al. 2009). Contradictory evidence, however, also exists in a study by Wagner et al. (2012) which suggested Swiss family members witnessing an assisted death were more likely to suffer complicated grief. Differing clinical practices, however, and the cultural ramifications of such deaths, including social stigmatisation (Gamondi et al. 2015), may have a bearing. This is, however, an area with limited studies (Fish 2017) and more research is warranted. There is also a possibility of a non-response bias as family members who are depressed or more adversely affected may not participate in research.

Palliative care and assisted dying

Whatever form it takes, nowhere is assisted dying more of a contested issue than within palliative care (PC) itself. Rejected as an option by Dame Cicely Saunders principally on moral grounds (Saunders 1959), palliative care associations are often opposed to its practice, with a notable exception being the Flemish Federation. Box 21.2 shows some of the current position statements of palliative care associations, federations and societies.

Box 21.2   Position statements on assisted dying from palliative care associations, federations and societies

- *European Palliative Care Association*: The official position is that euthanasia and PAS should not be included in PC, but there is no consensus 'due to incompatible normative frameworks that clash'.
- *The Australian and New Zealand Society of Palliative Medicine*: Adopts the stance of the World Medical Association that euthanasia is in 'conflict with ethical principles of medical practice'.
- *American Academy of Hospice and Palliative Medicine*: 'Physicians practicing in jurisdictions in which PAD is legally permitted should never

be obligated to participate in PAD if they hold moral or professional objections, nor should they be prohibited from participating within parameters defined by relevant statutes and terms of employment. Physicians who affirmatively respond to requests for PAD are obligated to ensure their actions are consistent with best available practices that limit avoidable suffering through end of life.'

- *The Canadian Hospice Palliative Care Association*: 'Euthanasia or assisted suicide is not a part of quality end-of-life care.'
- *Flemish Palliative Care Federation*: 'The palliative care team is available to all patients, even those who request euthanasia. Palliative care guarantees full and proper consideration of these requests for euthanasia.'
- *International Association for Hospice and Palliative Care*: 'Palliative care units should not be responsible for overseeing or administering these practices.'

Nonetheless, in some jurisdictions, palliative care services co-exist alongside active legislation. It needs to be acknowledged, however, that direct comparison of PC provision globally is problematical as, where it exists, there are variations in its configuration. Rarely, for example, does palliative care replicate the provision in the UK. American hospice programmes are most likely to focus on home care while Belgian palliative care teams often work in hospitals (Dierckx de Casterlé et al. 2010; National Hospice and Palliative Care Organization 2015). In the Netherlands, where palliative care is not a medical speciality, hospices are plentiful, but often do not provide the range of services expected of a hospice in the UK, focusing on end of life inpatient care. Such issues complicate the direct comparison of PC between jurisdictions with active legislation as it confounds the measurement of quality indicators, for example, resource allocation (Chambaere et al. 2011). In some jurisdictions such as Belgium and Luxembourg (Berghe et al. 2013; Thill 2015), palliative care is also a relatively new speciality being formally established at the same time as AD legislation. There is some evidence that AD has increased referrals and admission to hospice services in the USA (Wang et al. 2015).

Integrated models

Integrated models are said to exist in Belgium (Bernheim et al. 2008) and Luxembourg (Thill 2015). Here palliative care and AD exist side by side, supported by separate laws, such as the Belgian Act of Palliative Care (Adams 2008) and the Euthanasia Law (Kidd 2002). This dual legislation appeased opponents of AD with the Act of Palliative Care (2002) guaranteeing access to PC for all. The law, however, stops short of demanding that all AD patients are seen by a palliative care specialist, the so-called 'palliative care filter'. Patients do, however, need to be informed of all their options, and physicians and institutions may apply the palliative care filter anyway. In practice, PC teams, particularly in hospitals, are likely to know the patient and have a role in supporting the care team, but how many agree with it or actively participate is unknown (Berghe et al. 2013). Few papers exist regarding practice in Luxembourg (MS 2009) where theoretically a similar integrated model exists, but there are concerns that PC is under-resourced for the challenges it brings (Thill 2015). This is a serious issue as AD may increase workloads. In a study in the Netherlands, 50 per cent of the hospice patients admitted wanting to discuss AD and, although most requests were retracted, appraisal of their seriousness and of fears that could be alleviated was needed (Lewis, n.d.).

While some favour an integrated model (Bernheim et al. 2008), not all agree with this option (Materstvedt 2013). Disagreements include whether or not PC has been improved (Berghe et al. 2013) or can operate alongside AD, while maintaining its own principles (Randall 2013). Common values have been identified (Hurst and Mauron 2006), such as reducing human suffering, not reducing patients to a biological status, and the desire for a 'good death'. Practically, patient autonomy, valued by both sides of the debate (Hurst and Mauron 2006), means that some practitioners must not abandon patients despite their choices, particularly in the USA (Campbell and Cox 2010). Often participating staff have to cope, however, with limited professional and organisational guidance, which is often carefully worded. An Oregonian study (Campbell and Cox 2010), where 90.1 per cent of AD patients were enrolled in a hospice programme (Oregon Public Health Division 2016), highlighted that few hospice programmes (16 per cent) fully cooperated with the law. Staff were permitted to engage in neutral dialogue with patients (32 per cent) or could refer the patient to their physician (27 per cent), but few programmes reported providing, paying for, or assisting with lethal drug administration (Campbell and Cox 2010). In contrast, the majority of Dutch PC units (80 per cent) do permit assisted deaths (pers. comm. Onwuteaka-Philipsen 2015), with the exception of the religiously affiliated, who transfer patients to their family doctor or to a hospital where it is permitted.

Unexpected consequences of legislation

A consequence of AD legislation is the viewing of other palliative end of care options as potentially illegal (Berghe et al. 2013). This may result in raising the thresholds for sedation, withdrawing or withholding of treatment and the intensive alleviation of symptoms using drugs (Berghe et al. 2013). It is also suggested that palliative sedation or increasing opioid dosages will become more popular, as they are easier than the legal procedures for an assisted death (Rys et al. 2012).

Objective appraisal is, however, difficult. Research suggests intensive symptom alleviation has increased in the Netherlands (Onwuteaka-Philipsen et al. 2012), but this may be due to an improved knowledge of PC principles rather than a desire to hasten death. Palliative sedation has also come under scrutiny, but this care area is blighted by inconsistent terminology and elusive quantification of its ability to relieve distress (Rady and Verheijde 2012). Evidence from the Netherlands (Anquinet et al. 2013), however, suggests its use is lower than in the UK, with incidences of 8 per cent (hospitals) and

11 per cent (community) compared with 17 per cent and 19 per cent for the same settings in the UK (Anquinet et al. 2013). Dutch practitioners also have the benefit of very comprehensive sedation guidelines (KNMG 2009) which may discourage inappropriate use, but, as in the UK, appraisal of such matters is difficult as the prescriber's intention may be unknown (Douglas et al. 2008). Perhaps most helpful is Berghe et al.'s (2013) suggestion that end of life care options should not be seen as interchangeable, but as having their own indications, making them more or less appropriate with the overall aim being to ensure a peaceful death.

Learning exercise 21.1

Sue, a community nurse, has visited Simon, a 73-year-old independently minded gentleman with inoperable pancreatic cancer. He lives alone, but has a supportive friend Ann who lives locally.

Using the Internet to find out about his condition, and despite palliative chemotherapy, he is aware his long-term prognosis is not very good. He dislikes being ill and is worried about being a burden on Ann. Although they have had a long friendship and she is caring, the couple are not intimate.

He has watched several television programmes about the Swiss clinic Dignitas and asks you directly for your advice on assisted dying. What issues would you need to consider? Do you know of any sources of advice?

Clinical challenges: how to respond to a wish for an assisted death

It has long been appreciated that healthcare professionals will provide care for patients who wish to hasten death including nurses (Ganzini et al. 2002) and doctors (Griffiths et al. 2012). Clinical guidelines on dealing with a direct request are, however, much rarer.

Currently in the UK the practice of assisting dying is unlawful, but nonetheless the Royal College of Nursing (RCN) provides comprehensive guidance for responding to a request (RCN 2016). This clarifies the law in the UK, discusses why patients may request a hasten death and how to approach such a request. All requests for a hasten death have to be dealt with compassionately (Griffith et al. 2012), but in jurisdictions where assisted dying is not permitted, being clear about the law is essential.

In the UK it is unwise for nurses to supply information to patients relating to assisting dying such as naming, supplying details of such organisations or arranging travel (RCN 2016). Instead practitioners should 'Stop and think' (RCN 2016) and, in a nonjudgemental fashion, draw out the reason for a request. Such discussions can lead to the patients completing a new, or a revised, advance care plan providing it contains lawful options. Careful documentation of conversations is needed and, if in doubt, considering the involvement of senior colleagues is recommended (RCN 2016). Offering your personal stance on assisted dying is not recommended. Acknowledging the request empathetically, listening and checking the patient's concerns are helpful and may lead to establishing the reasons for a request (RCN 2016). It may also be possible to alleviate some fears when the patient's reasoning is established.

Multi-disciplinary discussion to consider the patient's needs should be undertaken. If not already known to palliative care services, referral may be instigated.

Depression may feature in 20 per cent of requests (Ganzini et al. 2000) so psychological review, including mental capacity, is strongly recommended (RCN 2016). Ongoing support of the patient needs to be considered, but staff will also need to consider their own needs with clinical supervision suggested as helpful.

Conclusion

This chapter has summarised the terminological issues, due care criteria and the practices occurring in jurisdictions globally which permit assisted dying. More research on the role of nurses is justified, particularly with the expanding role of nurses in some jurisdictions, but where it exists, an overview has been included. Although caring for patients who request to hasten death is not new, in the context of AD, the challenges may be considerable and nurses need to be clear about the legally permitted practices. In the context of a lack of organisational or professional guidance, this is particularly important. The role of palliative care in AD is controversial, contested and complicated by differing models of palliative care provision globally. Some of the salient issues related to models integrating PC and assisted dying are highlighted. The chapter ends with guidance for nurses on how to respond to a request for an assisted death.

References

Adams. M. (2008) Belgium and the Belgian health care system. In Griffiths, H., Weyers, H. and Adams, M. (eds) *Euthanasia and the Law in Europe*. Oxford: Hart Publishing.

American Academy of Hospice and Palliative Medicine (2016) Statement on physician assisted dying. Available at: http://aahpm.org/positions/pad (accessed 13 January 2017).

ANQ (2013) *Bill 52. An Act Respecting End-of-Life Care*. Available at: http://www.assnat.qc.ca/en/travaux-parlementaires/projets-loi/projet-loi-52-40-1.html (accessed 20 November 2016).

Anquinet, L., Raus, K., Sterckx, S. et al. (2013) Similarities and differences between continuous sedation until death and euthanasia – professional caregivers' attitudes and experiences: focus group study. *Palliative Medicine*, 27(6): 553–61.

Australian and New Zealand Society of Palliative Medicine, I. (2016) ANZSPM Position Statement (2013) on the Practice of Euthanasia and Assisted Suicide. Available at: http://www.anzspm.org.au/c/anzspm?a=da&did=1005077 (accessed 13 January 2017).

AVV, NU'91 and KNMG (2006) *Handreiking voor Samenwerking Artsen*, Verpleegkundigen en Verzorgenden bij Enthanasie [Guidelines to Support the Collaboration of Physicians, Nurses and Caretakers in Euthanasia Procedures] (4th edn). Utrecht, the Netherlands: AVV, Nu'91 and KNMG.

Berghe, P., Mullie, A., Desment, M. et al. (2013) Assisted dying: the current situation in Flanders: euthanasia embedded in palliative care. *European Journal of Palliative Care*, 20(6): 266–72.

Bernheim, J., Deschepper, R., Distelmans, W. et al. (2008) Development of palliative care and legalisation of euthanasia: antagonism or synergy? *BMJ*, 336: 864–7.

Bilsen, J., Robijn, L., Chambaere, K. et al. (2014) Nurses' involvement in physician-assisted dying under the euthanasia law in Belgium. *International Journal of Nursing Studies*, 51: 1696–7.

BioEdge (2016) Euthanasia tourism on the rise in Belgium. Available at: https://www.bioedge.org/bioethics/euthanasia-tourism-on-the-rise-in-belgium/11985 (accessed 28 January 2017).

Borasio, G.D. (2015) Point de vue médical sur le suicide assisté – la bienveillance négligée. *BMS*, 96: 889–91.

Bosshard, G. (2008) Switzerland. In Griffiths, J., Weyers, H. and Adams, M. (eds) *Euthanasia and Law in Europe*. Portland, OR: Hart Publishing.

Bosshard, G., Ulrich, E. and Bär, W. (2003) 748 cases of suicide assisted by a Swiss right-to-die organisation. *Swiss Medical Weekly*, 133: 310–17.

Bosshard, G., Ulrich, E., Ziegler, S.J. et al. (2008) Assessment of requests for assisted suicide by a Swiss right-to-die society. *Death Studies*, 32: 646–57.

Boudreau, J.D. and Somerville, M.A. (2013) Euthanasia is not medical treatment. *British Medical Bulletin*, 106: 45–66.

Brinkman-Stoppelenburg, A., Vergouwe, Y., van der Heide, A. et al. (2014) Obligatory consultation of an independent physician on euthanasia requests in the Netherlands: what influences the SCEN physicians' judgement of the legal requirements of due care? *Health Policy*, 115: 75–81.

CAD (2012) *The Commission on Assisted Dying*. London: Demos. Available at: https://www.demos.co.uk/project/the-commission-on-assisted-dying/ (accessed 20 November 2016).

California Department of Public Health (2016) End of Life Care Option Act AB -15. Available at: https://www.cdph.ca.gov/Pages/EndofLifeOptionAct.aspx (accessed 28 January 2017).

Campbell, C.S. and Cox, J.C. (2010) Hospice and physician-assisted death: collaboration, complicance and complicity. *Hastings Center Reports*, 40(5): 26–35.

Canadian Hospice Palliative Care Association (2014) Hospice Palliative Care in Canada. Available at: http://www.chpca.net/projects-and-advocacy/advocacy-strategy.aspx (accessed 31 January 2017).

Canadian Hospice Palliative Care Association (2016) Update on Medical Aid in Assistance in Dying (MAID). Available at: http://www.chpca.net/projects-and-advocacy/chpca-policy-alerts/chpca-policy-alert-bill-c-14-medical-assistance-in-dying-(maid)-update.aspx (accessed 31 January 2017).

Chambaere, K., Centro, C., Alejandro Hernandez, E. et al. (2011) *Palliative Care Development in Countries with a Euthanasia Law. Report for the Commission on Assisted Dying Briefing Paper.* Available at: http://www.commissiononassisted-dying.co.uk/wp-content/uploads/2011/10/EAPC-Briefing-Paper-Palliative-Care-in-Countries-with-a-Euthanasia-Law.pdf (accessed 13 February 2014).

Chapman, C. (2006) Swiss hospital lets terminally ill patients commit suicide in its beds. *BMJ,* 332: 7.

Colorado Government (2016) Colorado End of Life Options Act. Available at: https://www.sos.state.co.us/pubs/elections/Initiatives/titleBoard/filings/2015-2016/145Final.pdf (accessed 28 January 2017).

Commission for Assisted Dying (2017) Euthanasia in Columbia. Available at: http://www.commissiononassisteddying.co.uk/euthanasia-in-colombia/ (accessed 21 September 2017).

Dan, B., Fonteyne, C. and Clément de Cléty, S. (2014) Self-request euthanasia for children in Belgium. *Lancet,* 383: 671–2.

Death with Dignity Act of 2015, L21-0182 Effective from Feb. 18 2017, Council of the District of Columbia (2017).

Death with Dignity National Center (2016) *Death with Dignity Acts.* Available at: http://www.deathwithdignity.org/advocates/national (accessed 20 November 2016).

Dees, M.K., Vernooij-Dassen, M.J., Dekkers, W.J. et al. (2013) Perspectives of decision-making in requests for euthanasia: a qualitative research among patients, relatives and treating physicians in the Netherlands. *Palliative Medicine,* 27(1): 27–37.

Dembosky, A. (2016) Drug company jacks up cost of aid-in-dying medication. Available at: http://www.npr.org/sections/health-shots/2016/03/23/471595323/drug-company-jacks-up-cost-of-aid-in-dying-medication (accessed 28 January 2017).

Dierckx de Casterlé, B., Denier, Y., De Bal, N. et al. (2010) Nursing care for patients requesting euthanasia in general hospitals in Flanders, Belgium. *Journal of Advanced Nursing,* 2410–20.

Dignitas (2016) Dignitas: to live with dignity. Available at: http://www.dignitas.ch/ (accessed 5 January 2017).

Douglas, C., Kerridge, I. and Ankeny, R. (2008) Managing intentions: the end of life administration of analgesics and sedatives, and the possibility of slow euthanasia. *Bioethics,* 22(7): 388–96.

Dyer, O., White, C. and Garcia Rada, A. (2015) Assisted dying: law and practice around the world. *BMJ,* 351: h4481.

Emanuel, E. (1994) The history of euthanasia debates in the United States and Britain. *Annals of Internal Medicine,* 121(10): 793–802.

Emanuel, E., Onwuteaka-Philipsen, B., Unwin, J. et al. (2016) Attitudes and practice of euthanasia and physician-assisted suicide in the United States, Canada, and Europe. *JAMA,* 316(1): 79–80.

Exit Deutsche Schweiz (2014) GV stimmt pro Altersfreitod. Available at: https.www.exit.ch/news/news/details/kommen-sie-zur-gv/ Kommentar dazu (accessed 31 January 2017).

Federatie Palliative Zorg Viaanderen (2011) Over palliatieve zorg en euthana-sie [On palliative care and euthanasia]. Amsterdam: Federatie Palliative Zorg Viaanderen.

Fischer, S., Huber, C.A., Imhof, L. et al. (2009) Suicide assisted by two Swiss right-to-die organisations. *Journal of Medical Ethics,* 34: 810–14.

Fish, J. (2017) The experience of bereavement following a physician assisted suicide (PAS). What do we know about the needs of these bereaved? *Bereavement Care*, 36(1): 8–10.

Francke, A.L., Albers, G., Bilsen, J. et al. (2016) Nursing staff and euthanasia in the Netherlands: a nation-wide survey on attitudes and involvement in decision-making and the performance of euthanasia. *Patient Education and Counseling*, 99: 783–9.

Friedel, M. (2014) Does the Belgian law legalising euthanasia for minors really address the needs of life-limited children? *International Journal of Palliative Nursing*, 20(4): 265–7.

Gamondi, C., Borasio, G.D., Limoni, C. et al. (2014) Legalisation of assisted suicide: a safeguard to euthanasia? *Lancet*, 384: 127.

Gamondi, C., Borasio, G.D., Oliver, P. et al. (2016) Palliative care physicians' experiences of the Swiss model of assisted suicide: a qualitative interview study. Submitted for publication: June.

Gamondi, C., Pott, M., Forbes, K. et al. (2015) Exploring the experiences of bereaved families involved in assisted suicide in Southern Switzerland: a qualitative study. *BMJ Supportive and Palliative Care*, 5: 146–52.

Gamondi, C., Pott, M. and Payne, S. (2013) Families' experiences with patients who died after assisted suicide: a retrospective interview study in southern Switzerland. *Annals of Oncology*, 24(6): 1639–44.

Ganzini, L., Goy, E.R., Dobscha, S.K. et al. (2009) Mental health outcomes of family members of Oregonians who request physician aid in dying. *Journal of Pain Symptom Management*, 38(6): 807–15.

Ganzini., L., Harvath, T.A., Jackson, A. et al. (2002) Experiences of Oregon nurses and social workers with hospice patients who request assistanece with suicide. *New England Journal of Medicine*, 347(8): 582–8.

Ganzini., L., Nelson, H.D., Schmidt, T.A. et al. (2000) Physicians' experiences with the Oregon Death with Dignity Act. *New England Journal of Medicine*, 342(8): 557–63.

Gardner, D.B. (2012) Quality in life and death: can we have the conversation? *Nursing Economics*, 30(4): 224–32.

Gauthier, S., Mausbach, J., Reisch, T. et al. (2014) Suicide tourism: a pilot study on the Swiss phenomenon. *Journal of Medical Ethics*, doi:10.1136/medethics-2014-102091.

Goligher, E., De Sorbo, L., Cheung, A. et al. (2016) Why conscientious objection merits respect. *CMAJ*, 188: 822–3.

Griffiths, J.L., D' Silva, S. and Call, D. (2012) A commpassionate reponse to a request to die. *Psychiatric Annals*, 42(4): 127–32.

Griffiths, J., Weyers, H. and Adams, M. (2008) *Euthanasia and Law in Europe*. Portland, OR: Hart Publishing.

Hurst, S.A. and Mauron, A. (2006) The ethics of palliative care and euthanasia: exploring common values. *Palliative Medicine*, 20: 107–12.

International Association for Hospice and Palliative Care (2017) Position Statement: Euthanasia and Physician-Assisted Suicide. *Journal of Palliative Medicine*, 20(1): 8–14.

Jackson, G. and Bowman, M. (2011) Analysis of implications of the Baxter Case on potential criminal liability. Available at: http://leg.mt.gov/bills/2011/Minutes/Senate/Exhibits/jus32a41.pdf (accessed 20 November 2016).

Kidd, D. (2002) The Belgian Act on Euthanasia of May 28th. *Ethical Perspectives*, 9(2–3): 182–7. Available at: http://www.ethical- perspectives.be/viewpic.php?TABLE=EP&ID =59 (accessed 9 December 2016).

Kimsma, G. and van Leeuwen, E. (2012) Reviews after the Act: the role and work of Regional Euthanaia Review Committees. In Younger, S.J. and Kimsma G.K. (eds) *Physician-Assisted Death in Perspective: Assessing the Dutch Experience.* New York: Cambridge University Press.

KNMG (2009) *Guideline for Palliative Sedation.* Available at: https://www.knmg.nl/ contact/about-knmg.htm (accessed 21 September 2017).

KNMG (2011) *The Role of the Physician in the Voluntary Termination of Life.* Available at: https://www.knmg.nl (accessed 14 November 2016).

KNMG (2012) *Euthanasia in the Netherlands: The Facts.* Royal Dutch Medical Association. Available at: http://knmg.artsennet.nl/Over-KNMG/About-KNMG.htm (accessed 7 May 2015).

Levenseinde Clinic (2016) Available at: https://www.levenseindekliniek.nl/en/ (accessed 5 January 2017).

Lewis, D.A. (n.d.) Assisted dying in the Netherlands: What is the experience of Dutch healthcare professionals in a hospice and a chronic disease care centre? PhD thesis, Lancaster University.

Lewis, P. and Black, I. (2013) Reporting and scrutiny of reported cases in four jurisdictions where assisted dying is lawful: a review of the evidence in the Netherlands, Belgium, Oregon and Switzerland. *Medical Law International*, 13(4): 221–39.

Manning, M. (1998) *Euthanasia and Physician-Assisted Suicide: Killing or Caring?* New York: Paulist Press.

Materstvedt, L.J. (2013) Palliative care ethics: the problems of combining palliation and assisted dying. *Progress in Palliative Care*, 21(3): 158–64.

Materstvedt, L.J. and Bosshard, G. (2015) Euthanasia and palliative care. In Cherny, N., Fallon, M., Kaasa, S. et al. (eds) *Oxford Textbook of Palliative Medicine* (5th edn). Oxford: Oxford University Press.

Michlowski, S. (2009) Legalising active voluntary euthanasia through the courts: some lessons from Columbia. *Medical Law Review*, 17: 183–218.

Montana Supreme Court (2009) *Baxter v. State of Montana.* Available at: http://cases. justia.com/montana/supreme-court/2009-12-31-DA 09-0051 Published – Opinion.pdf? ts=1396129594 (accessed 31 January 2017).

Moyano, J.R. (2008) Ten years later, Columbia is still confused about euthanasia. Available at: http://www.bmj.com/rapid-response/2011/11/01/ten-years-later-colombia-still-confused-about-euthanasia (accessed 21 January 2017).

MS (2009) *Euthanasia and Assisted Suicide Law of 16th March.* Ministère de la Santé. Available at: http://www.sante.public.lu/fr/publications/e/euthanasie-assistance-suicide-questions-reponses-fr-de-pt-en/euthanasie-assistance-suicide-questions-en. pdf (accessed 24 January 2017).

National Hospice and Palliative Care Organization (2015) NHPCO's Facts and Figures: Hospice Care in America. Available at: http://www.nhpco.org/sites/default/files/public/Statistics_Research/2015_Facts_Figures.pdf

NL Gov (2012) Euthanasia, assisted suicide and non-resuscitation on request. Available at: https://www.government.nl/topics/euthanasia/contents/euthanasia-assisted-suicide-and-non-resuscitation-on-request (accessed 11 January 2017).

Oregon Legislature (1994) The Oregon Death with Dignity Act, 127.800. Available at: https://www.oregonlegislature.gov/bills_laws/ors/ors127.html (accessed 13 February 2017).

Oregon Public Health Division (2016) Oregon Revised Statute. Available at: http://www.worldrtd.net/sites/default/files/newsfiles/Oregon report 2015.pdf (accessed 31 January 2017).

Onwuteaka-Philipsen, B.D., Brinkman-Stoppelenburg, A., Penning, C. et al. (2012) Trends in end-of-life practices before and after the enactment of the euthanasia law in the Netherlands from 1990 to 2010: a repeated cross-sectional survey. *Lancet*, 380: 908–15. doi: 10.1016/s0140-6736(12)61034–4.

Pasman, H.R.W. (2012) When requests do not result in euthanasia or assisted suiside. In Younger, S.J. and Kimsma G.K. (eds) *Physician-Assisted Death in Perspective: Assessing the Dutch Experience*. New York: Cambridge University Press.

Pasman, H.R.W., Willems, D.L. and Onwuteaka-Philipsen, B.D. (2013) What happens after a request for euthanasia is refused? Qualitative interviews with patients, relatives and physicians. *Patient Education and Counseling*, 92: 313–18.

PoC (2016) Statutes of Canada. Chapter 3. Available at: http://www.parl.gc.ca/House-Publications/Publication.aspx?Language=E&Mode=1&DocId=8384014. (accessed 13 February 2017).

Radbruch, L., Leget, C., Bahr, P. et al. (2015) Euthanasia and physician-assisted suicide: a White Paper from the European Association for Palliative Care. *Palliative Medicine*, 30(2): 104–16.

Rady, M.Y. and Verheijde, J.L. (2012) Deep sedation at the end of life: life-shortening effect and palliative efficacy. *American Journal of Hospice and Palliative Medicine*, 30(1): 100–1.

Randall, F. (2013) Commentary on 'Assisted dying – the current situation in Flanders: euthanasia embedded in palltaive care'. *European Journal of Palliative Care*, 20(6): 273–6.

RCN (2016) *When Someone Asks for Your Assistance to Die* (2nd edn). London: Royal College of Nursing. Available at: https://www.rcn.org.uk/news-and-events/news/updated-guidance-on-assisted-suicide (accessed 10 February 2017).

Rosenfeld, B., Pessin, H., Marziliano, A. et al. (2014) Does desire for hastened death change in terminally ill cancer patients? *Social Science & Medicine*, 11: 35–40.

Rys, S., Deschepper, R., Mortier, F. et al. (2012) The moral difference or equivalence between continuous sedation until death and physician-assisted death: word games or war games? *Bioethical Enquiry*, 9: 171–83.

Saunders, C. (1959) Care of the dying 1: the problem of euthanasia. *Nursing Times*, 9 October, pp. 60–1.

Snijdewind, M.C., Willems, D.L., Deliens, L. et al. (2015) A study of the first year of the end-of-life clinic for physician-assisted dying in the Netherlands. *JAMA*, 175(10): 1633–40.

Starks, H., Back, A.L., Pearlman, R.A. et al. (2007) Family member involvement in hastened death. *Death Studies*, 31(2): 105–30.

Swarte, N.B., van der Lee, M.L., van der Bom, J.G. et al. (2003) Effects of euthanasia on the bereaved family and friends. *BMJ*, 327: 189–94.

Taylor, M. and Martin, S. (2014) Whose death is it anyway? Perspectives on end-of-life care in Canada. *HealthcarePapers*. 14(1): 7–19.

Thill, B. (2015) Euthanasia and assisted suicide in Luxembourg: the personal views of a palliative care physician. *European Journal of Palliative Care*, 22(1): 22–5.

TLRAS (2002) The Dutch Termination of Life on Request and Assisted Suicide (Review Procedures) Act. Available at: http://www.eutanasia.ws/documentos/Leyes/Internacional/Holanda%20Ley%202002.pdf (accessed 3 May 2016).

Tucker, K. (2015) Normalizing aid-in-dying within the practice of medicine. *Hasting Center Reports*, 45(5): 3.

van Bruchem-van de Scheur, G., van der Arend, A., Abu-Saad, H.H. et al. (2008) The role of nurses in euthanasia and physician-assisted suicide in The Netherlands. *Journal of Medical Ethics*, 34(4): 254–8.

Vermont General Assembly (2013) Patient Choice at End of Life, Vermont Statute, Title 18, Chapter 113. Available at: http://legislature.vermont.gov/statutes/chapter/18/113 (accessed 28 January 2017).

Vink, T. (2016) Self-euthanasia, the Dutch experience: in search for the meaning of a good death or Eu Thanatos. *Bioethics*, 30(9): 681–8.

Wagner, B., Keller, V., Knaevelsrud, C. et al. (2012) Social acknowledgement as a predictor of post traumatic stress and complicated grief after witnessing assisted suicide. *International Journal of Socal Psychiatry*, 58(4): 381–5.

Wang, S.-Y., Aldridge, M.D., Gross, C.P. et al. (2015) Geographic variation of hospice use patterns at the end of life. *Journal of Palliative Medicine*, 18(9): 771–80.

Washington State Department of Health (2016) Washington State Department of Health 2015 Death with Dignity Act Report Executive Summary. Available at: http://www.doh.wa.gov/portals/1/Documents/Pubs/422-109-DeathWithDignityAct2015.pdf (accessed 28 January 2017).

Washington State Death with Dignity Act (2008) Available at: http://www.doh.wa.gov/YouandYourFamily/IllnessandDisease/DeathwithDignityAct (accessed 28 January 2017).

Case cited

Baxter v. State of Montana 2009

Chapter

22

Facilitating change in palliative care

Laura Green and Sue Spencer

Introduction

Never doubt that a small group of thoughtful, committed citizens can change the world. Indeed, it is the only thing that ever has.

(Margaret Mead)

Contemporary palliative care faces unprecedented challenges. Changing demographics, political and economic uncertainty, and continued development of medical technology mean that caring for people at the end of life is becoming more complex, both in practical and ethical terms. Nurses are in key positions to effect change and service development, but historically have not always been empowered to do so. This chapter addresses the issue of facilitating change in palliative care. Four case studies in this chapter give help to root this in real-life situations.

The call for change: why is change needed in palliative and end of life care

Medical and technical knowledge relating to health and disease is expanding at speed globally, leading to increased longevity. But this also means that people often experience an extended prognosis with life-limiting illnesses, sometimes with a protracted dying phase. The point at which a person can be said to be dying is not clear, and interventions and treatments are often continued until close to death. In essence, these changes mean that more people are living to very old age but are also experiencing suffering associated with multiple morbidities, including dementia. A ten-year project in the United States has revealed great progress, for example, the recognition of palliative medicine as a distinct clinical field. But it has also highlighted issues of concern, such as reduced proportion of non-medical members of palliative care teams and on-going inequalities in access to specialist palliative care (Clark 2013).

The traditional palliative care approach proposed by Dame Cicely Saunders no longer meets the needs of *all* people at the end of life. There are inequalities of access to palliative care for people in different countries, with different diagnoses, from different cultural backgrounds and in different contexts of care. In resource-poor countries, additional challenges are faced in providing palliative care that often relate to political concerns and fragmented infrastructure. A recent evaluation by the Economist's Intelligence Unit ranked countries in terms of 'quality of death', which included consideration of the palliative and healthcare environment, human resources, the affordability and quality of care, and the level of community engagement. Palliative care provision is only available in a minority of countries. From a global perspective and particularly in countries without specific palliative care services, there are unprecedented challenges to facilitating good end of life care, and a pressing need to develop services that are effective, evidence-based and equitable (The Economist Intelligence Unit 2015).

Change refers to any act or process by which something shifts from one way of being or doing things to another. In this process, the identity of the original form is lost. This can present practical, emotional and political challenges to those involved, at all levels (Manley et al. 2005). Nurses are often close to patients and their families at the end of life, and this gives them a sensitivity to what is needed and gives insight into the complexity of care (Richer et al. 2013). Nurses are therefore well positioned to effect and enact change to improve, adapt and evolve palliative care. Becoming a change agent does not necessarily require a position of seniority. We suggest that facilitating change is a frame of mind, an approach, and an attitude available to all. Indeed, nurses cannot *fail* to be agents of change. It is a duty incumbent on nurses as professionals seeking to maintain patient-centred services.

However, this professional duty requires that nurses are adequately equipped to navigate and facilitate change in their clinical areas. Regrettably, nurses are often the passive recipients of changes to services rather than the instigators and catalysts. In part, this can be attributed to the legacy of traditional hierarchical models where nurses enact practices defined by physicians and service managers. However, it can also relate to a lack of deep understanding within the profession about the nature of change, and inadequate education about facilitating change in the real world. Change requires a range of social and political resources that are often not available to nurses who may often be preoccupied with the day-to-day demands of providing care to patients.

Traditional models of change tend to view both the agents and the recipients of change as rational beings. However, models of change offer at best a scaffold which offers insight into some of the various forces at play in the process of change; there is no tried and tested method to effect enduring change. We propose four key concepts that support nurses in facilitating change:

1   Transitions
2   Agency

3   Systems

4   Relationships.

This chapter is aimed at nurses working with people at the end of life, in generalist or specialist settings, and nurses who are in key positions of influence with regards to change, clinical nurse specialists, managers and leaders in all clinical areas. We do not offer an instruction manual for change. Rather, our aim is to consider the nature of change, and the kaleidoscope of factors that facilitate or inhibit effective and enduring change.

Transitions

The single biggest reason organisational changes fail is that no one has thought about endings or planned to manage their impact on people. Naturally concerned about the future, planners and implementers all too often forget that people have to let go of the present first.

(Bridges 2009, p. 37)

All change, whether for better or worse, is accompanied by transitions. This means an inevitable period of uncertainty or liminality (Kralik et al. 2006). Attitudes towards change are influenced by emotions and relate to what people think they are going to lose. The wish for order and predictability is at the heart of the human condition and people are often intolerant of change – particularly when this is associated with ambiguity (Obholzer and Roberts 2003). A person's tolerance of change is influenced by their cultural and social context, as well as the perceived impact of the change on their personal and professional well-being. It is important that emotional investment is considered a factor, particularly in larger changes such as organisational restructuring. There may also be fears over temporary incompetence if the change relates to practice, as well as to a perceived threat of being judged. Such anxieties may exacerbate resistance to change (Bridges 2009).

Change requires engagement from a range of stakeholders but anyone initiating change, whether it is at an individual level or an organisation-wide level, needs to be aware of potential obstacles. One significant obstacle is the assumption that people respond to change rationally, despite historical evidence that this is rarely the case.

Resistance to change is often perceived to be subversive and those who object are labelled as dissidents. Yet resistance is a natural response to threat, and awareness of this must be at the heart of any planned changes. One example might be initial objections of nurses to a planned change to single nurse administration of controlled drugs. If there are co-existing concerns about staffing levels, then an objection to this may be on the suspicion that the organisation is seeking to reduce the numbers of qualified nurses required on a shift. These kinds of suspicions require a level of engagement with staff, and reassurance about the rationale for the change, which acknowledges these concerns as valid and understandable in context.

Engaging people in change requires 'emotional intelligence' (Goleman 1995), that is, awareness of the consequences of one's actions on those around you, insight into one's own and others' responses (the latter is often referred to as empathy). An emotionally intelligent nurse will be able to manage emotions healthily and to hold the emotions of others in a compassionate way. Because change involving people often results in a sense of unease or instability and a move away from comfortable and familiar routines, emotionally intelligent change agents are able to assist people to develop resilience and to tolerate the insecurity that often accompanies the process of change.

Bridges' transition model has been widely used in leadership programmes and illuminates the emotional dimensions of the personal and professional responses. People experience numerous transitions along this journey, and often these points are accompanied by resistance. Resistance can take many forms, including changes in group dynamics, sabotage and disruption, and difficult communication (Chow and Chan 2015). Undermining of managers can take place and passive aggressive resistance can become normalised and tolerated (Atkinson 2016). Avoiding this is not necessarily always possible, but full involvement of all those affected by the change can go some degree towards minimising the likelihood of resistance. Time spent identifying those who may be affected by proposed changes is time well invested and often too many assumptions are made at the early stages of a project as to who might need to be involved in the process and proposed outcomes.

Transitions are often described as 'liminal' states, where the former situation no longer exists, but the envisaged future situation has not yet fully arrived. This state can be difficult and frustrating, particularly as different members of staff may adopt change at different speeds. Ongoing reassurance for staff of the value of the change is beneficial, and may be framed in terms of information, emotional support or reminders of the original impetus for the change. Meaningful on-going evaluations of the change can be helpful, as in the provision of adequate information about what is going on, why things are happening the way they are and information on whom the change impacts. Regular feedback, including anonymous evaluations and contributions to process reports, can help people feel involved and included in the process.

Bridges argues that new ways of working must be made explicit. Furthermore, he recommends acknowledgement that staff need to let go of previous ways of working before they are able to embrace change. It is important to identify roles and relationships in the new system of working, including checking whether people are feeling included and valued. Loss and grief are natural responses to change, and emotional responses to this can appear as resistance to change. For staff working in end of life care, these emotional responses can be suppressed in favour of presentation of kindness that in itself can limit change. One example of this is the resistance of nurses to the introduction of new technologies such as telemedicine to support end of life care (HURYK 2010; Taylor et al. 2014).

Dixon-Woods et al. (2014), drawing on the experience of the Health Foundation's evaluations of programmes it has supported, set out ten challenges facing those who aim to improve the quality (however defined, and whether large- or small-scale) of health service delivery (Health Foundation 2013). They conclude that 'there is no magic bullet in improving quality in healthcare'. Improvement requires multiple, often apparently contradictory, approaches: strong leadership alongside a participatory culture, direction and control and also flexibility in implementation according to local need, and critical feedback on performance without the attachment of blame (Health Foundation 2013, p. 882).

Publicly accountable healthcare services are required to be effective and efficient. In the UK, this means adopting management techniques, including performance measurement, the separation of service providers and commissioners, and the development of patient-reported outcomes measurements or PROMs. There is controversy over the role of measurement in palliative care. Some believe that end of life care is too complex and multidimensional to be reducible to measurable outcomes and that, even if these were quantifiable, it is difficult to pinpoint which interventions are causally associated with outcomes. In contrast, it has been argued that measurement of outcomes is not only possible but essential if services are to be developed appropriately (Bausewein et al. 2011; Collins et al. 2015; Higginson et al. 2015) and that what is required is the development of outcomes specific to palliative care that acknowledge the complexity of this care environment and of the experiences of patients facing the end of life. If palliative care is to be justified in a healthcare economy that requires demonstration of effectiveness and efficiency, the judicious use of outcomes measures is essential. Without measurement, it becomes impossible to prove what works, to demonstrate changes in patient conditions, and to ensure that patients receive the most appropriate interventions.

Outcome measures can be used in several ways. In the patient-specific sense, they can be used to ascertain a patient's baseline with regards to symptoms or distress or function, and subsequently to trace changes in the person's condition over time. This is the intended use for the iPOS that is currently being validated as part of the Outcome Assessment and Complexity Collaborative (OACC) suite of outcome measures (Higginson et al. 2015). Another use of measures is to examine change following a particular intervention, or to evaluate the effectiveness of a change in a service or treatment. An example of this might be to measure anxiety levels after participation in a multi-disciplinary breathlessness clinic, which might serve a dual purpose of both evaluating the effectiveness of the clinic, and as a means of comparing or benchmarking the impact of different services (Farquhar et al. 2014).

Palliative care research is relatively under-funded in comparison to other clinical areas. The evidence base is expanding but remains small, reflecting both pragmatic and ethical difficulties in researching this population and a lack of recognition by funders that it is possible to establish best practice in such a complex, diverse and multi-professional field. Further, research findings often fail to become integrated into practice. The 'theory–practice gap' in palliative care is a concern; services often evolve in silos, responding to good ideas rather than building on best evidence. Very few evidence-based healthcare improvements are actually put into practice, and it has been estimated that it takes, on average, around 17 years for knowledge to be applied (Colditz 2006). Reasons for failed innovations are complex and include the characteristics of the innovator and the organisation, the nature of the dissemination, and organisational patterns of communication. Yet palliative care is as much in need of demonstrating effectiveness and efficiency as other areas of clinical practice. It is therefore important to consider how to translate research findings into practice, and this requires awareness of change theory. Making enduring changes requires knowledge of the best methods for implementation to facilitate timely quality improvement. Current work in Australia is seeking to enhance the strength of palliative care research (Chan et al. 2014) in order to facilitate evidence-based change.

This emerging area of knowledge, known as improvement science, is neither audit nor research. Audit seeks to measure what is happening, against an agreed standard of best practice. Research seeks to discover new answers to problems or questions. Improvement science aims to bridge the space between these two, to reduce the gap between 'what is actual and what is possible'. It seeks to apply the principles of evidence-based practice to the 'science' of improvement, for example, through identification of potential barriers and facilitators to change. Implementation science examines the methods used in applying evidence to practice. The premise for implementation science is that it is just as important to know the best methods to apply evidence in practice as it is to establish that evidence base in the first place. As yet, there is relatively little in the way of empirical evidence to support improvement science (Health Foundation 2011) but this is gradually changing (see, for example, Kinley et al. 2014).

Agency

Change is inherently political (Van de Ven and Poole 1995) and success requires the engagement of all stakeholders. Indeed, Battilana suggests that all changes are 'an exercise in social influence' (Battilana and Casciaro 2012). An important influence on the success or failure of a planned change is the power, or agency, of the person facilitating the change. Agency refers to the capacity or power of a person to act in a given environment. It is the possibility of human choice influencing action, as contrasted to action occurring through natural forces.

Where a person possesses agency to bring about change, their motivations are *intrinsic*. Intrinsic factors engage people because they lead to pleasure or satisfaction at being involved in the change. *Extrinsic* motivations for change often mean that people engage in change activity for rewards, or more commonly to avoid punishment. Many changes in palliative care rely solely on extrinsic motivation, for example, auditing the use of end of life care pathways, or the numbers of people who develop pressure sores. Intrinsic factors may include the kind of satisfaction often described as the 'privilege' of being with people at the end of life. Religious or spiritual inclinations may also provide intrinsic motivation, as in the Christian roots of the hospice movement.

Agency refers to actions about which people have choices, compared to the influences of the environment and social structures that make choices impossible. This is contingent both on the individual's personal power, and on the environment in which they seek to act. Sometimes change arises out of a particular adverse event. These kinds of changes are usually implemented by people in authority, and are disseminated in a structured way such as through a programme of education – these are extrinsic motivations. Adoption of the change is not optional, and resistance may be high. However, other changes happen in a more organic and evolutionary fashion, perhaps from conversations with service users or from feedback/evaluation over time.

Learning exercise 22.1

A drug error has taken place on the ward. Root cause analysis seems to suggest that a breakdown in communication across nursing handover had taken place. Which of the following motivations for change are *instrinsic*, and which are *extrinsic*?

- Newly qualified nurse wants to know more about the different formulations of oxycodone, including modified-release and immediate-release, and generic forms.
- Managers are concerned about adverse publicity for the hospice.
- Nurses report feeling pushed for time during handover on the early shift.

How might this inform how practice is changed in response to the incident?

Change can be enabled through creating a sense of urgency, which will be more likely to lead to intrinsic motivations for change and a sense of agency among those likely to be most affected by potential change in practice. An example of creating urgency is shown in Case Study 22.1.

Case Study 22.1: Katie

Katie, the ward manager, has noticed that a lot of time is spent by nurses looking for the keys and/or a second nurse when patients are requesting oral morphine. It also often pulls qualified nurses away from tasks when they are incomplete. She finds some evidence that there is no legal requirement for double nurse checking of controlled drugs but it is something that has always been done. She works a couple of shifts to find out more about how much time is lost through double nurse checking. She asks some of the staff nurses what they would think if they did not need to find a second nurse every time a patient requested morphine.

'I think that would save so much time,' says one, 'it's silly anyway, because you always defer to the more senior nurse when you're double checking.' Another nurse, however, says, 'I would be really frightened of it, I think, these are potentially lethal medicines we are giving out and I don't have the confidence . . .'

The manager draws up an audit tool to measure through observation the time taken up by double nurse checking, and presents her findings to the team at the staff meeting. They are surprised to see that on each shift over an hour is spent waiting for a second checker or looking for the nurse with the drug cupboard keys. Over the following weeks, staff begin to discuss it more. A sense of urgency has been created through highlighting the issue of time and then leaving the team to observe their own practices and realise this for themselves.

Through presenting at the staff meeting, Katie has instigated the second stage of Kotter's model – the persuasion of stakeholders that change is necessary. Addressing the concerns of the nurses is key throughout the process, hence it is wise for Katie to now let the idea develop and be discussed within the team, so that at an appropriate time she can consult them to create a vision of change. If Katie is genuinely engaged with her staff, the implementation strategy is unlikely to be the same as what she may have envisaged at the start. Step 4 of Kottler's model involves communicating this vision of change. In step 5, Katie considers potential obstacles to this change, including nurses' worries about their competency in numeracy. Step 6 involves the creation of short-term wins for the team. Katie may, for example, repeat her observational audit to feed back to the team the time saved by the change in practice. Alternatively she may decide to hold a focus group to find out what staff think about the new routine. This would then be relayed to the remainder of the team. Kotter's final step will be to embed the change in the culture of the ward.

According to Kotter's model (Kotter 1995), the first step in successful change is to create a sense of urgency. The nurse as change agent is in a key position to communicate the key threats and opportunities offered by the change, and to construct hypothetical scenarios regarding future events. In so doing, the nurse can extend the sense of need for change to include colleagues at all levels of the professional hierarchy.

One highly influential mode of change is 'nudge theory' (Thayer and Sunstein 2008). Based on the influential book *Thinking Fast and Slow* (Kahneman 2011), it distinguishes between heuristics (the tendency to make rapid and automatic, and often mistaken decisions) and deliberation (a slower and more demanding process of conscious decision-making). It requires that we identify elements of the current situation that involve automatic thinking, and seek to perceive these as potential obstacles to change and to remove or mitigate them. Nudge theory suggests that we approach a problem by analysing the kinds of choices that could be made around that particular issue. Designing choices should, according to the theory, take into account knowledge of how people actually think (rapidly, automatically and often irrationally) rather than assuming that human thought is rational. Change innovations thus vary along a spectrum from those which essentially force change (such as banning smoking in a building) to those which involve the person being facilitated to actively choose the desired action. One of these core strategies is to create a shared norm, a mutually agreed ideal regarding what the vision of an organisation might be. This then makes changes within that framework more comprehensible to those affected by the change. Case Study 22.4 on p. 423 illustrates a real-life example of the use of nudge theory.

Learning exercise 22.2

Read Case Study 22.4 on p. 423.

- To fully understand nudge theory, it is important to be able to differentiate between automatic responses and a more deliberate response to the situation. Using Case Study 22.4, reflect on your responses to the project and identify where resistance might have originated. What 'nudges' might you initiate to enable people to retain agency and help raise awareness in relation to emotions?
- What support mechanisms might need to be available to help people process their feelings?
- What other resources might be required to help develop a sense of coherence and consistency in relation to identifying the processes people might be experiencing within the transition/change?

Systems

Healthcare organisations can work independently but are also dependent on wider stakeholders and insight into the referral systems or patterns of working within the system can provide enormous benefit in relation to commitment. Systems thinking allows us to find a way of making sense of the complexity and loosely connected actors involved in any context of healthcare delivery. Systems thinking is coupled with ecological models of thinking that incorporate the domains of environmental, social, psychological, emotional and physical determinants of organisational change (see, for example, Meadows and Wright 2015; Seddon 2008). Understanding the dynamics of care delivery helps make sense of what might be going on within the system at any one time. The impetus for change is a good starting point for examining the impact on the system, for example, it may be a national initiative requiring compliance for regulatory purposes (for example, the post-Francis Report duty of candour) or it may be an internal improvement initiative based on well-formed relationships and an evolution of understanding that requires a shift in patterns of communication (advance care planning conversations). Clarification of this starting point can help identify the system's components, helping to anticipate factors that may influence change.

Systems thinking provides a framework for agents to locate themselves. A systems approach and systems thinking change the focus from individual liability to collaborative accountability. Instead of blaming people for 'just not getting it' or rewarding early adopters of change, we analyse the whole inclusively, building relationships and growing involvement. A systems approach helps to explore the different levels of inter-related systems and the different levels that impact on the parts, for example, the macro-systems of policy and government initiatives, the meso-systems within and across organisations, and the micro-systems on a unit, a team or ward. Insight into the interlocking parts can facilitate where one part of the system may influence another – this may not be obvious until they are studied and listened to.

Relationships

Enabling engagement through the development of positive relationships is a very important factor in the success of change management (Hoogwerf et al. 2009). The practice development movement has enabled the profession to understand how nurses can lead change and improvement. Just as person-centred approaches in nursing benefit patients and relatives, person-based approaches towards stakeholders can foster inclusion and participation.

Collecting feedback is essential in evaluating services. What may appear to be a high quality service will only in fact be so if it is accessible, and if it meets people's needs. Patients, services users and carers are the most reliable sources. Such feedback may take a variety of forms, including satisfaction surveys or real-time interviews. Service user feedback is a valuable method of obtaining information on a service's performance, but it relies on sensitive and valid measures. Furthermore, its value depends on whether or not it leads to action. There is a gap between end of life care policy and people's experiences (Kinley et al. 2013; Borgstrom and Walter 2015). Service user involvement is therefore an essential aspect of any service improvement. Yet it risks being tokenistic unless engagement is with the populations who are most affected by the proposed changes. Meaningful involvement of users of palliative care services is often beset by practical challenges. For example, engaging with carers demands that carers have the time and resources to attend traditional modes of engagement such as focus groups or meetings.

Experience-based co-design (EBCD) is one approach to evaluating care that entails patients telling the story of their experience of care, and then working alongside staff to implement service improvement. Blackwell (2016) adopted an EBCD approach to understand and improve the experiences of patients with life-limiting illnesses attending Accident and Emergency (A&E) Departments. Findings from this work included the need for carers to be able to orientate themselves, to understand what was going on, and to see appropriate professionals during their visit. A film made by participants was expanded to include the experiences of A&E staff of providing care to patients with palliative care needs. The changes made in response to these concerns included regular visits by the hospital Specialist Palliative Care Team to the A&E Department and development of mandatory training for A&E staff. The King's Fund has produced a toolkit to guide experience-based co-design (available at: www.kingsfund.org.uk/projects/ebcd).

The rapid expansion of social media has meant that we have become ever more connected to one another, and to information. We are networked individuals with connections to family and friends, to colleagues and peers, and to organisations or information sources. When faced with a challenge, it is increasingly commonplace for us to turn to social media for solutions. However, the abundance of information that is available can also be a problem. Obtaining a balance between how one uses such networks is important to prevent them becoming burdensome, and to minimise any risks associated with disproportionate reliance on information obtained in this way. Mobilising social media for change can present both opportunities and obstacles (Moorley and Chinn 2014; 2015; Russell, Middleton-Green and Johnson 2015). However, there is general agreement that as the largest component of the healthcare workforce, it is incumbent on nurses to engage in change using multiple methods, and the existence of potential obstacles ought not to dissuade such engagement. Adherence to professional codes of conduct, awareness of potential multiple interpretations of tweets, and sensitivity to the public nature of the online community, mean that potential harms can be largely mitigated. Case Studies 22.2 and 22.3 present examples of real-life changes relating to social media.

Case studies

The following section describes some recent real-life changes in palliative and end of life care in Case Studies 22.2–22.6. We recommend that these are read with the above theoretical perspectives in mind, as they are illustrative of both enablers and barriers to change. Of particular significance is the source of the change, the change agent(s), and the broader context of urgency which gave rise to the change.

Case Study 22.2: Social media and engagement – #hpm and #WeEOLC

Nurses do not just occupy the structured, formal teams of which they are a part. They also frequently participate in a range of informal networks that may include nurses outside their immediate care setting, or those with whom they interact via social media. These informal networks are increasingly being recognised as crucial influences on organisations and can often lead to rapid dissemination of calls for change. We are more connected than ever before, with social media enabling communication across disciplines, countries and professional hierarchies. Yet this also means that we are bombarded with information regularly, and at times overwhelmingly. It is important for such information to be harnessed to enable it to serve the most useful purpose. The online community of practice @WeEOLC was developed as part of the suite of WeCommunities, established by an agency nurse who found herself isolated from the wider nursing community as she worked in a range of clinical settings without ever finding herself part of a team (Moorley and Chinn 2015). The online community has expanded rapidly in strength and diversity (see www.wecommunities.org/about) and now has around 56,000 followers worldwide, who participate in online 'Twitter chats' and various other modes of engagement. Within palliative care specifically, a similar forum for Twitter chats began in 2010 by authors of the palliative medicine blog 'Pallimed' (www.pallimed.org). The #hpm chat aims to bring clinicians and frontline workers together in an online forum where they can discuss issues of concern or interest within palliative care.

Case Study 22.3: Social media and change – #hellomynameis

A recent example is the Twitter campaign #HelloMyNameIs. The campaign, with a simple message at its core (for every healthcare or social care professional to introduce themselves by name to every patient), was launched in response to what is perceived to be depersonalising care (read more at http://hellomynameis.org.uk/) by Kate Granger, a doctor and also a terminally ill cancer patient. Purely through informal networks the campaign gathered momentum and has had worldwide influence in shaping healthcare organisation policies. Kate is included in this chapter because her experiences highlight three key characteristics of far-reaching and meaningful change. Had she been 'just' a doctor, her thoughtful words would have reached colleagues and health communities and potentially policy-makers; there are many articulate and passionate health professionals calling for change and compassionate care. Had she been 'just' a patient, her feelings of being ignored and invisible might have reached a patient experience forum, perhaps become a complaint that would have resulted in some local-level teaching and a change to the way in which staff were instructed in that area. Perhaps this change would have endured, and perhaps not. This would have depended on the culture of the ward, the institution, and the individuals within it. But Kate was both a health professional and a patient – as all health professionals will one day be – and for this reason the reach of her message has been global.

The success of the #hellomynameis campaign is a result, in part, of its simplicity. The very act of introducing oneself by name immediately challenges one of the key obstacles to compassionate care, which can be defined as being an 'us' and 'them' mentality, whereby health professionals (for self-protection, through busyness, or for other reasons) maintain a distance between themselves and the people for whom they are caring. The campaign was achievable, required no explanation, and emanated from one who had the experience of being on both sides of the bed, as it were.

This brings us to the final point regarding the success of Kate's campaign, and that is the value and power of social networks. Cutting across institutional and professional hierarchies, social media such as Twitter are an unmoderated forum for free speech. Of course, this requires great care. Tweets are comprised of just 140 characters and when talking about sensitive issues relating to end of life care, it is easy to inflame and ignite strong emotions and reactions. However, this brevity is also the strength of this medium of communication. It is possible to disseminate messages far and wide with great rapidity, often in real time, and for this communication to develop and evolve as new people become engaged and involved in the process.

Case Study 22.4: Using 'nudge' theory to mobilise change

One example of where nudge theory was used to gain momentum within a change movement is the Hospice Friendly Hospitals Programme (HFHP) in Ireland. This award-winning innovation was established in 2007, and since then has enrolled over 40 hospitals and around two hundred residential care settings in its programmes (read more at http://hospicefoundation.ie/healthcare-programmes/hospice-friendly-hospitals/). The HFHP recognises the complexity of the problems facing institutional care of the dying, and the programme targets multiple facets:

- *Attitudes and skills*: Training in communication at the end of life was set up for staff in acute hospitals ('final journeys'), staff in residential settings ('What matters to me') and for doctors and other healthcare professionals ('Dealing with bad news'). Trainer-training was provided to over 150 facilitators, who rolled the programme out to over 6000 staff.
- *Management and governance*: Most of the hospital partners have established end of life care committees, whose role is to look at a range of issues around end of life care. Committee membership includes clinical, support and administrative staff.
- *Physical environment*: Funding was secured to enhance the physical environment of hospitals, including the provision of family rooms and bereavement suites.
- *Engagement*: Through on-going communication with the media, the HFHP has ensured that the priorities the organisations seek to address are maintained in the public profile.
- *Ethical issues*: The HFHP has developed an ethical framework to guide end of life care.
- *Partnership*: There is recognition that such a broad scope of change requires engagement with stakeholders at multiple levels. To this end, the governance of the HFHP includes governmental health departments, third sector parties, professional bodies, educational institutions and political groups.

Case Study 22.5: Intrinsic motivation – 'Pushing Up Daisies'

'Pushing Up Daisies' (PUD) is a grassroots 'community-grown' festival in Todmorden in England, encouraging discussion of death and dying. The binding characteristic of those members of the community who established the group was that they found 'talking about and planning for end of life care pretty scary, and losing people pretty painful'. Their shared vision is of death becoming a more communal event, and 'not just in the hands of the professionals'. Through the mobilisation of social media (Facebook, Twitter) and a range of engagement events, the impact of their initiatives has spread beyond their immediate town. Increasing in popularity as well as in the diversity of those involved in the project, the group were awarded the National Council of Palliative Care's prize for best Dying Matters Initiative in 2016 (read more at www.pushingupdaisies.org). Each year, community involvement in the festival has grown rapidly, with the most recent Dying Matters week seeing over 70 separate events organised across the town, without any external funding or ownership by professional organisations. Encouraging the public to talk about death and dying was a core aim of the End of Life Care Strategy but most of these attempts have involved initiatives that are owned by institutions or organisations, such as hospices, healthcare services, or third sector groups. The unique feature of PUD is that it originated from within the community; this intrinsic motivation is arguably the secret of the group's extensive and diverse reach.

Case Study 22.6: Diffusion of innovation: The Gold Standards Framework

Everett Rogers' theory on the diffusion of innovation explains the spread and dissemination of new knowledge. Now we demonstrate through the use of a real-life example how this process can be seen. The Gold Standards Framework (GSF) was developed in the UK in 2000 as a grassroots initiative to improve primary palliative care from within primary care (Thomas 2003). Developed by Dr Keri Thomas, a GP with a special interest in palliative care, supported by a multi-disciplinary reference group of specialists and generalists, it was first piloted in Yorkshire in 2001, followed by a national phased programme supported by the NHS, Macmillan and more recently the DH End of Life Care Programme (Shipman et al. 2008). National spread was enabled through a strategic national cascade plan with the GSF Central Team supporting local facilitators, enabling best implementation of the work, overseeing training and audit plus developing further adaptations and resources.

- *Knowledge*: In the case of the GSF, the catalyst for change was ongoing concerns, articulated within the healthcare and social care professions and policies, and more broadly in the media, that the quality of end of life care in the community needed to improve. The initiative, introduced by Keri Thomas, a general practitioner (GP), was initially supported by a range of specialist and generalist palliative care professionals. The scheme was piloted in Yorkshire in 2001 and a book was published 2 years later (Thomas 2003).

- *Persuasion*: Timing was crucial in the success of the GSF. By the time the End of Life Care Strategy (EOLCS) was published in 2008, a series of internal and external evaluations of the framework had been undertaken, which included partnerships with diverse stakeholders with differing levels of influence. There was little doubt that the quality of end of life care needed to be improved, and the EOLCS not only confirmed this but also proposed that the GSF might be a useful innovation to adopt.

- *Decision*: Despite the recommendations from the EOLCS and then later in the NICE guidance, adoption of the GSF was initially patchy. In some areas, GSF facilitators were employed, whose role was to educate and support community teams wishing to adopt the framework. In other areas, this support was provided by specialist palliative care teams, who had a clear interest in promoting the framework's goals. Along the journey, changes were made. At first, the framework aimed to coordinate care provided by the primary care team, notably the general practitioners, to people living with advanced life-limiting disease at home. In 2004, this was adapted to include care provided at care homes, and more recently further adaptations. Research, commentary and discussion have increased in the years since the publication of the EOLC Strategy. Since 2010, more training programmes have become distance learning with e-supported group learning through the GSF Virtual Learning Zone and DVDs. The work is now based at the National GSF Centre in Shropshire, and led by Professor Keri Thomas (National Clinical Lead for the GSF Centre and Honorary Professor of End of Life Care at the University of Birmingham) with a small central team of very committed clinicians plus administrative support, Clinical Associates and reference groups. As well as primary care, GSF now provides training programmes on Care Homes (2004), Domiciliary Care (2012), Acute and Community Hospitals (2010), and Dementia Care (2012), with new developments including Spiritual Care and Clinical Skills. The GSF is currently at various stages of implementation in around 13 countries worldwide, including Australia, the USA, New Zealand, Canada, Belgium and China.

The impressive rate of adoption of the GSF depended on a number of factors: (1) a critical mass of engaged stakeholders in positions where they possess sufficient social and cultural power; (2) on-going external evaluations, originally using questionnaires and more recently the on-line After Death Analysis audit tool, plus several independent university-based evaluations; and (3) timing and readiness for change.

Conclusion

Palliative care does not stand still. Change and development are part of the terrain of end of life care, and as demographic, political and clinical factors change, so too must the shape of our services. The change process must remain open to ideas from stakeholders to enable on-going adaptation.

Overlooking the emotional aspect of change can lead to resistance. Involving and engaging all stakeholders, although time-consuming, can smooth the process and enhance organisational learning. High performing organisations often foster an attitude that accepts the flux and flow of change (Laloux and Wilber 2014). Nurses in palliative care who are agile when it comes to improving care, and who view change as normal, are assets for future care. Managers who understand emotional investment and ties will also have more success when it comes to working with people to improve care. Understanding roles and relationships using a system-wide perspective will widen the gaze and increase insight into how and why change might be resisted.

References

Atkinson, J. (2016) *Death by Passive Resistance*. Available at: www.heartoftheart.org (accessed 21 August 2016).

Battilana, J. and Casciaro, T. (2012) Change agents, networks, and institutions: a contingency theory of organizational change. *Academy of Management Journal*, 55(2): 1–42.

Bausewein, C., Simon, T.S., Benalia, H. et al. (2011) Implementing patient reported outcome measures (PROMs) in palliative care: users' cry for help. *Health and Quality of Life Outcomes*, 9: 27.

Blackwell, R. (2016) Improving the experiences of palliative care for older people, their carers and staff in the emergency department using experience-based co-design. PhD thesis, King's College London.

Borgstrom, E. and Walter, T. (2015) Choice and compassion at the end of life: a critical analysis of recent English policy discourse. *Social Science and Medicine*, 136–7: 99–105.

Bridges, W. (2009) *Managing Transitions: Making the Most of Change*. New York: De Capo Press.

Chan, R.J., Phillips, J. and Currow, D. (2014) Do palliative care health professionals settle for low-level evidence? *Palliative Medicine*, 28(1): 8–9.

Chow, K.M. and Chan, J.C.Y. (2015) Pain knowledge and attitudes of nursing students: a literature review. *Nurse Education Today*, 35(2): 366–72.

Clark, D. (2013) *Transforming the Culture of Dying: The Work of the Project on Death in America*. New York: Oxford University Press.

Colditz, G. (2006) The promises and challenges of dissemination and implementation research. In Brownson, R., Colditz, G. and Proctor, E. (eds) *Dissemination and Implementation Research*. New York: Oxford University Press.

Collins, E.S., Witt, J., Bausewein, C. et al. (2015) A systematic review of the use of the Palliative Care Outcome Scale and the Support Team Assessment Schedule in palliative care. *Journal of Pain and Symptom Management*, 50(6): 842–53, e19.

Dixon-Woods, M., Baker, R., Charles, K. et al. (2014) Culture and behaviour in the English National Health Service: overview of lessons from a large multimethod study. *BMJ Quality and Safety*, 23(2): 106–15.

Farquhar, M.C., Prevost, A.T., McCrone, P. et al. (2014) Is a specialist breathlessness service more effective and cost-effective for patients with advanced cancer and their carers than standard care? Findings of a mixed-method randomised controlled trial. *BMC Medicine*, 12(1): 337–413.

Goleman, D. (1995) Emotional intelligence. *Personality and Individual Differences*, 9(5): 1091–100.

Health Foundation (2011) *Evidence Scan: Improvement Science*. Available at: www.health.org.uk/sites/health/files/ImprovementScience.pd

Health Foundation (2013) Lining up: how do improvement programmes work? Available at: www.health.org

Higginson, I., Murtagh, F. and Daveson, B. (2015) *OACC: Measuring Outcomes to Improve Care*. London: King's College London.

Hoogwerf, L., Frost, D. and McCance, T. (2009) The ever-changing discourse of practice development: can we all keep afloat? In Manley, K., McCormack, B. and Wilson, V. (eds) *International Practice Development in Nursing and Healthcare*. Oxford: Blackwell.

Huryk, L.A. (2010) Factors influencing nurses' attitudes towards healthcare information technology. *Journal of Nursing Management*, 18(5): 606–12.

Kahneman, D. (2011) *Thinking, Fast and Slow*. London: Allen Lane.

Kinley, J., Froggatt, K. and Bennett, M.I. (2013) The effect of policy on end-of-life care practice within nursing care homes: a systematic review. *Palliative Medicine*, 27(3): 209–20.

Kinley, J., Stone, L., Dewey, M. et al. (2014) The effect of using high facilitation when implementing the Gold Standards Framework in Care Homes programme: a cluster randomised controlled trial. *Palliative Medicine*, 28(9): 1099–1109.

Kotter, J.P. (1995) *Leading Change: Why Transformation Efforts Fail*. Boston: Harvard Business School Press.

Kralik, D., Van Loon, A.M. and Van Loon, P. (2006) Transitional processes and chronic illness. In Kralik, D., Paterson, B. and Coates, V. (eds) *Translating Chronic Illness Research into Practice*. Adelaide: Flinders University.

Laloux, F. and Wilber, K. (2014) *Reinventing Organisations*. Brussels: Nelson Parker.

Manley, K., Hardy, S., Titchen, A. et al. (2005) *Changing Patients' Worlds Through Nursing Practice Expertise: A Research Report*. London: Royal College of Nursing.

Meadows, D. and Wright, D. (2015) *Thinking in Systems: A Primer*. New York: Chelsea Green.

Moorley, C. and Chinn, T. (2014) Nursing and Twitter: creating an online community using hashtags. *Collegian*, 21(20): 103–9.

Moorley, C. and Chinn, T. (2015) Using social media for continuous professional development. *Journal of Advanced Nursing*, 71(4): 713–17.

Obholzer, A. and Roberts, V. (2003) *The Unconscious at Work: Individual and Organizational Stress in the Human Services.* London: Routledge.

Richer, M.-C., Ritchie, J. and Marchionni, C. (2013) Appreciative inquiry in health care. *British Journal of Healthcare Management*, 16(4): 164–72.

Russell, S., Middleton-Green, L. and Johnson, B. (2015) Using social media to create discussion. *International Journal of Palliative Nursing*, 21(11): 525–6.

Seddon, J. (2008) *Systems Thinking in the Public Sector.* Axminster: Triarchy Press.

Shipman, C., Gysels, M., White, P. et al. (2008) Improving generalist end of life care: national consultation with practitioners, commissioners, academics, and service user groups. *BMJ (Clinical Research Ed.*, 337: a1720.

Taylor, J., Coates, E., Brewster, L. et al. (2014) Examining the use of telehealth in community nursing: identifying the factors affecting frontline staff acceptance and telehealth adoption. *Journal of Advanced Nursing*, 71(2): 326–37.

Thayer, R.T. and Sunstein, C.R. (2008) *Nudge: Important Decisions about Health, Wealth and Happiness.* New Haven, CT: Yale University Press.

The Economist Intelligence Unit (2015) *The 2015 Quality of Death Index: Ranking Palliative Care Across the World.* London: The Economist Intelligence Unit.

Thomas, K. (2003) *Caring for the Dying at Home.* Oxford: Radcliffe Publishing.

Van de Ven, A.H. and Poole, M.S. (1995) Explaining development and change in organizations. *Academy of Management Review*, 20(3): 510–40.

Preparing to work in palliative care: developing educational competence

John Costello

Introduction

The aim of this chapter is to focus attention on the need for education in palliative care. Specifically, the chapter considers the diversity of need among practitioners working in generic and specialist roles. With this in mind, the chapter will examine three areas: (1) the role of the practitioner; (2) education and scholarship; and (3) teaching and learning.

First, the role of practitioners working in hospital and community settings, who increasingly want to be updated and need information about palliative care to help fulfil their obligation to remain life-long learners. They may be unsure of the best way of developing their education and scholarship and may benefit from focusing on specific study days or education to meet a country-specific need, such as revalidation and NMC registration in the UK.

Education and scholarship focus on post-registration education and scholarship issues, evaluating key areas that teaching and learning should address for those who need education to help fulfil their role in meeting the needs of patients and families they encounter at work. This section will also include many issues of equal relevance to undergraduate education.

The teaching role of many specialist nurses in palliative care includes their professional responsibility to provide education to others as part of their role. This section examines the preparation required to fulfil this role effectively.

Throughout the chapter, learning exercises and practice points are used to encourage engagement with the ideas and to provide teaching strategies to be used in your own teaching. Emphasis is placed on the development of critical thinking and the need to remain linked and grounded to clinical practice. For this reason, case studies are used.

The role of the practitioner in palliative care

The primary purpose of all education is to improve practice and hence influence the behaviour of individuals, in this case, those working in a palliative care context. One of the key ambitions of the new National Partnership for Palliative and End of Life Care (2015) focuses on staff being prepared to provide effective end of life care, in terms of having appropriate knowledge, skills, attitude and support to care and to implement evidence-based practice.

Preparing to work in palliative care having gained experience in another area of healthcare can be daunting, and yet, at the same time, very rewarding. Those wishing to work in palliative care will have previously encountered patients in need of palliative care or at the end of life. Palliative care practice is different from other mainstream areas such as medicine and surgery because practitioners face more ethical and legal issues. This emanates from an important principle associated with palliative care, i.e. patient autonomy.

There are two other distinct areas that relate to but have greater prominence in palliative care. These are Quality of Life (closely related to pain management and symptom control) and practitioner relationships with the patient and family. The latter (family relationships) is particularly significant as this is an area where many practitioners feel challenged. When deciding upon the most appropriate type of education to enable you to become updated and competent in improving your knowledge of palliative care practice, two factors should be considered. The first is the importance of inter-professional education because, in palliative care, multi-disciplinary team work is a central feature of care provision (Head et al. 2014). Second, the need to develop confidence in any new area rests on becoming competent. Gamondi et al. (2014) in a White Paper for the European Association of Palliative Care (EAPC) have highlighted 10 core interdisciplinary competencies. Competency is defined by the EAPC (2016) as a cluster of knowledge, skills and attitudes that are all related to one's role or responsibility. These correlate with job performance and can be measured against accepted standards and improved through training and development. These are illustrated in Box 23.1.

Box 23.1   Palliative care key competencies

- Autonomy
- Dignity
- Relationship between patient and healthcare professionals

- Quality of life
- Position towards life and death
- Communication
- Public education
- Multi-professional approach
- Grief and bereavement

The EAPC competencies highlight the need for team work and also focus attention on the needs of the patient's family and friends. Because palliative care practitioners have expertise in inter-disciplinary practice and team-based care, it leads the way for them to create educational opportunities for students to learn the skills for team practice and provision of quality patient-centred care. At the same time, it is necessary for practitioners to be competent at communication and in educating others, notably patients, family members, the public and members of the healthcare team, such as students, medical and allied medical staff. In summary, developing your role to become a palliative nurse practitioner requires you to consider three areas which will require change and/or evaluation of your current skills. First, your knowledge base and your potential to learn more specialist knowledge. Second, a potential change in attitude to consider how your individual role as a nurse needs to include working closely with other disciplines. Finally, an increase in your interpersonal skills relating to demonstrating empathy and compassion to patients and family and developing therapeutic relationships.

The need for education and scholarship

As part of the preparation for working in palliative care, it is essential to focus on the type of education that will benefit those with limited experience. A good place to begin is by adopting a habit of reading about various topics related to palliative care using journals, government reports and web sites. This type of scholarship will help you to get a feel for the types of issues you can expect to encounter on your educational journey. Box 23.2 contains a list of popular professional and academic journals with up-to-date developments in palliative care practice, policy and research. You will see that there are a huge number of journals to choose from and this is not a complete list. Some journals refer to supportive care, a term used to denote the dual focus made when supporting the family and facilitating social changes to enable the family patient to experience quality of life. Some journals relate more to medicine than nursing and others focus more on cancer than non-cancer conditions. This reflects one of the key issues in palliative care, which is that it is not just about cancer but non-cancer medical conditions such as motor neurone disease (MND), dementia and HIV/AIDS.

Box 23.2 Journals focused on medical and nursing aspects of palliative care

BMC Palliative Care http://www.biomedcentral.com/bmcpalliatcare/

Current Opinion in Supportive and Palliative Care journals.lww.com/co-supportiveandpalliativecare

European Journal of Palliative Care (TOC, A) http://www.ejpc.eu.com/ejpchome.asp

Indian Journal of Palliative Care http://www.jpalliativecare.com/

Innovations in End-of-Life Care http://www2.edc.org/lastacts/

International Journal of Palliative Nursing http://www.ijpn.co.uk/

Internet Journal of Pain http://www.ispub.com/ostia/index.php?xmlFilePath=journals/ijpsp/front.xml

Journal of Hospice and Palliative Nursing http://www.jhpn.com/

Journal of Palliative Medicine (TOC, e-mail notice available) https://www.ncbi.nlm.nih.gov/labs/journals/j-palliat-med

Palliative Medicine (TOC) http://pmj.sagepub.com/

Palliative and Supportive Care http://journals.cambridge.org/action/displayJournal?jid=PAX

Progress in Palliative Care (TOC) https://www.ncbi.nlm.nih.gov/labs/journals/prog-palliat-care

Some journals are listed with information as to whether the site has tables of contents (TOC) and abstracts (A).

For post-registered nurses with limited time available and no funding for full-time study, part-time courses and study days may be a good alternative. University schools of nursing and some hospices with educational facilities attached provide a range of courses and study days. Identifying the most appropriate course of study is important. Gaining academic credits for work is also important not only because these can go towards revalidation but are necessary to help you develop your expertise and contribution to life-long learning. Based on the identified EAPC competencies, an introduction to palliative care education for those moving into palliative care could consist of study days focused on topics listed in Box 23.3.

Box 23.3 Introductory education topics in palliative care

- Law and ethics
- Communication skills for palliative care practice
- Pain management

- Symptom control
- Spirituality
- Grief and bereavement
- Team working

Your individual learning needs

One of the first steps any practitioner needs to take when embarking on the study of a different discipline is knowing the best way for them to learn. Research into teaching and learning highlights that people learn in a variety of different ways. Some of us prefer to listen and take note of what is being said, for example, via lectures. While these methods are useful for conveying information, they are not entirely appropriate for those of us who prefer more interactive teaching methods, such as small group work, discussion or problem-solving groups. These ensure greater engagement with the subject matter (Frankel 2009). However, apart from determining the areas in palliative care you wish to study, consider also the best way you learn. Frankel's research identified that nurses prefer visual or active learning. Active learning is where you, as a student, learn by being involved and engaged in your own learning. What Frankel found suggests that training programmes which focus on lecture-style teaching may not help those who prefer to be active in their learning. Knowing your preferred learning style or styles makes a difference when it comes to trying to develop individual competence. Before embarking on any educational course, consider that the way we learn is different from the methods used to teach.

Self-assessment of your learning style

Being aware of how you learn best can help you decide not only on the most appropriate teaching method but also how you can customise your study skills. Some nurses prefer listening to lectures but find that afterwards they cannot recall what was said. Others get bored in lectures and prefer group work. Kolb and Kolb's (2005) experiential learning model is a useful framework for identifying your learning style (see Box 23.4).

Box 23.4   Kolb and Kolb's (2005) styles of learning

Kolb and Kolb identified four styles of learning:

1   Activist
2   Reflector
3   Theorist
4   Pragmatist

Learning exercise 23.1

Look at the list below and identify which of the methods of learning fits your style of learning best. Are you an activist, reflector, theorist or pragmatist?

* Activists learn best when they are doing simulation-type activities, role play case studies and homework where they are involved and hands on.
* Reflectors learn best when they are able to think back or reflect on their observations, they see something and they make their own notes, keep a journal or are given a chance to brainstorm ideas.

Selecting teaching methods that help you learn

When considering the best way to help you learn, consider the following two areas in relation to what study days and courses are available. In reality, you may not have the opportunity to pick and choose, but it's worth considering ways to maximise your learning potential.

The learning environment

The learning environment is recognised by many teachers and students to have an impact in either encouraging or impeding a positive learning experience (D'Souza et al. 2015; Haraldseid et al. 2015; Phillips 2015). A range of learning theories, concepts and approaches can be used to build and manage effective learning environments.

Opportunities for discussion

It is useful to choose a study or course with others who are studying at your level of professional development. This may not necessarily include a group of your peers, but those with whom you can discuss ideas to generate and develop understanding. Peer teaching and learning in nursing are recognised as a significant means of enabling students to maximise their learning (Stone et al. 2013; Stenberg and Carlson 2015).

Many people prefer active learning that includes an emphasis on work-based learning rather than classroom-based teaching methods. Teaching and learning related to topics such as setting up a syringe driver have greater interest and appeal than learning about topics unrelated to your area of interest. Learning about how to manage a patient with a Hickman line or conducting a pain assessment can be undertaken by using simulation-based learning because it enables practitioners to learn about things that they will encounter on a day-to-day basis.

Summary

This section has considered assessment of your learning style and different ways of maximising your learning. In palliative care it is necessary to consider how you learn, the environment you are working in, and the influence of others. Small group and individual teaching strategies relevant to palliative care include patient-led teaching and student-led seminars. These are things that can help you to ensure not only that you learn more but that learning can be fun and enjoyable.

Education and scholarship related to practice

This section focuses on post-registration education and scholarship issues. In doing so, the section evaluates key areas of palliative care education and practice, highlighting certain educational topics that may require updating in order to help fulfil the role of meeting the needs of patients and families. This section also includes issues of equal relevance to undergraduate education.

Team working in palliative care

The illness trajectory of the patient from diagnosis to death is often described using the journey metaphor. The palliative journey can begin at diagnosis, continuing until after death and include bereavement support. At times, the focus of the practitioner's attention is on family members. Support for the family at times can take precedence over the patient (such as at the end of life, when the patient is unconscious or in a persistent vegetative state, PVS). This can seem hard to understand at times, but is a key feature of palliative care practice, when the practitioner's focus is more to do with providing emotional support to the family (Brown 2016, p. 80). One of the key differences in the way palliative care practitioners work with patients compared to other practitioners, is the extent to which multi-professional team working is a central feature of their work. By respecting the contribution others make and acknowledging its significance, team work can help make a substantive contribution to the quality of the patient's life and reduce the anxiety and distress of the family, particularly when the family is going through a crisis. These situations can occur at diagnosis, when deciding treatment, when stopping treatment or when moving into the palliative phase of care. Being able to work as a team player is important for palliative care practitioners. Consider your role as a member of the team and assess your strengths and weaknesses by carrying out Learning exercise 23.2.

Learning exercise 23.2

On a scale of 1 (poor) to 10 (excellent) self-assess your team working skills.

I consider myself to be a strong team player.

1_____10.

I invariably consult with others about patient care.

1_____10.

I enjoy working as a member of the multi-disciplinary team.

1_____10.

I respect the role of others in the multi-disciplinary team.

1_____10.

I consider the family and patient to be part of the multi-disciplinary team.

1_____10.

I often seek advice from others about patients I care for.

1_____10.

I use my active listening skills in my team working.

1_____10.

When working in a team I invariably try to develop team strategies to help others.

1_____10.

Adapted from Parsell and Bligh (1999).

If you scored 7 or over for each (total score 56 plus), you are a good team player, while scores of 40 and below indicate a need for you to work on your team working skills. To assist you, see Bragadóttir's et al.'s paper (2016), which reports results from an international survey of teamwork in nursing, highlighting ways in which you can improve your team work skills.

Law and ethics

One of the key aspects of healthcare that relates closely to palliative care is law and ethics relating to patients with life-limiting illness (Becker 2015). Palliative care practitioners need to be aware of the many and often complex ethical and legal issues that some patients and families face during the palliative care journey. This is particularly important when patients with cancer are making the transition between active treatment and supportive and palliative care. Research highlights that many practitioners are uncertain about legal and ethical issues. These include, for example, the patient's right to have treatment withdrawn and the distinction between palliation of symptoms, withdrawal of treatment and assisted death (Phelps et al. 2014; Cheon et al. 2015).

Giving information and truth telling

A key ethical issue in proving reassurance and comfort to all patients is the giving of information about diagnosis, treatment and prognosis, especially for those with a life-limiting illness (Noble et al. 2015; Glogowska et al. 2016) and those with unrealistic expectations (Pfeil et al. 2015). No one likes to be the bearer of bad news. Most physicians prefer to do more good and avoid creating harm. There is much debate in palliative care about how much truth patients and families should be told about the illness and prognosis (Huang et al. 2015). Fallowfield and Jenkins (2004) argue that the truth hurts but deception is even worse. However, despite professionals wishing to disclose information, it is not always easy to be completely open and truthful. In particular, telling the truth and being accurate are problematic because of not being able to accurately predict the prognosis. This is also due to the ambiguity of advanced cancer diagnosis, uncertainty about the patient's general health and their co-morbidities (Mishelmovich et al. 2016). Moreover, few can predict the patient's likely psychological response to grave news (Long et al. 2016). Physicians may claim it is part of their clinical freedom to withhold information from a patient if they are likely to become non-compliant, because of mental health issues, attempts at self-harm or suicide. It is the case, however, that some patients do not have the mental capacity to understand and respond to the truth about their situation, especially if the news is not good. These issues and many others relating to the promotion of psychological well-being are discussed in more detail in Chapter 9 in this volume.

Assessing mental capacity

An important aspect of palliative care is establishing the mental capacity of the patient to make independent decisions. In the UK, the Mental Capacity Act (MCA) (UK Parliament 2005) is based on protecting vulnerable people and enabling their voice to be heard when, for example, they have a life-limiting illness. In hospital and care homes, formal capacity assessment occurs when a patient's mental capacity to make decisions about their care and treatment is questionable. Under the MCA *Substitute Decisions Act*, many situations require capacity assessments to be conducted by specially qualified assessors who must follow specific guidelines.

However, in practice, medical staff, social workers and psychiatrists may conduct capacity assessments although they should be formally trained and certified. A patient may be temporarily unable to make an autonomous decision due to illness, trauma or infection. In other cases they can make their mind up about where they want to be cared for because they can understand and state preferences about the present, but fail to comprehend the complexities of further chemotherapy treatment. Therefore, for them to give informed consent may not be possible in all cases. Each instance needs to be carefully considered, especially in cases where the patient has mental impairment such as Alzheimer's disease. Where it is anticipated that the patient may lose capacity in future due to ill health, it is useful to assist them to document their wishes as part of an Advance Medical Decision (AMD).

The AMD process involves making decisions about feeding, cardio-pulmonary resuscitation (CPR) and withholding and stopping treatment. Case Study 23.1 considers a number of situations where, as staff nurses and ward managers, you need to be aware of the options available to patients who find themselves with a medical condition for which there is no curative treatment (see Chapter 20 in this volume on advance care planning and ethics).

Case Study 23.1: George

George, aged 74, was admitted to the surgical ward with a 3-week history of abdominal pain, nausea and vomiting. He was suspected of having pancreatitis due to his raised serum amylase level. His GP had pre-warned him that it might be cancer. In the operating theatre it was confirmed that he had a tumour in his pancreas as well as metastatic spread. His prognosis was poor, in terms of having weeks or months to live. The surgeon referred him immediately to the palliative care team for advice and support. George and his wife Emily were told by the surgeon after the operation that there was a tumour and that they were going to do some more investigations. George and Emily had discussed the possible outcome and optimistically told themselves that treatment would be made available and that they would fight the cancer. George was strong-willed and convinced himself that he would battle the tumour and trust in the doctors.

The role of the nurse as a patient's advocate

As the staff nurse who admitted George to the ward, you are given the responsibility for ensuring that he receives a high standard of care and that Emily is given appropriate emotional support. After making sure George is comfortable and his pain is well controlled, you ask the surgeon to plan a time when you can both discuss George's prognosis. The surgeon is reluctant to engage specifically with George, stating that he feels a bit out of his comfort zone dealing with dying patients, preferring instead to let the hospital palliative care team 'take things from here'. He explained that is what he has done in the past and it worked well. You do not feel happy about the situation, especially when the surgeon suggests that you can talk to them if you prefer, but he was going into theatre.

Practice point 1

In a situation like this what are the options for you in supporting George and Emily? Clearly, there is a role for you to advocate on behalf of the patient and be proactive in making sure they are aware of the prognosis. You could leave it up to the palliative care team but you feel this would negate the trust built up between you and George and lead to further distress. You could be more assertive with the surgeon and insist that you both see George together before the palliative care team. Advocating on a patient's behalf is seen as part of the nurse's role. However, the evidence suggests that advocacy is potentially useful, but it is also problematic, because it requires a lot of moral courage and can fracture the pre-existing relationships with the rest of the team (Bickhoff et al. 2016). Contacting the palliative care team in advance of the referral and explaining the situation would help, especially if they agreed to you being part of the discussion that included you, Emily and George and the palliative care team, with or without the surgeon. This strategy would enable you to learn from the team how such matters are dealt with. The palliative care team will listen to the patient's concerns and discuss George and Emily's preferences. This is likely to involve Advance Care Planning (ACP), an issue discussed in more detail in Chapter 20.

Developing skills in communication

There are numerous short one-day courses in communication training available in the UK at hospices with an educational facility, such as St Christopher's in London, St Luke's in Plymouth, Essex and Sheffield, and St Ann's in Manchester. Hospice courses often focus on communication courses such as 'I don't know what to say', and *challenging conversations at the end of life, as well as breaking bad news and advanced care planning and more specific areas like spiritual care and bereavement.* For most courses you do not have to have any experience or qualifications (but check in advance), nor is there a need for you to be a qualified nurse for many of the courses, as they are multi-disciplinary. St Christopher's in London is one such hospice with an extensive educational resource; see their website for more information (http://www.stchristophers.org.uk/).

Specific communication training

One way of developing your communication skills is by undertaking a short inexpensive and very useful 3-hour course called Sage and Thyme training. This course was developed by clinical staff at the University Hospital of South Manchester NHS Foundation Trust (UHSM) and a patient in 2006. The aim is to train all grades of staff in how to develop their interpersonal skills. The training is focused on enabling staff to appreciate how active listening and empathic responding can meet the needs of patients who are worried and concerned about their illness. The course is designed for hospital and community care staff, including those with limited or no direct contact with patients.

Advanced communication training

Training in advanced communication can be undertaken in a number of ways. The most widely available courses are aimed at senior practitioners, medical staff and nurses (band 7 and above). An example being the Maguire 2/3-day Advanced Communication Skills Training. It is based on the work of psychiatrist Peter Maguire and colleagues and focuses on the Advanced Communication Skills Training Course and is based at the Christie Hospital, Manchester, UK. This course and many others focus on developing communication skills in managing complex and emotive situations, such as breaking bad news and disclosing sensitive information such as stopping treatment. For details, see the website (https://3-day-advanced-comm.eventbrite.co.uk).

There are numerous courses similar to this one available via internet sources. The University Hospital of South Manchester NHS Foundation Trust also runs an advanced communication course (Sage and Thyme ACP). The aim of this training is to enable practitioners to develop more advanced skills in facilitating conversations about advance care planning (see Chapter 20 in this volume for more details on ACP). The course is aimed at healthcare practitioners, including senior nurses and medical staff, and those hospital and community staff with experience in advance care planning (http://www.sageandthymetraining.org.uk/ use of the Sage and Thyme model).

Teaching and learning strategies

This section focuses on the role of the nurse as a practice educator in the clinical setting, looking at various teaching and learning strategies that may be used by practitioners in clinical practice. Many nurses who work with patients and families in receipt of palliative care find themselves having to inform others (Quill and Abernethy 2013) and educate others (Yang et al. 2013), for example, staff, patients and caregivers about the role of palliative care. Part of this role Yang et al. (2013) point out involves formal teaching from Advanced Practice Nurses (APN), who have the responsibility for practice education. Much of the clinical education in palliative care settings is conducted informally through facilitation rather than formal teaching. Facilitation can involve problem-solving using medical notes, listening to student nurses' anxieties and providing pastoral support, as well as supporting other nurses in decision-making about clinical care (Leonard et al. 2016).

This section looks at how to use different types of education strategies such as microteaching (Cajkler and Wood 2016), which can involve one-to-one teaching or a small group of two or three patients, family members or students. It will also consider small group teaching. Small group teaching can take advantage of *teachable moments* that can occur in practice when a situation arises, such as a patient experiencing breakthrough pain, or experiencing an epileptic seizure as a result of a brain tumour. After the incident has been managed, time is set aside to go through what happened and discuss what can be learnt from it. This can also be used as an opportunity to debrief those involved and go through events logically to maximise on the learning potential.

Role modelling

Some nurses fail to appreciate the importance of role modelling in practice and its impact on teaching and learning (Mikkonen et al. 2015; Felstead and Springett 2016). Traditionally referred to as learning from Nelly, role modelling is where others, for example, students and patients take note of good (and sometimes poor) practice, by observing how you perform your role as an experienced practitioner. Learning through observation is a key part of learning. Students benefit from the experience of watching someone they can trust and learn from (Felstead and Springett 2016).

The process known as *shadowing* is a very similar strategy whereby novice nurses less experienced than others accompany more experienced colleagues. They may not contribute much but learn from observing the techniques and methods used by experienced others. This requires confidence on the part of the experienced practitioner and some courage! Practitioners who facilitate learning by allowing someone to shadow them as they engage with others require effective communication skills as well as self-confidence. It is often useful to explain that the practitioner has a *shadow*, and what their role is, pointing out that the shadow may not contribute to any discussion but is there to observe. It is also useful for the practitioner to debrief or provide feedback to the shadow after an observational session, asking them what they understood and what they learnt. This provides the opportunity for questions and discussion about things that were unclear.

It may therefore be argued that educating others as an experienced palliative care practitioner is often not just about standing in front of a group of others, although some palliative care nurses excel at this also. Undergraduate students on clinical placements often give feedback on how much they have learned about practice. Student nurses point out that they felt included in what was going on, because of the skills and style being used by the practitioner. This is a rich form of learning that experienced practitioners can use once they become aware of the value of role modelling.

Microteaching

Another form of teaching and learning that often takes place in clinical practice is microteaching. This can involve the experienced practitioner taking the lead with one or more others learning about practice in an informal way that can sometimes involve patient/clients receiving care and treatment (Cajkler and Wood 2016). Microteaching can take many forms, for example, it can be structured around changing the dressing of a patient with a fungating breast tumour, counselling a patient distressed by their impending death or applying a compression aid for a patient with lymphoedema following breast surgery. One of the key elements in this type of opportunistic teaching is to ensure that the patient is happy to have others be part of the experience. It is also important not to cause distress or delay to the patient's care. Having discussions about the procedure after you have completed the session is part of microteaching. In some cases, microteaching can be planned and structured just like a formal teaching session. Learning exercise 23.3 is an example of planned microteaching that took place on the ward and involved a patient, a staff nurse and two undergraduate students. See also the practice point following it to assess the importance of paying attention to the details.

Learning exercise 23.3

Eric, a 67-year-old with advanced pancreatic cancer, was admitted to the medical ward for pain and symptom control. Staff nurse Jenny was asked to set up a syringe driver for pain control, because the palliative care team had determined that his pain, nausea and vomiting could be managed more effectively this way. After the ward handover, Jenny decided to involve the two student nurses (Liz and Sue) to observe using it as a microteaching exercise. Jenny explained the patient's situation, and explained to Eric what would take place. She prepared the syringe driver and the syringe together with the prescribed medication, explaining the different types of available syringe drivers and the way the morphine was diluted with water and the anti-emetic medication was combined in order to combat the effects of the morphine as well as Eric's symptoms. She assessed their knowledge of the common symptoms of patients with pancreatic cancer and the side effects of morphine. The students were there to observe but also to listen to the explanation given by Jenny and to help reassure Eric by holding his hand and chatting to him during the procedure where appropriate.

Jenny explained that the syringe driver meant that Eric would not require frequent injections and would provide a steady amount of pain relief and also help to control his feelings of nausea. It was explained that he could also be given oral medication if he required it. Eric seemed to be happy to be the centre of attention. Jenny was able to take her time and explain each stage of a procedure she had carried out many times. Eric had a venflon in situ that was working well. Jenny explained to the students the importance of checking the dosage of the syringe driver and the identity of the patient just like any other when medication is administered to a patient. A label with Eric's details and the drug details was placed on the syringe driver as well.

There was also a need to ensure Eric could mobilise if required, carrying the syringe driver in a pouch. It was made clear that if Eric experienced any further pain or nausea, he should inform the nurse immediately. The microteaching went well and Eric did not complain of pain or nausea, nor did he feel too sedated that he could not stay awake.

Practice point 2

When planning microteaching in the way Jenny did, preparation was all important. She considered the following:

- The learners' level of understanding and their learning needs. Was this a procedure they were ready to observe and was it something they were likely to have to undertake in future? She also asked them about their knowledge of the drugs and the need to document and label the drug type, amount and time on the syringe driver.
- What theoretical knowledge did they have about the use of continuous morphine for pain relief? Was it part of their learning objectives? Jenny questioned them in advance of the procedure to assess their knowledge. The patient was told in advance that student nurses would be observing and gave his consent.
- Jenny got the students to play an active role in the procedure by ensuring that the line was not going to get in Eric's way and was not going to get kinked or trapped in his clothing.

- Patient safety was emphasised in terms of checking the medical notes, completing the prescription chart, having the use of the drug witnessed by another nurse and documenting the dose and time it started and obtaining agreement that Eric was aware of what the syringe driver was for.
- The procedure was fully documented in the nursing notes and it was made clear that the dose was charted on the patient's documentation.
- Opportunity was given after the procedure for discussion and explanation of the details to maximise learning.

This type of microteaching is not unusual and is often found by students and other staff to be an extremely useful way of learning. It can be applied to a wide range of situations, not all practical, for example, observing breaking bad news to patients and families. The latter often requires the nurse to feel confident in their communication skills as well as having a good relationship with the patient. Microteaching or *opportunistic teaching* of this type often appears to be informal but it requires a good deal of structure and thinking about as the practice point illustrates. Practitioners may find it useful to select the types of things they feel confident in having others observe. Involving patients in teaching and using them as part of teaching can have a therapeutic effect on them (Costello and Horne 2005). Patients can also learn from microteaching by understanding more about their treatment and care. Medical staff have been using patients in medical teaching for many years (Bashour et al. 2012). Prior to using patients in ward teaching, it is necessary, as Bashour et al. (2012) point out, to explain that they are not obliged to take part and to ensure they are fully informed of their role. Selection of the patient is therefore a key part of successful microteaching involving patients.

Small group teaching

Small group teaching is a popular and common way of teaching in a variety of palliative care contexts (Costello 2007). It can take place by the bedside, in a ward office or in a classroom and can involve 2–8 learners. It is an ideal starting point for practitioners wishing to develop their public speaking and preparing for more formal classroom teaching to larger audiences. Teaching small groups has the added advantage of being more intimate and allowing for greater interaction with those involved. Leading such groups is more like facilitation than formal teaching. Encouraging learning by inviting questions and having discussions about sensitive issues is a useful way of preventing people feeling inhibited. Participants may also be reluctant to disclose their anxieties because of embarrassment, especially if they do not know each other! Practitioners engaging in small group teaching can use a number of basic but effective ways to develop integration and improve cohesion, referred to as icebreakers to help participants relax and feel part of the group. Box 23.5 gives an illustration of what are called ice breakers. These techniques are used to ensure effective small group teaching.

Box 23.5   Ice breakers to use in small group teaching

- Sharing concerns (see the 'fear in a hat' game (Costello 2007)).
- Disclosing reasons for wanting to learn.
- Getting participants to talk to each other, share names and experiences, then introduce your partner to the rest of the group.
- Using story board narratives, disclosing incidents with patients relevant to the teaching topic.
- Brainstorming likes and dislikes about a given topic.
- Setting the agenda for the small group teaching by stating what participants would like to know.

Getting the group to share concerns is very helpful as it prevents others feeling intimidated by lack of knowledge and experience. Icebreakers can and do help participants feel relaxed and part of the group and can involve humour and fun. Try 'Hospitals' as an ice breaker before your teaching (see Costello 2007). Hospitals is an activity-based game with the group leader in the middle of a room with students all sitting on seats and no spare seats. Participants are asked to adopt a name or a topic and when their name is called, they have to stand up and change seats, the group leader finds a vacant seat leaving one person in the middle to be the name caller. It is designed to stimulate and warm up the group.

Once the participants feel relaxed and have a sense of shared understanding of what they wish to achieve, the small group facilitator can maximise the learning potential by engaging students and keeping the discussion lively, interesting and fun. Avoid teaching *at the group* for any longer than 20 minutes to avoid lapses in concentration. Wherever possible, have activities pre-planned like working in pairs or sets and sharing clinical experiences such as incidents with patients that caused concern. Having previously spent time building trust in the group, the facilitator can use individual experiences to illustrate key points.

Small group teaching can potentially help to develop good relations between participants, because in a palliative care context, they can involve discussion of a sensitive nature. Many nurses feel anxious, especially when they are new to palliative care and they lack confidence in their communication skills. It is important that the group facilitator is sensitive to the emotions of participants and does not allow learners to feel intimidated, as anxiety prevents learning. Box 23.6 illustrates some of the do's and don'ts of small group work.

Box 23.6   Do's and don'ts when facilitating small group work

Do

- Encourage involvement and sharing of ideas.
- Develop a positive learning environment.

- Get participants to share feelings.
- Introduce yourself and disclose details, encourage others to do the same to develop trust.
- Get to know the participants.
- Plan comfort breaks.
- Be observant for signs of poor concentration.
- Be aware of the needs and feelings of the group.
- Encourage discussion and debate.

Don'ts

- Put students on the spot and make them feel uncomfortable.
- Ask them to disclose very personal information.
- Teach *at them*, give them opportunities to ask questions and interact.
- Put students down by being judgemental about their ideas.
- Conduct the teaching in an area where you are likely to be disturbed.
- Go over the allocated time for teaching.

Conclusion

This chapter has explored some of the practical, legal and ethical issues associated with palliative care education. It was structured into three sections to provide a logical progression to palliative care education and scholarship. Practitioners wishing to expand their awareness and knowledge of palliative care need to assess, develop and maintain the strengths and weaknesses of their existing skills and consider how to improve the way they engage with patients and families. This has been a central feature of the chapter and one that will help any practitioner to make a difference in caring for patients and families in receipt of palliative care.

Those practitioners with existing knowledge of palliative care who wish to develop the essential role of educating others need to consider that they are very likely to be doing this already as role models. Moreover, this group of practitioners need to develop their role as facilitators of learning and consider how to achieve teaching competence. This chapter has argued that education is a central feature of the role of palliative care practitioners and as such they provide care and support, as well as education.

References

Bashour, H., Sayed-Hassan, R. and Koudsi, A. (2012) Involving patients in medical education: ethical issues experienced by Syrian patients. *Education for Health*, 25(2): 87–91.

Becker, R. (2015) Dealing with ethical dilemmas. In *Fundamental Aspects of Palliative Care Nursing* (2nd edn). London: MA Healthcare Ltd, pp. 61–90.

Bickhoff, L., Levett-Jones, T. and Sinclair, P.M. (2016) Rocking the boat: nursing students' stories of moral courage: a qualitative descriptive study. *Nurse Education Today*, 42: 35–40.

Bragadóttir, H., Kalisch, B.J., Smáradóttir, S.B. and Jónsdóttir, H.H. (2016) The psychometric testing of the Nursing Teamwork Survey in Iceland. *International Journal of Nursing Practice*, 22(3): 267–74.

Brown, M. (2016) *Palliative Care in Nursing and Health Care*. London: Sage.

Cajkler, W. and Wood, P. (2016) Lesson study and pedagogic literacy in initial teacher education: challenging reductive models. *British Journal of Educational Studies*. doi: 10.1080/00071005.2016.1164295 (accessed 27 July 2016).

Cheon, J., Coyle, N. and Wiegand, D.L. (2015) Ethical issues experienced by hospice and palliative nurses. *Journal of Hospice and Palliative Nursing*, 17(1): 7–13.

Costello, J. (2007) Teaching and learning in small groups. In Bee, W. and Hughes, N. (eds) *Teaching and Learning in Palliative Care*. Oxford: Oxford University Press.

Costello, J. and Horne, M. (2005) Patients as teachers: utilising patients in classroom teaching. In Warne, T. and McAndrew, S. (eds) *Using Patient Experience in Nurse Education*. London: Palgrave.

D'Souza, M.S., Karkada, S.N., Parahoo, K. and Venkatesaperumal, R. (2015) Perception of and satisfaction with the clinical learning environment among nursing students. *Nurse Education Today*, 35(6): 833–40.

European Association for Palliative Care (EAPC) (2016) EAPC core competencies in palliative care: a White Paper. Available at: http://www.eapcnet.eu/ (accessed 1 July 2016).

Fallowfield, L. and Jenkins, V. (2004) Communicating sad, bad, and difficult news in medicine. *Lancet*, 363(9405): 312–19.

Felstead, I.S. and Springett, K. (2016) An exploration of role model influence on adult nursing students' professional development: a phenomenological research study. *Nurse Education Today*, 37: 66–70.

Frankel, A. (2009) Nurses' learning styles: promoting better integration of theory into practice. *Nursing Times*, 105(2): 24–7.

Gamondi, C., Larkin, P. and Payne, S. (2014) Core competencies in palliative care: an EAPC White Paper on palliative care education: part 2. *European Journal of Palliative Care*, 20(3): 140–5.

Glogowska, P., Simmonds, R., McLachlan, S. et al. (2016) 'Sometimes we can't fix things': a qualitative study of health care professionals' perceptions of end of life care for patients with heart failure. *BMC Palliative Care*, 15: 3. doi: 10.1186/s12904-016-0074-y (accessed 6 July 2016).

Habeshaw, S., Habeshaw, T. and Gibbs, G. (1992) *53 Interesting Things to Do in Your Seminars and Tutorials*. Avon: Technical and Educational Services Ltd.

Haraldseid, C., Friberg, F. and Aase, K. (2015) Nursing students' perceptions of factors influencing their learning environment in a clinical skills laboratory: a qualitative study. *Nurse Education Today*, 35(9): 1–6.

Head, B.A., Schapmire, T., Hermann, T. et al. (2014) The Interdisciplinary Curriculum for Oncology Palliative Care Education (iCOPE): meeting the challenge of interprofessional education. *Journal of Palliative Medicine*, 17(10): 1107–14.

Huang, H.L., Cheng, S.Y., Yao. C.A. et al. (2015) Truth telling and treatment strategies in end-of-life care in physician-led accountable care organizations: discrepancies between patients' preferences and physicians' perceptions. *Medicine (Baltimore)*, 94(16): e657.

Kolb, A.Y. and Kolb, D.A. (2005) Learning styles and learning spaces: enhancing experiential learning in higher education. *Academy of Management Learning and Education*, 4(2): 193–212.

Leonard, L., McCutcheon, K. and Rogers, K.M.A. (2016) In touch to teach: do nurse educators need to maintain or possess recent clinical practice to facilitate student learning? *Nurse Education in Practice*, 16(1): 148–51.

Long, A.C., Downey, L., Engelberg, R.A. et al. (2016) Physicians' and nurse practitioners' level of pessimism about end-of-life care during training: does it change over time? *Journal of Pain and Symptom Management*, 51(5): 890–7.

Mikkonen, K., Kyngäs, H. and Kääriäinen, M. (2015) Nursing students' experiences of the empathy of their teachers: a qualitative study. *Advances in Health Sciences Education*, 20(3): 669–82.

Mishelmovich, N., Arber, A. and Odelius, A. (2016) Breaking significant news: the experience of clinical nurse specialists in cancer and palliative care. *European Journal of Oncology Nursing*, 21: 153–9.

National Partnership for Palliative and End of Life Care (2015) Ambitions for palliative and end of life care: a national framework for local action: 2015–2020. Available at: http://endoflifecareambitions.org.uk/ (accessed 30 June 2016).

Noble, H., Price, J.E. and Porter, S. (2015) The challenge to health professionals when carers resist truth telling at the end of life: a qualitative secondary analysis. *Journal of Clinical Nursing*, 24(7–8): 927–36.

Parsell, G. and Bligh, J. (1999) The development of a questionnaire to assess the readiness of health care students for interprofessional learning (RIPLS). *Medical Education*, 33: 95–100.

Pfeil, T.A., Laryionava, K., Reiter-Theil, S. et al. (2015) What keeps oncologists from addressing palliative care early on with incurable cancer patients? An active stance seems key. *The Oncologist*, 20(1): 56–61.

Phelps, K., Regan, E., Oliver, D. et al. (2014) Withdrawal of ventilation at the patient's request in MND: a retrospective exploration of the ethical and legal issues that have arisen for doctors in the UK. *BMJ Supportive and Palliative Care*. doi:10.1136/bmjspcare-2014-000826 (accessed 26 July 2016).

Phillips, J.M. (2015) Strategies for promoting student engagement. In Billings, D.M. and Halstead, J.A. (eds) *Teaching in Nursing*. St Louis, MO: Elsevier, pp. 245–62.

Quill, T.E. and Abernethy, A.P. (2013) Generalist plus specialist palliative care: creating a more sustainable model. *New England Journal of Medicine*, 368: 1173–5.

Stenberg, M. and Carlson, E. (2015) Swedish student nurses' perception of peer learning as an educational model during clinical practice in a hospital setting: an evaluation study. *BMC Nursing*, 14: 48. doi: 10.1186/s12912-015-0098-2 (accessed 1 August 2016).

Stone, R., Cooper, S., and Cant, R. (2013) The value of peer learning in undergraduate nursing education: a systematic review. *ISRN Nursing*, http://dx.doi.org/10.1155/2013/930901 (accessed 16 July 2016).

UK Parliament (2005) Mental Capacity Act (2005). Available at: www.legislation.gov.uk/ukpga/2005/9/contents (accessed 2 August 2016).

Yang, G.M., Ewing, G. and Booth, S. (2013) What is the role of specialist palliative care in an acute hospital setting? A qualitative study exploring views of patients and carers. *Palliative Medicine*, 26(8): 1011–17.

Building the evidence base for palliative care nursing: overcoming challenges in research, knowledge transfer and implementation

Morag Farquhar and Jane L. Phillips

Introduction

High quality research is fundamental to evidence-based clinical practice. Research is distinct from clinical audit or quality improvement activities which typically review service delivery against predetermined standards to generate information; research generates new knowledge. While clinical academic nursing roles exist, most nurses will not be in a position to design or conduct their own studies. However, this chapter is relevant to all palliative care nurses as it explores the challenges inherent in generating and disseminating that knowledge in palliative care, and strategies for overcoming them. Regardless of whether nurses are designing, conducting, inspiring, supporting or consuming research, understanding these challenges is fundamental to improve care outcomes.

Research challenges

There are six key palliative care research challenges, many of which are inter-related: (1) ethics; (2) recruitment; (3) attrition; (4) outcomes; (5) respondent burden; and (6) randomisation. Each of these will be examined in turn before we then consider issues related to translating research into practice in the following section of the chapter. Box 24.1 suggests two primers related to the challenges of palliative care research.

Box 24.1   Primers for the challenges of palliative care research

1   MORECare: Methods Of Researching End of life Care (Higginson et al. 2013). Developed through systematic review and expert consultation, MORECare's evidence-based guidance includes ethics (Gysels et al. 2013), mixed methods (Farquhar et al. 2013), and statistical issues (Preston et al. 2013), and provides an e-learning module (MORECare 2013). It provides guidance predominantly at the project level.

2   *Research in Palliative Care: Can Hospices Afford Not to Be Involved?* (Payne et al. 2013). Initiated by the Commission into the Future of Hospice Care, this 2013 report outlines major concerns of national and local importance on research related to hospice care and offers recommendations to inform the work of the Commission in relation to research and research capacity building. As such, it provides guidance for key stakeholders (e.g. hospices and universities, and national organisations supporting hospice care) and at both management and strategic levels and professional staff levels.

Both sources of guidance are useful to clinicians conducting palliative care research in a range of settings, as well as those seeking a better understanding of its challenges.

Ethics

Ethical concerns about conducting research with people with life-limiting illness, who are vulnerable, unable to provide consent (Duke and Bennett 2010; Agar et al. 2013) or recently bereaved (Buckle et al. 2010), abound. However, evidence is increasing that these patients, informal carers and families are willing to participate (Gysels et al. 2008a; White and Hardy 2010; Shelby-James et al. 2012). While altruism is a common motivation (Gysels et al. 2008a), participants also benefit from being involved (Buckle et al. 2010; White and Hardy 2010; Coombs and de Vries 2016), gaining from talking and accessing additional services or information (Gysels et al. 2008a). However, research must remain clinically relevant, address unanswered questions, be scientifically sound, feasible and acceptable.

Given the prevalence of cognitive impairment, clinical depression, delirium, severe symptoms and affective disorders (impairing understanding of risks and benefits), and potential changes over time, deficits in decision-making capacity create challenges for patient recruitment into palliative care clinical studies (Hosie et al. 2013). Those obtaining consent should be trained and able to assess capacity (Kavanaugh and Campbell 2014). Where a patient has fluctuating capacity, or may lose capacity, there are five ethically valid consenting approaches: (1) consent on enrolment, (2) in advance, or (3) delayed until after study-start, (4) proxy consent (or by legally authorised representative), or

(5) consent waiver (Agar et al. 2013). These approaches increase participation rates, expedite knowledge generation and increase generalisability by better reflecting the population (Agar et al. 2013).

Researchers may uncover unreported or unidentified issues, including clinical conditions or even suicidal ideas (Clark and Dunbar 2003). There should be a planned response for such events (e.g. Box 24.2).

Box 24.2 Example palliative care study depression protocol

Living with Breathlessness (Primary Care Unit) was a mixed method multiple-component, longitudinal research programme to improve care and support in advanced chronic obstructive pulmonary disease (COPD). One component administered the Hospital Anxiety and Depression Scale (HADS) (Zigmond and Snaith 1983) to patients and carers – a screening tool for anxiety or depression. The study's Standard Operating Procedure (v10/01 2015), developed with its multi-disciplinary Programme Advisory Group, included this 'depression protocol' (actioned for six patients and two carers):

1 If patient or carer HADS score for depression is 15+ (probable case), or we have concerns during interviews (expressed suicidal thoughts), and participant not obviously on medication for depression and not discussed depression recently with a clinician: ask permission to speak to their GP.

2 If patient expresses suicidal thoughts, even in absence of HADS depression score 15+, treat this as a red flag and ask permission to speak to their GP.

3 Use positive wording: 'We would really like to let your GP know . . .', 'Your GP would like to know . . .', 'You do not have to feel this way, you could feel better', 'Our guidance is that if anyone has a score of 15 or more and we are concerned, then we should let their GP know and we need your permission to let them know.'

4 Discuss with principal investigator*.

5 If patient refuses to let us inform GP, check with patient if carer knows they are feeling very low.

6 If patient refuses permission, still inform GP in order to minimise risk of possible harm; participant safety is paramount.

7 Record interaction and outcome in fieldnotes.

*A principal investigator (PI) is the lead researcher for a project, usually the holder of the project funding, e.g. an independent research grant administered by the lead institution such as a university or clinical institution.

Where it is unclear whether patients are aware of their advanced disease status, adopt research language relating to hopes, concerns and predictions regarding future health and needs (picking up on participant cues) (Fitzsimons and Strachan 2012). Awareness of participants' emotions is important: offer breaks and opportunities to end interviews. Researchers should be trained in bringing interviews to a close, leaving participants in a safe emotional state with access to external support (Kavanaugh and Campbell 2014).

At study end or in the case of withdrawal (through toxicity or disease progression), participants can feel loss or abandonment. Formally marking participation and feeding back findings helps (Wilson et al. 2007) but is challenging where lives are limited yet the slow research and peer review process means respondents are usually 'the last to know' results, if at all (Fernandez et al. 2007). There are, however, potential harms related to content or 'delivery' of feedback and possible upset for the bereaved: identifying feedback preferences on recruitment may alert participants and families that results will be delivered if requested.

MORECare's ethical recommendations (Gysels et al. 2013) provide further guidance. However, Duke and Bennett (2010) noted limited debates on the well-being of researchers themselves and data managers (e.g. in data entry or transcription): for further reading, see (Steinhauser et al. 2006; Kavanaugh and Campbell 2014; Penner et al. 2016).

Recruitment

Effective timely participant recruitment is essential: it has a significant impact on findings. Even with well-defined inclusion criteria, varying definitions of supportive, palliative and end of life care mean participant identification is challenging. Palliative populations are heterogeneous: functional trajectories vary across (and within) the four classic disease groups of cancer, organ failure, frail elderly and dementia, challenging recruitment. Study populations should reflect the real world. Pragmatic inclusion and, especially, exclusion criteria are key, e.g. not excluding co-morbid patients. Keeping criteria broad (Shelby-James et al. 2012) and including an explicit supplementary 'inclusive approach' statement guides clinicians facilitating recruitment, pre-empting inappropriate exclusions (e.g. Box 24.3).

Box 24.3 Example of an explicit 'inclusive approach' statement

The Living with Breathlessness Study (Primary Care Unit) recruited over 500 patients with advanced COPD from 123 UK primary care practices. Each practice completed a recruitment log, which listed inclusion and exclusion criteria and the following explicit 'inclusive approach' statement:

> Patients in this study are *expected* to be older individuals, have serious lung disease, and possibly be housebound, so GPs are asked not to exclude patients for these reasons.

Patients meeting the inclusion criteria were logged along with exclusion criteria that excluded patients met, or any other reason for exclusion. The principal investigator contacted practices to review cases where 'other' reasons were related to the inclusive statement.

Patients can be recruited from various settings (with approvals), depending on the research question, for example, healthcare settings (primary, community, secondary or tertiary care) or non-healthcare settings, such as support groups or online forums (although the latter may result in sampling bias, depending on the research question). Recruiting patients via clinicians is challenging. Time pressures and competing priorities (e.g. patients' immediate needs) deter clinicians from offering patients opportunities to participate. In palliative care, well-intentioned clinicians, families (Ling et al. 2000), ethics committees, managers, and even researchers themselves, intentionally or unintentionally 'gatekeep', 'protecting' patients from participation. Gatekeeping prolongs recruitment, impacting on validity and reliability through sampling bias (Ewing et al. 2004; White et al. 2008). It occurs despite growing evidence, noted above, that even very ill patients wish to participate (White and Hardy 2010) and some patients (Gysels et al. 2008a), carers (Hudson 2003) and bereaved relatives (Koffman et al. 2012) benefit. It raises issues of paternalism and loss of autonomy (Ewing et al. 2004) for those capable of deciding whether to participate and negotiating how they want this to happen (Gysels et al. 2008a).

Public and Patient Involvement (PPI) can develop recruitment strategies, materials and study designs to optimise participation (Kavanaugh and Campbell 2014). Daveson et al. (2015) provide guidance on PPI in palliative care research. To optimise participation, consider patients' clinical pathway, their treatment- or information-related burden and how that may impact on participation. Early engagement with clinicians (e.g. Box 24.4) facilitates this.

Box 24.4   Example of engagement with clinicians to optimise recruitment

Sharing Bad News was a qualitative study to inform development of an intervention to support patients to share their lung cancer diagnosis with family and friends (Ewing et al. 2016).

Patients were recruited from thoracic oncology clinics at two hospitals. Early discussions with clinicians identified three different palliative care pathways (palliative chemotherapy, palliative radiotherapy and supportive care) and optimum recruitment points on each, considering likely treatment- or information-related burden. Consequently, patients were invited to participate 4–6 weeks post-diagnosis. The required purposive sample was successfully recruited, facilitated by the clinicians.

Participants may also be carers, the bereaved, clinicians, other stakeholders, whole teams or sites. Defining and identifying most of these is relatively straightforward, but defining, identifying and recruiting carers presents challenges. Not all carers recognise the label 'carer'. Sampling frames are rare: carer registers are scarce within health systems and recording carers within patient records varies. Therefore, carer recruitment usually occurs via patients, requiring patient recruitment in the first place, patient recognition of their 'carer' and willingness to invite their carer to participate; thus patients become 'gatekeepers'. Successful recruitment of the bereaved requires additional sensitivity in timing (Bentley and O'Connor 2015), recruitment materials, and data collection, as well as a strategy for identification (DiGiacomo et al. 2013).

Recruitment is further challenged by deteriorating health (Addington-Hall 2007; Ling et al. 2000), or death, between identification, consenting and data collection. Whether recruiting patients, carers, or clinicians, flexibility optimises participation, e.g. offering choices in time, day, methods (e.g. telephone, face-to-face, electronic data collection), venues, and potential co-presence of others (e.g. see Box 24.5).

Box 24.5   Example of flexible approach to participation

Learning about Breathlessness (Farquhar et al. 2016a) was a qualitative study to develop an educational intervention for carers of patients with breathlessness in advanced disease. Carer workshops were planned to co-develop the intervention, based on carer and patient interviews and an expert workshop. Carers were recruited via posters, presentations and recruitment pack handouts in:

- primary care
- secondary care
- patient and carer support groups.

Interested carers contacted the research team. Several asked if they could 'bring the patient' to the workshop – as a support or simply as this was easier. The study protocol included free respite care to facilitate carer participation, but this was not taken up – carers preferred to bring the patient along.

Unexpectedly, including both patients and carers in the workshops proved empirically valuable as many carers wanted to learn 'with their patient'. Patient inclusion in carer workshops therefore facilitated both carer recruitment and development of a carer intervention appropriate for a co-present patient.

Monitoring reasons for exclusion helps identify unwarranted exclusions, enabling entry criteria modification (Shelby-James et al. 2012). Pilot work identifies feasibility of entry criteria, emergent gatekeeping issues, likely response rates and timelines for planning: Thabane et al. (2010) provide helpful guidance on pilot and feasibility studies.

Useful palliative care recruitment resources include systematic reviews (Boland et al. 2015), empirical studies (Sygna et al. 2015) and the growing number of population- or setting-specific recruitment 'lessons learned' papers, e.g. Campbell et al.'s (2016) case study of challenges and solutions to recruitment in a UK hospice.

Attrition

Attrition refers to participant loss through study withdrawal, non-response to follow-up, or protocol deviation, and affects any study involving follow-up (Steinhauser et al. 2006; Addington-Hall 2007; Fitzsimons and Strachan 2012; Shelby-James et al. 2012), e.g. longitudinal observational or intervention studies. Some attrition is inevitable in palliative care through deterioration or death, but can also result from respondent burden, circumstance (e.g. relocation) or contextual changes (e.g. in local services). Unavoidable attrition is sometimes addressed through proxies, but proxies bring validity and reliability issues (McPherson and Addington-Hall 2003; Higginson and Gao 2008). Evidence-based estimates of attrition inform sample size calculations (Shelby-James et al. 2012), therefore publishing attrition rates helps other researchers.

Attrition can impact on validity through data loss and needs reporting: it is data in itself. MORECare's taxonomy of palliative attrition types facilitates this: attrition due to death (ADD), attrition due to illness (ADI) and attrition at random (AAR) (Preston et al. 2013). Data can be missing at person- or item-levels. Establish an analysis plan before recruitment starts (*a priori*), which examines patterns of missing data and attrition and takes these into account in analysis (Preston et al. 2013). Methods for handling missing quantitative data include complete case analysis, modelling procedures, and imputation (e.g. last value carried forward, regression procedures, means), but can impact on subsequent summary statistics and analyses (Diehr and Johnson 2005; Fielding et al. 2006). Diehr and Johnson (2005) advise using methods that account for deaths and imputation methods for data missing for other reasons. Palliative-modified intention-to-treat analysis has been proposed for Phase III trials (Currow et al. 2012). Regardless of approach, clear reporting of the method used is paramount (Fielding et al. 2006).

Retention strategies (reduce avoidable attrition) include systematic tracking, check-in calls, minimising respondent burden (see below), maintaining interviewer-respondent dyads (caseloads), interviewer-respondent ethnicity matching, providing data collection timelines to participants, flexible data collection (modes, venues, timings), joint interviewer-respondent setting of follow-up dates, thank you letters, appropriately skilled and trained interviewers, participant information recall (e.g. pet's name), and incentives (Northouse et al. 2006; Steinhauser et al. 2006).

Outcomes

Palliative care predominantly seeks to improve quality of life and death: study outcomes may therefore be subjective and multi-dimensional (Steinhauser et al. 2006; Addington-Hall 2007; Cawley et al. 2011) and encompass multiple perspectives: patients, carers, (other) family members, and clinicians (as service providers or referrers). Identifying indicators of quality of life, death and care is complex: how to define concepts such as quality of life has long been debated (Farquhar 1995). Expected deterioration may also negate 'improvement' on scores and identifying whether adverse events result from an intervention or natural disease progression is challenging.

Outcome selection depends on the research question, intervention goals, and study population: patients, carers and clinicians may have different views on what is important to measure (Aspinal et al. 2006). Subsequent choice of measure depends on validity, reliability and acceptability. Reviews of palliative care outcome measures are useful (e.g. Mularksi et al. 2007; Agar and Luckett 2012; Stiel et al. 2012), including on specific outcomes, such as psychological distress (Kelly et al. 2006) and bereavement risk (Sealey et al. 2015), on specific populations, such as cancer carers (Shilling et al. 2016) and bereaved relatives (Mayland et al. 2008), and on specific symptoms, for example, breathlessness (Bausewein et al. 2007).

Research questions may lend themselves to quantitative or qualitative outcomes, or both (mixed methods). Qualitative data can encompass more, capturing a range of outcomes from several intervention components (Farquhar et al. 2016b) than even multi-dimensional quantitative outcomes; Rocker (2011) questions whether score change in response to a therapeutic intervention tells 'only part of the story'. Guidance exists on conducting qualitative interviews in palliative and end of life studies (Gysels et al. 2008b; Steinhauser and Barroso 2009), including in patients' homes (Sivell et al. 2015), with older people (Pleschberger et al. 2011) or carers (Funk and Stajduhar 2009), and joint patient-carer interviews (Swetenham et al. 2015).

A single quantitative 'primary' outcome is required for randomised controlled trials (RCTs). Although RCTs usually include additional secondary outcomes, determining a *primary* outcome is difficult in palliative care. The potentially different margins, and greater spread, of benefits in palliative care complex interventions make identifying a single primary outcome challenging (Farquhar et al. 2016b). Richards (2015) described gains from 'simple' nursing interventions which individually make only a marginal difference, but together reduce discomfort and anxiety. Cumulative benefit may be identified by combining several (quantitative) outcomes: it may simply be unrealistic to expect one (quantitative) measure to capture palliative care (Farquhar et al. 2016b).

Mixed method outcomes may be more relevant than quantitative outcomes alone, given palliative care's complex multi-dimensional objectives (Cawley et al. 2011), and have been used in palliative RCTs (Farquhar et al. 2014; Farquhar et al. 2016b). However, they are not a panacea (Flemming et al. 2008): their appropriateness depends on the research question. They can be costly and bring their own unique data collection, integration and dissemination challenges (Farquhar et al. 2011).

Varying service configurations limit the generalisability of study findings (external validity). Defining both intervention and standard care elements in RCTs is crucial (Dickson and Jack 2008), especially in multi-site studies (Shelby-James et al. 2012), but is challenging in palliative care where interventions are tailored to individual need (Grande and Todd 2000). Definitions maintain fidelity and inform future translation (discussed below). There are frameworks for identifying key concepts of palliative and end of life care (Ferrell 2005), and a checklist for patient and service characteristics reporting to help identify outcomes (Currow et al. 2012). Similarly, the European Association for Palliative Care's basic dataset describes palliative care cancer populations and variable recording (Sigurdardóttir et al. 2014).

Respondent burden

Minimising respondent burden is essential for patients with high symptom burden, intensive appointment schedules, and busy carers. Reviewing the length, complexity, location and timing of data collection is important (Kavanaugh and Campbell 2014). Collect the least amount of data necessary and use existing data wherever possible, accessing sub-groups for additional measurements (Shelby-James et al. 2012). Streamline consenting procedures to minimise burden (Sivell et al. 2015) and gain consent for secondary analysis of data to reduce need for new participants. Involving patients and carers in study design through PPI (e.g. reviewing recruitment, consenting and data collection plans) can facilitate burden-minimisation.

Participants undertake complex cognitive processes in answering questions, including interpretation, retrieving information from memory, decision processes to estimate answers and response formulation (Murtagh et al. 2007). Pilot work identifies participant (and researcher) time and effort: reviewing audio-recordings of questionnaire administration can reveal challenges participants face in responding that, in addition to suggesting burden, may actually question validity (Farquhar et al. 2010a). Similarly, cognitive interviewing can refine new questionnaires: Murtagh et al. (2007) is a good palliative example.

Interventions themselves can also cause burden if overly complex in content or duration. Developing interventions through a phased approach, as advocated by the Medical Research Council (MRC) (2000) framework for developing and evaluating complex interventions, enables both intervention and study protocol modification to reduce burden, e.g. Farquhar et al. (2009) reduced a palliative care intervention's duration by 4 weeks through a MRC Phase II pilot trial.

Randomisation

RCTs are the gold standard for clinical research, but randomisation as a control can be problematic in palliative care where it denies access to an intervention which participants, or their clinicians, consider beneficial (Grande and Todd 2000; Farquhar et al. 2009b). It can therefore impact on recruitment. Stepped-wedge (Brown and Lilford 2006) or fast track/waiting list trial designs (Grande and Todd 2000; Farquhar et al. 2009b; Higginson and Booth 2011) help, but the ability to use designs with a 'waiting' element depends on patients' location on those varying disease trajectories: those close to death may not have time to wait. Optimising intervention length minimises 'waits'.

Regardless of design, randomisation must be considered fair by patients, carers and clinicians, and participants should receive good care in all trial arms (Grande and Todd 2000). Providing rescue medication for control arm participants in drug trials may reduce clinician concerns about uncontrolled symptoms (Shelby-James et al. 2012).

High-quality rigorous RCTs are feasible (Shelby-James et al. 2012), but many palliative care questions can be answered through observational or quasi-experimental designs, sometimes rendering them more generalisable (Schildmann and Higginson 2011).

Translating research into practice

It is one thing to conduct robust research but another to use it. Translating what we know into everyday practice presents five key challenges: (1) evolving science; (2) time from discovery to practice; (3) premature translation vs lost in translation; (4) integrating implementation; and (5) clinical practicalities.

Evolving science

Translational research is an umbrella term encompassing a range of approaches including 'knowledge translation' and 'implementation research' (McKibbon et al. 2010).

Knowledge translation

'Knowledge translation' describes the generation, application and implementation of knowledge (Greenhalgh and Wieringa 2011). It occurs within a complex system of interactions between researchers and knowledge users, requiring action at system (community, government, policy, organisation), provider (clinicians) and consumer (patients and families) levels (Graham et al. 2006). Five key questions can guide knowledge translation:

- What should be transferred?
- To whom?
- By whom?
- How?
- And with what effect? (adapted from Lavis et al. (2005)).

It is best conceptualised as a cyclical 'knowledge to action' process (Graham and Tetroe 2007). The Delirium in Palliative Care Project used this approach to determine the best way to address system and clinical practice evidence gaps (Figure 24.1).

Implementation science

Implementation science seeks to ensure effective delivery of evidence-based strategies (Aldridge Carlson 2013). It uses methods that either: describe and/or guide translation of research into practice (process models), provide insight into understanding or explaining what influences implementation outcomes (determinant frameworks, classic theories, implementation theories), or evaluates implementation processes (evaluation frameworks) (Grol et al. 2005), by answering implementation questions (Box 24.6).

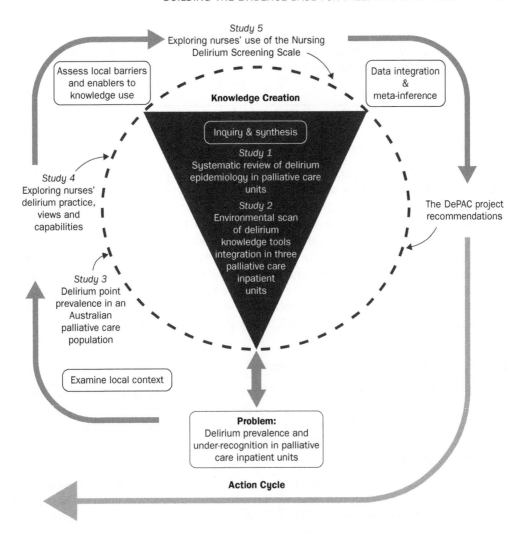

Figure 24.1 Application of knowledge to action process to improve delirium recognition and management in in-patient palliative care
Source: Hosie (2015, p. 74).

Box 24.6   Example implementation questions

- How does the real-world context influence sustained adoption and use of effective interventions?
- How do we accelerate adoption and sustained appropriate use of drugs, therapeutics, and diagnostics?
- How do we significantly increase uptake where there is low adoption?

> • How do we remove roadblocks preventing doctors, nurses, and families from adhering to delivery of highly beneficial treatments and practices?
> • What factors must be addressed to maximise sustainability?
>
> (National Heart Lung and Blood Institute 2014)

Time from discovery to practice

An early example of prolonged time from discovery to applying knowledge was the observation that daily citrus intake prevented scurvy (Doherty 2005). Many died and suffered in the 194 years it took to implement this evidence. Delays persist today, partly because of exponential growth since the first RCT in 1948 to around 150,000 in 2004 (Stolberg et al. 2004) and 832,620 at the last count (Cochrane Library 2015). Even within palliative care the increase is staggering: one in every 122 published RCTs in 2005 was in palliative or hospice care (Tieman et al. 2008). As our evidence base grows, we need to translate high-level evidence more rapidly into practice to reduce patient exposure to off-licence medications and/or unproven treatments, for which consent is rarely sought and there is potential harm (Pavis and Wilcock 2001; To et al. 2013).

Premature translation vs lost in translation

The rapid uptake and withdrawal of the Liverpool Care Pathway illustrates dangers in adopting interventions that have not been robustly tested (Neuberger et al. 2013; Chan et al. 2014) or may benefit from better implementation strategies. While this is an example of adverse impact of too rapid translation of low-level evidence, the opposite can occur with high-level evidence.

A double-blind placebo RCT of efficacy and toxicity of subcutaneous Ketamine for cancer pain found no difference between Ketamine (an anaesthetic dissociative hallucinogenic medication) and placebo (Hardy et al. 2012). Patients receiving Ketamine were more likely to experience more severe adverse effects daily: the number needed to treat for one additional patient to have a positive outcome was 25 (95% CI, six to ∞) (Hardy et al. 2012). Translating this evidence into practice may only occur with replication and evidence synthesis (Ioannidis 2006): release of the trial results in conjunction with best pain management for neuropathic cancer pain may enable practice improvement (Quibell et al. 2015). As translation of evidence into practice takes approximately 17 years, and only 14 per cent of discoveries are translated (Morris et al. 2011), this will require a targeted strategy.

Integrating implementation

Clinical practice based on 'tradition', as opposed to evidence, denies patients and families best palliative care, placing them at risk of harm (Phillips 2015). We must integrate implementation into research beyond traditional approaches of continuing medical education, pharmaceutical detailing, and guideline development, which largely fail to deliver change, particularly when used in isolation: alternatives include community-based participatory and public health research, and health policy analysis (Westfall et al. 2007). Adopting an integrated approach, with implementation elements at each phase, would also ensure implementation is budgeted for (Higginson et al. 2013).

Clinical practicalities

Palliative care clinicians and researchers need to identify interventions with sufficient evidence to be implemented, to adapt and test interventions in varied contexts, and accurately describe intervention elements, implementation components and effectiveness (Aldridge Carlson 2013). A number of web-based resources are available (Box 24.7).

Box 24.7   Web-based translational research resources

- Implementation Science: http://cancercontrol.cancer.gov/IS/ (accessed 25 September 2016)
- Knowledge Translation Canada: http://ktclearinghouse.ca/ktcanada (accessed 25 September 2016)
- *Implementation Science Journal*: http://www.implementationscience. com/about/access (accessed 25 September 2016)
- US Department of Veterans Affairs – Quality Enhanced Research Initiative: www.queri.research.va.gov/default.cfm (accessed 25 September 2016)
- US Agency for Healthcare Research and Quality: www.ahrq.gov/ (accessed 25 September 2016)
- Methods Of Researching End of life Care (MORECare) Statement, supporting topic-specific papers and e-learning module: https://www.kcl.ac.uk/ nursing/departments/cicelysaunders/research/studies/morecare.aspx (accessed 25 September 2016)
- CareSearch – Palliative Care Knowledge Network – Implementing Change: https://www.caresearch.com.au/caresearch/tabid/335/Default.aspx (accessed 25 September 2016)

As has been discussed elsewhere in this book, much of our existing evidence focuses on cancer rather than other chronic conditions, lacks methodological rigour, or health economic evaluation, which makes addressing these limitations crucial.

Learning exercise 24.1

Read a published research paper, or consider a new research question, relating to your area of practice or interest. Having read this chapter, reflect in your reading or thinking on the challenges we have outlined. The paper may not state the challenges encountered, or how they were overcome, but try to imagine that study actually being conducted in your clinical area. Or reflect on the challenges inherent in answering a new research question and potential solutions.

Consider:

- What might be the challenges relating to: ethics, recruitment, randomisation (if relevant), respondent burden, attrition (if relevant) and outcomes?
- How might they be overcome?
- How might the study findings be translated into practice?

Conclusion

There are inherent challenges in generating and disseminating new knowledge in palliative care which we have outlined, along with the strategies for overcoming them. The six key inter-related challenges of palliative care research relate to: (1) ethics; (2) recruitment; (3) attrition; (4) outcomes; (5) respondent burden; and (6) randomisation. The five key challenges of implementing the knowledge generated by research into everyday practice are related to: (1) working with evolving science; (2) time from discovery to practice; (3) premature translation vs losing knowledge in translation; (4) integrating implementation; and (5) clinical practicalities. Combining robust research designs, which acknowledge and address these inherent challenges, with well-developed implementation strategies has the best chance of success in building the required evidence base for high quality palliative and end of life care.

References

Addington-Hall, J. (2007) Introduction. In Addington-Hall, J.B., Higginson, I.J. and Payne, S. (eds) *Research Methods in Palliative Care*. Oxford: Oxford University Press.

Agar, M., Ko, D.N., Sheehan, C. et al. (2013) Informed consent in palliative care clinical trials: challenging but possible. *Journal of Palliative Medicine*, 16: 485–91.

Agar, M. and Luckett, T. (2012) Outcome measures for palliative care research. *Current Opinion in Supportive and Palliative Care*, 6: 500–7.

Aldridge Carlson, M.D. (2013) Research methods priorities in geriatric palliative medicine. *Journal of Palliative Medicine*, 16: 838–42.

Aspinal, F., Hughes, R., Dunckley, M. et al. (2006) What is important to measure in the last months and weeks of life? A modified nominal group study. *International Journal of Nursing Studies*, 43: 393–403.

Bausewein, C., Farquhar, M., Booth, S. et al. (2007) Measurement of breathlessness in advanced disease: a systematic review. *Respiratory Medicine*, 101: 399–410.

Bentley, B. and O'connor, M. (2015) Conducting research interviews with bereaved family carers: when do we ask? *Journal of Palliative Medicine*, 18: 241–5.

Boland, J., Currow, D.C., Wilcock, A. et al. (2015) A systematic review of strategies used to increase recruitment of people with cancer or organ failure into clinical trials: implications for palliative care research. *Journal of Pain and Symptom Management*, 49: 762–72. e5.

Brown, C.A. and Lilford, R.J. (2006) The stepped wedge trial design: a systematic review. *BMC Medical Research Methodology*, 6: 54.

Buckle, J.L., Dwyer, S.C. and Jackson, M. (2010) Qualitative bereavement research: incongruity between the perspectives of participants and research ethics boards. *International Journal of Social Research Methodology*, 13: 111–25.

Campbell, L.C., Bailey, C., Armour, K. et al. (2016) A team approach to recruitment in hospice research: engaging patients, close people and health professionals. *International Journal of Palliative Nursing*, 22: 324–32.

Cawley, D., Waterman, D., Roberts, D. et al. (2011) A qualitative study exploring perceptions and experiences of patients and clinicians of palliative medicine outpatient clinics in different settings. *Palliative Medicine*, 25: 52–61.

Chan, R.J., Phillips, J. and Currow, D. (2014) Do palliative care health professionals settle for low-level evidence? *Palliative Medicine*, 28: 8–9.

Clark, P.C. and Dunbar, S.B. (2003) Identifying possible depression in clinical research: ethical and outcome considerations for the investigator/clinician. *Applied Nursing Research*, 16: 53–9.

Cochrane Library (2015) *About the Cochrane Library* [Online]. Available at: http://www.cochranelibrary.com/about/about-the-cochrane-library.html (accessed 5 February 2015).

Coombs M.P.R. and Devries, K. (2016) Can qualitative research interviews have therapeutic benefit for participants in end-of-life and bereavement research? *European Journal of Palliative Care*, 23: 227–31.

Currow, D.C., Plummer, J.L., Kutner, J.S. et al. (2012) Analyzing phase III studies in hospice/palliative care. A solution that sits between intention-to-treat and per protocol analyses: the palliative-modified ITT analysis. *Journal of Pain and Symptom Management*, 44: 595–603.

Daveson, B.A., De Wolf-Linder, S., Witt, J. et al. (2015) Results of a transparent expert consultation on patient and public involvement in palliative care research. *Palliative Medicine*, 29: 939–49.

Dickson, R. and Jack, B. (2008) Best supportive care in lung cancer: do we know what it is? *Palliative Medicine*, 22: 413–14.

Diehr, P. and Johnson, L.L. (2005) Accounting for missing data in end-of-life research. *Journal of Palliative Medicine*, 8: s-50–s-57.

Digiacomo, M., Lewis, J., Nolan, M. et al. (2013) Transitioning from caregiving to widowhood. *Journal of Pain and Symptom Management*, Published online, 8 April 2013.

Doherty, S. (2005) History of evidence-based medicine: oranges, chloride of lime and leeches: barriers to teaching old dogs new tricks. *Emergency Medicine Australasia*, 17: 314–21.

Duke, S. and Bennett, H. (2010) Review: a narrative review of the published ethical debates in palliative care research and an assessment of their adequacy to inform research governance. *Palliative Medicine*, 24: 111–26.

Ewing, G., Ngwenya, N., Benson, J. et al. (2016) Sharing news of a lung cancer diagnosis with adult family members and friends: a qualitative study to inform a supportive intervention in cancer care. *Patient Education and Counseling*, 99: 378–85.

Ewing, G., Rogers, M., Barclay, S. et al. (2004) Recruiting patients into a primary care based study of palliative care: why is it so difficult? *Palliative Medicine*, 18: 452–9.

Farquhar, M. (1995) Definitions of quality of life: a taxonomy. *Journal of Advanced Nursing*, 22: 502–8.

Farquhar, M., Ewing, G. and Booth, S. (2011) Using mixed methods to develop and evaluate complex interventions in palliative care research. *Palliative Medicine*, 25: 748–57.

Farquhar, M., Ewing, G., Higginson, I.J. et al. (2010) The experience of using the SEIQoL-DW with patients with advanced chronic obstructive pulmonary disease (COPD): issues of process and outcome. *Quality of Life Research*, 19: 619–29.

Farquhar, M., Higginson, I.J. and Booth, S. (2009a) Fast-track trials in palliative care: an alternative randomized controlled trial design. *Journal of Palliative Medicine*, 12: 213.

Farquhar, M., Higginson, I.J., Fagan, P. et al. (2009b) The feasibility of a single-blinded fast-track pragmatic randomised controlled trial of a complex intervention for Breathlessness in Advanced Disease. *BMC Palliative Care*, 8: 9.

Farquhar, M., Penfold, C., Ewing, G. et al. (2016a) Developing an educational intervention on breathlessness in advanced disease. In *9th World Research Congress of The European Association for Palliative Care (EAPC)*. Dublin: Palliative Medicine.

Farquhar, M., Preston, N., Evans, C.J. et al. (2013) Mixed methods research in the development and evaluation of complex interventions in palliative and end-of-life care: report on the MORECare consensus exercise. *Journal of Palliative Medicine*, 16: 1550–60.

Farquhar, M., Prevost, A.T., Mccrone, P. et al. (2014) Is a specialist breathlessness service more effective and cost-effective for patients with advanced cancer and their carers than standard care? Findings of a mixed-method randomised controlled trial. *BMC Medicine*, 12: 194.

Farquhar, M., Prevost, A.T., Mccrone, P. et al. (2016b) The clinical and cost effectiveness of a Breathlessness Intervention Service for patients with advanced non-malignant disease and their informal carers: mixed findings of a mixed method randomised controlled trial. *Trials*, 17: 185.

Fernandez, C.V., Santor, D., Weijer, C. et al. (2007) The return of research results to participants: pilot questionnaire of adolescents and parents of children with cancer. *Pediatric Blood and Cancer*, 48: 441–6.

Ferrell, B.R. (2005) Overview of the domains of variables relevant to end-of-life care. *Journal of Palliative Medicine*, 8: s-22–s-29.

Fielding, S., Fayers, P., Loge, J. et al. (2006) Methods for handling missing data in palliative care research. *Palliative Medicine*, 20: 791–8.

Fitzsimons, D. and Strachan, P.H. (2012) Overcoming the challenges of conducting research with people who have advanced heart failure and palliative care needs. *European Journal of Cardiovascular Nursing*, 11: 248–54.

Flemming, K., Adamson, J. and Atkin, K. (2008) Improving the effectiveness of interventions in palliative care: the potential role of qualitative research in enhancing evidence from randomized controlled trials. *Palliative Medicine*, 22: 123–31.

Funk, L.M. and Stajduhar, K.I. (2009) Interviewing family caregivers: implications of the caregiving context for the research interview. *Qualitative Health Research*, 19: 859–67.

Graham, I.D., Logan, J., Harrison, M.B. et al. (2006) Lost in knowledge translation: time for a map? *Journal of Continuing Education in the Health Professions*, 26: 13–24.

Graham, I.D. and Tetroe, J. (2007) Some theoretical underpinnings of knowledge translation. *Academic Emergency Medicine*, 14: 936–41.

Grande, G. and Todd, C. (2000) Issues in research: why are trials in palliative care so difficult? *Palliative Medicine*, 14: 69–74.

Greenhalgh, T. and Wieringa, S. (2011) Is it time to drop the 'knowledge translation' metaphor? A critical literature review. *Journal of the Royal Society of Medicine*, 104: 501–9.

Grol, R., Wensing, M. and Eccles, M. (2005) *Improving Patient Care: The Implementation of Change in Clinical Practice*. Edinburgh: Elsevier.

Gysels, M., Evans, C.J., Lewis, P. et al. (2013) MORECare research methods guidance development: recommendations for ethical issues in palliative and end-of-life care research. *Palliative Medicine*, 27: 908–17.

Gysels, M., Shipman, C. and Higginson, I.J. (2008a) 'I will do it if it will help others': motivations among patients taking part in qualitative studies in palliative care. *Journal of Pain and Symptom Management*, 35: 347–55.

Gysels, M., Shipman, C. and Higginson, I.J. (2008b) Is the qualitative research interview an acceptable medium for research with palliative care patients and carers? *BMC Medical Ethics*, 9: 7.

Hardy, J., Quinn, S., Fazekas, B. et al. (2012) Randomized, double-blind, placebo-controlled study to assess the efficacy and toxicity of subcutaneous ketamine in the management of cancer pain. *Journal of Clinical Oncology*, 30: 3611–17.

Higginson, I.J. and Booth, S. (2011) The randomized fast-track trial in palliative care: role, utility and ethics in the evaluation of interventions in palliative care? *Palliative Medicine*, 25: 741–7.

Higginson, I.J., Evans, C.J., Grande, G. et al. (2013) Evaluating complex interventions in end of life care: the MORECare statement on good practice generated by a synthesis of transparent expert consultations and systematic reviews. *BMC Medicine*, 11: 111.

Higginson, I.J. and Gao, W. (2008) Caregiver assessment of patients with advanced cancer: concordance with patients, effect of burden and positivity. *Health and Quality of Life Outcomes*, 6: 42.

Hosie, A., Davidson, P.M., Agar, M. et al. (2013) Delirium prevalence, incidence, and implications for screening in specialist palliative care inpatient settings: a systematic Review. *Palliative Medicine*, 27: 486–98.

Hosie, A.M. (2015) Delirium epidemiology, systems and nursing practice in palliative care inaptient settings: a descriptive mixed methods project (DePAC Project). D.Phil., University of Notre Dame Australia.

Hudson, P. (2003) The experience of research participation for family caregivers of palliative care cancer patients. *International Journal of Palliative Nursing*, 9: 120–3.

Ioannidis, J.P. (2006) Evolution and translation of research findings: from bench to where? *PLoS Clinical Trials*, 1: e36.

Kavanaugh, K.L. and Campbell, M.L. (2014) Conducting end-of-life research: strategies for success. *Nursing Science Quarterly*, 27: 14–19.

Kelly, B., McClement, S. and Chochinov, H.M. (2006) Measurement of psychological distress in palliative care. *Palliative Medicine*, 20: 779–89.

Koffman, J., Higginson, I.J., Hall, S. et al. (2012) Bereaved relatives' views about participating in cancer research. *Palliative Medicine*, 26: 379–83.

Lavis, J., Hammill, A.C., Gildiner, A. et al. (2005) *A Systematic Review of the Factors that Influence the Use of Research Evidence by Public Policymakers: Report Submitted to the Canadian Population Health Initiative*. Hamilton: Government of Canada.

Ling, J., Rees, E. and Hardy, J. (2000) What influences participation in clinical trials in palliative care in a cancer centre? *European Journal of Cancer*, 36: 621–6.

Mayland, C., Williams, E. and Ellershaw, J. (2008) How well do current instruments using bereaved relatives' views evaluate care for dying patients? *Palliative Medicine*, 22: 133–44.

McKibbon, K.A., Lokker, C., Wilczynski, N.L. et al. (2010) A cross-sectional study of the number and frequency of terms used to refer to knowledge translation in a body of health literature in 2006: a Tower of Babel? *Implementation Science*, 5: 16.

McPherson, C. and Addington-Hall, J. (2003) Judging the quality of care at the end of life: can proxies provide reliable information? *Social Science and Medicine*, 56: 95–109.

Medical Research Council (2000) *A Framework for Development and Evaluation ef RCTs for Complex Interventions to Improve Health*. London: MRC Health Services and Public Health Research Board.

MORECare (2013) *Methods for Evaluating Service Delivery Models for End of Life Care (EOLC): Development of Best Practice Guidance (MORECare)* [Online]. London: King's College London. Available at: http://www.kcl.ac.uk/lsm/research/divisions/cicelysaunders/research/studies/morecare.aspx (accessed 10 October 2016).

Morris, Z.S., Wooding, S. and Grant, J. (2011) The answer is 17 years, what is the question? Understanding time lags in translational research. *Journal of the Royal Society of Medicine*, 104: 510–20.

Mularski, R.A., Dy, S.M., Shugarman, L.R. et al. (2007) A systematic review of measures of end-of-life care and its outcomes. *Health Services Research*, 42: 1848–70.

Murtagh, F.E., Addington-Hall, J.M. and Higginson, I.J. (2007) The value of cognitive interviewing techniques in palliative care research. *Palliative Medicine*, 21: 87–93.

National Heart Lung and Blood Institute (2014) New NHLBI Center focuses on translation research and implementation science [Online]. USA: National Institute of Health. Available at: http://www.nhlbi.nih.gov/news/spotlight/fact-sheet/new-nhlbi-center-focuses-translation-research-and-implementation-science (accessed 10 October 2016).

Neuberger, J., Guthrie, C., Aaronvitch, D. et al. (2013) *More Care, Less Pathway: A Review of the Liverpool Care Pathway*. London: Department of Health.

Northouse, L.L., Rosset, T., Phillips, L. et al. (2006) Research with families facing cancer: the challenges of accrual and retention. *Research in Nursing and Health*, 29: 199–211.

Pavis, H. and Wilcock, A. (2001) Prescribing of drugs for use outside their licence in palliative care: survey of specialists in the United Kingdom. *British Medical Journal*, 323: 484–5.

Payne, S., Preston, N., Turner, M. et al. (2013) *Research in Palliative Care: Can Hospices Afford Not to Be Involved? A Report for the Commission into the Future of Hospice Care*. London: Hospice UK.

Penner, J.L., Stevenson, M., Parmar, M.P. et al. (2016) The psychosocial needs of students conducting research with patients and their families in advanced cancer and palliative care: a scoping review. *Palliative and Supportive Care*, 15(2): 1–7.

Phillips, J.L. (2015) Implementing evidence-based palliative care. *International Journal of Palliative Nursing*, 21: 55.

Pleschberger, S., Seymour, J.E., Payne, S. et al. (2011) Interviews on end-of-life care with older people: reflections on six European studies. *Qualitative Health Research*, 21: 1588–600.

Preston, N.J., Fayers, P., Walters, S.J. et al. (2013) Recommendations for managing missing data, attrition and response shift in palliative and end-of-life care research: part of the MORECare research method guidance on statistical issues. *Palliative Medicine*, 27(10): 899–907.

Primary Care Unit. *Living with Breathlessness Study* [Online]. Cambridge: University of Cambridge. Available at: http://www.phpc.cam.ac.uk/pcu/research/research-projects-list/living-with-breathlessness-study/ (accessed 4 October 2016).

Quibell, R., Fallon, M., Mihalyo, M. et al. (2015) Ketamine. *Journal of Pain Symptom Management*, 50: 268–78.

Richards, D.A. (2015) Complex interventions and the amalgamation of marginal gains: a way forward for understanding and researching essential nursing care? *International Journal of Nursing Studies*, 52: 1143–5.

Rocker, G. (2011) Dyspnea: recent insights and innovations. *Progress in Palliative Care*, 19: 219–22.

Schildmann, E.K. and Higginson, I.J. (2011) Evaluating psycho-educational interventions for informal carers of patients receiving cancer care or palliative care: strengths and limitations of different study designs. *Palliative Medicine*, 25: 345–56.

Sealey, M., Breen, L.J., O'Connor, M. et al. (2015) A scoping review of bereavement risk assessment measures: implications for palliative care. *Palliative Medicine*, 29: 577–89.

Shelby-James, T.M., Hardy, J., Agar, M. et al. (2012) Designing and conducting randomized controlled trials in palliative care: a summary of discussions from the 2010 clinical research forum of the Australian Palliative Care Clinical Studies Collaborative. *Palliative Medicine*, 26: 1042–7.

Shilling, V., Matthews, L., Jenkins, V. et al. (2016) Patient-reported outcome measures for cancer caregivers: a systematic review. *Quality of Life Research*, 25(8): 1859–76.

Sigurdardóttir, K.R., Kaasa, S., Rosland, J.H. et al. (2014) The European Association for Palliative Care basic dataset to describe a palliative care cancer population: results from an international Delphi process. *Palliative Medicine*, 28(6): 463–73.

Sivell, S., Prout, H., Hopewell-Kelly, N. et al. (2015) Considerations and recommendations for conducting qualitative research interviews with palliative and end-of-life care patients in the home setting: a consensus paper. *BMJ Supportive and Palliative Care*. Published online first: bmjspcare-2015-000892.

Steinhauser, K.E. and Barroso, J. (2009) Using qualitative methods to explore key questions in palliative care. *Journal of Palliative Medicine*, 12: 725–30.

Steinhauser, K.E., Clipp, E.C., Hays, J.C. et al. (2006) Identifying, recruiting, and retaining seriously-ill patients and their caregivers in longitudinal research. *Palliative Medicine*, 20: 745–54.

Stiel, S., Pastrana, T., Balzer, C. et al. (2012) Outcome assessment instruments in palliative and hospice care: a review of the literature. *Supportive Care in Cancer*, 20: 2879–93.

Stolberg, H.O., Norman, G. and Trop, I. (2004) Randomized controlled trials. *American Journal of Roentgenology*, 183: 1539–44.

Swetenham, K., Tieman, J., Butow, P. et al. (2015) Communication differences when patients and caregivers are seen separately or together. *International Journal of Palliative Nursing*, 21: 557–63.

Sygna, K., Johansen, S. and Ruland, C.M. (2015) Recruitment challenges in clinical research including cancer patients and caregivers. *Trials*, 16: 428.

Thabane, L., Ma, J., Chu, R. et al. (2010) A tutorial on pilot studies: the what, why and how. *BMC Medical Research Methodology*, 10: 1.

Tieman, J., Sladek, R. and Currow, D. (2008) Changes in the quantity and level of evidence of palliative and hospice care literature: the last century. *Journal of Clinical Oncology*, 26: 5679–83.

To, T.H., Agar, M., Shelby-James, T. et al. (2013) Off-label prescribing in palliative care: a cross-sectional national survey of palliative medicine doctors. *Palliative Medicine*, 27: 320–8.

Westfall, J.M., Mold, J. and Fagnan, L. (2007) Practice-based research: 'Blue Highways' on the NIH roadmap. *JAMA*, 297: 403–6.

White, C., Gilshenan, K. and Hardy, J. (2008) A survey of the views of palliative care healthcare professionals towards referring cancer patients to participate in randomized controlled trials in palliative care. *Supportive Care in Cancer*, 16: 1397–405.

White, C. and Hardy, J. (2010) What do palliative care patients and their relatives think about research in palliative care? A systematic review. *Supportive Care in Cancer*, 18: 905–11.

Wilson, E., Elkan, R. and Cox, K. (2007) Closure for patients at the end of a cancer clinical trial: literature review. *Journal of Advanced Nursing*, 59: 445–53.

Zigmond, A.S. and Snaith, R.P. (1983) The hospital anxiety and depression scale. *Acta Psychiatrica Scandinavica*, 67: 361–70.

Chapter

25

Growing and developing palliative care worldwide: assessing and developing public health approaches to palliative care

Richard Harding, Mackuline Atieno and Julia Downing

Introduction

The provision of palliative care is a global challenge. WHO's 2014 Global Report revealed that only 58 per cent of countries have a palliative care service (Lynch et al. 2013). Only one in 10 of the 20 million people each year who require palliative care at the end of life actually receive it, and 80 per cent of the need is in low- and middle-income countries (LMIC) (Connor and Sepulveda 2014). In 2014, the World Health Assembly (WHA) passed its first resolution on palliative care, recognising that

> Palliative care, when indicated, is fundamental to improving quality of life, well-being, comfort and human dignity for individuals, being an effective person-centred health service that values patients' need to receive adequate, personally and culturally sensitive information on their health status, and their central role in making decisions about the treatment received.
>
> (WHA 2014)

Groups in need in LMIC

The following four groups in particular are worth highlighting due to the needs across LMIC: (1) cancer cases; (2) HIV cases; (3) children and young people; and (4) those suffering non-communicable diseases.

Cancer epidemiology

As populations age and societies industrialise, increasing numbers of people in LMIC will require cancer care. By 2020, 70 per cent of cancer cases will be in LMIC (Farmer et al. 2010). GLOBOCAN estimates 5.3 million cancer deaths in less developed regions during 2012 (Ferley et al. 2014). The lifetime risk of a woman in Africa dying of cancer is double that in developed countries (Parkin et al. 2008). This has led to palliative care being identified as an essential component of cancer control programmes in LMIC (Gelband et al. 2015). Also in Sub-Saharan Africa and indeed the majority of LMIC, individuals will present late and therefore have advanced incurable disease at the time of detection and diagnosis (Kanavos 2006). Many may even present too late to gain a meaningful diagnosis. This late presentation is often due to limited access to health, reliance on traditional healers, and stigma. For example, cancer stigma leads to late presentation among Arab women with gynaecological cancers (Ortashi 2013) and late breast cancer presentation in India (Babu, Lakshmi and Thiyagarajan 2013). In West Bengal, cancer is often believed to be infectious, and diagnosis is concealed to reduce stigma (Ray and Mandal 2004). Death taboo also leads to poor access to, and inappropriate provision of, end of life care (Bhatnagar and Joshi 2013).

HIV epidemiology

HIV and AIDS also remain a significant contributor to progressive illness in LMIC. Some 25.6 million people were living with HIV in Sub-Saharan Africa in 2015, with 1.55 million new infections in 2015 alone (190,000 of these in children under the age of 15 years) (UNAIDS 2015). Adolescent girls and young women aged 15–24 years are at particularly high risk of HIV infection, accounting for 25 per cent of new infections among adults in Sub-Saharan Africa (SSA) in 2015 (Kelley et al. 2016). Women accounted for more than half those living with HIV in SSA in 2014 (UNAIDS 2015). A Fast-Track approach to HIV treatment, concentrating on the hardest-hit countries (the majority of which are LMIC), has been instigated and reinforces the determination to achieve the 90-90-90 treatment target by 2010, that is 90 per cent of people living with HIV will know their status; 90 per cent of people who know their status are accessing treatment; and 90 per cent of people on treatment have suppressed viral load (UNAIDS 2014). However, there is a still a long way to go to achieve this with only 39 per cent of adults living with HIV in SSA accessing antiretroviral treatment in 2013 (Avert 2016). Other LMIC are impacted in similar ways, with the incidence of HIV being higher in poorer countries.

Children and young people

In 2014, children under the age of 15 years accounted for 26 per cent of the population worldwide, with that figure increasing to 40 per cent in the least developed nations (Human Rights Campaign. 2016). Nearly all child deaths occur in LMIC, and almost half of those in SSA. A recent estimation into the need for palliative care for children globally suggests that over 21 million children need palliative care annually, with an estimation of over 8 million with life-limiting and life-threatening diseases requiring some specialist palliative care service provision (Connor et al. 2016). This need was estimated by using an agreed list of ICD-10 diagnosis based on the Together for Short Lives four categories of children needing palliative care (2013), and modified in discussions with the WHO Department of Health Statistics. In general, the higher the income category for a country, the higher its Human Development Index (HDI) and the lower the need for children's palliative care (Connor et al. 2016).

Non-communicable diseases

In addition to the focus on cancer and HIV palliative care, there is a rising incidence of non-cancer-related non-communicable diseases (NCDs) that require palliative care (Powell et al. 2015). NCDs (which include cardiovascular diseases, diabetes, cancers and chronic respiratory diseases) are the leading causes of death globally (WHO 2014). Some 38 million of the 56 million deaths that occurred globally in 2012 (68 per cent) were due to NCDs and of these, almost 75 per cent (i.e. 28 million) occurred in LMIC (WHO 2014). In some LMIC, such as countries in Africa, it is projected that annual deaths due to NCDs will increase and become the leading cause of death by 2030 (Boutayeb and Boutayeb 2005; WHO 2010a; 2014). For example, the Uganda Heart Institute in Kampala saw a 500 per cent increase in outpatient attendance due to heart-related conditions between 2005 and 2009 and this continues to increase. However, it is only recently that palliative care has been considered a global health issue (Harding and Higginson 2014).

Global inequalities at the end of life

Access to palliative and end of life care

The quality of death within a country closely mirrors a country's Gross Domestic Product (GDP), i.e. the poorer the country's economy, the poorer the quality of death. The Economist's 'Quality of Death Ranking' is a summary assessment consisting of comprehensive national policies, the extent to which palliative care is integrated into the National Health Service, the strength of the hospice movement, and community engagement on the issue. The top five countries were identified as the UK, Australia, New Zealand, Ireland and Belgium. The bottom five countries were Myanmar, Nigeria, the Philippines, Bangladesh and Iraq. This evidence demonstrates that the health inequalities that persist throughout life are mirrored in death, despite palliative care being simple and cheap to provide, and is cost-saving. Likewise, the Global Atlas of Palliative Care at the End of Life, lists 75 countries in the world with no known palliative care activity, the majority of which are LMIC, while 18 out of the 20 countries with advanced integration are high-income countries, with just Uganda and Romania breaking the trend (Connor and Sepulveda 2014). Similarly, when looking at the provision of children's palliative care, a systematic review found that 65.6 per cent of countries globally had no known children's palliative care activity, with only 5.7 per cent having provision that was reaching mainstream providers, all of which were high-income countries, with the exception of South Africa, an upper middle-income country (Knapp et al. 2011).

Treatment access

Access to treatment contributes significantly to global inequalities at the end of life. In considering access to cancer treatment, there needs to be access to all three primary modalities such as surgery, chemotherapy (systemic therapy) and radiotherapy. While in LMIC patients often present late with advanced disease, limited access to affordable and quality cancer treatment has contributed to mortality-to-incidence ratios approximately 20 per cent higher than in other countries. Although approximately 60 per cent of cancer patients would benefit from radiotherapy at some point during the course of their disease, it is often not available to the 82 per cent of the world's population living in LMIC, which have only 32 per cent of the radiotherapy machines available globally. In Africa and Asia, there are at least 22 countries without radiotherapy services available (Levin, El Gueddari and Meghzifene 1999; Barton, Frommer and Shafiq 2006), and for some, such as in Uganda, there is one machine. This is currently not working, therefore impacting greatly on the treatment available to individuals in Uganda, Rwanda, Democratic Republic of Congo, Sudan and Burundi (The Cancer Atlas 2012) as it provides treatment for their patients too. Due to limited data in many LMIC, little is known regarding access to appropriate chemotherapy and surgery treatment, however, it is assumed that this too is low (Hanna and Kangolle 2010).

While the lack of accessibility and availability of treatment is a challenge, other challenges include a lack of diagnostic and screening facilities, as well as trained health personnel (The Cancer Atlas 2012). For example, in SSA, there is less than one pathologist per 500,000 population, with the exception of South Africa and Botswana, therefore accessing an accurate diagnosis is in itself a challenge, thus impacting on the treatment being given. In Uganda, the doctor-patient ratio is 1:24,725 against a WHO recommended level for Africa of 1:10,000, and a nurse-patient ratio of 1:11,000 against a WHO recommended level of 1:400 (Ministry of Finance 2013) (Table 25.1). This is reflected in the majority of LMIC, thus the actual number of health professionals is lower than within other countries. Many of these will not have had appropriate training for end of life care.

Table 25.1 Doctor-patient ratios by region

Region	Nurses and midwives per 1,000 people in 2011 (World Bank 2016a)	Physicians per 1,000 people in 2011 (World Bank 2016b)
High income	8.6	2.9
Upper middle income	3.0	2.0
Middle income	2.3	1.4
Lower middle income	1.7	0.8
Low income	–	0.1

The public health approach to palliative care

Public health is broadly defined as a tool used by society to protect, promote and restore people's health (Cohen and Deliens 2012). The aim of a public health approach is 'to protect and improve the health and quality of life of a community by translating new knowledge and skills into evidence-based, cost-effective interventions that will be available to everyone in the population who needs them' (Stjernswärd et al. 2007). In applying the public health approach to palliative care, it is important to view health, not just in terms of a curative approach to health, i.e. restoring an individual to full fitness, but to consider health in terms of a general feeling of well-being, psychosocial well-being, and aiming for the best possible situation within the current context. Thus, the public health approach looks less at the biomedical approach but more on social and economic aspects and aims to focus more on equity and attempting to break down barriers in both health professionals and the public. Cohen and Deliens (2012) describe public health at the end of life as 'the efforts organized by society to optimize the circumstances of the dying and all those involved through collective or social actions'. In other words, the public health approach to palliative care is concerned with the quality of palliative care for populations, not just the individuals within them, thus embracing a wider perspective than that of the medical and biomedical models in developing palliative care.

Public health approaches to palliative care have been emphasised over the past decade, and have been growing in importance and practice acceptance. The enhanced public health model for palliative care identified the components needed to effectively integrate palliative care into a society/system and improve access and availability of palliative care. Four components of this model were described: (1) appropriate policies; (2) adequate availability of medicine; (3) education of health workers; and (4) implementation of services (Stjernswärd et al. 2007). Appraisal of the WHO strategy has also advocated for a further underpinning additional activity – that of research – in order to inform and evaluate the drug/policy/education/implementation pillars (Harding et al. 2013). However, there are many challenges in implementing this public health approach. Kellehear and Sallnow (Sallnow et al. 2009) identified three key challenges: (1) the inability, reluctance or refusal to understand key health promotion concepts and apply these within palliative care; (2) training in the public health approach to palliative care is poor or absent; and (3) the public health sector needs to enter the palliative and end of life arena.

The role of nursing in a public health approach to palliative care

Nurses have a key role in the public health approach to palliative care, particularly in LMIC, where they can be found at all levels of the healthcare system. They have the broad range of skills needed for palliative care, they are more readily available than medical and clinical officers and have played a pivotal role in the on-going development of palliative care in LMIC such as across SSA (Downing et al. 2006; Mwangi-Powell et al. 2015). Thus. nursing is the hallmark of patient care in LMIC. With the doctor-patient ratio in low-income countries ranging from 0.014 per 1,000 population in Liberia to 0.209 per 1,000 people in Nepal, nurses represent the highest ratio of health professionals to patient care (0.274 per 1,000 in Liberia and 0.46 per 1,000 in Nepal).

Nurses and midwives in LMIC will have had access to a wide variety of nursing training programmes, thus, there will be different cadres of nurses such as nursing aides, Enrolled and Registered nurses who have undertaken a certificate in nursing, those with a diploma such as the Diploma in comprehensive nursing, and those with a degree such as the BSc Nursing. Often nurses and midwives will be dual trained and working interchangeably, particularly in the rural settings. Alongside the range in cadres, nursing practice in palliative care will vary from the palliative care approach, general palliative care to the specialist level, with nurses providing the palliative care approach having received palliative care training in their professional training. Those providing general palliative care are those involved in palliative care but do not provide it as the main part of their work – for example, those nurses working on a general hospital medical ward, where some patients will require palliative care, but not all of them. Finally, they may be working within palliative care at the specialist level – either for adults, children or both (De Vlieger et al. 2004; Gamondi, Larkin and Payne 2013a; 2013b; Downing et al. 2014b). The majority of nurses in LMIC will be working at the generalist level, with opportunities for specialist level education in palliative care being limited.

The principles of nursing support the holistic nature and philosophy of palliative care. Their role in palliative care is broad and will vary from country to country, however, in LMIC, where nurses not only provide nurse-led palliative care services, they also provide leadership in mentorship, advocacy, education and research, their role features the following core elements: integration of palliative care into all levels of service provision; development of team work; assessment; communication and counselling; treatment and prescribing as appropriate; training and supervision; advocacy and health promotion, all provided within a culturally appropriate and sensitive manner (Downing et al. 2006). Nurses work in the context of limited resources, systems where medicines are often out of stock, and thus they have to be innovative in providing services.

Appropriate policies

Advocating for appropriate policies, guidelines and legal frameworks is best undertaken together, as a palliative care community, whether locally, nationally or globally. While many nurses may not be working at the global level, they should all be advocating for palliative care at the local and, where possible, national level. This component of the WHO public health model focuses on appropriate policies, including palliative care in the national health plan, funding and models of service delivery and policies for essential medicines (Stjernswärd et al. 2007). The process of advocating for these things needs to take place at the different levels and by all those involved in palliative care.

Collaboration is key in this, and this was seen by the palliative care community coming together to advocate for the WHA resolution on palliative care (WHA 2014), which will impact the development of policies, guidelines and the inclusion of palliative care in health plans at the national level. Examples where collaboration has contributed greatly to advocacy attempts, and where nurses have been at the forefront of this advocacy, are found in Uganda and India. In Uganda, a draft national palliative care policy has been developed (Nabudere, Obuku and Lamorde 2014) and endorsed by the Senior Management Committee (SMC) of the Ministry of Health in 2015 and is now awaiting final ratification. Other LMIC are also following suit, for example, Zimbabwe, Swaziland and Namibia (Luyirika et al. 2016). In Kenya, policies have been decentralised, but palliative care has been included in several regional level health policies.

Preparing nurses to advocate and to lead within the field of palliative care is essential. Thus, an innovative palliative care nurse leadership fellowship programme has been implemented in Uganda (Downing et al. 2016b). The programme aims to develop palliative care nurse leaders through supporting and mentoring them in the implementation of best practices and participation in local and national palliative care related projects. Twenty nurses from across Uganda are undertaking the fellowship, which includes three taught weeks interspersed by time in their places of work and mentorship from both local and international nurse mentors. To date, this programme has enabled nurses to advocate for palliative care and bring about changes in their places of work and they are working together on national-level projects, including the evaluation of nurse prescribing in Uganda, which will develop data that will be used at the national and international levels. It is hoped that a similar nurse leadership programme can be implemented in other LMIC, and there are plans to implement a nurse leadership programme in India (LeBaron et al. 2016) in order to enact evidence-based policy and practice change.

Availability of medicines

The availability of palliative care medications is one of the main pillars in the WHO model to achieve a public health approach to palliative care (Stjernsward, Foley and Ferris 2007). There is evidence of high prevalence and burden of pain among people with advanced disease in LMIC. In Sub-Saharan Africa, people with advanced cancer report a prevalence of pain within the past 7 days of 87.4 per cent (Harding et al. 2011), among HIV patients 82.6 per cent (Harding et al. 2012), and among heart failure patients 91.3 per cent (Lokker et al. 2013). The focus on availability of opioids among LMIC has been a major focus for policy advocacy. Uganda provided enormous leadership, with a strategic approach to change law, enhance education, and improve supply of opioids for palliative care (Jagwe and Merriman 2007). Nurses are now able to attend specialist training that enables them to prescribe opioids (Merriman and Harding 2010).

An initial evaluation of the Uganda model to increase opioid availability found no diversion of morphine from the patient, and greater availability in district pharmacies (Logie and Harding 2005). A more comprehensive evaluation of nurse prescribing is currently underway in Uganda. This evaluation, approved by the World Health Organization, is being undertaken collaboratively by the Ministry of Health, Makerere Palliative Care Unit (MPCU), the Palliative Care Association of Uganda (PCAU), Hospice

Africa Uganda (HAU) and the African Palliative Care Association (APCA). It recognises the complexity of availability and accessibility to medications, and builds on previous work which addressed the barriers to pain-relieving medications in 12 African countries which included issues of: supply; legislation; education; and practical issues, including a lack of prescribers and the infrastructure available (Harding et al. 2010a). Thus, the conceptual framework for the evaluation takes into account the different component parts involved in the process of nurse prescribing and the evaluation is being conducted in three parts: (1) preparation of the nurses for their role, i.e. is the training fit for purpose? (Nabirye et al. 2016); (2) the actual process of assessing and managing patients' pain, including the prescription of oral morphine and patient outcomes (Dusabimana et al. 2016); and (3) the system in which the nurses are working through a rapid appraisal (Sekyondwa et al. 2016). The evaluation, being undertaken by nurses, is on-going with results and lessons learnt expected in 2017.

While working hard at the patient and service level to improve access to medicine for palliative care, nurses also have a role at the national and global level in inputting to and impacting advocacy to increase access. At the national level they are part of any national palliative care association and can work through them to advocate to the Ministry of Health and to participate in national and global campaigns such as World Hospice and Palliative Care Day Activities (WHPCD). WHPCD takes place on the first Saturday of October each year. The theme of the day will vary from year to year, for example: 'Hidden Lives, Hidden Patients' (Downing 2015) and 'Living and Dying in Pain: It doesn't have to happen' (Jackson 2016). Each year resources are developed that nurses can use in their advocacy activities – for example, the 'Living and Dying in Pain toolkit' gives clear rationale of the size of the problem, how it can be overcome, and makes recommendations for people and their families in need of pain relief, for healthcare workers and volunteers and to national governments. It also gives examples of different ways to mark WHPCD (Jackson 2016). These documents, along with resources such as the essential palliative care medicines list (De Lima and Doyle 2007), are available to nurses so that they can use them in order to increase access and availability to palliative care medications.

Education and capacity building

Education within the public health strategy is aimed at a wide audience, including the media and the public, healthcare providers and trainees, palliative care experts and family caregivers (Stjernswärd et al. 2007). While general nursing education is provided at various levels, it is important that palliative care educational programmes reflect this and enable nurses to gain an understanding and skills in palliative care, regardless of the type of training programme they are undertaking, e.g. certificate, diploma and degree programmes. Work has been undertaken in different parts of the world to identify the core competencies required for nurses working in both adult and children's palliative care and when and how they might achieve these. For example, the core competencies for different professions developed by the APCA (2012), the core competencies for children's palliative care developed by the Paediatric Task Force of the

European Association of Palliative Care (EAPC) (Downing et al. 2014b) and the guide for the development of palliative nurse education in Europe by the EAPC Task Force (De Vlieger et al. 2004).

Work is on-going to ensure that there are courses available at the three different levels of care provision discussed above, i.e. (1) the palliative care approach; (2) general palliative care; and (3) specialist palliative care. Over the past decade there has been an emphasis on trying to integrate palliative care into nurse training via the nursing teaching institutions and universities. The integration into such curricula is an essential element of the WHA resolution (WHA 2014) on palliative care and is key in ensuring that the nurses of the future are all well informed about palliative care. An example of this is the Kenya Medical Training College (KMTC), a state corporation under the Ministry of Health, which trains nurses across the country. They have integrated palliative care into their certificate, diploma and higher diploma courses for nurses, and have undertaken reviews into how this is working from the perspective of the teachers and the students as part of the teachers' own on-going development through the BSc in Palliative Care offered by the Institute of Hospice and Palliative Care in Africa (IHPCA), in affiliation with Makerere University, Kampala, Uganda. Other countries working on the integration of palliative care into undergraduate nursing training include Uganda, Kenya, Ghana, Tanzania, Malawi and Indonesia.

For the nurses working at the generalist level, i.e. providing palliative care but not as the main focus of their role, there are a wide variety of training programmes available. These include basic introductory courses supported by the national palliative care associations, donor-funded programmes and the Ministry of Health. For example, in Rwanda, the Rwanda Biomedical Center (RBC) has approved on-going basic training programmes which are being rolled out throughout the country. In Zambia, the Palliative Care Alliance of Zambia (PCAZ) worked alongside the Ministry of Health to develop national training materials on palliative care, as have a wide number of countries including Tanzania, South Africa, Kenya, Malawi, Uganda among others. There are a wide variety of training materials that can be used for basic-level training. Many, such as the palliative care toolkit (Bond et al. 2008) and trainers manual (Lavy 2009), are available in a wide number of languages, e.g. Kiswahili, Bengali and Vietnamese, and have been used globally in LMIC.

While knowledge of palliative care is important, so too is the development of skills and so the importance of mentorship and clinical placements is emphasised, with placements being seen as a core component of basic palliative care training. Training programmes may also be given in a variety of formats, including face-to-face programmes, blended courses and e-learning programmes. ecancer has collaborated with Cardiff University to develop and implement a palliative care e-learning course for healthcare professionals in Africa and India. The International Children's Palliative Care Network (ICPCN) also offers e-learning programmes on a variety of aspects of children's palliative care.

At the specialist level, there is less availability of courses for nurses to undertake specialist training in palliative care. In Sub-Saharan Africa, the IHPCA, based at HAU in Kampala, offers a variety of courses, including a Diploma in Clinical Palliative

Care, a Diploma and Degree in Palliative Care and are currently developing a Master's programme. The two Diploma programmes lead to nurses working in Uganda to be registered as nurse prescribers (as long as they have done the prescribers module). Similar specialist training is conducted and being developed in other countries in conjunction with supporting universities, such as Kenya, Tanzania and Malawi. Nurses are also able to join the Post Graduate Diploma and Master's Programme at the University of Cape Town (Gwyther and Rawlinson 2007) and can focus on either children's or adult palliative care. A diploma in children's palliative care is also available through Mildmay Uganda and is the first of its kind. Other programmes can be found in different parts of the world, often requiring funding or scholarships for nurses in LMIC to undertake. Thus, one of the major challenges for nurses in LMIC in undertaking specialist level training, both within and outside of their home countries, is that of funding. Often courses are not affordable on a nurse's salary and are not currently funded though the mainstream government programmes – which is a priority for the on-going sustainability of palliative care. Thus, nurses rely on sponsorship or donor-funded programmes, yet the donor base for palliative care in LMIC is dwindling with access for nurses becoming harder and harder. Thus, there is an urgent need to identify innovative ways of incorporating palliative care education within the public health approach and integrate it into the existing courses while developing specialist training.

Not only is the capacity building of nurses essential for the development of palliative care, nurses have a role in building capacity in others, and the role of educator is implicit in the unique function of the nurse (Henderson 1997). If palliative care is to be available to all who need it, then nurses need to build the capacity of community volunteers/ caregivers (or equivalent), nursing aides, accredited social health activists (ASHAs) (community health workers) and family members. Nurses need to train, mentor and supervise these carers to provide palliative care in order to roll palliative care out into the rural settings, in order to help identify and care for individuals needing palliative care in the community. Examples of effective use of volunteers can be found in India, for example, in Tata Memorial Hospital (Muckaden and Pandya 2016) and in community models (Kar et al. 2015) and in Uganda at Hospice Africa Uganda (Jack et al. 2011).

Implementation of services

There are a wide variety of models of palliative care service delivery in LMIC, ranging from stand-alone specialist palliative care programmes, integrated hospital-based services, home-based care programmes, to single practitioners struggling to provide services on their own, on top of full-time work. Integration into existing health systems is an integral part of the WHA resolution (WHA 2014) and a review of the evidence of models in SSA reported an urgent need to develop a public health approach that integrates care into national health systems, in order to increase accessibility of palliative care (Mwangi-Powell et al. 2013). Nurses have a central role in increasing the accessibility of palliative care through task shifting, providing quality palliative care services, running nurse-led programmes and the implementation of different models of care.

Task shifting is not a new phenomenon in LIMCs. It involves delegation of specially assigned duties from one person to another, usually of a different profession. The World Health Organization (WHO 2016) suggests that it involves the rational redistribution of tasks among health workforce teams where specific tasks are moved, where appropriate, from highly qualified health workers to health workers who may have less training and fewer qualifications in order to make more efficient use of available human resources. In order for palliative care to become accessible to all those who need it in LMIC, there needs to be an element of task shifting, both from medical officers to nurses and also from nurses to community volunteers/support workers, or from specialist to generalist nurses.

In palliative care, nurses are taking on the lion's share in task shifting, providing services involving the whole continuum of holistic care and total pain management. One of the most highlighted task shifting successes in nursing care is the allowance of specially trained nurses to prescribe oral morphine in Uganda (Jagwe and Merriman 2007), with other countries such as Rwanda, Malawi and South Africa soon to follow suit. Alongside this, task shifting from nurses to community workers has increased access to palliative care in numerous countries including Uganda, Malawi and India, through developing models of rural palliative care services that rely heavily on local volunteers or community caregivers (Kumar 2007; Defilippi and Cameron 2010; Downing et al. 2010; Jack et al. 2011; Grant et al. 2011). These volunteers are trained to work with the nurses and other health professionals in the identification and basic management of individuals requiring palliative care in their homes. The grafting of palliative care onto home-based care programmes, thus integrating it into existing structures, has been successful.

Other nurses have moved into administration, research and programme work, and where the nurses are trained as specialists in palliative care, more tasks are being undertaken by the nurses, and it is hoped that on-going documentation around these shifted tasks will instill confidence and accountability in practice. A variety of nurse-led programmes have been developed in different LMIC. A novel nurse-led pain education intervention has been delivered in Malawi (Nkhoma et al. 2013). In a randomised controlled trial, Nkhoma developed an educational intervention comprising a 30-minute face-to-face meeting, a leaflet, and a follow-up telephone call at 2 weeks (Nkhoma et al. 2015). The content of the educational intervention covered definition, causes, and characteristics of pain in HIV/AIDS; beliefs and myths about pain and pain medication; assessment of pain; and pharmacological and non-pharmacological management. The intervention reduced pain intensity and increased caregiver confidence to deliver care. It is important that palliative care provision is not reduced to pain management.

Communication and information have been identified as priority needs among people with advanced disease in Sub-Saharan Africa (Selman et al. 2009). The majority of the public also say they would wish to be told of a poor prognosis, in both Kenya (Downing et al. 2014a) and Namibia (Powell et al. 2014). A novel nurse-led intervention to enhance person-centredness was designed for the large numbers of people in Africa living with HIV infection and accessing treatment (Lowther et al. 2012). Mental health problems persist and are highly prevalent alongside antiretroviral treatment (ART)

(Lowther et al. 2014). Among people living with HIV in Africa, psychosocial problems are the most pressing concerns (Harding et al. 2014). Therefore, a huge number of people living with HIV are required to remain in care and adhere to therapy in what is an under-resourced health system. In response to this clinical and policy need to respond with appropriate care, a nurse-led palliative care intervention was developed (Lowther et al. 2012). Existing ART clinic nurses were provided with a two-week training course in palliative care, and a structured person-centred assessment form and care planning that followed principles of palliative care assessment. A local hospice provided weekly mentorship and case review, plus care for complex cases. The intervention improved psychological morbidity, mental health quality of life, and psychosocial concerns (Lowther et al. 2015).

A nurse-led palliative care service in South Africa has responded to the high proportion of hospital patients who have life-limiting illness (van Niekerk and Raubenheimer 2014). Evidence suggests that among acute beds in the Cape Metro area, 16.6 per cent of patients had active life-limiting illness (van Niekerk and Raubenheimer 2014). Similar studies at a national referral hospital in Uganda have shown between 37.7 per cent and 46 per cent of active life-limiting illness, with 96 per cent of these having palliative care needs (Lewington et al. 2012; Jacinto et al. 2014). This clearly poses a huge burden and potential cost. The 'Abundant Life' programme in a public hospital in South Africa was developed to ensure that all patients approaching the end of life can access palliative care. This nurse-led service provides a hospital-based palliative care service with community follow-up and family-based community support meetings. An evaluation of the service found that it reduced admissions and length of stay, increased the proportion of home deaths, and reduced costs (Desrosiers et al. 2014).

In hospitals in LMIC, a variety of different models of palliative care provision exist. Variations include where there are identified individuals around the hospital who work together to provide palliative care, a dedicated individual working in palliative care or a multi-disciplinary specialist palliative care team. In response to the 46 per cent of patients in the hospital having life-limiting illnesses (Lewington et al. 2012), a link-nurse programme was set up at Mualgo Hospital, the National Referral Hospital in Kampala, Uganda. Some 27 link-nurses were trained and mentored over a two-year programme in order to empower hospital nurses to provide generalist palliative care and refer on to the specialist palliative care team as needed. An evaluation of this programme demonstrated that it is a practical model for integrating palliative care into generalist services and increasing access to palliative care within a large hospital setting (Downing et al. 2016a). Since the initial evaluation, the link-nurse programme has been expanded to more than 10 other hospitals in Uganda, and to other countries.

Research

Research is a pillar to quality nursing practice. Evidence-based practice supports improvement of patient care in line with proven best practices (Gerrish and Lacey 2010). Despite using innovative solutions to patient care (i.e. frangipani for herpes zoster and pawpaw seeds for constipation), the amount of documented evidence of best practices is wanting. There is a need for research in children's palliative care in SSA (Harding et al. 2010) and the need for research in palliative care generally was recognised by the Declaration of Venice, which aims to develop a global palliative care research initiative, focusing on LMIC (Powell et al. 2008). Collaboration is key to the ongoing development of research in palliative care in LMIC, and nurses should play an important part in any research collaboration, whether a North-South or South-South collaboration, thus ensuring on-going capacity building for nurses in the field of research.

Nurses are increasingly finding new ways of improving palliative care and thus need support in actualising their findings through rigorous scientific processes. Various research networks have been instigated in order to develop local research capacity, including the MPCU research network, the African Palliative Care Research Network, the Lien collaborative for palliative care with the APHN, and the EAPC Research Network. Support for researchers from LMIC has enabled researchers to undertake RCTs, qualitative and quantitative research along with research into outcome measurement. Through these different networks, funds for fellowships and research grants will help with on-going development in palliative care research.

Research as an integral part of the public health strategy is being integrated into the work of many palliative care organisations – it is no longer seen as an 'added extra' or a 'luxury' but as an essential component of palliative care service provision. The importance of evidence-based practice has prompted the implementation of journal clubs and case conferences which provide updates on recent developments in palliative care as well as discuss complex patient issues. National and regional palliative care associations have also recognised the need for good quality palliative care research and are supporting members to review the evidence and take part in research as appropriate. Likewise nurses who are students on the different palliative care degree and Master's programmes will all be involved in undertaking research and need to be supported to present their research at conferences and for publication in appropriate journals.

A wide range of research is being encouraged, including needs assessments, palliative care standards audits, and evaluation – all of which will support quality improvement and development of palliative care sites. One of the more recent areas of research in LMIC is that of the use of technology in palliative care. The era of technologies is impacting on LMIC and on nursing practice. The introduction of digital gadgets for vital signs and patient monitoring will enhance nursing practice through saving time for other procedures as well as providing accurate information. The use of computers to record patient data has upgraded patient information and improved follow-up. Various studies have illustrated the benefit of the use of the telephone in patient follow-up and care, including studies on ARV adherence. Nurses are increasingly calling patients to monitor their use of opioids at home, to book home visit appointments as well as reminding patients to keep appointments. Mobile phones have also been used to alert healthcare workers on changing patient conditions and have helped. Early research into the use of m-health (using mobile phone technology) in Uganda focused on strengthening pharmaceutical systems for palliative care services across both urban and rural settings. Initial results demonstrated that an m-health approach could improve existing processes for strengthening palliative care medication supply management, e.g. patient record management, pharmacy for casting and supply planning (Namisango et al. 2016).

Challenges for nurses in developing and implementing a public health approach for palliative care

A wide range of challenges face nurses in LMIC in developing and implementing the public health approach to palliative care (Mwangi-Powell et al. 2015). Challenges include the following:

- *Delayed health-seeking behaviour* – in LMIC, many patients will delay seeking healthcare – whether because of the distance from which they live from a health centre, out of fear or because they will consult traditional healers first. Therefore, they present with advanced disease and complex symptoms.
- *Work overload* – often the nurses have limited time to give to palliative care patients as they are often deployed elsewhere and undertake palliative care as an addition or in their own time. Thus, palliative care is not integrated into their work and is often seen as extra work which can only be completed if there is time. Thus, workload, combined with low compensation of nurses, leads to demotivation, moving into other fields, and brain drain to other countries offering better terms and opportunities for professional development.
- *Lack of a career progression* – the development of a career pathway in palliative care is slow, and in many places there is no opportunity to work in a specialist role. While many palliative care nurses are recognised in their work places for their expertise, the majority of health systems in LMIC do not have provision for recognition and remuneration of specialist nurses. Thus, in some instances, nurses are even required to take a reduction in pay to specialise in palliative care as they no longer fit into the recognised pay structure. There also needs to be more liaison between the different ministries and professional bodies in order to recognise nurses further.
- *Lack of trained palliative care professionals* – in LMIC, the number of trained nurses in palliative care is minimal, both in terms of generalist and specialist palliative care, therefore, nurses are often working in isolation, or expected to work as a specialist but only have generalist training, but there is no one else.
- *Task shifting* – ensuring that the correct statements and codes of practice are in existence to enable task shifting. In some countries, for example, Kenya and Mozambique, any prescription by nurses will be countersigned by the doctors in order to retain responsibility and to cover the nurses legally. Another important issue in task shifting is ensuring that people are trained appropriately with proper training and mentorship, so that the nurses and/or community workers feel confident and are able to implement what they have learnt.
- *Logistics* – the times when medicines are not available and a lack of logistics for hospitals can deter the practice of quality palliative care, for example, in the instance of being out of stock of medications, leading to inefficient pain management.

- *Deployment of staff* – the deployment of nurses and allocation of duties do not take into account their specialisation but is done on a rotational roster, therefore, nurses who have been trained in palliative care can be moved to other settings where they are unable to put their palliative care skills into practice. While with the process of integration, palliative care programmes are being started in many hospitals in LMIC, there needs to be a way of allocating trained palliative care nurses to these programmes and then retaining them.
- *Finances* – most LMIC countries' budget for healthcare is below the 15 per cent country budget as recommended by the Abuja Declaration (WHO 2010b).
- *Sustainability* – this is a challenge for many palliative care programmes which have developed in parallel with existing structures. Thus, the integration of palliative care, as recommended by the WHA resolution, should help in the on-going sustainability of services through the engagement of relevant stakeholders and Ministries of Health.
- *The need for continuous advocacy* – this is essential if countries are to include palliative care in the mainstream government service providers and to ensure the inclusion of palliative care medicines in the essential country medications lists.
- *Lack of availability of palliative care medications* – this is a key issue for nurses and there is a need for on-going advocacy for the availability of low cost oral morphine solution/tablets. Often nurses are working in situations where opioids may not be available at all, or may only be available in limited situations.
- *Inclusion of palliative care indicators in the main Government Health Management Information System (HMIS)* – this is essential but is only just being realised in a few LMIC, e.g. in Uganda and Rwanda.
- *Other challenges* – these include a lack of rigorous research evidence showing the benefits of palliative care, poor public awareness and understanding, lack of government support and funding, cultural taboos surrounding death and the disclosure of diagnosis, providing palliative care in humanitarian and crisis situations.

Conclusion

While challenges do exist for nurses in LMIC to develop and implement palliative care services, there is also a range of opportunities on which they can build. The WHA resolution on palliative care (WHA 2014) clearly makes the case for integration of palliative care into existing structures, including the work of the multi-disciplinary team and nurses. The resolution provides a great opportunity for nurses to advocate with their national associations, nursing leaders, palliative care organisations and Ministries of Health for its integration across different sectors of the health system. Throughout the five foundation pillars essential for palliative care, nurses have a wide range of opportunities facing them, including the increasing availability of and access to technology such as m-health and e-learning. In LMIC, where the workforce is already strained, the workers may not have to leave their families to go for long study sessions and can continue providing services at their work places while learning new skills. Studies indicated that 75 per cent of the students studying online were employed (Strother 2002), thus e-learning is convenient, especially for adult learners, due to its flexibility and can be an opportunity for expanding nurse education in palliative care.

Nurses are increasingly being encouraged to lead and support palliative care programmes and quality improvement projects at their health facilities. This exposes them to evidence-based practice as well as managerial and leadership skills outside of clinical work. Nurses should therefore be encouraged to seek other related competencies within specialist practice in order to complement their clinical skills, for example, in research, management and leadership, social sciences and public health. Partnerships within and outside of the country are also essential in order to obtain and introduce innovative technologies and experiment with m-health. It is also important that palliative care education is not just provided in English, but in a variety of languages, so that any training can be delivered in the language appropriate to the nurses who are either receiving or facilitating the training. Nurses also need to take advantage of working where possible within a multi-disciplinary team, so that they not only can learn from others, but also so that the others can also learn from them. This chapter, within the broader aims of this book, provides a framework to enable nursing to advance palliative care as a public health priority throughout the world.

Recommended resources

African Palliative Care Research Network [Online]. African Palliative Care Association (APCA). Available at: https://www.africanpalliativecare.org/articles/african-palliative-care-research-network/ (accessed 12 October 2016).

Density of nursing and midwifery personnel (total number per 1000 population) [Online]. WHO Health Workforce. Available at: http://gamapserver.who.int/gho/interactive_charts/health_workforce/NursingMidwiferyDensity/atlas.htmlhttp://gamapserver.who.int/gho/interactive_charts/health_workforce/NursingMidwiferyDensity/atlas.html (accessed 10 October 2016).

Density of physicians (total number per 1000 population) [Online]. WHO Health Workforce. Available at: http://gamapserver.who.int/gho/interactive_charts/health_workforce/PhysiciansDensity_Total/atlas.htmlhttp://gamapserver.who.int/gho/interactive_charts/health_workforce/PhysiciansDensity_Total/atlas.html (accessed 10 October 2016).

Gwyther, L. and Rawlinson, F. (2007) Palliative medicine teaching program at the University of Cape Town: integrating palliative care principles into practice. *Journal of Pain Symptom Management*, 33: 558–62.

Palliative Care e-learning course for healthcare professionals in Africa [Online]. ecancereducation Available at: http://ecancer.org/education/course/1-palliative-care-e-learning-course-for-healthcare-professionals-in-africa.phphttp://

ecancer.org/education/course/1-palliative-care-e-learning-course-for-health-care-professionals-in-africa.php (accessed 12 October 2016).

Palliative Care Toolkits and Training Manual Files [Online]. Worldwide Hospice Palliative Care Alliance Available at: http://www.thewhpca.org/resources/category/palliative-care-toolkits-and-training-manualhttp://www.thewhpca.org/resources/category/palliative-care-toolkits-and-training-manual (accessed 11 October 2016).

Text-only version of the palliative care e-learning course for healthcare professionals in India [Online]. ecancereducation. Available at: http://ecancer.org/education/course/18-text-only-version-of-the-palliative-care-e-learning-course-for-healthcare-professionals-in-india.phphttp://ecancer.org/education/course/18-text-only-version-of-the-palliative-care-e-learning-course-for-healthcare-professionals-in-india.php (accessed 12 October 2016).

References

APCA (2012) *African Palliative Care Association Core Competencies: A Framework of Core Competencies for Palliative Care Providers in Africa*. Kampala: APCA.

Avert (2016) *HIV and AIDS in Sub-Saharan Africa Regional Overview*. Available at: http://www.avert.org/professionals/hiv-around-world/sub-saharan-africa/overview (accessed 4 December 2016).

Babu, G.R., Lakshmi, S.B. and Thiyagarajan, J.A. (2013) Epidemiological correlates of breast cancer in South India. *Asian Pacific Journal of Cancer Prevention*, 14: 5077–83.

Barton, M.B., Frommer, M. and Shafiq, J. (2006) Role of radiotherapy in cancer control in low-income and middle-income countries. *The Lancet Oncology*, 7: 584–95.

Bhatnagar, S. and Joshi, S. (2013) 'A good death'—sequence (not stigma), to an enigma called life: case report on end-of-life decision making and care. *American Journal of Hospice and Palliative Care*, 30(7): 626–7.

Bond, C., Lavy, V. and Wolldridge, R. (2008) *Palliative Care Toolkit: Improving Care from the Roots Up in Resource-Limited Settings*. London: Help the Hospices.

Boutayeb, A. and Boutayeb, S. (2005) The burden of non communicable diseases in developing countries. *International Journal for Equity in Health*, 4: 2.

Cohen, J. and Deliens, L. (2012) Applying a public health perspective to end-of-life care. In Cohen, J. and Deliens, L., *A Public Health Perspective on End of Life Care*. Oxford: Oxford University Press, pp. 3–18.

Connor, S. and Sepulveda, C. (eds) (2014) *Global Atlas of Palliative Care at the End of Life*. Geneva; WHPCA.

Connor, S.R., Downing, J. and Marston, J. (2016) Estimating the global need for palliative care for children: a cross-sectional analysis. *Journal of Pain and Symptom Management*, 53(2): 171–7.

Defilippi, K.M. and Cameron, S. (2010) Expanding the reach of palliative care to community-based home care programs. *Journal of Pain and Symptom Management*, 40: 3–5.

De Lima, L. and Doyle, D. (2007) The International Association for Hospice and Palliative Care list of essential medicines for palliative care. *Journal of Pain and Palliative Care Pharmacotherapy*, 21: 29–36.

De Vlieger, M., Gorchs, N., Larkin, P. and Porchet, F. (2004) *A Guide for the Development of Palliative Nurse Education in Europe: Palliative Nurse Education: Report of the EAPC Task Force*. Milan: European Association of Palliative Care.

Desrosiers, T., Cupido, C., Pitout, E. et al. (2014) A hospital-based palliative care service for patients with advanced organ failure in Sub-Saharan Africa reduces admissions and increases home death rates. *Journal of Pain Symptom Management*, 47: 786–92.

Downing, J. (2015) *Hidden Lives, Hidden Patients: 2015 World Hospice and Palliative Care Day Report*. London: Worldwide Hospice and Palliative Care Aliance and International Children's Palliative Care Network.

Downing, J., Batuli, M., Kivumbi, G. et al. (2016a) A palliative care link nurse programme in Mulago Hospital, Uganda: an evaluation using mixed methods. *BMC Palliative Care*, 15: 40.

Downing, J., Finsch, L., Garanganga, E. et al. (2006) *Role of the Nurse in Resource-Limited Settings. A Clinical Guide to Supportive and Palliative Care for HIV/AIDS in Sub-Saharan Africa*. Kampala: African Palliative Care Association.

Downing, J., Gomes, B., Gikaara, N. et al. (2014a) Public preferences and priorities for end-of-life care in Kenya: a population-based street survey. *BMC Palliative Care*, 13: 4.

Downing, J., Leng, M. and Grant, L. (2016b) Implementing a Palliative Care Nurse Leadership Fellowship Program in Uganda. *Oncology Nursing Forum*, 43: 395–8.

Downing, J., Ling, J., Benini, F. et al. (2014b) A summary of the EAPC White Paper on core competencies for education in paediatric palliative care. *European Journal of Palliative Care*, 21: 245–9.

Downing, J., Powell, R.A. and Mwangi-Powell, F. (2010) Home-based palliative care in Sub-Saharan Africa. *Home Healthcare Nurse*, 28: 298–307.

Dusabimana, M., Kelet, K., Yayeri, B. et al. (2016) Evaluation of nurse opioid prescribers in Uganda. Paper presented at APCA/WHPCA Palliative Care Conference: Hospice and Palliative Care: Resolution to Action., 17–19 August 2016, Kampala, Uganda.

Farmer, P., Frenk, J., Knaul, F.M. et al. (2010) Expansion of cancer care and control in countries of low and middle income: a call to action. *Lancet*, 376: 1186–93.

Ferlay, J., Soerjomataram, I., Ervik, M. et al. (eds) (2014) *Estimated Global Cancer Incidence, Prevalence and Mortality in Globocan 2012*. Lyon, France: IARC.

Gamondi, C., Larkin, P. and Payne, S. (2013a) Core competencies in palliative care: an EAPC White Paper on palliative care education: part 1. *European Journal of Palliative Care*, 20: 86–91.

Gamondi, C., Larkin, P. and Payne, S. (2013b) Core competencies in palliative care: an EAPC White Paper on palliative care education: part 2. *European Journal of Palliative Care*, 20: 140–5.

Gelband, H., Sankaranarayanan, R., Gauvreau, C.L. et al. (2015) Costs, affordability, and feasibility of an essential package of cancer control interventions in low-income and middle-income countries: key messages from Disease Control Priorities, 3rd edition. *Lancet*, 387: 2133–44.

Gerrish, K. and Lacey, A. (2010) *The Research Process in Nursing*. Chichester: John Wiley and Sons, Ltd.

Grant, L., Brown, J., Leng, M. et al. (2011) Palliative care making a difference in rural Uganda, Kenya and Malawi: three rapid evaluation field studies. *BMC Palliative Care*, 10: 8.

Gwyther, L. and Rawlinson, F. (2007) Palliative medicine teaching program at the University of Cape Town: integrating palliative care principles into practice. *Journal of Pain Symptom Management*, 33: 558–62.

Hanna, T.P. and Kangolle, A.C. (2010) Cancer control in developing countries: using health data and health services research to measure and improve access, quality and efficiency. *BMC International Health and Human Rights*, 10: 24.

Harding, R. and Higginson, I.J. (2014) Inclusion of end-of-life care in the global health agenda. *Lancet Global Health*, 2: e375–6.

Harding, R., Powell, R.A., Kiyange, F. et al. (2010a) Provision of pain- and symptom-relieving drugs for HIV/AIDS in Sub-Saharan Africa. *Journal of Pain and Symptom Management*, 40: 405–15.

Harding, R., Selman, L., Agupio, G. et al. (2011) The prevalence and burden of symptoms amongst cancer patients attending palliative care in two African countries. *European Journal of Cancer*, 47: 51–6.

Harding, R., Selman, L., Agupio, G. et al. (2012) Prevalence, burden, and correlates of physical and psychological symptoms among HIV palliative care patients in Sub-Saharan Africa: an international multicenter study. *Journal of Pain Symptom Management*, 44: 1–9.

Harding, R., Selman, S., Powell, R. et al. (2013) Research into palliative care in Sub-Saharan Africa. *Lancet Oncology*, 14: 183–8.

Harding, R., Sheer, L. and Albertyn, R. (2010b) *The Status of Paediatric Palliative Care in Sub-Saharan Africa: An Appraisal*. London: The Diana Princess of Wales Memorial Fund and King's College London.

Harding, R., Simms, V., Penfold, S. et al. (2014) Quality of life and wellbeing among HIV outpatients in East Africa: a multicentre observational study. *BMC Infectious Diseases*, 14: 613.

Henderson, V. (1997) *Basic Principles of Nursing Care*. Geneva: International Council of Nurses.

Human Rights Campaign (2016) *Healthcare Equality Index* [Online]. Available at: http://www.hrc.org/hei/patient-self-identification (accessed 6 October 2016).

Jacinto, A., Masembe, V., Tumwesigye, N.M. and Harding, R. (2014) The prevalence of life-limiting illness at a Ugandan National Referral Hospital: a 1-day census of all admitted patients. *BMJ Supportive and Palliative Care*, 5(2): 196–9.

Jack, B.A., Kirton, J., Birakurataki, J. and Merriman, A. (2011) 'A bridge to the hospice': the impact of a Community Volunteer Programme in Uganda. *Palliative Medicine*, 25: 706–15.

Jackson, K. (2016) Living and dying in pain: it doesn't have to happen. World Hospice and Palliative Care Day Toolkit 2016. London; Worldwide Hospice and Palliative Care Alliance.

Jagwe, J. and Merriman, A. (2007) Uganda: delivering analgesia in rural Africa: opioid availability and nurse prescribing. *Journal of Pain Symptom Management*, 33: 547–51.

Kanavos, P. (2006) The rising burden of cancer in the developing world. *Annals of Oncology*, 17(suppl. 8): viii15–viii23.

Kar, S.S., Subitha, L. and Iswarya, S. (2015) Palliative care in India: situation assessment and future scope. *Indian Journal of Cancer*, 52: 99–101.

Kelley, A.S., Covinsky, K.E., Gorges, R.J. et al. (2016) Identifying older adults with serious illness: a critical step toward improving the value of health care. *Health Services Research*, 52(1): 113–31.

Knapp, C., Woodworth, L., Wright, M. et al. (2011) Pediatric palliative care provision around the world: a systematic review. *Pediatric Blood and Cancer*, 57: 361–8.

Kumar, S.K. (2007) Kerala, India: a regional community-based palliative care model. *Journal of Pain and Symptom Management*, 33: 623–7.

Lavy, V. (2009) *Palliative Care Toolkit: Trainer's Manual*. London: Help the Hospices.

Lebaron, V., Maurer, M., Gilson, A. et al. (2016) Empowering nurses from low and middle income countries to enact evidence-based policy and practice changes to improve cancer pain management. Paper presented at 2016 World Cancer Congress. Mobilsing Action: Inspiring Change, November, Paris.

Levin, C.V., El Gueddari, B. and Meghzifene, A. (1999) Radiation therapy in Africa: distribution and equipment. *Radiotherapy and Oncology*, 52: 79–83.

Lewington, J., Namukwaya, E., Limoges, J. et al. (2012) Provision of palliative care for life-limiting disease in a low income country national hospital setting: how much is needed? *BMJ Supportive and Palliative Care*, 2: 140–4.

Logie, D.E. and Harding, R. (2005) An evaluation of a morphine public health programme for cancer and AIDS pain relief in Sub-Saharan Africa. *BMC Public Health*, 5: 82.

Lokker, M.E., Gwyther, L., Magona, P. et al. (2013) The prevalence and burden of physical and psychological symptoms in patients with advanced heart failure attending a South African public hospital. *European Journal of Heart Failure*, 12: S307.

Lowther, K., Selman, L., Harding, R. and Higginson, I.J. (2014) Experience of persistent psychological symptoms and perceived stigma among people with HIV on anti-retroviral therapy (ART): a systematic review. *International Journal of Nursing Studies*, 51: 1171–89.

Lowther, K., Selman, L., Simms, V. et al. (2015) Nurse-led palliative care for HIV-positive patients taking antiretroviral therapy in Kenya: a randomised controlled trial. *Lancet HIV*, 2: e328–34.

Lowther, K., Simms, V., Selman, L. et al. (2012) Treatment outcomes in palliative care: the TOPCare study. A mixed methods phase III randomised controlled trial to assess the effectiveness of a nurse-led palliative care intervention for HIV positive patients on antiretroviral therapy. *BMC Infectious Diseases*, 12: 288.

Luyirika, E.B., Namisango, E., Garanganga, E. et al. (2016) Best practices in developing a national palliative care policy in resource limited settings: lessons from five African countries. *ecancermedicalscience*, 10: 652.

Lynch, T., Connor, S. and Clark, D. (2013) Mapping levels of palliative care development: a global update. *Journal of Pain Symptom Management*, 45: 1094–96.

Merriman, A. and Harding, R. (2010) Pain control in the African context: the Ugandan introduction of affordable morphine to relieve suffering at the end of life. *Philosophy, Ethics and Humanities in Medicine*, 5: 10.

Ministry of Finance (2013) Health workers' shortage in Uganda: where should the government focus its efforts? [Online]. BMAU, Budget Monitoring Accountability Unit. Available at: http://www.finance.go.ug/dmdocuments/6-13%20Health%20Workers%20Shortage%20in%20Uganda%20May%202013.pdf (accessed 10 October 2016).

Muckaden, M. and Pandya, S.S. (2016) Motivation of volunteers to work in palliative care setting: a qualitative study. *Indian Journal of Palliative Care*, 22: 348–53.

Mwangi-Powell, F.N., Downing, J., Powell, R.A. et al. (2015) Palliative care in Africa. In Ferrell, B.R., Coyle, N. and Paice, J.A. (eds) *Oxford Textbook of Palliative Nursing*. Oxford: Oxford University Press.

Mwangi-Powell, F.N., Powell, R.A. and Harding, R. (2013) Models of delivering palliative and end-of-life care in Sub-Saharan Africa: a narrative review of the evidence. *Current Opinion in Supportive and Palliative Care*, 7: 223–8.

Nabirye, E.O., Ojera, A., Namwanga, R. et al. (2016) A review of the curriculum for nurse opioid prescribers: how competent in prescribing are they after their training? APCA/WHPCA Palliative Care Conference: Hospice and Palliative Care: Resolution to Action, 17–19 August 2016, Kampala, Uganda.

Nabudere, H., Obuku, E. and Lamorde, M. (2014) Advancing palliative care in the Uganda health system: an evidence-based policy brief. *International Journal of Technology Assessment in Health Care*, 30: 621–5.

Namisango, E., Ntege, C., Luyirika, E.B. et al. (2016) Strengthening pharmaceutical systems for palliative care services in resource-limited settings: piloting a mHealth application across a rural and urban setting in Uganda. *BMC Palliative Care*, 15: 20.

Nkhoma, K., Seymour, J. and Arthur, A. (2013) An educational intervention to reduce pain and improve pain management for Malawian people living with HIV/AIDS and their family carers: study protocol for a randomised controlled trial. *Trials*, 14: 216.

Nkhoma, K., Seymour, J. and Arthur, A. (2015) An educational intervention to reduce pain and improve pain management for Malawian people living with HIV/AIDS and their family carers: a randomized controlled trial. *Journal of Pain Symptom Management*, 50: 80–90, e4.

Ortashi, O. (2013) Gynecological cancer services in Arab countries: present scenario, problems and suggested solutions. *Asian Pacific Journal of Cancer Prevention*, 14: 2147–50.

Parkin, D.M., Sitas, F., Chirenje, M. et al. (2008) Part I: Cancer in indigenous Africans – burden, distribution, and trends. *Lancet Oncology*, 9: 683–92.

Powell, R., Downing, J., Radbruch, L. et al. (2008) Advancing palliative care research in Sub-Saharan Africa: from the Venice Declaration, to Nairobi and beyond. *Palliative Medicine*, 22: 885–7.

Powell, R.A., Ali, Z., Luyirika, E. et al. (2015) Out of the shadows: non-communicable diseases and palliative care in Africa. *BMJ Supportive and Palliative Care*, [000751]. doi: 10.1136/bmjspcare-2014-000751.

Powell, R.A., Namisango, E., Gikaara, N. et al. (2014) Public priorities and preferences for end-of-life care in Namibia. *Journal of Pain Symptom Management*, 47: 620–30.

Ray, K. and Mandal, S. (2004) Knowledge about cancer in West Bengal: a pilot survey. *Asian Pacific Journal of Cancer Prevention*, 5: 205–12.

Sallnow, L., Kumar, A. and Kellehear, A. (2009) Public health and palliative care: an historical overview. In Sallnow, L., Kumar, A. and Kellehear, A. (eds) *Proceedings of the 1st International Conference on Public Health and Palliative Care*. London: Institute of Palliative Medicine, pp. 18–27.

Sekyondwa, M., Kasirye, M., Amoris, J. et al. (2016) Rapid appraisal of the health system in Uganda in the context of palliative care nurse prescribing. Paper presented at APCA/WHPCA Palliative Care Conference: Hospice and Palliative Care: Resolution to Action, 17–19 August 2016, Kampala, Uganda.

Selman, L., Higginson, I.J., Agupio, G. et al. (2009) Meeting information needs of patients with incurable progressive disease and their families in South Africa and Uganda: multicentre qualitative study. *BMJ*, 338: b1326.

Stjernswärd, J., Foley, K.M. and Ferris, F.D. (2007) The public health strategy for palliative care. *Journal of Pain Symptom Management*, 33: 486–93.

Strother, J.B. (2002) An assessment of the effectiveness of e-learning in corporate training programs. *The International Review of Research in Open and Distributed Learning*, 3: 1.

The Cancer Atlas (2012) Global innovation in better-value cancer care is needed to face current challenges [Online]. Available at: http://canceratlas.cancer.org/taking-action/management-and-treatment/ (accessed 12 October 2016).

Together for Short Lives (2013) *A Core Pathway for Children with Life-Limiting and Life-Threatening Conditions* (3rd edn). Available at: http://www.togetherforshortlives.org.uk/professionals/childrens_palliative_care_essentials/approach (accessed 4 December 2016).

UNAIDS (2014) *90-90-90: An Ambitious Treatment Target to Help End the AIDS Epidemic*. Geneva: UNAIDS.

UNAIDS (2015) *Fact Sheet* [Online]. Available at: http://www.unaids.org/en/resources/fact-sheet (accessed 12 October 2016).

van Niekerk, L. and Raubenheimer, P.J. (2014) A point-prevalence survey of public hospital inpatients with palliative care needs in Cape Town, South Africa. *South African Medical Journal*, 104: 138–41.

WHA (World Health Assembly) (2014) Strengthening of palliative care as a component of comprehensive care throughout the life course [Online]. Available at: http://apps.who.int/gb/ebwha/pdf_files/WHA67/A67_R19-en.pdf (accessed 10 May 2016).

WHO (World Health Organization) (2010a) *Global Status Report on Noncommunicable Diseases*. Geneva: WHO.

WHO (World Health Organization) (2010b) *The Abuja Declaration: Ten Years On* [Online]. Available at: http://www.who.int/healthsystems/publications/Abuja10.pdf.

WHO (World Health Organization) (2014) *Global Status Report on Noncommunicable Diseases*. Geneva: WHO.

WHO (World Health Organization) (2016) *Treat, Train, Retrain HIV/AIDS. Task Shifting: Global Recommendations and Guidelines.* Geneva: WHO.

World Bank (2016a) Nurses and midwives per 1,000 people 2011 [Online]. Available at: http://data.worldbank.org/indicator/SH.MED.NUMW.P3 (accessed 4 December 2016).

World Bank (2016b) Physicians per 1,000 people (2011)[Online]. Available at: http://data.worldbank.org/indicator/SH.MED.PHYS.ZS (accessed 4 December 2016).

Index